Succinct Pediatrics

Evaluation and Management for Common and Critical Care

Editors

Leonard G. Feld, MD, PhD, MMM, FAAP
John D. Mahan, MD, FAAP

Associate Editor

Charles F. Willson, MD, FAAP

D1551755

American Academy of Pediatrics
141 Northwest Point Blvd
Elk Grove Village, IL 60007-1019
www.aap.org

American Academy of Pediatrics Publishing Staff

Mark Grimes, *Director, Department of Publishing*
Alain Park, *Senior Product Development Editor*
Carrie Peters, *Editorial Assistant*
Theresa Wiener, *Manager, Publishing and Production Services*
Linda Diamond, *Manager, Art Direction and Production*
Amanda Cozza, *Editorial Specialist*
Mary Lou White, *Director, Department of Marketing and Sales*
Linda Smessaert, *Brand Manager, Clinical and Professional Publications*

Library of Congress Control Number: 2015934991
ISBN: 978-1-58110-955-9
eBook: 978-1-58110-968-9
MA0763

The recommendations in this publication do not indicate an exclusive course of treatment or serve as a standard of care. Variations, taking into account individual circumstances, may be appropriate.

Brand names are furnished for identification purposes only. No endorsement of the manufacturers or products mentioned is implied.

Every effort has been made to ensure that the drug selection and dosages set forth in this text are in accordance with the current recommendations and practice at the time of publication. It is the responsibility of the health care professional to check the package insert of each drug for any change in indications and dosages and for added warnings and precautions.

The publishers have made every effort to trace the copyright holders for borrowed material. If they have inadvertently overlooked any, they will be pleased to make the necessary arrangements at the first opportunity.

9-370/1015

1 2 3 4 5 6 7 8 9 10

Contributors

Marco A. Arruda, MD, PhD
Glia Institute
Ribeirão Preto, São Paulo
Brazil

Jeffrey R. Avner, MD, FAAP
Chief, Division of Pediatric Emergency Medicine
Professor of Clinical Pediatrics
Children's Hospital at Montefiore
Albert Einstein College of Medicine
Bronx, NY

Dwight M. Bailey, DO
Medical Director, Pediatric Intensive Care Unit
Pediatric Specialty Care Division
Levine Children's Hospital
Carolinas HealthCare System
Charlotte, NC
Associate Professor of Pediatrics
University of North Carolina School of Medicine
Chapel Hill, NC

Russell C. Bailey, MD
Assistant Professor of Neurology and Pediatrics Director
Pediatric Epilepsy Monitoring Unit
Department of Neurology
University of Virginia
Charlottesville, VA

Marcelo E. Bigal, MD, PhD
Vice President, Global Clinical Development
Migraine and Headaches
Teva Pharmaceuticals
Frazer, PA
Department of Neurology
Albert Einstein College of Medicine
Bronx, NY

Mary Jo Bowman, MD, FAAP
Department of Pediatrics
Division of Emergency Medicine
Nationwide Children's Hospital
The Ohio State University
Columbus, OH

Brian K. Brighton, MD, MPH
Department of Orthopaedic Surgery
Attending Pediatric Orthopaedic Surgeon
Levine Children's Hospital at Carolinas Medical Center
Charlotte, NC

Jeana Bush, MD
Levine Children's Hospital at Carolinas Medical Center
Charlotte, NC

Ricardo A. Caicedo, MD, FAAP
Department of Pediatrics
Division of Gastroenterology, Hepatology, and Nutrition
Levine Children's Hospital at Carolinas Medical Center
Charlotte, NC

Kevin S. Carter, MD
Department of Pediatrics
Levine Children's Hospital at Carolinas Medical Center
Charlotte, NC

Suzette Surratt Caudle, MD, FAAP
Pediatric Specialties Care Division
Section on Inpatient Pediatrics
Carolinas HealthCare System
Vice Chair for Education, Department of Pediatrics
Levine Children's Hospital at Carolinas Medical Center
Charlotte, NC

Nicole L. Chandler, MD
Assistant Professor
University of North Carolina School of Medicine
Chapel Hill, NC

Margaret A. Chase, MD
Department of Pediatrics
Division of Critical Care Medicine
Nationwide Children's Hospital
Columbus, OH

Lay Har Cheng, MD, MSPH
Department of Pediatrics
Division of Gastroenterology, Hepatology, and Nutrition
Levine Children's Hospital at Carolinas Medical Center
Charlotte, NC

Christine B. Cho, MD
Department of Pediatrics
Division of Pediatric Allergy and Clinical Immunology
National Jewish Health
Denver, CO

Richard J. Chung, MD, FAAP
Department of Pediatrics and Internal Medicine
Duke University School of Medicine
Durham, NC

Daniel M. Cohen, MD, FAAP
Department of Pediatrics
Section of Emergency Medicine
Nationwide Children's Hospital
Columbus, OH

Edward E. Conway, Jr, MD, MS, FAAP, FCCM
Milton and Bernice Stern Department of Pediatrics
Division of Pediatric Critical Care
Mount Sinai Beth Israel Medical Center
New York, NY

Timothy E. Corden, MD, FAAP
Associate Professor, Department of Pediatrics
Division of Critical Care Medicine
Policy Codirector, Injury Research Center
Medical College of Wisconsin
Associate Director, Pediatric Critical Care Unit
Children's Hospital of Wisconsin
Milwaukee, WI

Cheryl D. Courtlandt, MD, FAAP
Faculty, Division of General Pediatrics
Direction, Pediatric Asthma Program
Levine Children's Hospital
Carolinas HealthCare System
Charlotte, NC

Jennifer Crotty, MD, FAAP
Assistant Professor of Pediatrics
Brody School of Medicine at East Carolina University
Greenville, NC

Amanda W. Dale-Shall, MD, MS
Division of Pediatric Nephrology and Hypertension
Levine Children's Hospital
Carolinas HealthCare System
Charlotte, NC

Rachel Dawkins, MD, FAAP
Louisiana State University
Baton Rouge, LA

Kristi S. Day, MD
Internal Medicine/Pediatrics Hospital Medicine
Central Baptist Hospital
Lexington, KY

Scottie B. Day, MD, FAAP
Associate Professor
University of Kentucky
Chief, Heinrich A. Werner Division of Pediatric Critical Care
Director, Pediatric Transport and Outreach
Kentucky Children's Hospital/UK Healthcare
Lexington, KY

Jason E. Dranove, MD
Department of Pediatrics
Division of Gastroenterology, Hepatology, and Nutrition
Levine Children's Hospital at Carolinas Medical Center
Charlotte, NC

Marlie Dulaurier, MD, FAAP
Department of Pediatrics
Division of Emergency Medicine
Nationwide Children's Hospital
The Ohio State University
Columbus, OH

Leonard G. Feld, MD, PhD, MMM, FAAP
President, Physician Enterprise
Pediatric Specialists of America
Miami Children's Health System
Miami, FL

Steven L. Frick, MD
Chair, Department of Orthopaedic Surgery
Nemours Children's Hospital
Professor of Orthopaedic Surgery
University of Central Florida College of Medicine
Orlando, FL

Beng Fuh, MD
Assistant Professor of Pediatrics
Department of Pediatrics
Division of Hematology and Oncology
East Carolina University
Greenville, NC

John S. Giuliano, Jr, MD
Associate Professor of Pediatrics
Pediatric Critical Care
Yale University School of Medicine
New Haven, CT

David Goff, MD, FAAP
Department of Pediatrics and Department of Internal Medicine
Brody School of Medicine at East Carolina University
James and Connie Maynard Children's Hospital at Vidant Medical Center
East Carolina University
Greenville, NC

Delia L. Gold, MD, FAAP
Department of Pediatrics
Division of Emergency Medicine
Nationwide Children's Hospital
Columbus, OH

Andrew Z. Heling, MD, FAAP
Department of Pediatrics
University of North Carolina Hospitals
Chapel Hill, NC

Laurie Hicks, MD, FAAP
Pediatric Palliative Medicine Physician
Medical Director, Pediatric Advanced Care Team
Levine Children's Hospital at Carolinas Medical Center
Charlotte, NC

Karin Hillenbrand, MD, MPH, FAAP
Associate Professor
Vice Chair for Education, Department of Pediatrics
Brody School of Medicine at East Carolina University
Greenville, NC

Richard Hobbs, MD, FAAP
Department of Pediatrics and Internal Medicine
University of North Carolina School of Medicine
Chapel Hill, NC

Lacy C. Hobgood, MD, FAAP, FACP
Department of Pediatrics
Medical Director
East Carolina University Adult and Pediatric Health Care
Greenville, NC

Chad Thomas Jacobsen, MD, MS
Department of Pediatrics
Division of Pediatric Hematology/Oncology
Levine Children's Hospital at Carolinas Medical Center
Charlotte, NC

Laurie H. Johnson, MD
Department of Pediatrics
Division of Emergency Medicine
Cincinnati Children's Hospital Medical Center
Cincinnati, OH

Douglas T. Johnston, DO, FAAAAI, FACAAI
Assistant Professor of Internal Medicine and Allergy and Immunology
Edward Via College of Osteopathic Medicine, Carolina Campus
Physician, Asthma and Allergy Specialists
Charlotte, NC

Colleen A. Kraft, MD, FAAP
Department of Pediatrics
Division of General Pediatrics
Virginia Tech Carilion School of Medicine and Research Institution
Roanoke, VA

Ada T. Lin, MD, FAAP
Department of Pediatrics
Division of Critical Care
Nationwide Children's Hospital
Columbus, OH

Jacob A. Lohr, MD
Department of Pediatrics
University of North Carolina Hospitals
Chapel Hill, NC

Elizabeth H. Mack, MD, MS, FAAP
Division of Pediatric Critical Care
Associate Professor, Pediatrics
Medical Director, GME Quality and Safety
Medical University of South Carolina
Charleston, SC

John D. Mahan, MD, FAAP
Professor, Department of Pediatrics
Section of Nephrology
Nationwide Children's Hospital
Columbus, OH

Indrajit Majumdar, MD, MBBS
Assistant Professor of Pediatrics
Division of General Pediatrics
Division of Pediatric Endocrinology and Diabetes
State University of New York at Buffalo
Women and Children's Hospital of Buffalo
Buffalo, NY

Kimberly Marohn, MD
Assistant Professor of Pediatrics
Pediatric Critical Care
Baystate Children's Hospital
Springfield, MA

Keri A. Marques, MD, FAAP
Department of Pediatrics
Division of Neonatology
Neonatal-Perinatal Fellow
Vermont Children's Hospital at University of Vermont
Burlington, VT

Mark J. McDonald, MD, FAAP
Associate Professor
Division of Pediatric Critical Care
Department of Pediatrics
University of Louisville School of Medicine
Medical Director, Just for Kids Critical Care Center
Kosair Children's Hospital
Louisville, KY

Kenya McNeal-Trice, MD, FAAP
Department of Pediatrics
Division of General Pediatrics and Adolescent Medicine
University of North Carolina School of Medicine
Chapel Hill, NC

Alan J. Meltzer, MD, FAAP
Pediatric Program Director
Director, Division of General Pediatrics
Goryeb Children's Hospital–Atlantic Health System
Assistant Professor of Clinical Pediatrics
Rutgers University New Jersey Medical School
Morristown, NJ

Leslie Mihalov, MD, FAAP
Department of Pediatrics
Division of Emergency Medicine
Nationwide Children's Hospital
Columbus, OH

William Mills, MD, MPH
Department of Pediatrics
Division of Pediatric Emergency Medicine
University of North Carolina School of Medicine
Chapel Hill, NC

Patricia D. Morgan, MD, FAAP
Department of Pediatrics
Medical Director, Child Maltreatment Section
Faculty, General Pediatrics Division
Levine Children's Hospital at Carolinas Medical Center
Charlotte, NC

Heidi Murphy, MD, FAAP
Louisiana State University
Baton Rouge, LA

Suresh Nagappan, MD, MSPH
Associate Professor
University of North Carolina School of Medicine
Chapel Hill, NC

Ryan A. Nofziger, MD, FAAP
Department of Pediatrics
Division of Critical Care Medicine
Nationwide Children's Hospital
Columbus, OH

Nicole O'Brien, MD
Department of Pediatrics
Division of Critical Care Medicine
Nationwide Children's Hospital
The Ohio State University
Columbus, OH

John M. Olsson, MD, FAAP
Department of Pediatrics
Division of General Pediatrics
Brody School of Medicine at East Carolina University
Greenville, NC

Vandana Kudva Patel, MD, FAAAAI, FACAAI
Physician, Asthma and Allergy Specialists
Charlotte, NC

Amber M. Patterson, MD, FAAP
Department of Pediatrics
Section of Allergy/Immunology
Nationwide Children's Hospital
The Ohio State University College of Medicine
Columbus, OH

Betsy Pfeffer, MD, FAAP
Assistant Professor of Pediatrics
Columbia University Medical Center
New York, NY

Victor M. Piñeiro, MD
Department of Pediatrics
Division of Gastroenterology, Hepatology, and Nutrition
Levine Children's Hospital at Carolinas Medical Center
Charlotte, NC

Lauren Piper, MD, MS, FAAP
Department of Pediatrics
Division of Pediatric Critical Care
Levine Children's Hospital at Carolinas Medical Center
Charlotte, NC

Kathleen V. Previll, MD, FAAP
Department of Pediatrics General Division
Brody School of Medicine at East Carolina University
Greenville, NC

Renee P. Quarrie, MBBS
Department of Pediatrics
Section of Emergency Medicine
Nationwide Children's Hospital
Columbus, OH

Teresa Quattrin, MD, FAAP
University at Buffalo Distinguished Professor
A. Conger Goodyear Professor
Chair, Department of Pediatrics
State University of New York at Buffalo
Pediatrician in Chief
Chief, Division of Diabetes/Endocrinology
Women & Children's Hospital of Buffalo
Buffalo, NY

Usha Ramkumar, MBBS, FAAP
Department of Pediatrics
General Pediatrics Division
Levine Children's Hospital at Carolinas Medical Center
Charlotte, NC

Suzanne M. Reed, MD
Department of Pediatrics
Division of Hematology/Oncology
Nationwide Children's Hospital
Columbus, OH

Melissa Rhodes, MD
Department of Pediatrics
Division of Hematology/Oncology
Nationwide Children's Hospital
Columbus, OH

Kenneth B. Roberts, MD, FAAP
Professor Emeritus of Pediatrics
University of North Carolina School of Medicine
Chapel Hill, NC

Carl J. Seashore, MD, FAAP
Department of Pediatrics
University of North Carolina Hospitals
Chapel Hill, NC

Kristina Simeonsson, MD, MSPH
Department of Pediatrics
Brody School of Medicine at East Carolina University
Greenville, NC

Joseph Stegman, MD, FAAP
Medical Director
Developmental and Behavioral Pediatrics at the Carolinas
Adjunct Assistant Professor
Department of Pediatrics, School of Medicine
University of North Carolina
Chapel Hill, NC

Michael J. Steiner, MD, FAAP
Department of Pediatrics
Division of General Pediatrics and Adolescent Medicine
North Carolina Children's Hospital at the University of North Carolina
Chapel Hill, NC

John Stephens, MD, FAAP
Departments of Internal Medicine and Pediatrics
Division of General Pediatrics and Adolescent Medicine and General Internal
   Medicine
North Carolina Children's Hospital at the University of North Carolina
Chapel Hill, NC

Erin H. Stubbs, MD, FAAP
Department of Pediatrics
Division of General Pediatrics
Levine Children's Hospital at Carolinas Medical Center
Charlotte, NC

Kristin Stukus, MD, FAAP
Assistant Professor
Division of Pediatric Emergency Medicine
Nationwide Children's Hospital
The Ohio State University College of Medicine
Columbus, OH

Nicole Sutton, MD, FAAP, FACC
Department of Pediatrics
Division of Cardiology
Children's Hospital at Montefiore
Albert Einstein College of Medicine
Bronx, NY

Randi Teplow-Phipps, MD, FAAP
College Health Physician
Purchase College, State University of New York
Purchase, NY

Nathan E. Thompson, MD, PharmD
Assistant Professor of Pediatrics–Critical Care
Medical College of Wisconsin
Wauwatosa, WI

Philip T. Thrush, MD
Department of Pediatrics
The Heart Center
Nationwide Children's Hospital
The Ohio State University
Columbus, OH

William T. Tsai, MD, FAAP
Department of Pediatrics
Critical Care Medicine
Advocate Children's Hospital Park Ridge
Park Ridge, IL

Deanna Todd Tzanetos, MD, MSCI, FAAP
Department of Pediatrics
Division of Pediatric Critical Care
University of Louisville
Louisville, KY

Scott Vergano, MD, FAAP
Assistant Professor of Pediatrics
Eastern Virginia Medical School
Attending Pediatrician
Children's Hospital of The King's Daughters
Norfolk, VA

Martin Wakeham, MD, FAAP
Assistant Professor, Department of Pediatrics
Division of Critical Care Medicine
Associate Director, PCCM Fellowship
Medical College of Wisconsin
Associate Medical Director
Pediatric Critical Care Unit
Children's Hospital of Wisconsin
Milwaukee, WI

Christine A. Walsh, MD, FAAP, FACC
Department of Pediatrics
Division of Cardiology
Children's Hospital at Montefiore
Albert Einstein College of Medicine
Bronx, NY

April Wazeka, MD, FAAP
Department of Pediatrics
Respiratory Center for Children
Goryeb Children's Hospital
Morristown, NJ

Donald J. Weaver, Jr, MD, PhD, FAAP
Department of Pediatrics
Division of Nephrology and Hypertension
Levine Children's Hospital at Carolinas Medical Center
Charlotte, NC

Melinda A. Williams-Willingham, MD, FAAP
Pediatrician, Private Practice
Decatur Pediatric Group, PA
Clarkston, GA

Charles F. Willson, MD
Clinical Professor of Pediatrics
Brody School of Medicine at East Carolina University
Greenville, NC

Andrew R. Yates, MD, FAAP
Department of Pediatrics
The Heart Center
Nationwide Children's Hospital
The Ohio State University
Columbus, OH

Nader N. Youssef, MD, FAAP, FACG
Digestive Healthcare Center
Hillsborough, NJ
NPS Pharmaceuticals Inc.
Bedminster, NJ

Dedication

We are most appreciative for the long-term support and understanding from our families, who have born a great deal as we have toiled through this and many other projects.

To our loved ones: Barbara, Kimberly, Mitchell, Greg, Whitney (LF), and Ann, Chas, Mary, Christian, Emily, Elisa, Erika, Aileen, and Kelsey (JM).

Contents

Part 2
Critical and Emergency Care

Preface

The practice of pediatrics requires rapid access to evidence-based information to make timely diagnoses and offer accurate treatment for common conditions. This is our deliverable to you in *Succinct Pediatrics*. Starting with this volume, *Succinct Pediatrics* will be an ongoing series covering the entire scope of pediatric medicine. Each volume is envisioned to include short chapters with key figures and invaluable tables, allowing physicians the opportunity to deliver the highest quality of care to their patients in the most direct way possible.

As senior editors, we were fortunate to have wonderful associate editors who were able to select an excellent group of authors for the 286 chapters that will eventually encompass the entire series. Those editors are Charles Willson, Jack Lorenz, Warren Seigel, James Stallworth, and Mary Anne Jackson. In *Succinct Pediatrics: Evaluation and Management for Common and Critical Care*, our first book in the series, the authors have provided discussions on 72 topics with key points and detailed therapies. The book starts with an overview of the core knowledge needed for medical decision-making, authored by Jeffrey Avner. Understanding medical decision-making is the foundation for making the right decisions at the right time for patients. We have also provided evidence-based levels of decision support (as appropriate) throughout the book to permit physicians insight into the level of evidence for diagnostic tests as well as the selection of different treatment modalities. Selected readings have been provided for the print version of this book, with full reference lists for each chapter provided online at www.aap.org/SuccinctPediatrics.

The first part of this book addresses common problems in general pediatric practice. Seeing as it would be difficult to include every disease process and still be "succinct," we decided rather for a "top 50" approach, which would then be supported by the forthcoming sections and volumes of *Succinct Pediatrics*, the series. Chuck Willson used his wealth of experience to help guide us in the selection of chapters included in this volume.

Critical care and emergencies cross into general and specialty pediatrics and, as such, have been included in this book. Part 2, Critical and Emergency Care, covers 2-dozen key conditions seen as urgent or pediatric emergencies that may require intensive care expertise. This part actually serves as a bridge to the forthcoming volumes of *Succinct Pediatrics*, in which the focus will shift to pediatric specialties and other entities vital for the practice of general pediatrics.

We truly appreciate the wonderful guidance and assistance from the American Academy of Pediatrics. Our senior product development editor, Alain Park, was our superb director who helped choreograph every aspect of the book.

We sincerely hope that you will find *Succinct Pediatrics* an indispensable handbook and guide to the evaluation and management of your patients.

Leonard G. Feld, MD, PhD, MMM, FAAP, and John D. Mahan, MD, FAAP

Levels of Evidence

For *Succinct Pediatrics*, we asked each author to rank, where appropriate and feasible, evidence supporting the effectiveness of the different evaluation and treatment options detailed in the book. To this end, we suggested using the ranking system outlined in the 1989 US Preventive Services Task Force guidelines[1] and summarized as follows:

- ▶ Level I: Evidence obtained from at least one properly designed randomized controlled trial.
- ▶ Level II-1: Evidence obtained from well-designed controlled trials without randomization.
- ▶ Level II-2: Evidence obtained from well-designed cohort or case-control analytic studies, preferably from more than one center or research group.
- ▶ Level II-3: Evidence obtained from multiple time series with or without the intervention. Dramatic results in uncontrolled trials might also be regarded as this type of evidence.
- ▶ Level III: Opinions of respected authorities, based on clinical experience, descriptive studies, or reports of expert committees.

Reference

1. *Guide to Clinical Preventive Services: Report of the U.S. Preventive Services Task Force.* Darby, PA: Diane Publishing; 1989

Core Knowledge for Medical Decision-Making

Jeffrey R. Avner, MD

Key Points

- Rational medical decision-making requires knowledge of cognition, inherent biases, knowledge of disease prevalence and risk, and an understanding of pretest and posttest probabilities.

- Medical decision-making is influenced by clinical (ie, history and physical examination) and nonclinical (eg, patient, clinician, practice) factors.

- Clinicians need to learn and recognize the shortcomings and biases that may be part of their own decision-making.

- The hierarchy of study validity can provide a means of interpreting the level of evidence a study provides.

- Evidence-based medicine in the form of systematic reviews is a useful way of obtaining the best available data on a specific research question.

Overview

Medical decision-making is the cornerstone of diagnostic medicine. It is a complicated cognitive process by which a clinician sorts through a variety of clinical information to arrive at a likely diagnosis among many possibilities. This diagnostic impression then forms the basis of patient management with the ultimate goal of improved health.

However, any medical decision-making contains some inherent element of uncertainty. Furthermore, the ability of a clinician to obtain all necessary information and ensure its accuracy is time-consuming and often impractical in most clinical settings. Many turn to heuristics, an intuitive understanding of probabilities, to drive cognition and arrive at an "educated guess," one that is based on the recognition of specific patterns in clinical findings associated with a particular diagnosis and gleaned from years of experience. With this knowledge, the clinician can quickly sort through a limited set of historical and physical examination findings to support the decision. However, this type of "pattern recognition" is usually not data driven from the literature and therefore may contain bias, ultimately leading to many possible diagnostic errors (Box 1).

Box 1. Common Biases in Decision-Making

Anchoring (Premature Closure)	Overly relying on a few initial clinical findings and failing to adjust diagnosis as new information is gathered; non-supporting findings are devalued inappropriately.
Attribution Bias	Determining a diagnosis based on incomplete evidence such as overemphasizing personality or behavioral characteristics
Availability Bias	Overestimating the likelihood of what comes to mind most easily, often a recent experience, therefore neglecting the true rate (prior probability) of the illness and overestimating the unusual or remarkable
Confirmation Bias	Tending to favor evidence that supports the considered diagnosis and devaluing or not seeking any evidence to the contrary
Diagnostic Momentum Error	Allowing the effect of a preexisting diagnostic label to constrain unbiased reasoning

Failure to appreciate the changing epidemiology of disease (eg, the decline in occult bacteremia prevalence after universal pneumococcal vaccination) may lead to an overestimation of illness. Not knowing accurate pretest probability or how to apply it can lead to inappropriate testing. Personal experience with patients with similar presenting findings also causes bias. For example, a clinician who has been sued for missing a particular diagnosis is likely to overestimate the prevalence of that diagnosis in the future. Alternatively, a clinician who has not seen a relatively rare event (eg, meningitis in a well-appearing 2-week-old febrile newborn) or not seen a particular diagnosis (eg, Lemierre syndrome) may underestimate the prevalence of or not even consider that illness. Furthermore, if symptoms supporting the educated guess are found early in decision-making, the clinician may settle on a diagnosis before gathering other important, and possibly conflicting, findings (see "Anchoring (Premature Closure)" in Box 1). Thus, rational medical decision-making requires knowledge of cognition, inherent biases, knowledge of disease prevalence and risk, and an understanding of pretest and posttest probabilities. Additionally, it is often helpful for clinicians to practice *metacognition*, a process to reflect on their decision-making approaches and resultant patient outcomes to ascertain why they may have missed a diagnosis or whether they should modify their management in the future. By becoming more aware of their cognitive process, clinicians may be able to reduce errors and increase efficiency in diagnosis.

Other strategies of medical decision-making are often used, each with particular advantages and disadvantages. An *algorithmic* approach is often favored in busy settings where rapid management or critical decisions must be made. Flowcharts or clinical pathways direct decision-making into a stepwise process based on preestablished criteria, allowing for rapid assessment and standardization of care. While clearly valuable for many situations (eg, advanced life support, head trauma), algorithms tend to be applied rigidly and limit independent thinking. Other decision-making approaches may focus on "ruling out the worst case" such that management overly focuses on rare but high morbidity diagnoses or "making sure we don't miss it" by entertaining an exhaustive array of rare and perhaps esoteric diagnoses. These strategies generally overuse resources and testing.

In practice, clinicians generally use a combination of cognitive approaches adjusted for the practice setting, time limitation, available resources, and other factors. Furthermore, in the era of family-centered care, most management plans should take into account not just the clinician's clinical impression but also the patient's feelings about his health and disease in question. Still, the basis of medical decision making must lie in scientific reasoning, using the best available data and systematic observations to develop an effective approach to the patient and his symptoms. This requires the clinician to incorporate evidence-based medicine (EBM) into decision-making to derive the best answer to the clinical question. Evidence-based medicine focuses on clinically relevant research and takes into account the validity of study methodology, the power of predictive markers, the accuracy of diagnostic tests, and the effectiveness and safety of treatment options to answer a specific clinical question concerning the individual patient. Although it is difficult for a clinician to find, analyze, and assimilate information from a multitude of journals, the development of systematic reviews, databases, and information systems allows for a rapid incorporation of EBM into clinical practice, aiding the clinician in keeping pace with new advances (Table 1).

Table 1. The Steps of Evidence-Based Medicine

Step 1	Define the question.	Frame the need for specific information into an answerable clinical question.
Step 2	Find the evidence.	Systematically retrieve the best evidence to answer the question.
Step 3	Assess the evidence.	Critically evaluate the evidence for validity and application.
Step 4	Apply the evidence.	Integrate the evidence with clinical experience in the framework of patient-specific factors (biological and social) and patient values.
Step 5	Evaluate effectiveness.	Follow the patient's clinical course with regard to the desired outcome, and use it as a basis for similar strategies in the future.

Evaluation
· · · · · · · · · ·

In evaluation of a child, the clinician is continuously gathering new information to change the likelihood (or probability) of the child having a particular disease. Often this takes the form of Bayes theorem, in which new data are applied to a degree of uncertainty (prior probability) to yield a new, updated degree of certainty (posterior probability) (Figure 1).

Clinician's Thought Process

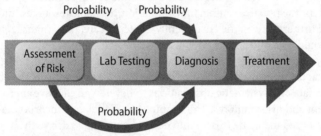

Figure 1. Clinician's thought process.

Because clinical research usually involves studies of groups of patients, the clinician must be able to apply those data to a specific patient who may or may not share characteristics with the study group. Thus, evaluation of any patient begins with the acquisition of factors that make the patient unique. In considering how likely a child is to have a particular disease, specific historical factors (eg, age, duration of symptoms, time of year), as well as physical examination findings (eg, clinical appearance, presence of fever, focal finding), allow the clinician to adjust the risk assessment by changing the pre-assessment probability. For example, risk of a urinary tract infection in a febrile 6-month-old may be 4% (pre-assessment probability). However, for a febrile uncircumcised boy with temperature above 39°C for more than 24 hours and no other source on examination, that risk rises to 15% (post-assessment probability). For some patients, the increase in probability may lead the clinician to further hone risk assessment by ordering laboratory or radiologic testing. In other scenarios, the post-assessment probability alone might be sufficient to begin preliminary treatment and further management. For example, a febrile 2-year-old who is ill appearing and has petechiae on the extremities has a high probability of having a serious bacterial illness (eg, meningococcemia) just on risk assessment alone. For this patient, further testing may be done with the caveat that administration of empiric antibiotics should not be delayed. The clinician should not weigh the probability of having a disease in isolation but must also take into account the morbidity of a delay in diagnosis. In a sense, the clinician needs to weigh risks and benefits relative to the certainty of diagnosis to determine what level of probability testing or management should be initiated.

Testing
. . . .

Laboratory tests should always complement but not replace clinical judgment. Generally, testing is used in 2 ways. In screening, an asymptomatic patient is tested to determine her risk of a particular disease. In diagnostic testing, the patient already has a symptom and the test is used to help reduce ambiguity of the underlying diagnosis. After the patient is assessed, and if there is still sufficient uncertainty of diagnosis or resultant management strategy, the clinician should use laboratory testing to increase or decrease the patient-specific probability of disease. This is determined by characteristics inherent in the test as well as the manner in which the test is being used.

Some tests provide continuous results and a wide range of numeric values, with the magnitude of the increments in value being significant and consistent. Continuous tests include those for white blood cell count, erythrocyte sedimentation rate, and C-reactive protein concentration. As no single value will rule in or rule out a diagnosis, a selected cutoff is often used. However, this cutoff is somewhat arbitrary, as it only gives rise to increasing or decreasing the probability of disease. Other tests have dichotomous results such as positive or negative. A positive result (eg, a positive blood culture) usually confirms or eliminates a disease from consideration. However, every test has its limitations, including false-positive and false-negative results.

Test results in the clinical arena are often used as predictors of disease. For example, the predictive value of a positive test is what percentage of patients with this positive test has the disease, while the negative predictive value is how many patients with a negative test do not have the disease. These predictive values are useful because clinicians often have the test result and seek to determine who has or does not have the disease. However, predictive values depend on the incidence of the disease. Tests used to predict rare events (eg, bacteremia in a well-appearing febrile infant) will usually have low positive and high negative predictive values solely because the incidence of disease is so low. On the other hand, sensitivity (ie, what percentage of patients with the disease have a positive test result) is independent of incidence. Clinicians need to consider which testing characteristic is most relevant to the clinical situation being evaluated. This often depends on the risks and benefits of testing versus the morbidity and mortality of missing the illness in the context of disease prevalence.

One of the best statistical approaches to decision-making is the use of likelihood ratios. A likelihood ratio provides an estimate of how much a test result will change the probability of the specific patient having a disease (percentage of ill children with a test result versus percentage of well children with a test result). The higher the likelihood ratio of a positive test result, the more effect the test will have in increasing the probability of disease (ie, it will lead to a higher posttest probability). Similarly, the lower the likelihood ratio (ie, below 1), the less likely the child has the disease. A likelihood ratio of 1 has no effect; likelihood ratios of 5 to 10 or 0.1 to 0.2 have moderate effect; and likelihood ratios of greater than 10 or less than 0.1 have large effect. These data allow the clinician to estimate the likelihood of the patient having or not having a disease. This must then be integrated into the clinician's medical decision-making by taking into account the risk and benefit of performing the test and its resultant effect on the probability of illness.

Management

Ultimately, the clinician's approach to the patient determines the health outcome. In that regard, the clinician decides on a specific probability threshold above which management is indicated. Effectiveness of a particular outcome is best determined by prior studies looking at risk factors, interventions, and outcomes in a similar population, the strength of which usually depends on study design (Table 2).

Descriptive studies, such as case reports or case series, report on a particular occurrence or outcome. Because a case study describes only an event, it is difficult to show causation. While the cases may be instructive, care must be taken in generalizing the results. Explanatory studies have stronger, hypothesis-driven study designs. *Randomized controlled trials* have the highest level of scientific rigor. This type of design starts with a study group, randomizes subjects into intervention and control groups, and measures the effect of an intervention on the outcome in each group, limiting systemic differences between the groups. A *cohort study* begins with a study population that is free of the outcome, classifies the group based on presence or absence of the risk factor, and measures the outcome in each group. In this type of design, subjects already had the risk factor, rather than it being imposed on them. However, it is impossible to be sure that the groups are comparable in terms of confounding variables. A *case-control study* begins with a group of patients with a disease and a matched group of control patients without the disease and compares the presence of a risk factor. Although this study design is very common, especially if the outcome is rare, the retrospective design may not take into account other factors that can lead to the outcome. Finally, *cross-sectional studies* compare the presence of a risk factor in groups of patients with and without the disease at a single point in time. While this is also a common methodology, especially in epidemiologic investigation of a disease outbreak, it is a very weak method of establishing causality.

Because it is often difficult for the clinician to synthesize information from available studies, the use of *systematic reviews* has become a useful means of summing up the best available data on a specific research question. After an exhaustive review of the literature, each study is screened for quality in a transparent manner to avoid bias and, if possible, the results are combined. These studies are generally readily available online (eg, The Cochrane Collaboration, available at www.cochrane.org) and provide a practical means for clinicians to practice EBM.

Table 2. Hierarchy of Study Validity

Validity (Level of Evidence)	Study Type	Sampling	Advantages	Disadvantages	Statistics
Higher	Systematic reviews	Literature search with objective assessment of methodological quality	Provide an exhaustive summary of relevant literature	May vary in standards and guidelines used	Meta-analysis
	Randomized controlled trials	Prospective	Allow for determination of superiority or non-inferiority of an intervention; can use intent to treat design	Limit systematic differences between groups	Incidence, relative risk
	Cohort studies	Prospective or retrospective	Allow for determination of causality	Make it difficult to ensure that groups are comparable	Incidence, relative risk
	Case-control studies	Retrospective	Are inexpensive, efficient; are practical for rare disorders	Are prone to sampling and recall bias	Odds ratio
	Cross-sectional studies	Single occasion	Are inexpensive	Present no clear evidence of causality; are not practical for rare disorders	Prevalence, odds ratio
Lower	Case reports or series	Retrospective	Are inexpensive, efficient	Present no statistical validity	None

Adapted from Perry-Parrish C, Dodge R. Research and statistics: validity hierarchy for study design and study type. *Pediatr Rev.* 2010;31(1):27–29.

Understanding different levels of design allows the stratification of evidence by quality (Box 2). This popular hierarchy permits a standard approach to quality and was selected as a method of assessing the evidence for this publication. However, the clinician is still required to assess not just the type of study design but also how well the study was conducted (internal validity) and the adequacy of the conclusions. For example, a poorly conducted randomized control trial with an insufficient sample size may not be of better quality than a well-designed case-control study. Other categorizations may be useful to assess levels of certainty regarding net benefit (Table 3) and recommendations for practice (Table 4).

Box 2. Levels of Evidence Used in This Publication

Level I	Evidence obtained from at least one properly designed randomized controlled trial
Level II-1	Evidence obtained from well-designed controlled trials without randomization
Level II-2	Evidence obtained from well-designed cohort or case-control analytic studies, preferably from more than one center or research group
Level II-3	Evidence obtained from multiple time series with or without the intervention. Dramatic results in uncontrolled trials might also be regarded as this type of evidence.
Level III	Opinions of respected authorities, based on clinical experience, descriptive studies, or reports of expert committees

Adapted from Harris RP, Helfand M, Woolf SH, et al. Current methods of the US Preventive Services Task Force: a review of the process. *Am J Prev Med*. 2001;20(3 Suppl):21–35, with permission.

Cause results are generally reported as relative risk or odds ratios. These statistical tests are used to determine the probability of having a particular outcome based on presence (or absence) of a particular test result. *Relative risk* is risk of an outcome in an intervention group divided by risk of the same outcome in the control group and is used in prospective cohort studies to determine the probability of a specific outcome. *Odds ratio* is the odds of an outcome in an intervention group divided by the odds of the same outcome in the control group and is used in case-control, retrospective studies to determine the "odds" of having an outcome. If there is no difference between the groups, the relative risk is 1 or the odds ratio is 1. If the intervention lowers the risk, the value is less than one, and if it increases the risk, the value is greater than 1. In an effort to incorporate factors related to an intervention in assessing effectiveness of that intervention to achieve a desired outcome, some studies report results in terms of the *number needed to treat* (NNT). This is the number of patients you need to treat to prevent one bad outcome or cause one good outcome. An NNT of 1 means that the treatment is effective in all patients (ie, as the NNT increases, effectiveness decreases). A high NNT needs to be weighed against the morbidity of the outcome being studied. For example, if 8 children would have to be treated continuously with phenobarbital for 2 years to prevent 1 febrile seizure, the NNT is 8. The clinician can then decide if the consequence of treating these children justifies the prevention of one febrile seizure. A higher NNT may be acceptable in situations in which the outcome is, for example, bacterial meningitis because there are potentially devastating consequences and the clinician might be willing to accept treating many children unnecessarily to prevent even one case.

Table 3. US Preventive Services Task Force Levels of Certainty Regarding Net Benefit

Level of Certainty	Description
High	The available evidence usually includes consistent results from well-designed, well-conducted studies in representative primary care populations. These studies assess the effects of the preventive service on health outcomes. This conclusion is therefore unlikely to be strongly affected by the results of future studies.
Moderate	The available evidence is sufficient to determine the effects of the preventive service on health outcomes, but confidence in the estimate is constrained by such factors as • The number, size, or quality of individual studies • Inconsistency of findings across individual studies • Limited generalizability of findings to routine primary care practice • Lack of coherence in the chain of evidence As more information becomes available, the magnitude or direction of the observed effect could change, and this change may be large enough to alter the conclusion.
Low	The available evidence is insufficient to assess effects on health outcomes. Evidence is insufficient because of • The limited number or size of studies • Important flaws in study design or methods • Inconsistency of findings across individual studies • Gaps in the chain of evidence • Findings not generalizable to routine primary care practice • Lack of information on important health outcomes More information may allow estimation of effects on health outcomes.

From Agency for Healthcare Research and Quality, US Preventive Services Task Force. *The Guide to Clinical Preventive Services 2014: Recommendations of the U.S. Preventive Services Task Force.* Available at: www.ahrq.gov/professionals/clinicians-providers/guidelines-recommendations/guide. Accessed September 3, 2014.

With the availability of sophisticated health information systems, the use of clinical decision-support tools is becoming a useful new technology to enhance care and reduce errors. Interactive computer software can be used by the clinician, in real time, to provide automated reasoning that takes into account the patient's clinical findings and the latest medical knowledge. By entering patient-specific information, preset rules of logic based on scientific evidence can help the clinician make a diagnosis or analyze patient data in a way that, in some ways, the clinician may not be able do on his own. To be sure, this technique cannot account for those non-clinical factors that may affect decision-making, but it may provide the clinician an efficient, inexpensive process to consider other diagnoses, reduce medical errors, and direct the most EBM approach.

Table 4. US Preventive Services Task Force Recommendation Definitions and Suggestions for Practice

Grade	Definition	Suggestions for Practice
A	The USPSTF recommends the service. There is high certainty that the net benefit is substantial.	Offer or provide this service.
B	The USPSTF recommends the service. There is high certainty that the net benefit is moderate, or there is moderate certainty that the net benefit is moderate to substantial.	Offer or provide this service.
C	The USPSTF recommends against routinely providing the service. There may be considerations that support providing the service in an individual patient. There is at least moderate certainty that the net benefit is small.	Offer or provide this service only if other considerations support the offering or providing of the service in an individual patient.
D	The USPSTF recommends against the service. There is moderate or high certainty that the service has no net benefit or that the harms outweigh the benefits.	Discourage the use of this service.
I Statement	The USPSTF concludes that the current evidence is insufficient to assess the balance of benefits and harms of the service. Evidence is lacking, of poor quality, or conflicting, and the balance of benefits and harms cannot be determined.	Read the clinical considerations section of USPSTF recommendation statement. If the service is offered, patients should understand the uncertainty about the balance of benefits and harms.

Abbreviation: USPSTF, US Preventive Services Task Force.

From Agency for Healthcare Research and Quality, US Preventive Services Task Force. *The Guide to Clinical Preventive Services 2014: Recommendations of the U.S. Preventive Services Task Force.* Available at: www.ahrq.gov/professionals/clinicians-providers/guidelines-recommendations/guide. Accessed September 3, 2014

Ultimately, the clinician must decide how to apply the best evidence to the patient. As noted previously, this is a very complicated process that should take into account clinical decision-making but may also be affected by nonclinical influences, be they patient related (eg, socioeconomic status, ethnicity, attitudes, preferences), clinician related (eg, time constraints, professional interactions), or practice related (eg, organization, resource allocation, cost). These factors are often integrated into medical decision-making, consciously or subconsciously, and may have a positive influence (eg, increasing patient compliance) or negative influence (eg, creation of health disparities) on health outcome. It is essential that clinicians be aware of these nonclinical factors to account for a patient's specific interest, thereby optimizing management.

Suggested Reading

Agency for Healthcare Research and Quality, US Preventive Services Task Force. *The Guide to Clinical Preventive Services 2014: Recommendations of the U.S. Preventive Services Task Force.* http://www.ahrq.gov/professionals/clinicians-providers/guidelines-recommendations/guide. Accessed September 3, 2014

Finnell SM, Carroll AE, Downs SM; American Academy of Pediatrics Subcommittee on Urinary Tract Infection. Diagnosis and management of an initial UTI in febrile infants and young children. Pediatrics. 2011;128(3):e749–e770

Hajjaj FM, Salek MS, Basra MK, Finlay AY. Non-clinical influences on clinical decision-making: a major challenge to evidence-based practice. *J R Soc Med.* 2010;103(5):178–187

Harris RP, Helfand M, Woolf SH, et al. Current methods of the US Preventive Services Task Force: a review of the process. *Am J Prev Med.* 2001;20(3 Suppl):21–35

Kianifar HR, Akhondian J, Najafi-Sani M, Sadeghi R. Evidence based medicine in pediatric practice: brief review. *Iran J Pediatr.* 2010;20(3):261–268

MacKinnon RJ. Evidence based medicine methods (part 1): the basics. *Paediatr Anaesth.* 2007;17(10):918–923

MacKinnon RJ. Evidence based medicine methods (part 2): extension into the clinical area. *Paediatr Anaesth.* 2007;17(11):1021–1027

Onady GM. Evidence-based medicine: applying valid evidence. *Pediatr Rev.* 2009;30(8):317–322

Papier A. Decision support in dermatology and medicine: history and recent developments. *Semin Cutan Med Surg.* 2012;31(3):153–159

Perry-Parrish C, Dodge R. Research and statistics: validity hierarchy for study design and study type. *Pediatr Rev.* 2010;31(1):27–29

Raslich MA, Onady GM. Evidence-based medicine: critical appraisal of the literature (critical appraisal tools). *Pediatr Rev.* 2007;28(4):132–138

Sandhu H, Carpenter C, Freeman K, Nabors SG, Olson A. Clinical decisionmaking: opening the black box of cognitive reasoning. *Ann Emerg Med.* 2006;48(6):713–719

CHAPTER 1

Abdominal Pain, Acute

John Stephens, MD, and Michael J. Steiner, MD

Key Points

- The major causes of acute abdominal pain in childhood are benign and self-limited. However, specific signs and symptoms and the clinical site of patient presentation can dramatically change the potential for severe disease.

- In most cases, history and physical examination findings can establish the diagnosis without further testing.

- Observation of indirect signs in small children, such as comfort in their parents' laps, can be helpful in narrowing the differential diagnosis.

- The most helpful diagnostic tests for appendicitis are clinical scoring systems that incorporate a variety of signs and symptoms, although in the right clinical setting the presence of some individual signs, such as rebound tenderness, dramatically increase the likelihood of appendicitis.

- Laboratory tests and radiologic imaging should be ordered in limited cases, particularly when history and examination findings suggest causes of pain that need urgent surgical intervention. These tests should be directed at the likely diagnosis.

Overview

Abdominal pain is a common concern in the pediatric population in all clinical settings. Clinicians and research studies define acute abdominal pain as the onset of pain within 72 hours to one week of presentation. In this chapter, acute abdominal pain is differentiated from recurrent abdominal pain (repeated episodes of similar abdominal pain over a more prolonged period of time) and chronic abdominal pain (pain that is usually or always present over a prolonged period of time) (see Chapter 2). Both recurrent and chronic abdominal pain can originate from diagnoses that overlap with acute abdominal pain. However, once abdominal pain has recurred or persisted for a prolonged period, the most likely causes are different from the differential diagnoses associated with acute abdominal pain.

Most cases of acute abdominal pain will prove to be from benign and self-limited conditions. Some patients, however, will present with urgent and occasionally life-threatening conditions causing their symptoms.

Knowledge of the most common causes of abdominal pain in patients within certain age ranges can help focus preliminary diagnostic efforts (Table 1-1). A diagnostic challenge is that abdominal pain can be caused by a wide variety of sources within and outside of the abdominal cavity.

Additionally, serial examination in many cases of diagnostic uncertainty is a reasonable and cost-effective approach.

Causes and Differential Diagnosis

The differential diagnosis of abdominal pain is extremely broad but can be narrowed dramatically based on patient age, historical factors, and the preliminary physical examination (Table 1-1). The most common diagnoses in emergency department settings are upper respiratory tract illnesses, including viral upper respiratory tract infections, acute otitis media, and group A streptococcal pharyngitis. Abdominal pain of unclear etiology, viral syndrome, and gastroenteritis are the most frequent diagnoses. The most common diagnosis requiring surgical intervention is appendicitis.

Clinical Features/Signs and Symptoms

Fever will raise or lower the probability of a number of conditions. In infants, this should raise level of suspicion for urinary tract infection or gastroenteritis. In toddlers, fever will also raise suspicion of urinary tract infection, along with respiratory infections, including lower lobe pneumonia, even in the absence of obvious respiratory symptoms. School-aged children with fever have similar diagnostic considerations but should be considered for group A streptococcal pharyngitis too. Fever in female adolescents with abdominal pain should also raise the possibility of ascending sexually transmitted infections. In addition, fever can be associated with appendicitis and other conditions causing peritonitis. Absence of fever lowers the probability of appendicitis.

Emesis is an extremely important symptom to assess. In infants, particular emphasis should be placed on presence or absence of bilious emesis, as bile-stained vomitus suggests an obstructive process in the proximal small bowel and is highly suggestive of a surgical and morbid cause of pain. Bilious emesis in the neonate should immediately prompt evaluation with an upper gastrointestinal tract series and discussion with a pediatric surgeon. In older children, emesis is less likely to be caused by intestinal obstruction and most frequently will be from acute gastroenteritis. Older children and adolescents can occasionally have bilious emesis after prolonged vomiting in the setting of a non-obstructive process. Classically, emesis will precede abdominal pain in gastroenteritis.

Table 1-1. Differential Diagnosis of Acute Abdominal Pain Based on Age and Important Symptoms

	Infant	Toddler	School-aged Child	Adolescent
Specific symptoms	• Fever • Emesis: bilious or not • Stool pattern: frequency and quality of stool • Decreased feeding • Peritoneal symptoms or signs	• Fever • Emesis • Stool pattern: frequency and quality of stool • Decreased appetite • Dysuria • Peritoneal symptoms or signs	• Fever • Emesis • Stool pattern: frequency and quality of stool • Decreased appetite • Dysuria • Pain character: colicky or dull • Peritoneal symptoms or signs	• Fever • Emesis • Stool pattern: frequency and quality of stool • Decreased appetite • Dysuria • Menstrual history/ pregnancy status • Pain character: colicky or dull • Peritoneal symptoms or signs
Common nonsurgical abdominal diagnoses	• Urinary tract infection • Gastroenteritis • Colic • Infantile dyschezia • Milk protein allergy	• Nonspecific abdominal pain • Gastroenteritis • Constipation • Mesenteric adenitis	• Nonspecific abdominal pain • Gastroenteritis • Constipation • Mesenteric adenitis	• Nonspecific abdominal pain • Gastroenteritis • Constipation • Ruptured ovarian cyst • Pelvic inflammatory disease
Common surgical diagnoses	• Pyloric stenosis • Volvulus • Hernia • Trauma • Intussusception • Hirschsprung disease	• Intussusception • Appendicitis • Trauma • Swallowed foreign body	• Appendicitis • Trauma	• Appendicitis • Trauma • Ovarian/ testicular torsion • Ectopic pregnancy
Non-abdominal or systemic causes	• Upper respiratory tract infection	• Upper respiratory tract infection • Pneumonia • Henoch-Schönlein purpura • Discitis	• Upper respiratory tract infection • Pharyngitis, group A streptococcal pharyngitis • Abdominal migraine • DKA • Pneumonia • Henoch-Schönlein purpura	• Upper respiratory tract infection • DKA • Pneumonia

Abbreviation: DKA, diabetic ketoacidosis.

This is in contrast to surgical causes of pain, which tend to have pain preceding emesis, though this pattern is not reliably consistent.

The stooling pattern can also provide important history. A common history in young infants is straining with apparent discomfort during defecation, resultant soft stools, and normal appearance in between. This pattern is seen with infantile dyschezia, a benign condition in infants learning coordination of abdominal contractions with relaxation of rectal and pelvic floor musculature. Bloody stools in infants are most frequently from medical causes such as milk protein allergy, but if the infant is distressed or ill appearing, more serious causes, including intussusception, should be considered. Bloody stools in older children with abdominal pain should raise level of suspicion for bacterial enteritis, although bowel necrosis from an urgent surgical diagnosis needs to be considered as well. Intussusception is most commonly seen in children during the second year of life and will typically cause episodic severe pain, often associated with crying and drawing of legs up to the abdomen. Diarrhea in all age ranges is associated with gastroenteritis but can accompany other conditions causing abdominal pain. Lack of stool output can indicate constipation but may also reflect ileus or anatomic intestinal obstruction and can be a subtle symptom of developing peritonitis.

Anorexia in older children is associated with appendicitis. It can also be associated with bacterial disease such as streptococcal pharyngitis and pneumonia, as well as any severe systemic disease.

Peritoneal symptoms tend to be subtle in children, especially younger ones. They often manifest by the child being less active. A history of increased pain with movement, such as while driving in a car over rough roads, is important and may need to be asked specifically of parents to be elicited.

Older children can have the same patterns as observed in infants and toddlers. In older children, pain preceding emesis is somewhat more suggestive of surgical pathology than the reverse.

Evaluation

In most settings, physicians approach the diagnosis of abdominal pain by simultaneously approaching 2 goals. First, physicians look for a constellation of symptoms and signs to confirm that one of the common relatively benign syndromes is present, such as gastroenteritis or nonspecific, self-limiting abdominal pain. Second, physicians are also continuously assessing for severe or red-flag findings that could suggest serious illnesses, particularly illnesses that need urgent surgical intervention.

Physical examination should begin with the child in a position of comfort away from the examiner. Overall comfort and appearance should be noted as well as if the patient is walking or moving normally, moving frequently, or lying still. For most children, this should be followed by a complete examination, focusing on the abdomen toward the end of the physical examination but before other uncomfortable examination elements. It is particularly important to focus on the anatomic structures located near the abdomen, including the lung bases superior to the abdomen and the genitalia and hips inferior to the abdomen. Specific examination of the abdomen may start with auscultation of bowel sounds and be followed by palpation of the abdomen. A rectal examination is usually not needed to diagnose the cause of abdominal pain. Similarly, gynecologic examination is rarely needed, but if vaginal discharge or lower abdominal pain and fever in an adolescent are present, pelvic examination can be critical. The most common diagnosis of acute abdominal pain that requires surgical intervention for all ages except infancy is appendicitis. In some case series in emergency departments, up to 10% of children with abdominal pain are reported to have appendicitis, even higher if certain historical elements are present. However, in a large case series with more than 1,000 children presenting to either an urgent care setting or emergency department at a large children's hospital, slightly less than 1% of children older than 2 years with a chief concern of abdominal pain had appendicitis. History and physical examination findings are most helpful when grouped in a clinical scoring system. The most commonly studied system is the Alvarado score (Box 1-1), which applies points for specific signs and symptoms as follows:

Box 1-1. Alvarado Score for Appendicitis (Note mnemonic of MANTRELS for criteria.)

		Value
Symptoms	Migration	1
	Anorexia-acetone	1
	Nausea-vomiting	1
Signs	Tenderness in right lower quadrant	2
	Rebound pain	1
	Elevation of temperature	1
Laboratory	Leukocytosis	2
	Shift to the left	1
Total score[a]		10

[a] Scores ≥7 points have a positive likelihood ratio that approximates 4.0 (confidence interval of 3.2 to 4.9) and scores ≤4 dramatically decrease the likelihood of appendicitis with a likelihood ratio of 0.05 (confidence interval of 0.0 to 0.85).
From Alvarado A. A practical score for the early diagnosis of acute appendicitis. *Ann Emerg Med.* 1986;15(5):557–564. Reprinted with permission.

In cases of diagnostic uncertainty, laboratory tests for complete blood count, erythrocyte sedimentation rate, and C-reactive protein concentration, and urinalysis, are usually the first tests ordered. Other laboratory tests evaluating for liver inflammation, pancreatic inflammation, genitourinary tract infections, or pregnancy should be used in appropriate clinical scenarios. Radiologic imaging should be focused on diagnosing or excluding specific conditions, rather than as a broad diagnostic tool in the undifferentiated patient.

Infant

Laboratory Tests

Catheterized urinalysis should be ordered for the febrile infant to exclude urinary tract infection. Stool antigen testing for rotavirus can be diagnostic in the setting of acute diarrheal illness, though management of disease is not altered by this result.

Radiologic Imaging

A plain abdominal radiograph, particularly with a supine and also an upright or lateral view, is helpful to evaluate for suspected obstructive processes or if signs of peritonitis are present to exclude a perforated viscus. It can suggest an intussusception but is generally not diagnostic. Ultrasound in experienced centers can diagnose intussusception; however, air or contrast (preferably water-soluble) enema will be both diagnostic and therapeutic. Upper gastrointestinal tract contrast study should be ordered when malrotation with volvulus or other proximal intestinal obstruction is suspected, usually in the presence of bilious emesis. Contrast enema is the test of choice when Hirschsprung is suspected in the acute setting. Guidelines suggest that anorectal manometry is a preferred diagnostic method for Hirschsprung disease in non-acute situations but cannot be immediately obtained in most centers. An abnormal contrast enema will reveal a transition point from a normal-sized rectum to a dilated sigmoid colon. This test should be done with no rectal manipulation in the preceding 24 hours to avoid temporarily dilating the transition point.

One to 5 Years

Laboratory Tests

Urinalysis should still be considered for the febrile patient. Group A streptococcal pharyngitis testing should also be considered. Rotavirus testing is a consideration in patients with diarrheal illness. Blood tests can be useful as an adjunct in diagnosis of acute appendicitis. A peripheral white blood cell count of less than 10,000/µL lowers posttest odds of appendicitis by 80% (likelihood ratio of 0.22), whereas one greater than 10,000/µL doubles posttest odds (likelihood ratio of 2.0).

Radiologic Imaging

Plain radiographs of the abdomen may be helpful to evaluate for constipation or when history or physical examination findings suggest obstruction or peritonitis. A plain radiograph of the chest should be considered for febrile patients, with or without respiratory symptoms, to exclude lower lobe pneumonia if no other cause of fever is apparent. Ultrasound may be utilized in experienced centers to look for intussusception. Additionally, ultrasound performs well with experienced operators in evaluation for appendicitis. Upper gastrointestinal tract contrast study should be performed when malrotation with volvulus or other proximal intestinal obstruction is suspected. Air or contrast enema will diagnose and treat cases of intussusception. Computed tomography can diagnose acute appendicitis reliably but is time-consuming and expensive and involves significant radiation exposure to the patient.

School-aged Child

Considerations are very similar to those for preschool-aged children, except that volvulus and intussusception are much less common, and patients can generally provide more detailed history and are more tolerant of physical examination.

Adolescent

Additional considerations include pregnancy and its complications, sexually transmitted infections, menstrual- and ovulation-related pain, and gonadal torsion.

Laboratory Tests

Urinalysis should be considered with symptoms of urinary frequency, dysuria, or hematuria. A urine pregnancy test should be considered for girls who are post-menarche. Urine can be sent for testing for sexually transmitted infections, and purulent urethral or vaginal discharge should be sent for gonorrheal and chlamydial disease testing.

Radiologic Imaging

Ultrasound with views of vascular structures when appropriate is often critical to diagnoses of genitourinary tract issues, including ovarian torsion, ectopic pregnancy, and testicular torsion.

Management

Treatment will depend on the underlying diagnosis. A firm diagnosis may not be obvious even after careful history, physical examination, and directed ancillary testing. In this case, serial abdominal examinations may be the best course. Several indications call for pediatric surgical consultation. These include signs or symptoms of peritonitis; intestinal obstruction, especially bilious or feculent emesis; incarcerated inguinal hernia; and any suggestion of surgical cause of abdominal pain on radiologic imaging, such as free air in the peritoneum. Suspected appendicitis is a frequent referral reason for surgical consultation.

Withholding pain medications in children with severe acute abdominal pain for fear of "masking" is not supported by medical evidence, and, in fact, adequate pain control may enhance diagnostic accuracy by allowing a more thorough physical examination. Acetaminophen is a reasonable choice in patients who can take oral medications and have mild to moderate pain, while weight-based intravenous morphine or fentanyl (not to exceed an adult dose) is safe and effective for patients who are unable to tolerate oral dosing or those who have more severe pain.

Suggested Reading

Bundy DG, Byerley JS, Liles EA, Perrin EM, Katznelson J, Rice HE. Does this child have appendicitis? *JAMA*. 2007;298(4):438–451

Green R, Bulloch B, Kabani A, Hancock BJ, Tenenbein M. Early analgesia for children with acute abdominal pain. *Pediatrics*. 2005;116(4):978–983

Ross A, LeLeiko NS. Acute abdominal pain. *Pediatr Rev*. 2010;31(4):135–144

Saito JM. Beyond appendicitis: evaluation and surgical treatment of pediatric acute abdominal pain. *Curr Opin Pediatr*. 2012;24(3):357–364

Scholer SJ, Pituch K, Orr DP, et al. Clinical outcomes of children with acute abdominal pain. *Pediatrics*. 1996;98(4):680–685

CHAPTER 2

Abdominal Pain, Functional

Nader N. Youssef, MD

Key Points

- Celiac disease should be screened for in any child with persistent gastrointestinal concerns.

- Coping strategies including guided imagery and hypnotherapy should be considered first-line therapy in the treatment of children with functional abdominal pain.

- Functional abdominal pain can be diagnosed based on the validated Rome criteria and utilization of a limited laboratory investigation panel to rule out metabolic or structural disease.

- A thorough explanation to the family that functional abdominal pain is a diagnosis that involves altered sensation and perception should be offered.

- Functional abdominal pain should be treated aggressively early in childhood, as evidence suggests that if left untreated, it may cause these patients to have irritable bowel syndrome and be susceptible to depression in adulthood.

- Regular scheduled follow-up visits at suggested intervals of every 2 to 3 months for these patients is essential during the early course of the treatment to build an alliance with patient and family.

Overview

Recurrent abdominal pain, or what is now commonly referred to as functional abdominal pain (FAP), is described as pain syndrome consisting of at least 3 episodes of abdominal pain over a period of 3 or more months and severe enough to affect activities. Only 5% to 10% of children with recurrent abdominal pain have an underlying organic process that contributes to their pain. Recent criteria have been developed to subdivide recurrent abdominal pain into different criteria depending on additional associated features such as nausea, bloating, or urgency with defecation and to be considered part of a group of functional gastrointestinal disorders with definitive, symptom-based diagnostic criteria known as the Rome criteria. Despite the differences in terminology, FAP and irritable bowel syndrome (IBS) are two closely related disorders.

Rome III Criteria for Diagnosis: Overlap of FAP and IBS

Rome III criteria for FAP require that abdominal pain is present at least once per week for 2 consecutive months in the absence of any metabolic, structural, or inflammatory process. Irritable bowel syndrome is defined as abdominal discomfort or pain associated with 2 or more of the following effects at least 25% of the time: improvement with defecation, onset associated with a change in frequency of stools, or onset associated with a change in form of stools. Symptoms that support the IBS diagnosis include (a) abnormal stool frequency (≥4 stools per day or ≤2 stools per week), (b) abnormal stool form (lumpy/hard or loose/watery stools), (c) abnormal passage of stools (ie, straining, urgency, or feeling of incomplete evacuation), (d) passage of mucus, and (e) bloating or feeling of abdominal distension. Adolescents may present with constipation (IBS-C), diarrhea (IBS-D), or a mix of the two (IBS-M).

Causes and Differential Diagnoses

The etiology of FAP is largely unknown. Pathophysiologic evidence would suggest 3 potential mechanisms for abdominal pain in functional bowel disorders: altered intestinal motility, altered intestinal sensory thresholds, and psychosocial factors.

Evaluation

A suggested set of laboratory investigations to aid in screening for intestinal inflammation and malabsorption are listed in Box 2-1. A comprehensive metabolic panel may help identify patients with potential conditions such as liver disorders. Celiac disease needs to be screened for with total IgA level and tissue transglutaminase and anti-endomysial antibodies. An abdominal radiograph can reveal occult constipation as a cause of recurrent abdominal pain. A hydrogen breath test will evaluate for lactase deficiency as a cause of symptoms. Stool testing for parasites (eg, *Giardia, Cyclospora,* and *Isospora*) and infections (eg, *Clostridium difficile, Salmonella, Shigella, Campylobacter jejuni*) should also be included in the work-up. In addition to determining sedimentation rate or C-reactive protein concentration to screen for systemic inflammation, a novel stool investigation known as fecal calprotectin has been developed to look at inflammation within the intestine and may be considered for initial screening to help differentiate IBS versus inflammatory conditions such as Crohn disease. However, history consistent with diarrhea accompanied by weight loss, blood in the stools, or suspected nutritional deficiency should prompt investigation for intestinal disease, including endoscopy, to rule out infection or mucosal pathology, such as inflammatory bowel disease, including Crohn disease or ulcerative colitis.

Box 2-1. Limited Evaluation for Functional Abdominal Pain

- Abdominal radiograph
- Anti-endomysial level
- C-reactive protein concentration
- Complete blood count
- Comprehensive metabolic panel
- Erythrocyte sedimentation rate
- Fecal calprotectin level
- Stools for infection including ova, parasite, and *Helicobacter pylori*
- Tissue transglutaminase level
- Total IgA level

Management

Conventional Approach

Current treatment for children with FAP is to reassure the child and family that no serious progressive disease is present, that she will eventually outgrow the symptoms, and that she must learn to cope with it. Pharmaceutical treatments are commonly used in an attempt to manage symptoms of FAP in childhood despite the lack of data supporting their efficacy. These approaches include fiber, antacids, and antispasmodics.

Innovative Approaches

In adults, low-dose antidepressants have been useful in the management of IBS. The role of amitriptyline as a monotherapy for FAP in children continues be unclear, is currently reserved for those who may have overlap anxiety or depression associated with significant disabling pain, and is used in combination with psychological intervention to emphasize more meaningful coping as part of their recovery.

Integrative Medicine Intervention

Studies have shown that many children (36%) presenting for the first time to a gastroenterologist are already on a complementary alternative medicine regimen (CAM). Symptomatic improvements were attributed to CAM by 73% of the parents of children given these therapies. Interventions include over-the-counter products, spiritual practices, visits to alternative practitioners, and dietary modifications. Over-the-counter products and dietary modifications ranked moderate on patient satisfaction scales, while spiritual practices and alternative practitioner visits ranked highest. Other CAM practices such as oral supplementation, acupuncture, aromatherapy, and osteopathic manipulation are popular among adult patients with FAP.

Guided Imagery or Hypnotherapy

Conventional treatment of FAP is largely unsatisfactory. Increasing evidence shows that mind/body approaches are quite useful in the treatment of FAP in children. These approaches are safe, inexpensive, and easy to administer. Children, with their inherent imaginative abilities, find them easy to learn and use. Guided imagery often becomes self-guided in children, especially with the use of reinforcement audiotapes in the evening during bedtime. These therapies have become first-line therapies for most pediatric gastroenterologists who are asked to evaluate children with FAP. These therapies are applicable to the whole range of children with FAP regardless of severity.

Mind/body approaches such as hypnotherapy, guided imagery, and relaxation techniques have been efficacious in the treatment of visceral pain disorders in children and are used for adults with FAP or IBS. Children were able to return to school and showed improvement in their quality of life on validated measures.

Long-term Considerations

Evidence shows that FAP is rarely a self-limiting condition, and after 5 years, one-third of children with it will continue to experience symptoms (Figure 2-1). Children with FAP can have significant school absence, family disruption, and social withdrawal with tendencies toward anxiety and depression. Such morbidity can result in impaired quality of life. Children with FAP continue to have increased health care utilization in young adulthood.

Children with FAP may have symptoms for more than one year until adequate relief is achieved. Patients with functional gastrointestinal disorders may additionally have sleep difficulties, headaches, dizziness, and fatigue.

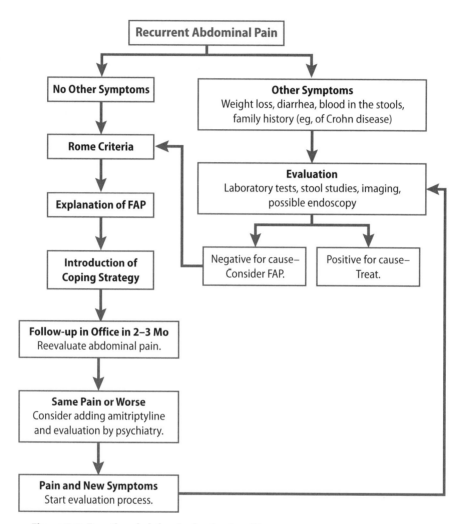

Figure 2-1. Functional abdominal pain algorithm.

Abbreviation: FAP, functional abdominal pain.

Suggested Reading
· · · · · · · · · · · · · · · · · ·

Chitkara DK, Talley NJ, Weaver AL, et al. Incidence of presentation of common functional gastrointestinal disorders in children: a cohort study. *Clin Gastroenterol Hepatol.* 2007;5(2):186–191

Di Lorenzo C, Youssef NN, Sigurdsson L, Scharff L, Griffiths J, Wald A. Visceral hyperalgesia in children with functional abdominal pain. *J Pediatr.* 2001;139(6):838–843

Hyams JS, Burke G, Davis PM, Rzepski B, Andrulonis PA. Abdominal pain and irritable bowel syndrome in adolescents: a community-based study. *J Pediatr.* 1996;129(2): 220–226

Saps M, Youssef N, Miranda A, et al. Multicenter, randomized, placebo-controlled trial of amitriptyline in children with functional gastrointestinal disorders. *Gastroenterology.* 2009;137(4):1261–1269

Varni JW, Lane MM, Burwinkle TM, et al. Health-related quality of life in pediatric patients with irritable bowel syndrome: a comparative analysis. *Dev Behav Pediatr.* 2006;27(6):451–458

Vlieger AM, Menko-Frankenhuis C, Wolfkamp SC, Tromp E, Benninga M. Hypnotherapy for children with functional abdominal pain or irritable bowel syndrome: a randomized controlled trial. *Gastroenterology.* 2007;133(5):1430–1436

Youssef NN, Murphy TG, Langseder AL, Rosh JR. Quality of life for children with functional abdominal pain: a comparison study of patients' and parents' perceptions. *Pediatrics.* 2006;117(1):54–59

Youssef NN, Rosh JR, Loughran M, et al. Treatment of functional abdominal pain in childhood with cognitive behavioral strategies. *J Pediatr Gastroenterol Nutr.* 2004;39(2):192–196

CHAPTER 3

Allergic Rhinitis

Christine B. Cho, MD; David Goff, MD; and Amber M. Patterson, MD

Key Points

- Rhinitis refers to symptoms of nasal itching, sneezing, congestion, rhinorrhea, or a combination thereof resulting from inflammation or neural activation of the mucosa lining the nasal cavities. A detailed history is the best initial tool for investigating whether these symptoms are caused by allergy.

- Allergy tests are not diagnostic themselves; they are used in correlation with the clinical history for diagnosing allergy. To diagnose allergic rhinitis, specific IgE to allergens detected through skin or blood testing must correlate with symptoms.

- Allergen avoidance, medication, and immunotherapy (in that order) are the mainstay of treatment for allergic rhinitis.

- Nasal corticosteroids are the first-line medication choice for allergic rhinitis.

Overview

Rhinitis refers to symptoms of nasal itching, sneezing, congestion, rhinorrhea or a combination thereof resulting from inflammation or neural activation of the mucosa lining the nasal cavities. Posterior nasal drainage may cause cough. The general public typically assumes rhinitis to be allergic, and colloquially, rhinitis is known as "hay fever" or "allergies." To diagnose allergic rhinitis, however, specific IgE to allergens through skin or blood testing must correlate with symptoms. Rhinitis can be categorized in multiple ways, including by duration, etiology, and severity. Allergic rhinitis can be further defined as seasonal or perennial, depending on the allergen and time course of symptoms. The ARIA (Allergic Rhinitis and its Impact on Asthma) classification system (Box 3-1) developed out of the work produced from a World Health Organization workshop and divides rhinitis by severity and frequency of symptoms. This method of categorization is a validated measure of severity and may be more clinically relevant than categorization by season (Evidence Level II-2).

Box 3-1. ARIA Rhinitis Classification

Intermittent	Persistent
■ <4 days/week	■ >4 days/week
■ or <4 weeks	■ and >4 weeks
Mild **Normal sleep and** ■ No impairment of daily activities, sports, leisure ■ Normal school and work ■ No troublesome symptoms	**Moderate/Severe** **One or more items** ■ Abnormal sleep ■ Impairment of daily activities, sports, leisure ■ Abnormal school and work ■ Troublesome symptoms

Abbreviation: ARIA, Allergic Rhinitis and its Impact on Asthma.

Allergic rhinitis is associated with other atopic conditions: allergic conjunctivitis, asthma, atopic dermatitis, food allergy, and oral allergy syndrome. Oral allergy syndrome, or pollen-food allergy syndrome, causes oropharyngeal swelling and pruritus when a pollen-allergic person eats foods whose proteins cross-react with specific pollens to which he or she is allergic. The food proteins involved in oral allergy syndrome are heat labile, so patients do not have symptoms when those foods are cooked. Examples include peach, apple, or cherry cross-reacting with birch tree pollen and melon or banana cross-reacting with ragweed pollen. Comorbid conditions for allergic rhinitis include recurrent or refractory acute otitis media and sinusitis.

Causes and Differential Diagnosis

Allergies are caused by a dysfunctional immune response to nonpathogenic proteins in the environment. They develop in genetically predisposed children after repeated exposure to allergens over time. When a person develops sufficient allergy antibodies (IgE) to a specific allergenic protein, symptoms arise. Allergic rhinitis is caused by mast cell degranulation in the nasal cavities after allergen binds to specific IgE on mast cells. Perennial allergens include dust mite, cockroach, and animal dander. Seasonal allergies vary by regional climate, and generally, tree pollen is present in the spring, grass pollen in the summer, and weed pollen in the fall. Molds can be found outdoors and indoors in damp, dark areas but are not prevalent when the temperature is below freezing. Smoke, particulates, and strong odors trigger a neural response, so they are considered irritants, not allergens.

Many potential risk factors for allergic rhinitis have been studied. The strongest risk factors for developing allergic rhinitis are allergen exposure, having another atopic condition (ie, the atopic march), and an atopic family history

(Evidence Level II-2, Evidence Level III). Atopy is seen more in first-born children, in industrial societies, among those of higher socioeconomic status, in non-white children, and with ozone or tobacco smoke exposure (Evidence Level II-2, Evidence Level III).

Many conditions aside from allergies can cause rhinitis and therefore be confused with allergic rhinitis. The major categories of these other conditions are anatomic abnormalities, non-allergic inflammatory rhinitis, non-allergic noninflammatory rhinitis, and medication-induced rhinitis (Table 3-1). Most anatomic etiologies demonstrate persistent, refractory, and static congestion in the absence of pruritus. If symptoms are persistently unilateral, the primary cause will likely be anatomic. Non-allergic rhinitis is dominated by congestion, rhinorrhea, or both; triggers are usually irritating in nature or cannot be identified. Many patients experience symptoms in response to both allergic and irritant triggers; this is called mixed rhinitis. Non-allergic rhinitis with eosinophilia syndrome presents as perennial pruritus, sneezing, and watery rhinorrhea with eosinophils in the mucosa but no elevation in total or specific IgE. Rhinitis medicamentosa is rebound congestion after discontinuing topical (alpha agonist) decongestants used for more than 5 consecutive days.

Table 3-1. Differential Diagnosis of Allergic Rhinitis

Structural/ Anatomic	Non-allergic Inflammatory	Non-allergic Non-inflammatory	Drug-Induced
Adenoid hypertrophy	Occupational	Gustatory	Rhinitis medicamentosa
Turbinate hypertrophy	Infectious	Vasomotor	Aspirin/NSAIDs
Deviated septum	NARES	Emotional	Antihypertensives
Foreign body	...	Hormonal (premenstrual, pregnancy, hypothyroidism)	Oral contraceptives
Tumor	...	Atrophic	Psychiatric medications (alprazolam, amitriptyline, chlorpromazine)
Choanal atresia	...	Nasopharyngeal reflux	Immunosuppressants (cyclosporine, mycophenolate)
Cerebrospinal fluid leak[a]	...	Idiopathic	...
Nasal polyps	...	...	...

Abbreviations: NARES, non-allergic rhinitis with eosinophilia syndrome; NSAID, nonsteroidal anti-inflammatory drug.

[a] Unilateral rhinorrhea in setting of facial trauma.

Clinical Features

· · · · · · · · · · · · · · ·

Symptoms of allergic rhinitis are similar to those of non-allergic rhinitis, but in general "itch" is a dominant feature of pediatric allergy, whereas persistent nasal congestion or runny nose without itch are more suggestive of non-allergic causes (Box 3-2, Table 3-2, Figures 3-1 and 3-2). Consider allergic rhinitis when any of these symptoms are persistent, which may be intermittent, recurrent, or chronic in nature.

Box 3-2. Symptoms of Allergic Rhinitis

- Itching (nose, eyes, ears, throat)
- Sneezing
- Runny nose (clear, watery) or other drainage
- "Stuffed up"/nasal congestion
- Postnasal drip ± cough, throat clearing, or sore throat
- Watery eyes
- Red eyes
- Headache
- Daytime somnolence or poor concentration

Table 3-2. Signs and Physical Examination Findings of Allergic Rhinitis

General	Eyes	Ears	Nose	Throat/Neck
Allergic salute (rubbing nose)	Puffy eyelids	Otosclerosis from history of recurrent acute otitis media[a]	Nasal/allergic crease[b] (hyperpigmented line across nose from chronic nose rubbing)	Posterior pharyngeal cobblestoning
Nasal speech	Bilateral conjunctivitis without exudate	Otitis media with effusion[a]	Turbinate edema[c]	Shotty cervical lymphadenopathy
Scratching (nose, eyes, ears, skin)	Cobblestoning of conjunctiva (lymphoid hyperplasia)	...	Pale mucosa[c,d] (bluish hue)	...
Nose picking	Infraorbital/ allergic shiners[b]	...	Boggy[c] (wet)	...
Snoring or mouth breathing	Dennie-Morgan lines[b] (accentuated lines or folds on lower eyelid)	...	Rhinorrhea or nasal discharge	...

[a] Allergic rhinitis and recurrent otitis media often coexist, but no causal relationship has been established.
[b] See Figure 3-2.
[c] See Figure 3-3.
[d] Nasal turbinates may appear erythematous, rather than pale, in patients with non-allergic or mixed rhinitis.

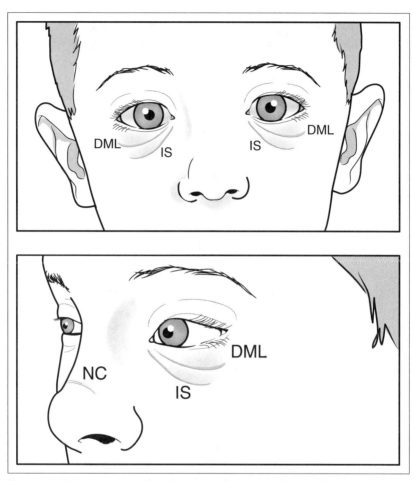

Figure 3-1. Common presenting signs in patients with allergic rhinitis.

Abbreviations: DML, Dennie-Morgan lines; IS, infraorbital/allergic shiners; NC, nasal/allergic crease.

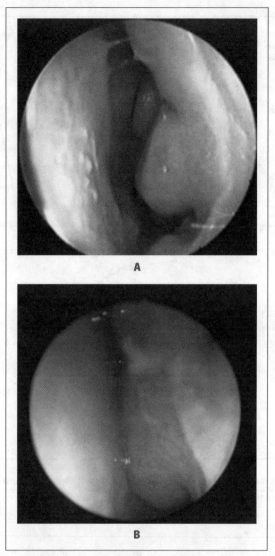

Figure 3-2. Nasal examination findings.
Views of left nasal vestibules with turbinates shown on
right and nasal septums (on left of images). Both exhibit
pale, boggy (wet), edematous nasal turbinates. **A,** Middle
nasal turbinate seen partially obstructing nasal cavity
(in background). **B,** Inferior turbinate completely
obstructing nasal cavity.

Evaluation

History

A thorough focused history is the best diagnostic tool for evaluating rhinitis. Allergy-specific history should include inquiry about nasal and ocular symptoms experienced, frequency, severity, timing, seasonality, duration, symptom triggers, and response to medication (Box 3-3). Patients that can identify an allergen as a trigger for their symptoms (Evidence Level II-3) or have a personal or family history of atopy have a significantly increased likelihood of allergy (Evidence Level II-2). Common allergens are listed in Box 3-4. It is also helpful to ask about non-allergic triggers. Examples of mucosal irritants include cigarette smoke, strong odors (eg, perfume, cleaning chemicals), or particulates (eg, dusty surroundings, fresh-cut grass) (see Box 3-3). Abrupt changes in temperature and humidity can also irritate the nasal mucosa.

Box 3-3. Questions to Elicit Allergy History

- What is your main symptom? (Check for itchy nose; rhinorrhea; sneezing; nasal congestion, obstruction, or both; and watery or itchy eyes.)
- Has a doctor ever diagnosed that you have hay fever, allergic rhinitis, asthma, or eczema?
- How long have you had these symptoms?
- Do you have the symptoms all the time, or do they come and go? For how long are you symptom-free?
- Are you aware of anything that seems to bring the symptoms on, such as being outdoors, being around animals, or something you handle at school, work, or home?
- Do you have a family member with allergy, asthma, or eczema problems?
- What medications have you already tried for these symptoms? Effects?
- Do you have other medical conditions, or are you on other medication?

Adapted with permission from Bousquet J, Khaltaev N, Cruz AA, et al. Allergic Rhinitis and its Impact on Asthma (ARIA) 2008 update (in collaboration with the World Health Organization, GA(2)LEN and AllerGen). *Allergy.* 2008;63(Suppl 86):8–160.

Allergic rhinitis symptoms are known to contribute to problems with cognitive functioning, sleep, and self-esteem, all of which can result in poor concentration and learning deficits (independent of medication side effects [Evidence Level I]). It is essential to ask parents and patients with suspected allergic rhinitis about these quality of life issues to ensure they are addressed and monitored as part of the overall allergic rhinitis treatment plan.

Box 3-4. Common Rhinoconjunctivitis Triggers

Allergic Triggers	Irritant Triggers
Perennial <ul><li>Furry animals/pets (cat, dog, guinea pig, hamster, rabbit, mouse, farm animals)</li><li>Dust mites</li><li>Cockroach</li><li>Indoor mold</li></ul> **Seasonal** <ul><li>Pollen from tree, grass, or weed</li><li>Outdoor mold</li></ul>	<ul><li>Cigarette smoke</li><li>Strong scents (perfume, cologne, cleaning chemicals)</li><li>Excessive dust (made up of dirt, hair, skin, which may or may not contain dust mites)</li><li>Fresh-cut grass/grass clippings</li><li>Extreme changes in temperature or weather</li></ul>

By identifying the most bothersome symptom and its frequency, treatment can be tailored accordingly. A general medical and surgical history is also important in the evaluation, ensuring to address history of recurrent infections or otolaryngological procedures (ie, ear tubes, turbinate reduction, tonsillectomy, adenoidectomy, or a combination thereof). Those with rhinitis may experience more acute otitis medias, urinary tract infections, or sinus (when developmentally present) infections than typical peers.

Abnormal physical examination findings (described above) support the diagnosis but are not specific for allergic rhinitis. Conversely, if symptoms are not acutely present during evaluation, allergic rhinitis should not be excluded as the cause of intermittent symptoms. By combining a detailed history and physical examination findings, one can gauge the type and severity of rhinitis the patient is experiencing and offer basic avoidance and treatment recommendations.

Allergy Testing

Testing for allergies measures IgE-mediated reactions to specific allergens by skin or blood tests and is most useful when tests and patients are properly selected. Good candidates for testing include patients whose symptoms are difficult to control, who desire allergy immunotherapy, or who have persistent asthma. Children of any age can undergo either form of testing, though it should be considered that allergies result from allergen exposure over time and that very young infants (<9 mo) are unlikely to have developed naso-ocular symptoms from IgE-mediated environmental allergy. Selecting specific allergens based on likely relevance for each patient is preferred over large, batch testing to avoid confusion from false-positive or extraneous results. Positive results that identify allergens and correlate with timing of symptoms are considered clinically relevant, and these are extremely useful for clarifying avoidance measures and prescribing immunotherapy. Negative results prevent unnecessary avoidance measures.

Skin testing is the traditional and preferred method of allergy testing. It provides a simple, immediate, in vivo test of IgE-mediated sensitivity to specific allergens that is reliable and strongly associated with nasal symptoms (Evidence Level II-1). Skin testing must be done under the direction of a physician with specialized training in allergy tests and their interpretation.

Current allergen-specific IgE blood assays are an improvement from radio-allergosorbent methods and have good specificity and negative predictive value when compared to skin testing (Evidence Level III). Positive predictive values of these assays have not been established for environmental allergens, but very high or negative serum allergen-specific IgE levels could be useful.

Pulmonary Function Testing

Asthma often coexists with and is exacerbated by allergic rhinitis. Objective pulmonary function tests should be considered in patients presenting with concern for allergies, recurrent cough or wheeze, recurrent bronchitis, or other persistent respiratory symptoms. Spirometry with flow-volume loop is a method commonly used for evaluating lung function. To properly perform the test, patients must be cooperative, follow directions, and coordinate forced vital capacity breaths as instructed; children generally acquire this ability by age 5 to 7 years.

Referral to Allergist

When avoidance of known triggers and empiric treatment fail to adequately alleviate rhinitis symptoms, referral to an allergy-trained subspecialist is warranted for further evaluation and consideration of allergy immunotherapy.

Management

The goals of therapeutic intervention are to minimize symptoms of allergic rhinitis by reducing nasal and other local edema and inflammation, improving asthma control if indicated and overall improving the patient's quality of life. The steps include avoidance, medication, and allergen immunotherapy in appropriately selected patients.

The pillar of management for the allergic person is avoidance of known allergens and irritants that trigger his or her symptoms. The clinical assessment of rhinitis as allergic, non-allergic, or mixed allows the clinician to recommend appropriate avoidance measures (Box 3-5).

The second step of management is pharmacologic. Treatment for allergic and non-allergic rhinitis is similar, and guidance of therapy by symptom pattern (frequency and predominant symptom) can be used for both conditions (Figure 3-3, Table 3-3). Patient and parental preference for nasal versus oral medication should be considered to enhance compliance.

Box 3-5. Allergen Avoidance Measures (Evidence Level I for Indoor Allergens)

Pollen

For symptoms worse in spring, summer, or fall,
- Follow local pollen counts from the National Allergy Bureau.[a]

When pollen counts are high,
- Limit outdoor exposure.
- Use air conditioning when inside.
- Bathe before bedtime to remove pollen from hair/skin.

Dust Mites

For symptoms year-round, often worse in morning or when humid,
- Focus on the bedroom, where most dust mite exposure occurs, and use all of these measures for maximal effect.
- Limit stuffed animals and clutter.
- Control humidity (keep below 50%)/avoid humidifiers.
- Encase bedding in impermeable covers (mattress, box spring, and all pillows). Vinyl crib/toddler mattresses do not need to be covered.
- Wash bed linens/blankets (with favorite stuffed animal) weekly in 130°F (54.5°C) water.
- Vacuum carpet weekly with HEPA vacuum.
- Consider hard flooring and blinds instead of carpeting and curtains.

Furry Animals/Pets

For symptoms worse around cat, dog, or other specific animal,
- Remove animal from home.

If unable to remove from home,
- Wash pet at least weekly.
- Keep pet out of bedroom.
- Use HEPA air purifier.

Cockroaches

If present in home
- Exterminate.
- Avoid locations with infestation.

Fungi (Outdoor)

For symptoms worse when outside during rainy/damp seasons,
- Follow local mold spore counts from the National Allergy Bureau.[a]
- Avoid decaying plant matter, jumping in leaf piles.

Box 3-5 *(cont)*

Fungi (Outdoor)

When spore counts are high,

- Limit outdoor exposure.
- Use air conditioning when inside.

Fungi (Indoor)

If present in home

- Remedy leaks/other moisture.
- Replace contaminated articles.
- Apply dilute bleach to moldy, nonporous surfaces.
- Dispose of moldy food.
- Use dehumidifier in damp areas.
- Use HEPA air purifier.

Abbreviation: HEPA, high-efficiency particulate air.
[a] At http://pollen.aaaai.org (regional pollen and mold spore counts).

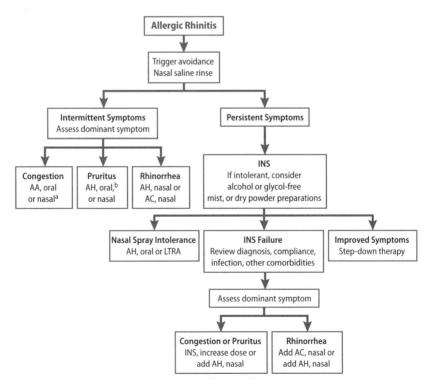

Figure 3-3. Therapeutic algorithm for allergic rhinitis.

Abbreviations: AA, alpha agonist; AC, anticholinergic; AH, antihistamine; INS, intranasal corticosteroids; LTRA, leukotriene receptor antagonist.

[a] Topical alpha agonists should not be used for more than 5 consecutive days.

[b] Second-generation H1 antihistamines are preferred over first generation.

Table 3-3. Select Medications for Allergic Rhinitis

Trade Name	Compound	Strength	Age (y)	Dose
Nasal steroids				
Flonase	Fluticasone propionate	50 mcg	≥4	1–2 sprays every day
Nasacort AQ	Triamcinolone	55 mcg	2–5	1 spray every day
			≥6	1–2 sprays every day
Nasonex	Mometasone	50 mcg	2–11	1 spray every day
			≥12	2 sprays every day
Omnaris	Ciclesonide	50 mcg	≥12	2 sprays every day
Qnasl powder aerosol	Beclomethasone	80 mcg	≥12	2 sprays every day
Veramyst	Fluticasone furoate	27.5 mcg	≥2	1–2 sprays every day
Zetonna	Ciclesonide	37 mcg	≥12	1 spray every day
Antihistamines				
Allegra	Fexofenadine	30 mg/5 mL	2–11	30 mg twice a day
		30, 60 mg	≥12	60 mg twice a day
		180mg	≥ 12	180 mg every day
Claritin	Loratadine	1 mg/mL	2–5	5 mg every day
		10 mg	≥6	10 mg every day
Zyrtec	Cetirizine	1 mg/mL	6–23 mo	2.5 mg every day–twice a day
		5/10 mg	≥6	5–10 mg every day
Nonsteroidal sprays				
Astelin	Azelastine	0.1%	5–11	1 spray twice a day
		0.1%	≥12	1–2 sprays twice a day
Astepro	Azelastine	0.15%	≥12	1–2 sprays every day–twice a day
Atrovent	Ipratropium	0.03%	≥5	2 sprays twice a day–3 times a day
Patanase	Olopatadine	665 mcg	6–11	1 spray twice a day
			≥12	2 sprays twice a day
Combination (antihistamine/steroid) spray				
Dymista	Azelastine/ fluticasone	137 mcg/50 mcg	≥12	1 spray twice a day

Modified from Allergy Med Card, Nationwide Children's Allergy Clinic (A. Patterson, J. Seyerle, P. Mustillo).

Intranasal Corticosteroids

Nasal steroids are the most effective monotherapy for allergic rhinitis (Evidence Level I), and most forms of non-allergic rhinitis. They work best when used daily (Evidence Level II-1), although they can be used intermittently (onset of action is within 12 h) (Evidence Level II-1). Nasal steroids alone can treat both nasal and ocular symptoms and are equal or superior than H1 antihistamines combined with leukotriene antagonists in the treatment of seasonal allergic rhinitis (Evidence Level I). Currently available nasal steroids are equally effective (Evidence Level I). Newer formulations (ie, fluticasone, mometasone, budesonide) are preferred to first generations because of decreased systemic bioavailability, though growth suppression was never demonstrated with the older generation in short-term (1-year) studies (Evidence Level III). Ciclesonide is a steroid pro-drug that is activated in the nasal mucosa, virtually eliminating systemic bioavailability. The most common adverse effects are nasal irritation and nose bleeds, which can usually be mitigated by administering with proper technique (Figure 3-4).

Antihistamines

Oral H1 antihistamines are inferior to intranasal corticosteroids (INS) (Evidence Level I); however, they can be used if nasal sprays are not tolerated or desired. Combining an antihistamine with INS may be considered, although supporting studies are limited and many studies demonstrate no additional effect (Evidence Level I). Second-generation H1 antihistamines are preferred to first-generation because they are less sedating (less lipophilic), particularly relevant for any child

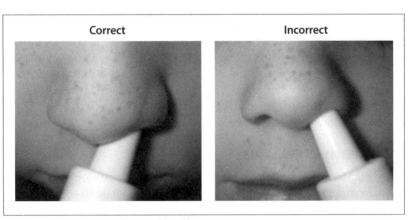

Figure 3-4. Proper use of a nasal medication.
1. Blow nose to remove mucous.
2. Look down toward toes as if reading a book.
3. Gently insert nozzle straight back into nostril (using opposite hand).
4. Aim nozzle away from midline septum (toward ipsilateral eye).
5. Spray as directed (usually 1 or 2 sprays).
6. Avoid blowing nose or sniffing after spraying to allow medicine to stay in the nose.

Photos courtesy of Amber M. Patterson, MD.

in an educational setting or operating a motor vehicle (Evidence Level I). Cetirizine, levocetirizine, fexofenadine, desloratadine, and loratadine have comparable effects, though individual patients may respond better to one over another (Evidence Level III). Unlike the other second-generation products, cetirizine and levocetirizine may cause drowsiness at recommended doses (Evidence Level I). Oral antihistamines work within 2 hours of dosing and are most effective for concerns of ocular or nasal itching. Antihistamines can have effects on the cholinergic receptor, though this is less so with second-generation products. These anticholinergic adverse effects can alleviate non-allergic rhinitis symptoms in some patients but may also lead to dryness of the mouth and eyes. In general, choices other than antihistamines are typically better for non-allergic or mixed rhinitis.

Antihistamine Nasal Sprays

Azelastine and olopatadine are available by prescription and are indicated for both non-allergic and allergic rhinitis. They improve nasal congestion with rapid onset in 5 to 15 minutes and thus can be used as needed. Because of anticholinergic effects, they also can be used for rhinorrhea or postnasal drip. Their effectiveness is equal or superior to oral second-generation antihistamines (Evidence Level I). They are generally less effective than monotherapy with INS (Evidence Level I), but when combined, nasal steroid plus nasal antihistamine provide more benefit than nasal steroid plus oral antihistamine (Evidence Level I).

Leukotriene Receptor Antagonist

Montelukast, available generic since 2012, is approved for the treatment of allergic rhinitis and asthma; however, it is inferior to INS (Evidence Level I) and no different than oral antihistamines (loratadine being the common comparator) (Evidence Level I). It provides an option for treating a younger child with allergic rhinitis and asthma who is not requiring inhaled corticosteroid controller. The safety profile is good, but the clinician must be aware of the reported neuropsychiatric effects that sometimes occur with this agent, including insomnia, anxiety, depression, and rarely suicide.

Anticholinergic Nasal Sprays

When rhinorrhea is a predominant symptom and first-line treatments have failed, ipratropium bromide is a good choice for drying up the nose. It is not a first-line therapy for allergic rhinitis.

Non-pharmacologic Treatment

Evidence supports that topical saline is beneficial for the symptoms of chronic rhinorrhea and rhinosinusitis when used as monotherapy or adjunctive therapy (Evidence Level I). Nasal saline drops in infants or saline rinses in older children should be considered in those with more mild, episodic symptoms or as adjunctive therapy.

Adjusting Treatment

As with asthma treatment management, step-up therapy should be considered if the patient's symptoms are not well-controlled (see Figure 3-5). If step-up therapy is not helpful, consider referral to an allergy specialist. In contrast, if good control is achieved after 4 to 6 weeks, a reduction in therapy should be considered to minimize medication use.

Ocular Treatment

Some cases of allergic rhinoconjunctivitis may not have adequate response to nasal corticosteroids or nonsedating antihistamines, and eye drops may be indicated. For acute or intermittent allergic conjunctivitis, over-the-counter ocular drops containing an antihistamine/vasoconstrictor (eg, naphazoline/pheniramine) combination are more effective than either agent alone (Evidence Level I). For recurrent or chronic ocular symptoms, mast cell stabilizers combined with antihistamines are most effective (Evidence Level I).

Immunologic

Subcutaneous allergen immunotherapy (SCIT) is effective in the treatment of allergic rhinitis and allergic asthma (Evidence Level II-2). It is appropriate therapy for children (usually ≥5 y) and adults. Though it has mainly been studied in adults, SCIT is thought to benefit children most, as it may prevent the development of new allergen sensitizations and asthma in patients with allergic rhinitis (Evidence Level II-1). Good candidates are those with allergic rhinitis that fails or does not tolerate pharmacologic therapy, those who prefer not to use pharmacologic therapy, or those who want to begin SCIT as a potential permanent solution to chronic allergies. Serious systemic allergic reactions can occur. Successful SCIT requires at least 3 to 5 years of treatment, and some patients require longer treatment.

If administering allergist-prescribed immunotherapy for patients in the office, it is important to observe patients for 30 minutes after each injection for rare, life-threatening anaphylactic reactions, which typically occur within this time frame. Abrupt discontinuation of weekly injections requires a reduction in allergen dilution, which the allergist determines in the immunotherapy dosing schedule.

SCIT has been used for more than 100 years and continues to be the most common method of administering aeroallergen immunotherapy. In 2014, the US Food and Drug Administration approved sublingual immunotherapy tablets as another option for treating grass and ragweed pollen allergy. Sublingual treatment offers self-administration at home; efficacy depends on not missing daily doses. Future options for aeroallergen immunotherapy under research include alternative routes of administration (eg, intralymphatic), recombinant extracts, and use of adjuvants to boost the immune response.

Long-term Monitoring

The patient's goal for treatment should be used to direct management and follow-up. To maintain adequate symptom control long-term, review allergen avoidance measures at each visit. Assess medication compliance, and if using a nasal medication, have the patient demonstrate proper technique. Correcting poor nasal spray technique can often alleviate symptoms without escalating therapy. Consider tapering medications if symptoms are well-controlled or during off-allergy season, and ask about medication adverse effects. Periodically assess allergy symptom effects on quality of life because issues such as missed school or work, poor sleep quality, diminished smell or taste, or fatigue can indicate lingering subclinical symptoms.

If symptoms are not well-controlled and avoidance measures and medication compliance have been addressed, consider other medication options. Surgical revision of anatomic abnormalities or medication-resistant nasal turbinate hypertrophy should be considered if maximal medical therapy and avoidance measures are suboptimally improving symptoms. Atopic individuals can acquire additional environmental allergies over time, and those with worsening, previously controlled symptoms warrant reevaluation to identify potential new triggers. Allergen immunotherapy should be considered for persistent or worsening symptoms if allergies are the primary cause of symptoms. If the patient is already on IT, assessment of treatment effect and deciding when to discontinue IT should be regularly assessed by the patient's allergist.

Cooperative management and good communication between primary care physician and subspecialist is essential for maximizing the allergy patient's overall well-being.

Suggested Reading

Bernstein IL, Li JT, Bernstein DI, et al. Allergy diagnostic testing: an updated practice parameter. *Ann Allergy Asthma Immunol.* 2008;100(3 Suppl 3):S1–S148

Bousquet J, Reid J, van Weel C, et al. Allergic rhinitis management pocket reference 2008. *Allergy.* 2008;63(8):990–996

Calabria C, Dietrich J, Hagan L. Comparison of serum-specific IgE (ImmunoCAP) and skin-prick test results for 53 inhalant allergens in patients with chronic rhinitis. *Allergy Asthma Proc.* 2009;30(4):386–396

Droste JH, Kerhof M, de Monchy JG, Schouten JP, Rijcken B. Association of skin test reactivity, specific IgE, total IgE, and eosinophils with nasal symptoms in a community-based population study. The Dutch ECRHS Group. *J Allergy Clin Immunol.* 1996;97(4):922–932

Gergen PJ, Turkeltaub PC. The association of individual allergen reactivity with respiratory disease in a national sample: data from the second National Health and Nutrition Examination Survey, 1976-80 (NHANES II). *J Allergy Clin Immunol.* 1992;90(4 Pt 1):579–588

Kulig M, Bergmann R, Klettke U, Wahn V, Tacke U, Wahn U. Natural course of sensitization to food and inhalant allergens during the first 6 years of life. *J Allergy Clin Immunol.* 1999;103(6):1173–1179

Montoro J, Del Cuvillo A, Mullol J, et al. Validation of the modified allergic rhinitis and its impact on asthma (ARIA) severity classification in allergic rhinitis children: the PEDRIAL study. *Allergy.* 2012;67(11):1437–1442

Murray AB, Milner RA. The accuracy of features in the clinical history for predicting atopic sensitization to airborne allergens in children. *J Allergy Clin Immunol.* 1995;96(5 Pt 1):588–596

Vuurman EF, van Veggel LM, Uiterwijk MM, Leutner D, O'Hanlon JF. Seasonal allergic rhinitis and antihistamine effects on children's learning. *Ann Allergy.* 1993;71(2):121–126

Wallace D, Dykewicz M, Bernstein D, et al. The diagnosis and management of rhinitis: an updated practice parameter. *J Allergy Clin Immunol.* 2008;122(2 Suppl):S1–S84

CHAPTER 4

Anemia

Suzanne M. Reed, MD, and Melissa Rhodes, MD

Key Points

- Normal values for hemoglobin are age and gender dependent. To diagnose anemia in a child, it is important to evaluate the hemoglobin level in reference to those values.

- The complete blood count (with indices), platelet count, peripheral smear, and reticulocyte count form the basis for the initial evaluation of anemia in a child. The reticulocyte count is particularly important because it allows the clinician to distinguish disorders of low production (low or inappropriately normal reticulocyte count) from those of increased destruction (elevated reticulocyte count).

- Iron deficiency is the most common cause of anemia in the pediatric population and must be differentiated from thalassemia to avoid unnecessary and potentially harmful iron therapy.

- Many anemias are inherited; family history is essential in approaching the differential diagnosis of a child with anemia.

- Anemia associated with another cytopenia should alert a physician to a potential bone marrow disease.

Overview

Anemia is a common hematologic abnormality in children. It is defined as a reduction in hemoglobin concentration or in red blood cell (RBC) mass compared to normal (reference) ranges. The lower limit of the normal range is considered to be 2 standard deviations below the mean for a specific population. It is important to note that normal ranges differ based on age and gender, with lower mean values in younger children compared to older and in females compared to males (Table 4-1). Anemia should be thought of as a symptom, not a disease, and a specific cause must always be sought. The list of conditions that cause anemia is extensive, but with an organized approach, the differential can be substantially narrowed. One way to begin to classify a patient's anemia is by considering whether the anemia is a *production* or a *destruction* problem. Within each of these broad categories, a patient's history, family history, physical examination, and laboratory evaluation will, together, help uncover the diagnosis.

Table 4-1. Normal Mean and Lower Limits of Normal for Hemoglobin, Hematocrit, and Mean Corpuscular Volume

Age (yr)	Hemoglobin		Hematocrit (%)		Mean Corpuscular Volume (µM³)	
	Mean	Lower limit	Mean	Lower limit	Mean	Lower limit
0.5–1.9	12.5	11.0	37	33	77	70
2–4	12.5	11.0	38	34	79	73
5–7	13.0	11.5	39	35	81	75
8–11	13.5	12.0	40	36	83	76
12–14 female	13.5	12.0	41	36	85	78
12–14 male	14.0	12.5	43	37	84	77
15–17 female	14.0	12.0	41	36	87	79
15–17 male	15.0	13.0	46	38	86	78
18–49 female	14.0	12.0	42	37	90	80
18–49 male	16.0	14.0	47	40	90	80

From Brugnara C, Oski FA, Nathan DG. Diagnostic approach to the anemic patient. In: Orkin SH, Nathan DG, Ginsburg D, et al, eds. *Nathan and Oski's Hematology of infancy and Childhood*. 7th ed. Philadelphia, PA: Elsevier Saunders; 2009:456, with permission.

Causes

The absolute value to define a child as "anemic" depends on age and gender (see Table 4-1). The causes of anemia in children are many, but a classification schema based on production problems versus increased destruction is a useful method to conceptualize evaluation and treatment of anemia in children (Box 4-1).

Box 4-1. Etiologies of Anemia in Children

Production Problems	Increased Destruction Problems
■ Bone marrow failure: aplastic anemia, dyserythropoiesis (eg, Diamond-Blackfan anemia) ■ Transient erythroblastopenia of childhood ■ Iron deficiency anemia ■ B12 deficiency ■ Folate deficiency ■ Thalassemia ■ Anemia of chronic disease	■ Autoimmune-mediated hemolysis ■ Hereditary spherocytosis ■ Microangiopathic anemia ■ G6PD deficiency ■ Pyruvate kinase deficiency ■ Sickle cell disease ■ Unstable hemoglobin variants ■ Hereditary pyropoikilocytosis ■ Paroxysmal nocturnal hemoglobinuria

Abbreviation: G6PD, glucose-6-phosphate dehydrogenase.

Based on information available from the complete blood count (CBC) (including RBC indices), peripheral smear and reticulocyte count, decreased production (low reticulocyte count or inappropriately normal reticulocyte count) versus increased destruction (elevated reticulocyte count) can easily be discerned. The peripheral smear and RBC indices can further aid in the differential analysis and help guide further diagnostic testing.

Evaluation and Management

Production Problems

Anemia caused by defective RBC production can be the result of dysfunctional erythropoiesis or an insufficient rate of erythropoiesis (Table 4-2). The bone marrow is the site where RBCs are produced, and anemia occurs when either the supplies (dietary nutrients and proteins coded for in DNA) are lacking or the production is insufficient. Most of these disorders will be related to nutritional deficiencies, thalassemias, and a range of bone marrow failure syndromes. We will discuss nutritional deficiencies and thalassemias, as bone marrow failure syndromes are outside the scope of this chapter.

Nutritional Deficiencies

Iron deficiency is the most common nutritional deficiency that causes anemia. It can develop from decreased dietary intake or from iron loss (ie, blood loss), and a detailed patient history is critical to distinguish between these two causes. This includes particular attention to the child's daily milk, meat, and vegetable consumption, as well as any bleeding from the nose, mouth, urine, or stool or bleeding with cough or vomiting. A detailed menstrual history should be obtained in post-menarchal girls. While an overall iron-poor diet can lead to iron deficiency, a particularly common concurrent nutritional problem is excessive cow's milk consumption in toddlers. The mechanism of this particular anemia is twofold: decreased dietary iron intake (because milk contains very little iron, and because it is filling, there is minimal intake of actual food) and irritation of the intestinal wall, causing microscopic gastrointestinal tract blood loss. While officially "malnourished," these children have good growth due to the high caloric content of milk.

Table 4-2. Laboratory Evaluation for a Child With Anemia

Mechanism of Anemia	Decreased Production	Increased Destruction
Common tests		
...	CBC, platelet count, peripheral smear, reticulocyte count	CBC, platelet count, peripheral smear, reticulocyte count
Specific tests		
Iron deficiency	Ferritin level, serum iron level, TIBC	...
Folate/B6 deficiency	RBC folate level, serum B12 level	...
Thalassemia	Hemoglobin electrophoresis	...
Anemia of chronic disease	CRP, ESR, ferritin level, serum iron level, TIBC	...
Autoimmune-mediated hemolysis	...	Coombs, specific RBC antibody levels
Hereditary spherocytosis	...	Specific RBC membrane function and structure tests (osmotic fragility)
Microangiopathic anemia	...	Peripheral smear
G6PD deficiency	...	RBC G6PD assay
Pyruvate kinase deficiency	...	RBC PK enzymatic assay
Sickle cell disease	...	Hemoglobin electrophoresis
Unstable hemoglobin variants	...	Peripheral smear (Heinz body), hemoglobin HPLC, stability tests
Hereditary pyropoikilocytosis	...	Peripheral smear, osmotic fragility tests
Paroxysmal nocturnal hemoglobinuria	...	Expression of granulocyte GPI-linked proteins

Abbreviations: CBC, complete blood count; CRP, C-reactive protein; ESR, erythrocyte sedimentation rate; G6PD, glucose-6-phosphate dehydrogenase; GPI, glycosylphosphatidylinositol; HPLC, high-performance liquid chromatography; PK, pyruvate kinase; RBC, red blood cell; TIBC, total iron-binding capacity.

The laboratory evaluation of a patient with concerns for iron deficiency should include a CBC, reticulocyte count, and iron studies, including ferritin level, serum iron level, and total iron-binding capacity (TIBC) (see Table 4-2). The CBC of a patient with iron-deficiency anemia demonstrates a *microcytic* anemia with elevated RBC distribution width and, commonly, thrombocytosis. The degree of microcytosis is proportional to the degree of anemia: the lower the hemoglobin, the lower the mean corpuscular volume (MCV). Reticulocyte count should be inappropriately normal or low. Iron studies should be reflective of low iron stores: decreased ferritin level, decreased serum iron level, and elevated TIBC. Note that the serum iron level can be within range in iron deficiency if the child has recently had an iron-containing meal or has recently started iron supplementation.

Proper diagnosis and correction of iron deficiency is important, as chronic iron deficiency can cause long-term cognitive impairment (Evidence Level II-2). Treatment is with iron supplementation, 3 to 6 mg/kg/d of elemental iron (note: iron preparations have varied concentrations of elemental iron), depending on severity of iron deficiency (Evidence Level I). With proper treatment, patients typically feel better within 1 to 2 days and have appropriate reticulocytosis in about 1 week, and hemoglobin (Hgb) will increase about 2 g/dL for the 3 subsequent weeks. Hemoglobin should normalize within 6 to 8 weeks. Treatment should continue until ferritin levels normalize and inciting factors are corrected.

Vitamin B12 and folate deficiencies are uncommon causes of anemia, specifically megaloblastic anemia, in children. Deficiencies develop from inadequate intake (usually from a vegan diet or an infant exclusively breastfed by a vegan mother) or from defective absorption (from small bowel disease). In addition to classic symptoms of anemia, B12 and folate deficiencies can also be associated with gastrointestinal symptoms, especially glossitis. Vitamin B12 deficiency is also associated with neurologic symptoms. The anemia caused by these deficiencies is macrocytic compared to the microcytic anemia of iron deficiency. It can also be associated with neutropenia and thrombocytopenia. Serum B12 level and RBC folate (serum folate is less reliable) level can be used to diagnose these deficiencies. Treatment of megaloblastic anemia is vitamin supplementation and may include further investigation of the mechanism of deficiency, such as evaluating for pernicious anemia or other intestinal or systemic diseases. It is important to note that patients can have combined nutritional deficiencies, which can result in a normocytic anemia.

Thalassemias

Just as certain nutritional deficiencies cause ineffective erythropoiesis and anemia, so do deficiencies of other elements essential for RBC and Hgb production. Thalassemias are inherited anemias that are caused by deficiencies of essential globin proteins, most commonly α- and β-globin proteins. These disorders are most often found in people with Mediterranean, Middle Eastern, African, or Asian ancestry. Thalassemia is a spectrum of disease, with severity of the anemia—and thus severity of symptoms—dependent on the specific genetic defect and subsequent amount of globin protein produced.

Laboratory evaluation demonstrates a microcytic anemia, similar to iron-deficiency anemia, but iron study findings are within the normal range. Oftentimes, the RBC will be elevated in thalassemia. The Mentzer Index (MCV/RBC) can be used to help distinguish between iron deficiency and thalassemia: a value greater than 13 suggests iron deficiency, while a value less than 13 suggests thalassemia. On Hgb electrophoresis, Hgb A2 is elevated in β-thalassemia. The newborn screening is also an important method for diagnosis. In α-thalassemia, Hgb Barts is present on the newborn screening. Hgb Barts will disappear over the subsequent several months, and Hgb H will become present in 3-gene deletion α-thalassemia. Newborn screening findings will be normal in β-thalassemia trait, but will show Hgb F only (complete absence of Hgb A) in β-thalassemia major. Genetic testing is available in specialized laboratories to identify specific gene defects, but this is often not necessary if all other laboratory findings are consistent with thalassemia. It is important to distinguish between thalassemia and iron deficiency when evaluating a microcytic anemia so that unnecessary iron therapy can be avoided and appropriate family planning counseling can be offered.

Treatment for thalassemia depends on severity of the disease. Defects that cause mild anemia or isolated microcytosis with within-range Hgb are termed *trait*, as in α- or β-thalassemia trait. No treatment is necessary for these patients. More severe globin deficiencies may necessitate intermittent or ongoing transfusion support. The most severe thalassemias that are compatible with extrauterine life (total absence of α-globin is not compatible with life) can be cured with bone marrow transplant.

Other RBC Production Problems

While nutritional deficiencies and thalassemia are the most common causes of impaired Hgb and RBC production, several other causes are noteworthy. Chronic diseases (eg, renal disease, hypothyroidism, rheumatologic disease, other chronic inflammation) typically cause a normocytic anemia. Transient erythroblastopenia of childhood is an idiopathic, self-resolving, isolated anemia typically occurring in a previously healthy child between ages 1 to 3 years. The MCV is normocytic to slightly macrocytic depending on when in the course of the condition it is diagnosed, and degree of anemia can range from mild to severe. Lead intoxication causes microcytic anemia, usually related to concomitant iron deficiency. Finally, any infiltrative bone marrow process, such as leukemia or metastatic solid tumors, can impair RBC production.

Destruction Problems

Anemias caused by RBC destruction (or hemolysis) can be further grouped into immune-mediated and non–immune-mediated etiologies. Symptoms of hemolytic anemias depend on the degree of anemia; however, in addition to general symptoms of anemia, symptoms that suggest a hemolytic process include jaundice, scleral icterus, and splenomegaly. Various laboratory values will also help identify RBC destruction compared to deficient production and also can help identify more specific etiologies.

Immune-Mediated Hemolytic Anemia

Immune-mediated hemolysis occurs when antibodies are produced and directed against RBCs. Most often, autoimmune hemolytic anemia (AIHA) occurs in otherwise healthy children, but can also occur in the presence of other systemic diseases and infections and with certain medications. Symptoms of AIHA are often dramatic as compared with those of patients who have anemia that has developed slowly over time, as in iron deficiency. Patients may have hours to days of headache, lightheadedness, syncope, and jaundice. In laboratory evaluation, patients will have varying degrees of anemia, which generally is normocytic. Laboratory values that point toward hemolysis are an appropriately elevated reticulocyte count (suggesting a healthy bone marrow) and elevated indirect bilirubin and lactate dehydrongenase. An important distinguishing laboratory test for AIHA is a Coombs test, also called a direct antiglobulin test. This test detects the presence of antibodies directed against RBCs and can also help distinguish between warm and cold AIHA.

In warm AIHA, antibodies are typically IgG, and they react with RBCs at body temperature. This is the more common kind of AIHA, and it results in an extravascular hemolysis and thus is more likely to be associated with hepatomegaly and splenomegaly. First-line treatment for warm AIHA is corticosteroids. In cold AIHA, antibodies are typically IgM and react with RBCs at below body temperature. This hemolysis is intravascular and thus more likely to cause hemoglobinuria rather than hepatosplenomegaly. While much less common in pediatrics, cold AIHA is important to identify in these patients because blood products must be warmed prior to administration. In addition, corticosteroids are not helpful in cold AIHA, and treatment is supportive care with blood products (if needed) until antibody resolves.

Non–immune-Mediated Hemolytic Anemia

Hemolysis can also be caused by inherited structural defects in the RBC membrane and by RBC enzyme deficiencies. Hereditary spherocytosis (HS) is the most common inherited membrane structural defect in which the RBC shape is spherical rather than a biconcave disc, and therefore it is more fragile and likely to hemolyze. Hereditary spherocytosis has a spectrum of clinical severities, ranging from episodic normocytic anemia associated with fever/infection to significant chronic hemolysis requiring frequent blood transfusions. Symptoms, examination findings, and laboratory evaluation are similar to those for immune-mediated hemolysis discussed previously, except the Coombs test is negative. One of the often overlooked RBC indices is the mean corpuscular hemoglobin concentration, which is usually elevated in HS. The definitive laboratory test is the osmotic fragility test, but it should be noted that this is an unreliable test in children younger than 1 year. Sometimes HS can present in the neonatal period with prolonged or pronounced jaundice, but it can also present later in infancy or childhood. Hereditary spherocytosis is inherited in an autosomal dominant fashion 70% of the time, so family history of the disease is important to elicit. Treatment for the disease is symptomatic. Blood transfusions can be needed often, during acute illness only, or never. Folic acid supplementation should be used in patients with chronic hemolysis. Splenectomy is essentially curative and in the past was done routinely regardless of clinical severity of disease. Currently, management is more conservative, and the risks and benefits of splenectomy should be carefully considered with each patient.

Red blood cell enzyme defects also cause hemolytic anemia. The most common are glucose-6-phosphate dehydrogenase (G6PD) deficiency and pyruvate kinase deficiency. G6PD deficiency is an X-linked hemolytic anemia most often found in people of African, Asian, and Middle Eastern descent. In G6PD deficiency, RBCs are exquisitely sensitive to oxidative stress, and hemolytic anemia can result from triggers including infections, certain medications (including acetaminophen, aspirin, dapsone, nitrofurantoin, primaquine, and sulfa drugs, among others), and ingestion of fava beans. Along with other hemolysis laboratory values, serum G6PD level can be used to diagnose G6PD deficiency. It is important to check a G6PD level in a patient's healthy state after the hemolytic episode has resolved. In acute hemolysis and subsequent reticulocytosis, detectable G6PD level can increase because reticulocytes have more of the enzyme than mature RBCs. Treatment is preventive and symptomatic. Families should be counseled on appropriate food and medication avoidance and also on signs and symptoms of hemolytic crisis, as a blood transfusion may be necessary.

Pyruvate kinase deficiency is a less common RBC enzyme defect that causes hemolytic anemia. Its signs and symptoms are similar to that of G6PD deficiency. Pyruvate kinase deficiency is inherited in an autosomal recessive pattern and is most often found in people of northern European ancestry. Like G6PD deficiency, it has a spectrum of clinical severities and is diagnosed by hemolysis laboratory values and specific enzyme levels. Treatment is supportive, with some patients requiring monthly transfusions.

Other RBC Destruction Problems

Several other etiologies of RBC destruction should be kept in mind when evaluating a patient with hemolytic anemia. Sickle cell disease should not be overlooked, especially when evaluating someone of African descent. Although most patients are diagnosed in the neonatal period by newborn screening, some may be missed, and children born outside the United States are often not screened. When in doubt, a Hgb electrophoresis should be obtained. In addition, other etiologies of RBC destruction include unstable hemoglobin variants, rarer RBC enzyme deficiencies, hereditary pyropoikilocytosis, paroxysmal nocturnal hemoglobinuria, and systemic infections.

Summary
· · · · · · · · · ·

Anemia in the pediatric population has many distinct causes, and sometimes multiple etiologies are operative at the same time. A thorough patient history is the first step. Key patient and family history clues are listed in Table 4-3.

Once a proper history and physical examination are obtained, laboratory evaluation can aid in the narrowing of your differential. Figure 4-1 is one algorithm by which to evaluate anemia using specific laboratory findings.

Table 4-3. Essentials of Patient and Family History in Evaluation of Anemia

Patient History	
Ask about…	**Be thinking…**
Diet • Iron-containing veggies, meat, *milk* (be specific about quantity!), exclusive breastfeeding w/o iron supplementation	Iron deficiency
• Vegan, very restrictive	B12 or folate deficiency
• Goat's milk	Folate deficiency
Bleeding • Epistaxis, gum bleeding, bloody stool, hematuria	Iron deficiency
Jaundice or icterus (neonatal or episodic) If so, specific triggers	Hemolysis (eg, HS, G6PD, PK)
Family History	
Ask about…	**Be thinking…**
Anemia Often families with undiagnosed thalassemia will report family history of iron deficiency.	Any inherited anemia
Ethnic background	Thalassemias, G6PD deficiency
Blood transfusions	Inherited hemolytic anemia, thalassemia
Jaundice or cholecystectomy	Inherited hemolytic anemia
Splenectomy	HS

Abbreviations: G6PD, glucose-6-phosphate dehydrogenase; HS, hereditary spherocytosis; PK, pyruvate kinase; w/o, without.

42   Succinct Pediatrics

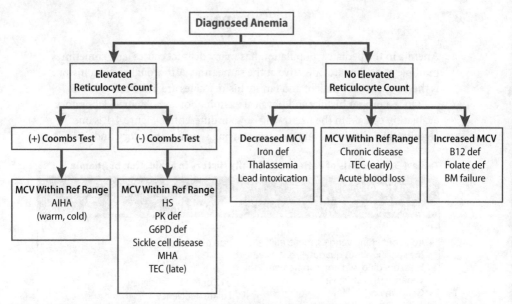

Figure 4-1. Algorithm for anemia based on reticulocytosis and MCV.

Abbreviations: AIHA, autoimmune hemolytic anemia; BM, bone marrow; def, deficiency; G6PD, glucose-6-phosphate dehydrogenase; HS, hereditary spherocytosis; MCV, mean corpuscular volume; MHA, microangiopathic hemolytic anemia; PK, pyruvate kinase; ref, reference; TEC, transient erythroblastopenia of childhood.

[a] In general, hemolytic anemias are normocytic. If signs of hemolysis are present and MCV is increased or decreased, think of a combined process.

Suggested Reading

Arceci R, Hann I, Smith O, eds. *Pediatric Hematology.* Oxford, United Kingdom: Blackwell Publishing; 2006

Janus J, Moerschel SK. Evaluation of anemia in children. *Am Fam Physician.* 2010;81(12):1462–1471

Lanzkowsky P, ed. *Manual of Pediatric Hematology and Oncology.* 5th ed. San Diego, CA: Academic Press; 2011

Lozoff B, Jimenez E, Hagen J, Mollen E, Wolf AW. Poorer behavioral and developmental outcome more than 10 years after treatment for iron deficiency in infancy. *Pediatrics.* 2000;105(4):e51

Nathan D, Ginsburg D, Orkin S, Look AT, eds. *Nathan and Oski's Hematology of Infancy and Childhood.* 6th ed. Philadelphia, PA: WB Saunders Company; 2003

Pineda O, Ashmead HD. Effectiveness of treatment of iron-deficiency anemia in infants and young children with ferrous bis-glycinate chelate. *Nutrition.* 2001;17(5):381–384

Sills RH. *Practical Algorithms in Pediatric Hematology and Oncology.* New York, NY: Karger; 2003

Walters MC, Abelson HT. Interpretation of the complete blood count. *Pediatr Clin North Am.* 1996;43(3):599–622

CHAPTER 5

Asthma

Cheryl D. Courtlandt, MD

Key Points

- The primary care clinician has a vital role in the diagnosis and management of children with asthma.

- Inhaled corticosteroids are the most effective treatment for persistent asthma in children. In spite of the use of inhaled corticosteroids, lung remodeling may still occur.

- Inhaled corticosteroids are safe in low and medium doses, and adverse effects are rare but do occur. As soon as control is established, a step down in therapy should occur.

- Dedicated asthma visits are effective in management; they are opportunities for reinforcement of education and assessment of control.

Overview

Asthma is the most common chronic illness of childhood, affecting more than 7 million children in the United States and millions more children internationally. Since the establishment of the first National Asthma Education and Prevention Program guidelines (NAEPP) (Evidence Level III), more than 20 years ago, significant advances have addressed the unique needs of the pediatric asthma patient. Asthma remains a major cause of pediatric hospitalizations and emergency department and urgent care visits, results in poor school attendance, and accounts for numerous lost days of work for parents. Children with poorly controlled asthma have decreased school performance, interrupted sleep, and difficulty in performing the work of childhood (eg, active play). The effect of the disease has a widespread effect on the patient and the family; this effect can be experienced in all or any of the social, financial, or psychological domains.

Definition

Asthma is most commonly described as a chronic inflammatory disorder of the airways, characterized with a reversible and an irreversible component. Asthma triggers cause inflammatory reactions that lead to airway hyperreactivity, airflow obstruction, and mucus production, which cause the respiratory tract symptoms of cough and wheeze.

Signs and Symptoms

In children, the most common symptom of asthma is cough; other common symptoms are shortness of breath and either an audible or auscultated wheeze. The cough is often described as dry and hacking, although it can produce eosinophil-filled sputum. Obstruction of airflow in the airways causes air hunger. Episodes of wheezing in asthma are usually associated with airflow obstruction, which may be intermittent, reversible, or irreversible.

Asthma Triggers

Exacerbating factors or triggers are common in patients with asthma. Patients may report a seasonal or cyclic pattern to their symptoms, and these changes may be associated with weather or exposure to cold or environmental irritants. In most pediatric patients, especially young children, viral infections are the trigger for most exacerbations. The most common viruses associated with exacerbations are respiratory syncytial virus, influenza, and rhinovirus. Despite recommendations from NAEEP and the American Academy of Pediatrics that all patients with asthma receive an annual influenza vaccine, little evidence shows that this intervention affects outcomes (Evidence Level III). Bacterial infections are rare causes of asthma, but chronic bacterial sinusitis may cause exacerbations of asthma symptoms. Recently, *Mycoplasma* species and *Chlamydia pneumoniae* have also been implicating factors in asthma exacerbations. Exposure to tobacco smoke remains the principle preventable environmental factor that causes asthma symptoms and aids the progression of symptoms. Environmental allergens play a more significant role in patients older than 3 years, but food allergies can be a factor in exacerbations of symptoms in infants, especially those with a history of atopy.

Exercise-induced asthma is usually characterized by acute onset of symptoms 10 to 15 minutes after the start of exercise. In patients with difficult-to-control exercise-induced asthma, those who do not respond quickly and completely to bronchodilators, an alternative diagnosis should be entertained; the most common diagnosis is poorly controlled asthma.

Diagnosis

Primary care clinicians caring for children are essential to confirm the diagnosis and initiate future management of asthma. Ideally, the diagnosis of asthma is made after careful consideration of history and physical examination findings coupled with assessment of asthma risk factors and objective pulmonary function testing if possible. A complete detailed history can be obtained using numerous tools or questions adapted from the NAEEP guidelines (Box 5-1). Asthma is a multifactorial disease with variable expression even within an individual child over time. A constellation of symptoms exist, namely cough, wheezing, and shortness of breath, that appear to have many divergent etiologies in the underlying pathogenesis. The newest evidence, using well-controlled prospective studies, reveals several general subgroups of children presenting with the clinical symptoms of wheezing and cough, but all of these phenotypes have different ages of presentation, duration, and persistence of symptoms and, most importantly, prognosis of future lung function (Evidence Level II-2).

Box 5-1. Detailed Assessment of Medical History

Presenting symptoms	▪ Cough ▪ Wheeze ▪ Shortness of breath ▪ Poor feeding ▪ Rapid breathing ▪ Chest tightness ▪ Sputum production ▪ Poor sleep or restless sleep (especially for infants)
Patterns of symptoms	▪ Seasonal variation ▪ Continuous ▪ Episodic ▪ Intermittent with severe exacerbations ▪ Relationship to exercise ▪ Onset, duration, frequency (number of days or nights per week or month) ▪ Daytime and nighttime symptoms ▪ Early morning symptoms

Box 5-1 *(cont)*

Triggers	<ul><li>Viral respiratory infections</li><li>Environmental indoor allergens</li><li>Pollen and grass</li><li>Home environment</li><li>Smoking (by patient, parents, other caregivers)</li><li>Exercise</li><li>Parent or caregiver occupations</li><li>Emotions and stress</li><li>Drugs</li><li>Food, food additives, and preservatives</li><li>Changes in weather, exposure to cold air</li><li>Endocrine factors</li><li>Gastroesophageal reflux disease</li><li>Sinusitis</li></ul>
Progression of symptoms	<ul><li>History of prematurity</li><li>History of neonatal lung injury</li><li>History of early RSV infection</li><li>Age of onset and progression of symptoms</li><li>Present management of symptoms</li><li>Frequency of short-acting beta$_2$-agonist use</li><li>Oral corticosteroids and frequency of use</li></ul>
Family history	<ul><li>History of atopy</li><li>History of asthma, allergy, sinusitis, rhinitis, nasal polyps in parents or siblings</li></ul>
Social history	<ul><li>Social barriers to adherence: parent or patient drug use, lack of education, lack of insurance, chaotic home situation, homelessness, lack of family support or support system</li><li>Day care</li><li>Multiple school-aged siblings</li></ul>

Box 5-1 *(cont)*

History of symptom exacerbations	<ul><li>Usual prodromal signs and symptoms</li><li>Rapidity of onset</li><li>Duration and frequency</li><li>Severity of exacerbation (ie, level of medical attention: doctor visit vs intensive care)</li><li>Sudden or life-threatening exacerbations</li><li>Any intubations</li><li>Any intensive care admissions</li><li>In the last year: number of<ul><li>– Hospitalizations</li><li>– ED visits</li><li>– Courses of oral steroids</li><li>– Exacerbations</li></ul></li><li>Most recent treatment strategy</li></ul>
Domain effect (social/financial/psychological)	<ul><li>Number of days missed from school/work</li><li>Limitation of activity, especially sports and strenuous work</li><li>History of nocturnal awakening</li><li>Effect on growth, development, behavior, school, or work performance, as well as lifestyle</li><li>Effect on family routines, activities, or dynamics</li><li>Economic effect</li></ul>
Family and patient perception	<ul><li>Current patient or parent knowledge of asthma, treatment options, adverse effects of medication, chronic disease management</li><li>Current level of family support</li><li>Use of alternative or complementary therapy</li><li>Economic resources</li><li>Sociocultural beliefs</li></ul>

Abbreviations: ED, emergency department; RSV, respiratory syncytial virus.

Adapted from National Asthma Education and Prevention Program. *Expert Panel Report 3: Guidelines for the Diagnosis and Management of Asthma. Full Report 2007.* Bethesda, MD: National Institutes of Health; 2007. NIH publication 07-4051. Available at: www.nhlbi.nih.gov/files/docs/guidelines/asthgdln.pdf. Accessed May 13, 2015.

Diagnosis in Children Younger than 5 Years

In children younger than 5 years, diagnosing asthma without an atopic history may be particularly taxing. Many infants or preschool-aged children can wheeze, usually in association with viral infections.

Although the symptoms of cough and wheeze are present in all subgroups of children with wheezing, children with a history of atopy appear different from non-atopic children. An abundance of available evidence now points to a combination of genetics, exposure to viral infections, and environment interactions as important in the expression of asthma. An IgE-mediated response and a genetic tendency to react to common allergens is the strongest identifiable predisposing factor for developing asthma. Common viral upper respiratory tract infections are one of the most important triggers of wheezing in the pediatric patient and may also contribute to development of asthma. An increasing body of evidence points to the individual's response to viral exposure and the adaptation of his immune system as possibly holding the key to development of wheezing with viral illness and subsequent progression to asthma (Evidence Level I).

The asthma predictive index (API) was updated and expanded by the Prevention of Early Asthma in Kids study group. This work resulted in the modified API (mAPI) that includes sensitization to allergens (Box 5-2). The modifications take into account that allergic sensitization to aeroallergens, such as dust mites, mold, or dander, have been postulated in several studies to be important factors in toddlers at risk for developing asthma. In addition, because of their increasing frequency in early childhood, allergies to milk, egg, or peanuts were also added to the index (Evidence Level II-2). The mAPI is recommended by NAEPP as a tool to aid in making the diagnosis of asthma in younger children and may be the best indicator of pediatric asthma and most sensitive for identifying those in need of the most aggressive treatment with inhaled corticosteroids.

The mAPI is positive for patients with 4 or more episodes of wheezing in a year with physician confirmation and either one major criteria or two minor criteria with a positive predictive index of 76%.

Very young patients with asthma, because of their size and developmental stage, are incapable of performing the necessary maneuvers for most formal objective testing of airflow obstruction. Newer experimental diagnostic testing for the infant and young child, such as nitric oxide determination and impulse oscillometry, are available in research and specialist settings but have limited availability in most primary care settings.

Box 5-2. Modified Asthma Predictive Index (mAPI)

History of 4 or more wheezing episodes with physician confirmation
And
Major criteria (one)

- Parental history of asthma
- Physician-diagnosed atopy
- Allergic sensitization to at least one aeroallergen

Minor criteria (two)

- Allergic sensitization to milk, egg, or nuts
- Wheezing not associated with viral URI
- Blood eosinophilia ≥4%

Abbreviation: URI, upper respiratory infection.

From Guilbert TW, Morgan WJ, Zeiger RS, et al. Atopic characteristics of children with recurrent wheezing at high risk for the development of childhood asthma. *J Allergy Clin Immunol.* 2004;114(6):1282–1287, with permission.

Diagnosis in Children Older than 5 Years

Details of the episodes of cough and wheeze and established patterns and triggers can aid in making an asthma diagnosis (Box 5-3). Spirometry may be useful in establishing objective criteria for the presence of airway obstruction of those patients older than 5 to 6 years. Response to albuterol can be documented by spirometry or improved clinical parameters (eg, respiratory rate, decreased cough, and wheeze) in children unable to perform for spirometry. Office-based spirometry is recommended by the NAEPP guidelines to be offered in all practices that care for patients with asthma.

Box 5-3. Environmental Factors Linked to Asthma Exacerbation

Household/Day Care/School/Parents' Home

- Tobacco smoke exposure (by parents, grandparents, siblings, teachers, other caregivers)
- Parental or caregiver occupations (eg, flour, dust, pesticides, mold, cleaning fluids, feathers, fibers)
- Exposure to cleaning chemicals and pesticides
- Household use of fireplaces, wood-burning stoves, kerosene heaters
- Poor air circulation
- Exposure to sick contacts, especially siblings and peers in day care
- Patient's sleeping area: shared spaces, cots, mattresses, couches, bedding, flooring, stuffed animals
- Animal exposure: cats, dogs, birds, unusual pets in the home/day care/school
- Mold and mildew: poor plumbing, leaking pipes, standing water
- Aerosols and sprays: cleaners, air fresheners, perfume or body sprays, aromatic oils
- Exposure to allergens
- Heating and cooling systems in the school/day care/parents' home

Spirometry measurements include forced vital capacity (FVC) and forced expiratory volume in one second (FEV1). Airflow obstruction is defined as FEV1 reduced to less than 80% of the predicted airflow in a healthy child and an FEV1/FVC ratio of less than 85%. There are reference tables that are based on age, height, sex, and race. Both of these parameters may be helpful, but FEV1/FVC appears to be a more sensitive measure of impairment than FEV1, whereas FEV1 may be a more useful measure of risk for future exacerbations.

Forced expiratory volume in one second has been noted to have a direct relationship to not only severity but also future symptoms and utilization of health care resources. In the pediatric patient, significant reversibility of airflow obstruction is diagnostic of asthma. A 9% increase of FEV1 after administration of a bronchodilator has been the established threshold (Evidence Level II-1). Many pediatric patients will have spirometry with the reference range but still have moderate to severe disease. Evidence from cross-sectional studies shows that spirometry alone does not adequately categorize severity of asthma in children and that assessments of symptoms, especially at nighttime, are better correlated (Evidence Level II-2). According to the NAEPP guidelines, this assessment of severity, along with spirometry, is optimal for diagnosing asthma (Table 5-1).

Table 5-1. Asthma Severity Classification at Diagnosis

Category	Exercise	Intermittent	Mild Persistent	Moderate Persistent	Severe Persistent
Daytime symptoms	None (except while exercising)	Less than 2 times per week	More than 2 times per week, not daily	Daily symptoms	Continuous symptoms throughout the day
Nighttime symptoms	None	Less than 2 times per month	2 to 4 times per month	Greater than 4 times per month, not nightly	More than 2 times per week, or nightly
FEV1	>90%	>80%	>80%	60%–80%	<60%

Abbreviation: FEV1, forced expiratory volume in one second.

Adapted from National Asthma Education and Prevention Program. *Expert Panel Report 3: Guidelines for the Diagnosis and Management of Asthma. Full Report 2007.* Bethesda, MD: National Institutes of Health; 2007. NIH publication 07-4051. Available at: www.nhlbi.nih.gov/files/docs/guidelines/asthgdln.pdf. Accessed May 13, 2015.

Peak flow meters are an objective measure of airflow used for comparison to an individual's personal best or as a response to changes in maintenance therapy (eg, stepping up or stepping down). These meters have variability and are dependent on patient effort. Consequently, these assessments are valuable in management strategies but not appropriate as the sole objective indicator in the diagnosis of asthma.

Although according to the latest NAEPP guidelines, allergy testing (of the skin or by serum) is currently recommended, this testing should not be used to confirm the diagnosis of asthma but rather to aid in the control of symptoms in patients with moderate to severe symptoms that are not well-controlled with the use of conventional treatments (Evidence Level III). The rationale for allergy testing in even young children is to educate families about avoidance of potential allergens. However, 2 extensive Cochrane Reviews found no evidence of benefit from avoidance in using single steps (eg, just mattress covers, just air filters) to avoid allergens. In all cases studied, numerous modalities of avoidance are suggested (Evidence Level I).

Asthma severity is determined best at the time of diagnosis, before initiation of therapy (see Table 5-1). There are 4 categories of asthma severity: intermittent, mild persistent, moderate persistent, and severe persistent. The severity assessment categorizes symptoms and level of impairment. In addition, a risk assessment should be performed based on the number of previous exacerbations requiring oral steroid intervention. In younger patients, risk factors for developing asthma are also factored into severity assessment (Table 5-2). There is an important distinction between intermittent and persistent asthma because all individuals who have persistent asthma should be started on long-term controller medication.

Table 5-2. Initial Exacerbation Risk Assessment

Age Group, y	Intermittent	Mild Persistent	Moderate Persistent	Severe Persistent
0–4	Less than 2 episodes per year requiring oral steroids	2 or more episodes in 6 months or 4 or more episodes of wheezing in a year with risk factors for asthma (see Box 5-2 or 5-3)	2 or more episodes in 6 months or 4 or more episodes of wheezing in a year with risk factors for asthma (see Box 5-2 or 5-3)	2 or more episodes in 6 months or 4 or more episodes of wheezing in a year with risk factors for asthma (see Box 5-2 or 5-3)
5–11	Less than 2 episodes per year	2 or more episodes in a year	2 or more episodes in a year	2 or more episodes in a year
12 and older	Less than 2 episodes per year	2 or more episodes in a year	2 or more episodes in a year	2 or more episodes in a year

Adapted from National Asthma Education and Prevention Program. *Expert Panel Report 3: Guidelines for the Diagnosis and Management of Asthma. Full Report 2007.* Bethesda, MD: National Institutes of Health; 2007. NIH publication 07-4051. Available at: www.nhlbi.nih.gov/files/docs/guidelines/asthgdln.pdf. Accessed May 13, 2015.

Differential Diagnosis

Cough and wheezing is a common concern among pediatric patients. Cough as the sole symptom of asthma is unusual in younger children, and subsequently careful consideration must be given to an alternative diagnosis even in patients previously labeled as having asthma. Most children, especially the youngest ones, who cough without any apparent symptom of wheezing probably do not have asthma. The singular symptom of cough is a poor indicator of asthma, particularly without any other key features of asthma. Other causes of cough and wheezing can be associated with bacterial infection, foreign body aspiration, and anatomic abnormalities, as well as other organic disease such as gastroesophageal reflux disease (Box 5-4).

Box 5-4. Differential Diagnosis of Wheezing and Cough

Disease/clinical condition	Additional symptoms or considerations that make the diagnosis of asthma less likely
Anatomic abnormalities ■ Tracheomalacia ■ Bronchomalacia ■ Vascular rings ■ Tracheoesophageal fistula	■ Noises change with position ■ Well-auscultated over trachea ■ Failure to respond to asthma treatment ■ Coughing with feeding
Bronchiolitis	■ May be difficult to distinguish ■ Poor response to treatment
GERD	■ Feeding difficulties ■ Neurologic abnormalities ■ Prematurity
Chronic cough ■ Allergic rhinitis ■ Bacterial sinusitis	■ Nasal congestion ■ Rhinorrhea ■ Headache and fever
Foreign body aspiration	■ Acute symptoms after choking episode ■ Localized wheezing
Recurrent aspiration	■ Failure to thrive ■ Neurologic abnormalities
Cystic fibrosis	■ Failure to thrive ■ History of pneumonia ■ Clubbing
Congestive heart failure	■ Cardiac murmur ■ Hepatosplenomegaly ■ Failure to thrive

Box 5-4 *(cont)*

Chronic lung disease of prematurity	■ Prematurity ■ Slow growth
Vocal cord dysfunction	■ Flattened PFT loops ■ Poor response to treatment
Chronic lung disease	■ Clubbing

Abbreviations: GERD, gastroesophageal reflux disease; PFT, pulmonary function test.

However, there is a small subset of patients, usually older children who have cough as their only or predominate symptom of asthma, whose cough is associated with airway hypersensitivity and who find relief of obstruction with a trial of bronchodilators. The diagnosis of cough-variant asthma may be complicated by cough associated with an acute viral illness. Often a patient will discontinue bronchodilator therapy after the acute illness has resolved only for the symptoms of cough to return in an otherwise well child. If the cough resolves after restarting bronchodilators, the diagnosis of asthma is more likely.

Management

Pediatric asthma is a multifactorial disease that requires multiple strategies which leverage the close relationship between pharmacologic intervention, environmental control, and patient education and self-management to control asthma symptoms.

Pharmacologic Intervention

The primary pharmacologic agents used in asthma therapy were directed at smooth muscle relaxation via bronchodilation. The latest NAEPP update, in recognition of the diversity of disease manifestation among the pediatric age group, has further divided management into 2 groups: birth to 5 years and 5 to 11 years. Current research has demonstrated that not only is the medication effect different in these age groups but there is extreme variability in their disease and, more importantly, its progression.

Numerous controlled and population studies have clearly demonstrated that although inhaled corticosteroids (ICS) are the first line of controller medication therapy for pediatric asthma and to prevent exacerbations, these medications have not been effective in stopping the progression of pediatric asthma. Several studies have demonstrated that, even with early treatment, the natural history of asthma may not be altered (Evidence Level I).

Previously, the guidelines have focused on assessment of severity at diagnosis and initial treatment. Updated guidelines emphasize these factors and introduce the concept of control of asthma symptoms while stepping up and down therapy. Although corticosteroids are considered safe, several studies have pointed to a slowing of linear growth attributed to use of ICS. Most studies have determined there is little effect on final adult height from low and medium dose ICS; a more recent study has shown there is an effect of ICS on final adult height (Evidence Level II-1). The main goals of asthma therapy are to decrease symptoms of impairment, reduce risk of exacerbation, prevent loss of lung function, and avoid adverse effects of medications. Studies have shown physicians often use evidence-based criteria to increase medications but are reluctant to step patients down once control has been achieved.

Inhaled corticosteroids are the treatment of choice for persistent asthma. Studies have demonstrated improved asthma symptoms, decreased exacerbations, and a decreased risk of sudden death, as well as improved lung function (Evidence Level I). Inhaled corticosteroids are most effective for secondary phase symptoms and have little or no direct effect on bronchospasm.

The therapeutic effects of inhaled corticosteroid peak after several weeks of use; however, some relief of symptoms may be seen after one week of daily therapy. In general, ICS are safe medications when administered at recommended dosages; many of the adverse effects reported in adults have not been demonstrated in children. There is a stepwise progression for initiating ICS therapy recommended by NAEEP (Table 5-3), which is aligned with severity assessment of impairment and risk of future exacerbations. This stepwise progression can be used for all inhaled corticosteroids, combination inhaled steroids, and long-acting beta$_2$-agonists and with oral corticosteroids. This same progression can be used by physicians to step down therapy from higher doses of ICS. Several effective delivery systems are available for use in the pediatric population including nebulizers, dry-powder inhalers, or metered-dose inhalers. Although younger children use nebulizers more frequently, evidence exists that demonstrates metered dose inhalers can be an effective delivery system in the youngest patients with asthma (Evidence Level I). Adverse effects of ICS can be minimized with use of a spacer device and by rinsing the mouth after administration. To limit systemic absorption, avoid oral candidiasis and ensure proper technique. A spacer device should always be used.

Leukotriene modifiers are recommended for use as adjunctive therapy for patients younger than 12 years whose asthma is not well-controlled with medium-dose ICS. Physicians often use these agents for mild persistent asthma; however, evidence demonstrates they are less effective and should only be used as an alternative if ICS are not tolerated. Cromolyn sodium and nedocromil are other anti-inflammatory agents used in asthma therapy and are primarily used as second-line therapy for patients with mild persistent asthma. These medications have an excellent safety profile but are less effective than ICS and therefore are not a preferred medication strategy. Theophylline, a bronchodilator with a small anti-inflammatory effect, has toxicity and requires monitoring. Omalizumab, a monoclonal anti-IgE antibody, has been utilized in patients with severe asthma not controlled by conventional therapy; allergists or pulmonologists usually supervise use of this drug. Further information about these medications and their indications are contained in the NAEEP guidelines (Evidence Level I).

Table 5-3. Stepwise Initiation of Asthma Therapy

Age Group, y	Intermittent	Mild Persistent	Moderate Persistent	Severe Persistent
0–4	Step 1 SABA as needed	Step 2 Low-dose ICS	Step 3 Medium-dose ICS	Step 5 High-dose ICS + LABA or LTM
			Step 4 Medium-dose ICS + LABA or LTM	Step 6 High-dose ICS + OCS + LABA or LTM
5–11	Step 1 SABA as needed	Step 2 Low-dose ICS	Step 3 Low-dose ICS + LABA or LTA or Medium ICS dose	Step 5 High-dose ICS + LABA
			Step 4 Medium-dose ICS + LABA	Step 6 High-dose ICS + OCS + LABA
12 and older	Step 1 SABA as needed	Step 2 Low-dose ICS	Step 3 Low-dose ICS + LABA or Medium ICS dose	Step 5 High-dose ICS + LABA or LTM
			Step 4 Medium-dose ICS + LABA	Step 6 High-dose ICS +OCS + LABA

Abbreviations: ICS, inhaled corticosteroids; LABA, long-acting beta$_2$-agonist; LTA, leukotriene receptor antagonist; LTM, leukotriene modifier; OCS, oral corticosteroids; SABA, short-acting beta$_2$-agonist.

Adapted from National Asthma Education and Prevention Program. *Expert Panel Report 3: Guidelines for the Diagnosis and Management of Asthma. Full Report 2007.* Bethesda, MD: National Institutes of Health; 2007. NIH publication 07-4051. Available at: www.nhlbi.nih.gov/files/docs/guidelines/asthgdln.pdf. Accessed May 13, 2015.

Long-acting beta$_2$-agonists similar to short-acting beta$_2$-agonists (SABA) are recommended for stepped-up control when ICS alone are not effective. In pediatrics, these medications should be used in combination therapy only: studies have implicated long-acting beta$_2$-agonist monotherapy with more severe exacerbations of asthma. These medications should be clearly labeled as controller medications and not for quick relief; they provide 12 hours of bronchodilation, but the onset of action is more than 1 hour.

Short-acting beta$_2$-agonists are used as quick relief medications for exacerbations of symptoms; the onset of action is 15 to 30 minutes, and the effects dissipate after 4 hours. Excessive use of these medications is linked to poorly controlled asthma. Short-acting beta$_2$-agonists are the mainstay of therapy for mild intermittent asthma and exercise-induced asthma (EIA). The symptoms of EIA can be prevented by pretreatment 15 to 20 minutes prior to physical activity. Exercise-induced asthma that is not easily controlled may be a sign of poorly controlled chronic asthma. In patients with mild intermittent asthma, if SABA are needed more than 2 times per week and if there are any nighttime symptoms, the diagnosis of persistent asthma is more likely.

In the stepwise progression, oral corticosteroids are used in the setting of poorly controlled symptoms or moderate to severe exacerbations. Oral administration has been shown to be as effective as intravenous, with onset of action in approximately 4 hours (Evidence Level I). Most studies have noted a few adverse effects from short bursts (<10 days of oral steroids). More than 2 bursts per year are associated with poorly controlled asthma, and more frequent use is associated with higher incidence of adverse effects (Evidence Level I)

Environmental Control

Tobacco smoke is the single most preventable cause of asthma exacerbations. Numerous studies among children with asthma have shown tobacco exposure is associated with increased severity of asthma and decreased lung function (Evidence Level I). Smoking cessation must be a priority for patients and their families. Using motivational interviewing techniques, readiness to quit smoking should be assessed at each visit. Numerous free and low-cost tobacco cessation programs are available in communities.

Almost 75% of children with asthma have been sensitized to at least one aeroallergen. Common indoor allergens include house dust mites, cockroach debris, pet dander, and molds. For children with hard-to-control asthma, prick skin testing or blood testing should be considered to determine evidence of allergic sensitization. Evidence supports that patients with persistent asthma and documented allergies can benefit from immunotherapy (Evidence Level II). The most successful interventions to reduce indoor allergens target all potential irritants. They include frequent vacuuming, laundering bedding in hot water, using of dust covers, cleaning all surfaces, removing food to eliminate roaches, and removing items that trap dust from sleeping areas. For children sensitized to pet dander, pets should be removed from the home. Dried saliva from pets is also a significant allergen, so pet removal from a patient's sleeping area alone will not alleviate symptoms.

Patient Education/Self-management

Patient education is a cornerstone in asthma care, and review is necessary at every visit. It is imperative that patients can adequately explain their disease and its management, especially the use of controller medications. Teach-back or other health literacy techniques should be used in each encounter. Self-management plans, such as asthma action plans or home maintenance plan of care, should be reviewed and updated at every visit.

The Planned Visit

Scheduling a planned visit is an opportunity for clinicians to encourage self-management, monitor symptoms, review treatment plans, and assess the need for ongoing therapy. Complementary and alternative therapies are commonly used by patients with asthma and their parents. A shared vision of treatment with specific goals may be helpful to both clinician and patient and family.

Often in the setting of an acute illness, it is difficult to make a global assessment and set appropriate goals. The current guidelines recommend these planned visits center around 4 components of asthma care.

1. Measures to assess and monitor asthma
2. Patient education
3. Control of environmental factors and other conditions that can worsen asthma
4. Medication use

During these visits, the clinician needs to assess level of control based on impairment and risk. If control is poor for no apparent reason, after assessment of medication adherence and environmental factors, therapy should be stepped up. After 2 weeks, the patient should be reassessed. When a patient has been well-controlled for 3 months, a step down in therapy should occur with a reassessment within 6 weeks. More active monitoring of symptoms and peak flow assessment should occur when therapy is stepped up or down. The recommended timing for these visits is at least every 3 months for moderate to severe patients and every 6 months for patients whose asthmas is well-controlled with mild symptoms. Patients with EIA can be assessed yearly if their symptoms are well-controlled. Medication compliance is an important factor in the assessment of control. If possible, pharmacy records in patients whose symptoms are not well-controlled should verify compliance.

Specialty Consultation

In spite of optimal management and compliance, some patients may have asthma that is difficult to control. These patients may require consultation with an allergist or a pulmonologist when stepwise control has not been achieved and impairment continues. The NAEPP guidelines suggest specialty referral for patients with a history of inpatient intensive care therapy, frequent hospitalizations, multiple courses of oral corticosteroids for exacerbations, or comorbidities that make the underlying asthma more difficult to manage; for candidates for immunotherapy; for patients that adhere to escalating treatment without any change in symptoms; and when additional diagnostic testing is warranted.

Suggested Reading

Bukutu C, Le C, Vohra S. Asthma: a review of complementary and alternative therapies. *Pediatr Rev.* 2008;29(8):e44–e49

Castro-Rodriquez JA, Holberg CJ, Wright AL, Martinez FD. A clinical index to define risk of asthma in young children with recurring wheezing. *Am J Respir Crit Care Med.* 2000;162(4 Pt 1):1403–1406

The Childhood Asthma Management Program Research Group. Long-term effects of budesonide or nedocromil in children with asthma. *N Engl J Med.* 2000;343(15):1054–1063

Guilbert TW, Morgan WJ, Zeiger RS, et al. Long-term inhaled corticosteroids in preschool children at high risk for asthma. *N Engl J Med.* 2006;354(19):1985–1997

Hill VL, Wood PR. Asthma, epidemiology, pathophysiology and initial evaluation. *Pediatr Rev.* 2009;30(9):331–335

Kelly HW, Sternberg AL, Lescher R, et al. Effect of inhaled glucocorticoids in childhood on adult height. *N Engl J Med.* 2012;367(10):904–912

National Asthma Education and Prevention Program. *Expert Panel Report 3: Guidelines for the Diagnosis and Management of Asthma. Full Report 2007.* Bethesda, MD: National Institutes of Health; 2007. NIH publication 07-4051. Available at: www.nhlbi.nih.gov/files/docs/guidelines/asthgdln.pdf. Accessed May 13, 2015.

Wood PR, Hill VL. Practical management of asthma. *Pediatr Rev.* 2009;30(10):375–385

CHAPTER 6

Attention-Deficit/ Hyperactivity Disorder

Rachel Dawkins, MD, and Heidi Murphy, MD

Key Points

- Attention-deficit/hyperactivity disorder (ADHD) is a common behavioral condition involving symptoms of hyperactivity, inattention, and impulsivity.
- Evaluation of ADHD, using ADHD specific rating scales, should take place in multiple settings.
- Children with ADHD commonly have coexisting comorbid conditions.
- Treatment of ADHD may involve behavioral therapies, educational interventions, or medications.

Overview

Attention-deficit/hyperactivity disorder (ADHD) is a common behavioral disorder of childhood and adolescence characterized by symptoms of hyperactivity, inattention, and impulsivity. Along with affecting behavior and altering each patient's developmental course, symptoms of ADHD interfere with the affected child's functionality in multiple settings, including school, home, and social encounters.

Causes

No single, specific cause for ADHD has been identified; however, the cause is likely multifactorial. Research has indicated a possible biological basis for ADHD involving the complex systems that control attention and regulate inhibition. Deficits in executive functions, such as memory, response inhibition, and concentration, are present in most patients with ADHD, and studies now suggest a genetic etiology in some cases. Though no specific genetic phenomenon has been found to be causative, several studies have suggested evidence of association with 8 particular genes. Research has investigated possible causality in association with severe early neglect and deprivation in infancy, maternal smoking during pregnancy, and traumatic brain injury.

The differential diagnoses for ADHD is wide and may include the following diagnoses: developmental variations, neurologic conditions, developmental conditions, emotional/psychological pathologies, medical conditions, or behavioral pathologies. Often, many of these diagnoses may coexist with ADHD (Box 6-1).

Signs and Symptoms

Three core symptoms—hyperactivity, inattention, and impulsivity—help define ADHD and its 3 subtypes.

Predominantly inattentive ADHD. Inattention, or a decreased ability to focus along with impaired cognitive processing, is the primary deficit noted in this subtype of ADHD.

Predominantly hyperactive-impulsive ADHD. Hyperactivity and impulsivity define this subtype. Inattention may be absent, but patients often have the inability to sit still or inhibit behaviors.

Combined subtype ADHD. Patients with combined subtype ADHD have all 3 core symptoms: hyperactivity, inattention, and impulsivity.

Because symptoms of ADHD may be secondary to a comorbid diagnosis, this must be considered when evaluating a patient for ADHD. For example, patients with learning disability should not have impulsivity or hyperactivity that imparts functional impairment. Additionally, patients with learning disabilities may have academic trouble in the specific domain of their disability but not in other areas. That is, a student with mathematical learning disability should not have difficulties with language skills. Children with ADHD will have functional impairment evident in all academic domains. The most common coexisting illness is oppositional defiant disorder and is found in up to 54% to 84% of patients with ADHD. Psychiatric disorders and behavioral problems commonly coexist with ADHD, as well as learning and language disorders (see Box 6-1).

Box 6-1. Common Comorbid Diagnoses

- Oppositional defiant disorder
- Conduct disorder
- Affective disorder
- Anxiety disorder
- Tic disorder
- Obsessive compulsive disorder
- Obsessive compulsive personality mania
- Major depressive disorder
- Learning disorder
- Language disorder (expressive or receptive)
- Pervasive developmental disorder
- Substance abuse
- Sleep apnea

Diagnosis

· · · · · · · · · ·

The *Diagnostic and Statistical Manual of Mental Disorders, Fifth Edition* (*DSM-5*) has defined specific criteria for the diagnosis of ADHD and its subtypes (Box 6-2).

Box 6-2. Attention-Deficit/Hyperactivity Disorder Diagnostic Criteria

---

A. **Persistent pattern of inattention or hyperactivity-impulsivity that interferes with functioning or development, as characterized by (1) or (2):**

    1. **Inattention: six or more of the following symptoms for at least 6 months**

        a. Often fails to give close attention to details or makes careless mistakes in schoolwork, at work, or during other activities
        b. Often has difficulty sustaining attention in tasks or play activities
        c. Often does not seem to listen when spoken to directly
        d. Often does not follow through on instructions and fails to finish schoolwork or chores
        e. Often has difficulty organizing tasks and activities
        f. Often avoids, dislikes, or is reluctant to engage in tasks that require sustained mental effort
        g. Often loses things necessary for tasks or activities
        h. Is often easily distracted by extraneous stimuli
        i. Is often forgetful in daily activities

    2. **Hyperactivity and impulsivity: six or more of the following symptoms for at least 6 months**

        a. Often fidgets with or taps hands or feet or squirms in seat
        b. Often leaves seat in situations when remaining seated is expected
        c. Often runs about or climbs in situations where it is inappropriate
        d. Often unable to play quietly
        e. Is often "on the go" as if "driven by a motor"
        f. Often talks excessively
        g. Often blurts out an answer
        h. Often has difficulty waiting his or her turn
        i. Often interrupts or intrudes on others

B. **Several inattentive or hyperactive-impulsive symptoms were present prior to age 12 years.**

C. **Several inattentive or hyperactive-impulsive symptoms are present in two or more settings.**

D. **There is clear evidence that the symptoms interfere with, or reduce, the quality of social, academic, or occupational functioning.**

E. **The symptoms do not occur exclusively during the course of schizophrenia/ psychosis and are not better explained by another mental disorder.**

---

*Source: Diagnostic and Statistical Manual of Mental Disorders, 5th Edition

Evaluation
· · · · · · · · · · ·

An evaluation for ADHD should be initiated by the primary care physician in any patient 4 to 18 years of age when the patient presents with symptoms of inattention, hyperactivity, or impulsivity. Likewise, academic or behavioral problems should prompt ADHD evaluation in this same cohort (Evidence Level III). The sheer number of patients with ADHD far exceeds capacity of the mental health system currently, and the initial evaluation for ADHD is within the general pediatricians' purview. Historically, ADHD diagnosis was limited to those patients who demonstrated the core symptoms of ADHD prior to age 7. However, with new diagnostic criteria from the *DSM-5*, the diagnosis of ADHD is no longer relegated to primary school-aged children but is now appropriate for adolescents and preschool-aged children as well. As such, the number of patients will likely continue to increase, further emphasizing the need for ADHD evaluation to be completed by the primary care physician.

To make the diagnosis of ADHD, primary care physicians should ensure that the patient meets the criteria for ADHD diagnosis as outlined by the *DSM-5* (see Box 6-2). It is imperative that impairment in more than one major setting be documented as well as information pertaining to the diagnosis gathered from those individuals (eg, parents, day-care providers, school teachers) involved in the child's care. All 18 symptoms of ADHD listed in the *DSM-5* should be discussed specifically. Rating scales such as the Vanderbilt diagnostic parent and teacher scales or similar evidence-based questionnaires may be helpful in gathering the information necessary to make the diagnosis. Additionally, alternative causes for symptoms prompting ADHD evaluation must be ruled out (Evidence Level III) and, again, the pediatrician should be aware that many conditions may coexist with ADHD (see Box 6-1). Evaluation must include assessment for these comorbid diagnoses (Evidence Level III).

Strictly speaking, in a patient with an unremarkable medical history, no laboratory or formal neurologic testing is indicated to diagnose ADHD, though these tests may be useful in some instances to rule out other diagnoses that may mimic ADHD or coexist with ADHD. Unless cognitive delays or learning disabilities are suspected, no formal psychological or neuropsychological testing is needed. However, if the physician is unable to differentiate a learning disability from ADHD or to determine if these coexist, formal psychological or neuropsychological testing may be indicated. Disorganized home routines, poor academic skills, or poorly structured academic environments may lead to symptoms that mimic ADHD, and evaluation for ADHD should specifically address these points.

Attention-deficit/hyperactivity disorder is a chronic, medical condition and must be addressed by the primary care physician as such. This requires pediatricians and health care providers for children and adolescents to use the model for a medical home when treating these patients (Evidence Level III), keeping in mind that current treatment options for ADHD address only the symptoms of ADHD and are not curative.

Management
· · · · · · · · · · · ·

For all patients with ADHD, a realistic, comprehensive, and evidence-based management plan should be developed in cooperation with the patient and his family.

Stimulant therapy, in most cases, is the criterion standard, and the US Food and Drug Administration (FDA) agreed that stimulants, amphetamines, and methylphenidates have been shown to be equally efficacious after rigorous study. Other medications including atomoxetine, long-acting clonidine, and guanficine may be considered as second-line therapies (Table 6-1).

The "Clinical Practice Guideline for the Diagnosis, Evaluation, and Treatment of ADHD in Children and Adolescents" published by the American Academy of Pediatrics divides the pediatric and adolescent populations into cohorts by age to address specific treatment recommendations: preschool-aged children (4–5 years), elementary school-aged children (6–11 years), and adolescents (12–18 years).

In preschool-aged patients, the American Academy of Pediatrics recommends evidence-based parent- or teacher-administered behavior therapy. Methylphenidate is a second-line treatment in this age group for patients with moderate-to-severe impairment in whom behavior interventions alone have not provided significant improvement in functionality. If evidence-based behavior treatment is unavailable, case-by-case consideration should be given to the risks versus benefits for initiating treatment with methylphenidate or delaying diagnosis and treatment (Evidence Level I). It is important to note that no stimulants or α_2-adrenergic antagonists have been FDA approved for the preschool-aged cohort. Typically, short-acting medications are utilized in this age group, as these patients may be more sensitive to dose-related adverse effects and have a slower metabolism of methylphenidate than older children. In addition, longer-acting agents are not typically available in the low-dose range necessary for this age group.

For elementary school-aged children, FDA-approved ADHD medications are first-line therapy (see Table 6-1) (Evidence Level I). Medication therapy should be in conjunction with parent- or teacher-administered behavior therapy (Evidence Level I). Evidence demonstrates stimulants to be the best first-line therapy, though atomoxetine, extended-release guanfacine, and extended-release clonidine can also be considered (Evidence Level II-1).

The FDA-approved medications for ADHD should be prescribed to the adolescent-aged patient (Evidence Level I) and the best treatment plan for these patients again includes concurrent behavior therapy (Evidence Level II-2).

In all age groups, if medications are used, the dose should be titrated to achieve maximum benefit with minimal side effects (Evidence Level III).

As the primary care physician to a patient with ADHD, you must take multiple factors into consideration when picking the initial medication for treatment: desired duration of medication effect, the subtype of ADHD (functional domain in which improvement is desired), adverse effects, and coexisting psychiatric or emotional conditions. Additionally, such considerations as the child's ability to swallow a pill, avoidance of school time administration, expense, and substance abuse among household members must also be addressed. Amphetamine and dexmethylphenidate, as above, are equally efficacious. Likewise, immediate-release and long-acting formulations are equally effective, and a decision

Table 6-1. Medications Approved by the US FDA for ADHD (Alphabetical by Class)

Generic Class/ Brand Name	Dose Form	Typical Starting Dose	FDA Max per Day
Amphetamine preparations			
Short acting			
Adderall	5, 7.5, 10, 12.5, 15, 20, 30 mg tab	3–5 y: 2.5 mg every day ≥6 y: 5 mg every–twice a day	40 mg
Dexedrine	5 mg	3 y: 2.5 mg every day	
DextroStat	5, 10 mg cap	≥6 y: 5 mg every–twice a day	
ProCentra	5 mg/5 mL	3–5 y: 2.5 mg every day ≥6 y: 5 mg every–twice a day	
Long acting			
Dexedrine Spansule	5, 10, 15 mg cap	≥6 y: 5–10 mg every–twice a day	40 mg
Adderall XR	5, 10, 15, 20, 25, 30 mg cap	≥6 y: 10 mg every day	30 mg
Vyvanse (lisdexamfetamine)	30, 50, 70 mg cap	30 mg every day	70 mg
Methylphenidate preparations			
Short acting			
Focalin	2.5, 5, 10 mg cap	2.5 mg twice a day	20 mg
Methylin	5, 10, 20 mg tab	5 mg twice a day	60 mg
Ritalin	5, 10, 20 mg	5 mg twice a day	60 mg
Intermediate acting			
Metadate ER	10, 20 mg cap	10 mg every day	60 mg
Methylin ER	10, 20 mg cap	10 mg every day	60 mg
Ritalin SR	20 mg	10 mg every day	60 mg
Metadate CD	10, 20, 30, 40, 0, 60 mg	20 mg every day	60 mg
Ritalin LA	10, 20, 30, 40 mg	20 mg every day	60 mg

Table 6-1 *(cont)*

Generic Class/ Brand Name	Dose Form	Typical Starting Dose	FDA Max per Day
Methylphenidate preparations			
Long acting			
Concerta	18, 27, 36, 4 mg cap	18 mg every day	72 mg
Daytrana Patch	10, 15, 20, 30 mg patch	10 mg every day	30 mg
Focalin XR	5, 10, 15, 20 mg cap	5 mg every day	30 mg
Quillivant XR	5 mg/mL liquid	≥6 y: 20 mg every day	60 mg
Selective norepinephrine reuptake inhibitor			
Atomoxetine			
Strattera	10, 18, 25, 40, 60, 80, 100 mg cap	<70 kg: 0.5 mg/kg/d for 4 days then 1 mg/kg/d for 4 days then 1.2 mg/kg/d	Lesser of 1.4 mg/kg or 100 mg
α_2-adrenergic antagonist			
Guanfacine ER			
Intuniv	1, 2, 3, 4 mg	1 mg every day for 1 week, may increase 1 mg per week	Lesser of 0.14 mg/kg or 4 mg

Abbreviations: ADHD, attention-deficit/hyperactivity disorder; cap, capsule; max, maximum; tab, tablet.
Adapted from Pliszka S. Practice parameter for the assessment and treatment of children and adolescents with attention-deficit/hyperactivity/disorder. *J Am Acad Child Adolesc Psychiatry.* 2007;46(7):894–921, with permission.

between which preparation to use should be based on the duration of therapy desired. Long-acting medications have the benefit of being less likely to cause addiction; however, they may not be available in a sufficiently low dose for some cohorts.

If comorbid diagnoses exist with ADHD, each diagnosis must be addressed individually, and these diagnoses and their treatment should be considered when medications for ADHD treatment are selected.

Three stages of medication use are described in the context of ADHD treatment: titration (typically 1–3 months), maintenance (variable duration), and termination. No therapeutic window has been identified for any ADHD medication; therefore, the goal of titration is to reduce core symptoms by 40% to 50% while avoiding unacceptable adverse effects. Once an effective dose is identified, maintenance therapy begins, and patients should be monitored every 3 to 6 months. During maintenance therapy, physicians should review adherence, monitor for adverse effects, and monitor the need for dose adjustments. Rating scales, such as the Vanderbilt, may be useful once again to monitor the effectiveness of treatment. Teacher feedback is paramount during both the titration and maintenance phases, as they are often the supervising adults for the patient during the period of dose effect. Termination of medications can be considered in patients who have had prolonged stable improvement in core ADHD symptoms. If desired, medications can be discontinued to identify whether medication is still needed, though it is imperative to note that ADHD is a chronic condition.

Stimulants have a response rate of approximately 70%. In children or adolescents who do not respond to one type of stimulant, at least one-half will respond to another stimulant. Thus, a systematic trial of stimulants must be undertaken by physicians. Failure of a second stimulant may indicate the patient needs an extended-release preparation or a nonstimulant medication such as clonidine. However, review of alternative causes of treatment failure such as poor adherence, medication misuse, or comorbid conditions should be completed. Beyond improving the core symptoms of ADHD, medications improve parent-child interactions, aggressive behaviors, and academic productivity and accuracy. Though stimulants will not treat any coexisting conditions, they may allow for better evaluation and treatment of comorbid conditions.

Adverse effects of stimulants have been well studied. Commonly, patients will experience decreased appetite (which may lead to poor growth), mood lability, sleep disturbance or nightmares, dizziness, rebound symptoms, and, in rare cases, psychosis. Primary care physicians should monitor height and weight of all patients on treatment medications for ADHD. Rigorous study has shown that stimulant medications may cause some minimal growth retardation in regard to height; however, ultimate reductions in adult height have never been shown to occur. Should patients on stimulant medications for ADHD cross more than 2 percentile lines on a growth chart, a medication "holiday" or medication change should be considered. Cardiovascular events have, historically, been a concern with regard to ADHD treatment medications. In patients with no medical histories of cardiovascular disease, no routine cardiac evaluation is necessary. However, if a patient with ADHD has a history of palpitations, congenital heart disease, or exercise intolerance or family history of sudden death, a cardiac evaluation may be warranted prior to starting stimulant therapy. Cardiovascular adverse effects of stimulant medications include minimal increases in pulse and blood pressure. Particularly in older children and adolescents, misuse of stimulants may be a concern. Medication holidays (ie, short periods of time, such as a weekend, during which patients abstain from medication use) may be considered for specific adverse effects; however, these are not routinely recommended and should be considered on a case-by-case basis.

Other Therapies

Behavior therapies, as mentioned above, play an integral role with medications in the treatment of ADHD. Making environmental changes, whether in the classroom or the home environment, can also help modify behaviors. These changes may include maintenance of a strict daily schedule, limiting choices presented to the patient, maintenance of a distraction-free environment, and setting small reachable goals. In school-aged children, individualized educational plans and school accommodations should be instituted. Evidence-based interventions use a reward and non-punitive consequence system to change problem behaviors in patients with ADHD. These therapies may include techniques such as positive reinforcement, time-out, response cost (ie, withdrawal of reward in response to problem behaviors), or token economy.

Alternative treatment options such as cognitive-behavior therapy, formal social skills training, and dietary modifications may be used in conjunction with pharmacologic and behavior modification therapies, but these options alone are not recommended for the treatment of ADHD.

Referral

Some circumstances may necessitate referral to a specialist such as a psychiatrist, neurologist, or developmental/behavioral pediatrician. Physicians are being asked to make the diagnosis of ADHD in very young patients, but many physicians do not feel comfortable making this diagnosis or starting medications in children who are not yet in kindergarten. Input from a specialist may also be useful for patients with serious or severe comorbid conditions such as psychosis, oppositional defiant disorder, and depression, as well as medical conditions such as autism or seizure disorder. The American Academy of Child and Adolescent Psychiatry recommends referral to a psychologist or neuropsychologist for any patient with a history showing significantly low general cognitive ability or for a patient with low achievement in language or mathematics relative to the patient's intellectual ability, as these conditions may confound the diagnosis (Table 6-2). Referral is also appropriate for patients with poor response to medication, with apparent treatment failure, or who do not obviously meet diagnostic criteria for ADHD but who display inattentive, hyperactive, or impulsive behaviors that interfere with their functionality.

Families of patients with ADHD should be made aware of resources in their community that may be of help, and patient and parent education should be provided.

Long-term Monitoring and Implications

Because growth restriction is a concern with regard to height, both height and weight should be followed regularly in patients on medications for treatment of ADHD. Up to 15% to 19% of patients with ADHD in childhood or adolescence will go on to begin smoking cigarettes or develop other substance abuse disorders. Additionally, data suggests that patients with ADHD have a greater risk of intentional and unintentional injuries, and some (especially female patients with ADHD) may be more likely to attempt suicide. Patients with ADHD are more likely than their peers to have motor vehicle accidents, and academic performance will likely continue to be impaired throughout schooling. Even in patients with childhood-diagnosed ADHD who do not continue to meet diagnostic criteria for ADHD as adolescents, school performance is impaired compared with their peers without ADHD. However, studies show that 60% to 80% of patients diagnosed with ADHD in childhood continue to meet criteria for ADHD through adolescence and into adulthood.

Table 6-2. Common Behavior Rating Scales Used in the Assessment of ADHD and Monitoring of Treatment

Name of Scale	Description (Reference/Source)
Academic Performance Rating Scale	19-item scale for determining a child's academic productivity and accuracy in grades 1–6 (Barkley RA, ed. *Attention-Deficit Hyperactivity Disorder: A Handbook for Diagnosis and Treatment*. New York, NY: Guilford; 1990)
ADHD Rating Scale-IV	18-item scale using *DSM-IV* criteria (DuPaul GJ, PowerTJ, Anastopoulos AD, Reid R, eds. *ADHD Rating Scales-IV: Checklists, Norms, and Clinical Interpretation*. New York, NY: Guilford; 1998)
Brown ADD Rating Scales for Children, Adolescents, and Adults	(Brown TE. *The Brown Attention-Deficit Disorder Scales*. San Antonio, TX: Psychological Corporation; 2001)
Child Behavior Checklist	Parent-completed CBCL and teacher-completed report form
Conners Parent Rating Scale-Revised	Parent and adolescent self-report versions available (Conners CK. *Conners Rating Scales-Revised*. Toronto, Canada: Multi-Health Systems; 1997)
Conners Teacher Rating Scale-Revised	(Conners CK. *Conners Rating Scales-Revised*. Toronto, Canada: Multi-Health Systems; 1997)
Conners-Wells Adolescent Self-report Scale	(Conners CK, Wells K. *Conners-Wells Adolescent Self-report Scale*. Toronto, Canada: Multi-Health Systems; 1997)
Home Situations Questionnaire-Revised, School Situations Questionnaire- Revised	HSQ-R, a 14-item scale designed to assess specific problems with attention and concentration (Barkley RA, ed. *Attention-Deficit Hyperactivity Disorder: A Handbook for Diagnosis and Treatment*. New York, NY: Guilford; 1990)
Inattention/Overactivity With Aggression Conners Teacher Rating Scale	10-item scale developed to separate the inattention and overactivity ratings from oppositional defiance (Loney J, Milich M. Hyperactivity, inattention, and aggression in clinical practice. In: *Advances in Behavioral and Developmental Pediatrics*. Vol 3. Wolraich M, Routh DK, eds. Greenwich, CT: JAI Press; 1982:113–147)
Swanson, Nolan, and Pelham and SKAMP Internet site ADHD.net	SNAP-IV, 26-item scale that contains *DSM-IV* criteria for ADHD and screens for other *DSM* diagnoses (Swanson JM. *School-Based Assessments and Intervention for ADD Students*. Irvine: KC Publishing; 1992) SKAMP, 10-item scale that measures impairment of functioning at home and at school (Wigal SB, Gupta S, Guinta D, Swanson JM. Reliability and validity of the SKAMP rating scale in a laboratory school setting. *Psychopharmacol Bull*. 1998;34[1]:47–53)

Table 6-2 *(cont)*

Name of Scale	Description (Reference/Source)
Vanderbilt ADHD diagnostic parent and teacher scales	Teachers rate 3 symptoms and 8 performance items measuring ADHD symptoms and common comorbid conditions. The parent version contains all 18 ADHD symptoms, with items assessing comorbid conditions and performance. (Wolraich ML, Lambert EW, Baumgaertel A, et al. Teachers' screening for attention-deficit/hyperactivity disorder: comparing multinational samples on teacher ratings of ADHD. *J Abnorm Child Psychol.* 2003;31[4]: 445–455)

Abbreviations: ADD, attention-deficit disorder; ADHD, attention-deficit/hyperactivity disorder; CBCL, Child Behavior Checklist; DSM, *Diagnostic and Statistical Manual of Mental Disorders*; HSQ-R, Home Situations Questionnaire-Revised; SKAMP, Swanson, Kotlin, Agler, M-Flynn, and Pelham; SNAP, Swanson, Nolan, and Pelham.

Adapted from Pliszka S. Practice parameter for the assessment and treatment of children and adolescents with attention-deficit/hyperactivity-disorder. *J Am Acad Child Adolesct Psychiatry.* 2007;46(7):894–921, with permission.

As adults, patients with childhood- or adolescent-diagnosed ADHD are more likely to have antisocial personality disorders or behaviors, and though employment rates are comparable to control groups, patients with ADHD often have lower-status jobs and tend to perform more poorly than their counterparts.

Few studies have been done on the implications of long-term medication use for ADHD. However, studies suggest that long-term medication use continues to reduce the number of teacher-reported ADHD symptoms. Patients on ADHD treatment medications continue to have improved functionality over their medication-free baseline.

Suggested Reading

American Academy of Pediatrics Subcommittee on Attention-Deficit/Hyperactivity Disorder, Steering Committee on Quality Improvement and Management. ADHD: clinical practice guidelines for the diagnosis, evaluation, and treatment of attention-deficit/hyperactivity disorder in children and adolescents. Pediatrics. 2011;128(5):1007–1022

American Psychiatric Association. *Diagnostic and Statistical Manual of Mental Disorders.* 5th ed. Arlington, VA: American Psychiatric Association; 2013

Floet AMW, Scheiner C, Grossman L. Attention-deficit/hyperactivity disorder. *Pediatr Rev.* 2010;31(2):56–68

National Institute for Children's Health Quality; American Academy of Pediatrics. *Caring for Children with ADHD: A Resource Toolkit for Clinicians.* http://www.nichq .org/childrens-health/adhd/resources/adhd-toolkit. Accessed February 2, 2015

Pliszka S. Practice parameter for the assessment and treatment of children and adolescents with attention-deficit/hyperactivity disorder. *J Am Acad Child Adolesc Psychiatry.* 2007;46(7):894–921

Stein MT, Perrin JM. Diagnosis and treatment of ADHD in school-aged children in primary care settings: a synopsis of the AAP practice guidelines. *Pediatr Rev.* 2003;24(3):92–98

CHAPTER 7

Autism Spectrum Disorder

Joseph Stegman, MD

Key Points

- Autism spectrum disorder is not a specific disorder but a pattern of developmental delay, defined by social deficits, communication impairments, and restrictive, repetitive, and stereotyped patterns.

- Autism spectrum disorder is a neurologic disorder associated with seizures.

- Under *DSM-5, autism spectrum disorder* is the only diagnostic term used. The terms *Asperger syndrome* and *pervasive developmental delay* are incorporated under autism spectrum disorder.

Overview

Autism spectrum disorder (ASD) is not a specific disorder but a pattern of developmental delay defined by 3 cardinal features: 1) social deficits, 2) communication impairments, and 3) restrictive, repetitive, and stereotyped patterns. No biological etiology identifies ASD. It is thought to result from a collection of different causes that present with this specific pattern of developmental delay.

Social Deficits

Of the list of social deficits in the *Diagnostic and Statistical Manual of Mental Disorders, Fifth Edition (DSM-5)*, lack of joint attention is the most consistent sign. Joint attention is the ability to spontaneously seek or share interests, enjoyments, and achievements with another person. Eye contact, although very important, is often variable and, as the basis of the parents' perception, may not always be clinically significant. Understanding the development of peer relationships is essential for understanding this disorder; however, prior to the age of 3 years, peer relations are difficult to define. Social reciprocity (the ability to observe that another person has thoughts, feelings, and different perspectives) is difficult to assess in toddlers. A clinician must sort out these subtle features to make accurate diagnoses at an early age.

Communication Delays

Lack of speech is one of the 3 cardinal signs of ASD, yet language delay alone is not sufficient for a diagnosis. There are primary speech disorders that must be considered as alternate explanations for language delay. In the child with ASD, language may be absent or, if present, the child may lack the ability to carry on conversation typical for his or her age. Toddlers with typical development have some speech by 18 months and reciprocal conversation by 24 months. There are odd, repetitive, and scripted forms of language that indicate ASD. Echolalia, or the use of repetitive vocalizations that lack meaning, is often present, but it is not necessary for the diagnosis of ASD.

Restrictive, Repetitive, and Stereotyped Behaviors

Children with ASD may demonstrate odd mannerisms with nonfunctional behaviors such as rocking, spinning, twirling, hand flapping, finger wiggling, and pacing. These behaviors are not limited to children with ASD; children with intellectual disabilities commonly demonstrate these same stereotyped behaviors. As the child gets older, focused areas of interest can become intrusive.

Regression

Approximately 25% of children with ASD will demonstrate typical communication and social development but are unable to retain the skills already acquired. This regression typically occurs between 15 and 24 months of age.

Associations

Intellectual Disability

Cognitive impairment has always been considered prevalent in ASD, although recent studies estimate that the association is below 50%, and in some reports, as low as 26% to 29%. The increased recognition of children with less severe symptoms or use of early intervention may be reasons for more recent reports of a lower prevalence of cognitive impairment.

Sensory Integration Dysfunction

Children with developmental delays and disabilities may overreact or underreact to environmental stimuli such as noise, smells, texture, pain, or touch. Reactions vary widely, however, and are not reliable as a collection of symptoms for the diagnosis of ASD.

Seizures

Autism spectrum disorder is a neurologic disorder associated with seizures. The risk of seizure directly correlates to the severity of neurodevelopmental delay. The most current data suggest that approximately 25% of affected individuals will have an associated seizure disorder over their life span. All types of seizures have been associated with ASD; lack of responsiveness to one's name, non-purposeful eye gaze, and motor stereotypies can be mistaken for seizures. Electroencephalograms are useful when there is a concern for seizure disorder but need not be part of the routine ASD work-up.

Self-injurious Behaviors

Self-injurious behaviors are stereotyped behaviors that occur with frustration caused by unsuccessful communication attempts, transitions, adaptations to new environments, boredom, depression, fatigue, sleep deprivation, or pain. They may include head banging, skin picking, eye poking, and hand biting. These behaviors provoke stress within the family and prevent the child with ASD from participating in community activities. The more severe the ASD and the more significant the intellectual disability, the worse these features tend to be.

Diagnostic and Statistical Manual of Mental Disorders, Fifth Edition

The *Diagnostic and Statistical Manual of Mental Disorders, Fifth Edition* (*DSM-5*) diagnostic criteria for ASD (www.autismspeaks.org/what-autism/diagnosis /dsm-5-diagnostic-criteria), published by the American Psychiatric Association in 2013, now define ASD as the only possible autism diagnosis. Disorders such as Asperger syndrome and pervasive developmental disorder–not otherwise specified are now incorporated into the diagnosis of ASD.

Asperger Syndrome

People formerly diagnosed with Asperger syndrome have the same social deficits and restrictive, repetitive, and stereotyped behaviors but no communication impairments. Restrictive behaviors are expressed as restrictive and intrusive interests. In many respects, this is an artificial selection of a subgroup of people who are considered in *DSM-5* to have ASD.

Pervasive Developmental Disorder–Not Otherwise Specified

Pervasive developmental disorder–not otherwise specified was used to define a population who have many of the symptoms of ASD and in many domains. They are considered in *DSM-5* to have an ASD. These individuals typically change with regard to their primary symptoms over time, with some developing more severe ASD symptoms and others developing without long-term impairments.

Rett Syndrome

Most children with Rett syndrome present with features of ASD, typically including fine motor delays, a hand-wringing stereotyped behavior, and regression. It is associated with severe seizures, microcephaly, and moderate to severe cognitive impairment. Positive DNA test results for the *MECP2* gene abnormality confirm the diagnosis.

Differential Diagnosis

The etiology of ASD is unknown. It is a biologically based, neurodevelopmental disorder that is believed to have a high degree of heritability. Family studies suggest that if one child has ASD, there is a 5% to 6% chance that a subsequent child will also have ASD. Current data suggest that ASD may be genetically based with an unknown environmental epigenetic factor that activates the genetic mechanism.

In 10% of people with ASD, a biological cause or association can be identified. There are biological conditions with ASD symptoms as the primary presentation. Some examples include fragile X syndrome, Down syndrome, Prader-Willi syndrome, Angelman syndrome, tuberous sclerosis complex, and phenylketonuria. A medical work-up should be considered in all children with ASD.

Fragile X Syndrome

Fragile X syndrome is the most common genetic condition that leads to intellectual disabilities. It is associated with macrocephaly, large ears, large testes, and joint hyperextensibility. Fragile X syndrome is familial, and there are medical implications for carriers. It is important that it be diagnosed.

Down Syndrome

Down syndrome, or trisomy 21 syndrome, is the most widely recognizable genetic disorder, and pediatricians expect a specific pattern of development delay. Because a number of children with Down syndrome will develop ASD, pediatricians need to monitor for its varied presentations.

Prader-Willi Syndrome

Prader-Willi syndrome presents with hypotonia and failure to thrive as an infant. It is characterized by overeating, small hands and feet, almond-shaped eyes, and mild cognitive impairments. It is caused by a microdeletion of the 15q chromosome and often associated with ASD features.

Angelman Syndrome

Angelman syndrome is also a microdeletion of the 15q chromosome. The difference between Prader-Willi syndrome and Angelman syndrome is based on uniparental disomy. Angelman syndrome presents with severe global developmental delay, ASD, lack of language, hypotonia, wide-based gait, progressive spasticity, and seizures.

Tuberous Sclerosis Complex

Tuberous sclerosis complex is associated with ASD behaviors, cognitive impairments, and seizures. It has a dominant inherited pattern, but most cases result from spontaneous mutations. The hallmark of the complex is hypopigmentated macules that may require a Wood lamp to be seen.

Phenylketonuria

Phenylketonuria is a readily identifiable cause of ASD. It now rarely develops due to widespread newborn screening and subsequent preventive therapies.

Clinical Features

The cardinal triad of clinical features for ASD are social deficits, impaired communication, and repetitive and restrictive behaviors and interests. The most common symptoms include poor eye contact, inability to form relationships, lack of response to one's name, lack of joint attention, lack of social reciprocity, lack of pretend play and imitation, delayed language development, limited conversation ability, scripting of memorized statements, echolalia, stereotypies and repetitive behaviors, obsessive and intrusive interests, lack of joyful expressions, or lack of recognition of parent's voice.

Surveillance and Screening

The American Academy of Pediatrics (AAP) recommends that all children be screened and monitored for development disorders, including ASD. The AAP has published an algorithm for pediatricians to use (Figure 7-1). The Modified Checklist for Autism in Toddlers (M-CHAT) is the best tool and best predictor of the development of ASD. It is a simple questionnaire completed by parents which is then is scored, with positive answers validated.

Evaluation

After completion of a detailed medical work-up for ASD, an abnormal result (etiology) is typically found 0% to 25% of the time. This wide range does not obviate the need for a thorough evaluation of any child with ASD for a definable cause. If comorbid intellectual disability occurs, there is greater likelihood of having an abnormal work-up.

Because more genetic abnormalities have been identified and associated with ASD, the completion of genetic testing is a reasonable approach. Chromosome analysis, DNA testing for fragile X syndrome, and a microarray analysis for microdeletions and micro-duplications would be typical genetic screenings. Magnetic resonance imaging of the brain should be completed if there is an associated microcephaly, macrocephaly, or any neurologic finding. Electroencephalogram testing is reserved for the child with significant language regression and signs suspicious for seizures.

Hearing screening should be completed on all children who have any language delay. This should be done regardless of a normal newborn hearing screen.

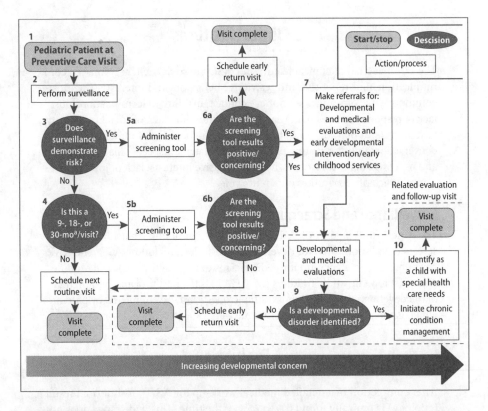

Figure 7-1. Developmental surveillance and screening algorithm within a pediatric preventive care visit.

Does surveillance demonstrate risk?

3 The concerns of both parents and child health professionals should be included in determining whether surveillance suggests the child may be at risk of developmental delay. If either parents or the child health professional express concern about the child's development, a developmental screening to address the concern specifically should be conducted.

Is this a 9-, 18-, or 30-mo[a]/visit?

4 All children should receive developmental screening using a standardized test. In the absence of established risk factors or parental or provider concerns, a general developmental screen is recommended at the 9-, 18-, and 30 month[a] visits. Additionally, autism-specific screening is recommended for all children at the 18-month visit.

Administer screening tool

5a and **5b** *Developmental screening* is the administration of a brief standardized tool aiding the identification of children at risk of a developmental disorder. Developmental screening that targets the area of concern is indicated whenever a problem is identified during developmental surveillance.

Are the screening tool results positive/ concerning?

6a and **6b** When the results of the periodic screening tool are normal, the child health professional can inform the parents and continue with other aspects of the preventive visit. When a screening tool is administered as a result of concerns about development, an early return visit to provide additional developmental surveillance should be scheduled even if the screening tool results do not indicate a risk of delay.

Make referrals for: Developmental and medical evaluations and early developmental intervention/early childhood services

7–8. If screening results are concerning the child should be scheduled for developmental and medical evaluations. *Developmental evaluation* is aimed at identifying the specific developmental disorder or disorders affecting the child. In addition to the developmental evaluation, a *medical diagnostic evaluation* to identify an underlying etiology should be undertaken. *Early developmental intervention/early childhood services* can be particularly valuable when a child is first identified to be at high risk of delayed development, because these programs often provide evaluation services and can offer other services to the child and family even before an evaluation is complete. Establishing an effective and efficient partnership with early childhood professionals is an important component of successful care coordination for children.

Developmental and medical evaluations

Is a developmental disorder identified?

9 If a developmental disorder is identified, the child should be identified as a child with special health care needs and chronic condition management should be initiated (see No. 10 below). If a developmental disorder is not identified through medical and developmental evaluation, the child should be scheduled for an early return visit for further surveillance. More frequent visits, with particular attention paid to areas of concern, will allow the child to be promptly referred for further evaluation if any further evidence of delayed development or a specific disorder emerges.

Identify as a child with special health care needs

Initiate chronic condition management

10 When a child is discovered to have a significant developmental disorder, that child becomes a child with special health care needs, even if that child does not have a specific disease etiology identified. Such a child should be identified by the medical home for appropriate chronic condition management and regular monitoring and entered into the practice's children and youth with special health care needs registry.

Figure 7-1 *(cont)*

[a] Because the 30-month visit is not yet part of the preventive care system and is often not paid by third-party payers at this time, developmental screening can be performed at 24 months of age.

From American Academy of Pediatrics Council on Children With Disabilities, Section on Developmental Behavioral Pediatrics, Bright Futures Steering Committee, Medical Home Initiatives for Children With Special Needs Project Advisory Committee. Identifying infants and young children with developmental disorders in the medical home: an algorithm for developmental surveillance and screening. *Pediatrics*. 2006;118(1):405–420.

Management

Developmental Therapies

Speech Therapy
Speech therapy offers specific approaches to speech production and language development and is essential for children who have not had speech and language develop at the appropriate age. It is the single most important therapy for a child to receive (Box 7-1).

Box 7-1. Autism Spectrum Disorder Management Approaches

Developmental Therapies	Behavior Therapies
■ Speech therapy	■ Applied behavior analysis
■ Occupational therapy	■ Social skill training
Educational Programs	**Psychopharmacotherapy**
■ Preschool programs	■ Stimulants and ADHD medications
■ School-based programs	■ SSRIs
■ Transitional programs to adulthood	■ Neuroleptics or atypical antipsychotics
■ Structured teaching (eg, TEACCH)	■ Alpha$_2$-agonists
	■ Sleep aids

Abbreviations: ADHD, attention-deficit/hyperactivity disorder; SSRI, selective serotonin reuptake inhibitor.

Occupational Therapy
Occupational therapy is controversial, especially when considering treatment for sensory integration dysfunction. Most families benefit from occupational therapy because it is a child-centered and goal-oriented approach to functionality. Occupational therapists provide support for parents learning to cope with their child's disability.

Educational Programs

Preschool Programs
Early intervention ends at the age of 3 years when children are transitioned into the school system for treatment. A diagnosis of ASD does not guarantee services. Exceptional children's services can vary from weekly consultations to more direct daily services. The extent of services depends on how ASD affects learning. Most exceptional children's programs incorporate preschool for its advantage of exposure to peers who do not have developmental delays.

School-Based Programs

The long-term prognosis for a child with ASD is directly tied to the educational level that the child is able to achieve. Children do best when afforded the least restrictive environment possible. School-based programs are similar to preschool programs; options include mainstreaming with resources and self-contained, specialized classrooms for the more severely affected. All children with ASD should have school-based assessment and an Individualized Educational Program.

Transitional Programs to Adulthood

Once a child with ASD reaches high school, a team will perform an assessment to determine appropriate educational expectations and develop a plan to meet those expectations. Adolescents who need group home living and occupational workshops, for example, are given a different educational plan than those capable of higher education.

Structured Teaching

The Treatment and Education of Autistic and Related Communication-Handicapped Children (TEACCH) program, developed by Schopler at the University of North Carolina, is an approach to teaching children with ASD. The environment is highly structured with a predictable sequence of activities, use of visual schedules, and routines.

Behavior Therapies

Applied Behavior Analysis

Applied behavior analysis is the process of applying psychological research-based interventions to change behavior and improve learning experiences. Interventions or positive reinforcements are used to maintain desirable adaptive behaviors.

Social Skill Training

Social skills help children to navigate different social situations. For children with ASD, these skills do not develop naturally and training is necessary. Classes can be held at school, mental health agencies, or private therapy offices. Social skill training may allow children with ASD to live more typical lives.

Psychopharmacotherapy

Medications are prescribed for comorbid conditions that occur with ASD but do not treat the primary condition. The following examples are not meant to be a full exploration of the medical management of ASD but outline medication types most commonly prescribed and their indications.

Stimulants and Attention-Deficit/Hyperactivity Disorder Medications

When children with ASD are hyperactive, impulsive, and inattentive, stimulants can be used. The criteria used to diagnosis attention-deficit/hyperactivity disorder (ADHD) should be applied before prescribing ADHD medication in children with ASD. Dosing, expected benefits, and side effects would not vary in a child with ASD and a child with ADHD.

Selective Serotonin Reuptake Inhibitors

Individuals with ASD struggle with adaptability and anxiety. Therefore, selective serotonin reuptake inhibitors are commonly prescribed. Because individuals with ASD have different targeted symptoms, research and development of standardized protocols is difficult.

Neuroleptics or Atypical Antipsychotics

Risperidone and aripiprazole are US Food and Drug Administration approved to treat repetitive self-stimulatory behaviors, aggression, and mood dysregulation in children with ASD. These are very potent medications with long-term risks, including the development of obesity, diabetes, and tardive dyskinesia.

Alpha$_2$-Agonists

Children with ASD are often hyperactive and over-aroused. Alpha$_2$-agonists, including guanfacine and clonidine, work well for overarousal. They are used to control blood pressure in adults, but there has been minimal effects on blood pressure in children treated with alpha$_2$-agonists. The most common side effect in children is drowsiness.

Sleep Aids

Besides guanfacine and clonidine, melatonin in over-the-counter preparations can be used to improve the initiation of sleep. It is considered safe and effective, is administered 2 hours prior to going to bed, and works best with dim ambient lighting.

Long-term Monitoring or Implications

For many individuals with ASD, there will be lifelong impairments often requiring lifelong assistance. It is difficult to predict the course of ASD in early childhood, but some predictors include cognitive ability, severity of symptoms, presence of joint attention, and play skills. Lack of language by the age of 5 years predicts more severe lifelong impairments. For those individuals who have associated biological disorders, their prognosis will more closely align with the biological disorder than ASD. Early intervention has been correlated with improved long-term prognosis. The percentage of children diagnosed with ASD between 2 and 5 years of age who may develop with minimal long-term disabilities has been estimated to be 30%.

Suggested Reading
· · · · · · · · · · · · · · · · · ·

Autism and Developmental Disabilities Monitoring Network Surveillance Year 2000 Principal Investigators; Centers for Disease Control and Prevention. Prevalence of autism spectrum disorders—Autism and Developmental Disabilities Monitoring Network, six sites, United States, 2000. *MMWR Surveill Summ.* 2007;56(1):1–11

Autism and Developmental Disabilities Monitoring Network Surveillance Year 2002 Principal Investigators; Centers for Disease Control and Prevention. Prevalence of autism spectrum disorders—Autism and Developmental Disabilities Monitoring Network, 14 sites, United States, 2002. *MMWR Surveill Summ.* 2007;56(1):12–28

Coplan J, Jawad AF. Modeling clinical outcome of children with autistic spectrum disorders. *Pediatrics.* 2005;116(1):117–122

Johnson CP, Myers SM; American Academy of Pediatrics Council on Children With Disabilities. Identification and evaluation of children with autism spectrum disorders. *Pediatrics.* 2007;120(5):1183–1215

Myers SM, Johnson CP; American Academy of Pediatrics Council on Children With Disabilities. Management of children with autism spectrum disorders. *Pediatrics.* 2007;120(5):1162–1182

Schaefer GB, Lutz RE. Diagnostic yield in the clinical genetic evaluation of autism spectrum disorders. *Genet Med.* 2006;8(9):549–556

Wetherby AM, Watt N, Morgan L, Shumway S. Social communication profiles of children with autism spectrum disorders late in the second year of life. *J Autism Dev Disord.* 2007;37(5):960–975

Wetherby AM, Woods J, Allen L, Cleary J, Dickinson H, Lord C. Early indicators of autism spectrum disorders in the second year of life. *J Autism Dev Disord.* 2004;34(5):473–493

CHAPTER 8

Back Pain

Brian K. Brighton, MD, MPH

Key Points

- Nonspecific lower back pain in children and adolescents is more common than previously thought and can initially be managed conservatively.

- The history and physical examination are essential for identifying "red flags" such as pain at rest or night, fever, recent history of trauma, neurologic symptoms (such as bladder dysfunction or leg pain), and progressive neurologic deficits on examination.

- Initial imaging with plain radiographs may help aid in the diagnosis, but magnetic resonance imaging and single-photon emission computed tomography bone scan can help identify specific problems.

Overview

The concern of back pain in children and adolescents is very common and can be caused by a number of conditions. Pediatric back pain in many cases, contrary to previous teachings, does not have a definitive diagnosis and is often described as nonspecific back pain or mechanical back pain. There are, however, instances in which an obvious structural or radiographic abnormality can be ascribed to an "organic" cause of the back pain. Therefore, pediatric patients with concerns of back pain require a systematic approach to the evaluation and treatment of back pain, by identifying pertinent elements of the history and physical examination that can lead to the appropriate diagnostic imaging without missing specific diagnoses.

Causes

The cause of back pain in children has been broadly classified as organic versus mechanical back pain. Within each of these categories are associated risk factors, and elements of the history and physical examination can help guide appropriate use of diagnostic tests and imaging. Table 8-1 provides a list of etiologies of back pain in children and adolescents.

Table 8-1. Etiology of Back Pain in Children and Adolescents

Common Etiologies	Other Etiologies
• Mechanical lower back pain • Muscle strain • Spinal deformity (eg, Scheuermann kyphosis, scoliosis) • Spondylolysis and spondylolisthesis • Intervertebral disc herniation	• Infectious (eg, discitis, osteomyelitis, tuberculosis) • Benign neoplasms (eg, osteoid osteoma, eosinophilic granuloma, osteoblastoma, aneurysmal bone cyst) • Malignant neoplasm (eg, leukemia, spinal cord tumor, osteosarcoma, metastatic disease) • Traumatic (eg, compression fractures, vertebral fractures) • Inflammatory (eg, juvenile rheumatoid arthritis, juvenile idiopathic arthritis, ankylosing spondylitis) • Psychogenic causes

Evaluation

In the clinical evaluation of patients who present with concerns of lower back pain, elements of the history and physical examination can lead to the appropriate diagnosis and treatment plan (Figure 8-1). In the history, concerns of neurologic deficits such as weakness, significant leg pain, and bowel or bladder concerns (such as urinary or stool incontinence) are red flags that require further investigation. Additionally, the location, frequency, and characteristics of the pain, as well as onset, duration (eg, acute traumatic events, less or greater than 6 weeks), and relieving and aggravating factors are important in distinguishing the cause of back pain. Fever, malaise, weight loss, and night pain may be associated with more concerning causes of back pain, such as tumor or infection.

Examinations

The physical examination should include a focused musculoskeletal examination of the spine as well as a neurologic examination. Patients should be examined in a gown to allow full visualization of the spine to evaluate for any deformity in the coronal plane, such as scoliosis, as well as sagittal deformities, such as kyphosis. Inspection of the skin allows for assessment of any associated cutaneous abnormalities, such as midline defects or hairy patches, which can be seen in myelomeningocele, or café au lait spots, which can be seen in neuro-fibromatosis. Palpation along the course of the spinous process of the posterior spine as well as the paraspinal musculature allows for appreciation of an associated tenderness or muscle spasm. Forward bending allows for assessment of any potential scoliosis but also allows for assessment of range of motion.

In addition to the musculoskeletal examination, a neurologic examination should be performed that includes the evaluation of motor and sensory function of the upper and lower extremities, the presence of ankle clonus or a Babinski sign, symmetry, and presence of abdominal reflexes as well and knee and ankle jerk reflexes. Additonally, the assessment of a straight-leg raise (positive with disc herniation), hamstring tightness assessed by popliteal angles (associated with

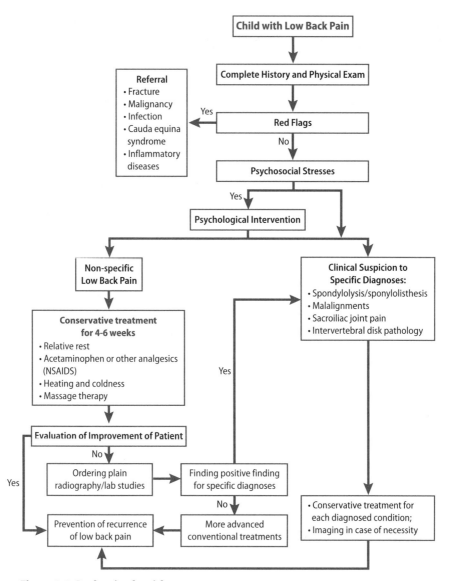

Figure 8-1. Back pain algorithm.

Abbreviations: exam, examination; lab, laboratory; NSAID, nonsteroidal anti-inflammatory drug.

From Kordi R, Rostami M. Low back pain in children and adolescents: an algorithmic clinical approach. *Iran J Pediatr.* 2011;21(3):259–270, with permission.

spondylolysis or spondylolisthesis), and a FABER (for flexion, abduction, and external rotation) test (sacroiliac joint pathology) should be performed.

Imaging

Imaging modalities such as plain radiographs, magnetic resonance imaging (MRI), and single-photon emission computed tomography (SPECT) bone scan are the most common studies used to evaluate back pain in children. There are no evidence-based practice guidelines regarding imaging of back pain in children; however, several authors have proposed imaging algorithms. Plain radiographs including anteroposterior and lateral views of the spine are indicated to diagnose bony conditions that may be seen in acute high-energy trauma or spinal deformity. While oblique views are commonly performed, their value has recently been studied and questioned in the pediatric population (Evidence Level II-2). Several authors have suggested an approach to advanced imaging in the setting of normal plain radiographs. Advanced imaging with MRI or SPECT bone scan should be considered for children with greater than 6 weeks of symptoms or neurologic deficits, night pain, or constitutional symptoms. The proper imaging study is selected for the probable diagnosis (ie, MRI for suspected disc herniation, SPECT bone scan for infection or tumor in cases when a spondylolysis is suspected).

Laboratory Tests

When infection or neoplasm is suspected, laboratory tests for a complete blood count with differential, erythrocyte sedimentation rate, and C-reactive protein concentration can be used to screen for such etiologies. Rheumatologic laboratory tests for antinuclear antibodies, rheumatoid factor, and HLA-B 27 may be indicated when the specific inflammatory diagnosis is suspected.

Management

Mechanical Lower Back Pain

Lower back pain or mechanical back pain caused by a muscle strain may present as new onset pain after an acute injury or strenuous activity. It may also be seen in the setting of more chronic pain associated with mild scoliosis or decon-ditioning related to obesity or sedentary activity. Physical examination may demonstrate paraspinal tenderness or limited painful motion with forward bending during a normal neurologic examination. Radiographs are reserved for patients who have persistent symptoms greater than 6 weeks' time. Treatment is usually a brief period of rest in combination with analgesics such as acetamino-phen or anti-inflammatory medications. In chronic situations, physical therapy with emphasis on core muscle strengthening and stretching and trunk stabiliza-tion along with other modalities such as heat and ice may improve the symptoms.

Spondylolysis and Spondylolisthesis

Spondylolysis is a fracture of the pars interarticularis in the posterior portion of the vertebral lamina. Spondylolisthesis is a fracture or developmental defect in the pars with varying degrees of forward slippage of the vertebral body typically occurring at the L5-S. Patients with spondylolisthesis may present with acute onset of lower back pain with radiation into the pelvis or buttocks. They may also present with a history of chronic lower back pain worsened by injury. A pertinent portion of the history is the patient's involvement with activities that result in repetitive hyperextension of the lumbar spine, such as gymnastics, weight lifting, or football. Examination may reveal paraspinal tenderness or spasm with limited and painful lumbar range of motion. Pain may be elicited and exaggerated with hyperextension of the spine. Often there are associated findings of hamstring tightness. Radiographs may reveal a defect at the level of the pars with no slippage in the setting of spondylolysis. SPECT bone scan and MRI can be used to make the diagnosis of spondylolysis (Figures 8-2 and 8-3). Treatment modalities include rest, anti-inflammatory medications, activity restrictions, physical therapy with emphasis on core strengthening, lumbosacral stretching, hamstring stretching, and avoiding hyperextension exercises. Additionally, a soft corset lumbosacral orthosis may be prescribed.

Infection

Children presenting with back pain, physical examination findings of back stiffness, and loss of lumbar lordosis may have discitis or osteomyelitis. Discitis and osteomyelitis can arise from hematogenous spread of bacteria across the vertebral end plates or into the vertebral bodies. This usually presents in children younger than 10 years. Laboratory values and MRI are diagnostic of the problems. Treatment consisting of antibiotics and surgical intervention is rarely required.

Tumors

While benign and malignant tumors of the spine are rare compared to other causes of back pain, some elements of the history and physical examinations can help lead to the diagnosis. Concerns of chronic pain, especially associated with pain at night; anorexia and weight loss; and occasional findings of atypical spinal deformity may raise level of suspicion for a tumor. Osteoid osteoma is a benign tumor of the spine and may present with localized back pain, which is worse at night and characteristically relieved by nonsteroidal anti-inflammatory drugs. Localized back pain with radiographs demonstrating vertebral plana are characteristic for eosinophilic granuloma. Bone pain as well as back pain is a frequent phenomena in children with leukemia. Lytic lesions or osteopenia may be seen on radiographs. Laboratory values on an index of suspicion may aid in diagnosis of leukemia.

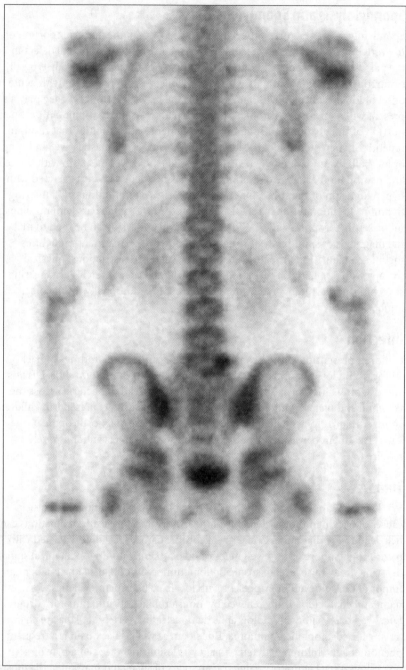

Figure 8-2. Positive single-photon emission computed tomography bone scan of 11-year-old male with back pain and right-sided L5 spondylolysis.

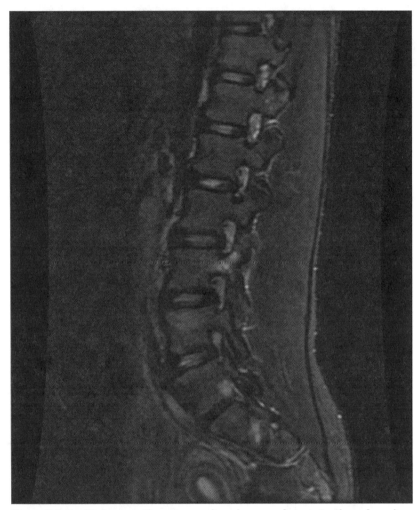

Figure 8-3. Sagittal magnetic resonance imaging scan demonstrating edema in the pars interarticularis consistent with spondylolysis in a 15-year-old gymnast with back pain.

Suggested Reading

Auerbach JD, Ahn J, Zgonis MH, Reddy SC, Ecker ML, Flynn JM. Streamlining the evaluation of low back pain in children. *Clin Orthop Relat Res.* 2008;466(8):1971–1977

Beck NA, Miller R, Baldwin K, et al. Do oblique views add value in the diagnosis of spondylolysis in adolescents? *J Bone Joint Surg Am.* 2013;95(10):e65, e61–67

Bhatia NN, Chow G, Timon SJ, Watts HG. Diagnostic modalities for the evaluation of pediatric back pain: a prospective study. *J Pediatr Orthop.* 2008;28(2):230–233

Fernandez M, Carrol CL, Baker CJ. Discitis and vertebral osteomyelitis in children: an 18-year review. *Pediatrics.* 2000;105(6):1299–1304

Klein G, Mehlman CT, McCarty M. Nonoperative treatment of spondylolysis and grade I spondylolisthesis in children and young adults: a meta-analysis of observational studies. *J Pediatr Orthop.* 2009;29(2):146–156

Kordi R, Rostami M. Low back pain in children and adolescents: an algorithmic clinical approach. *Iran J Pediatr.* 2011;21(3):259–270

Rogalsky RJ, Black GB, Reed MH. Orthopaedic manifestations of leukemia in children. *J Bone Joint Surg Am.* 1986;68(4):494–501

CHAPTER 9

Breastfeeding

Jennifer Crotty, MD

KEY POINTS

- Human milk is the criterion standard for infant feeding.
- Breastfeeding has numerous health benefits for mother and child.
- Pediatricians should educate and inform women about the benefits of breastfeeding.
- Treatment of complications associated with breastfeeding should be aimed at treating mother and child as a dyad.

Overview

Human milk is the criterion standard for nutrition for infants in the first year of life. Breastfeeding is the best way for a woman to feed her infant; however, it is not always perceived as being the easiest route. In view of all the benefits to the infant, mother, and society, the pediatrician has the important role of supporting breastfeeding to help these dyads attain long-term success.

Definitions

Terminology for types of breastfeeding is important to know when counseling on the benefits of each type. *Exclusive* breastfeeding refers to an infant for whom human milk is the only nutritional source with no other nutritional supplements or liquids. *Almost exclusive* refers to an infant who receives no milk other than human milk, with minimal amounts of other substances provided infrequently; this might refer to a 1-month-old who gets an ounce of water intermittently for constipation. *Partial* breastfeeding is a continuum, with *high partial* breastfeeding being greater than or equal to 80% of all feedings being human milk, *medium partial* being 20% to 80% of nutritional intake being human milk, *low partial* being less than 20% of nutritional intake being human milk, and *token partial* meaning breastfeeding is only for comfort, with no nutritionally significant intake from human milk.

Human milk is the perfect nutritional source because it changes as the infant grows. For several days after birth, the breast produces colostrum, a high protein, low carbohydrate fluid, with high concentrations of antibodies and live cells and a lower fat content than mature milk. By the time a newborn is 2 weeks of age, mature milk is produced in the mother, and the main protein is casein. Per liter, human milk has more calories, fat, and cholesterol but less protein, calcium, phosphorus, and vitamin D than commercially prepared formulas.

Recommendations

The American Academy of Pediatrics (AAP) 2012 policy "Breastfeeding and the Use of Human Milk" reaffirmed recommendations for exclusive breastfeeding for the first 6 months of life and breastfeeding for at least one year or longer if mother and child desire. Very few contraindications to breastfeeding exist (Box 9-1). In general, breastfeeding is not recommended when mothers are receiving chemotherapy, amphetamines, ergotamines, and statins. Maternal street drug use is a contraindication to breastfeeding; however, narcotic-dependent mothers enrolled in a supervised methadone maintenance program should be encouraged to breastfeed, as evidence shows their infants have fewer sequelae of neonatal abstinence syndrome than infants in similar situations who are formula fed (Evidence Level II-2).

Box 9-1. Contraindications to Breastfeeding

Infant Conditions

- Classic galactosemia (galactose 1-phosphate uridyltransferase deficiency)
- Maple syrup urine disease
- Phenylketonuria (Partial breastfeeding is possible with careful monitoring.)

Maternal Conditions

- Human immunodeficiency virus 1 infection (if replacement feeding is acceptable, feasible, affordable, sustainable, and safe)
- Human T-cell lymphotropic virus 1 and 2 infections (Varies by country; in Japan, breastfeeding is initiated.)
- Tuberculosis (active, untreated pulmonary tuberculosis, until effective maternal treatment for the initial 2 weeks or the infant is receiving isoniazid)
- Herpes simplex virus infection on a breast (until lesions on the breast are cleared)
- Medications (those of concern)
  - Most medications are considered safe because little gets into the milk.
  - A few select compound drugs of abuse and some radioactive compounds that have long half-lives require cessation of lactation.

From Lawrence R, Lawrence R. Breastfeeding: more than just good nutrition. *Pediatr Rev.* 2011;132(7):267–280.

Benefits

The benefits of breastfeeding have been studied extensively in recent literature. For a child who was ever breastfed, there is a reduced risk of acute otitis media, gastrointestinal tract infections, asthma, type 2 diabetes mellitus (DM), childhood leukemia, and sudden infant death syndrome (Evidence Level I). In addition, infants who were exclusively breastfed for greater than 4 months have reduced risk of hospitalization due to lower respiratory tract infections. Infants exclusively breastfed for at least 3 months have a decreased risk for developing atopic dermatitis. There are also many well-documented benefits for the mother such as reduced risk of developing breast or ovarian cancer and reduced risk of developing type 2 DM if the mother did not have gestational DM (Evidence Level II-2). The psychosocial benefits of maternal-infant bonding are present but are more difficult to quantify. In addition, the benefits to premature infants are indisputable and include decreasing the risk of common complications of infants born prematurely, such as respiratory syncytial virus, bronchiolitis, and necrotizing enterocolitis (Evidence Level I).

The Role of the Pediatrician

Ideally, the decision to breastfeed should be discussed at the prenatal pediatrician visit. Medical professionals should educate on the benefits of breastfeeding, and common problems should also be explained. Evidence shows that mothers who are vacillating about a feeding decision for their infants will often choose to breastfeed if encouraged by a medical professional (Evidence Level III). The role of the physician in encouraging breastfeeding is especially important in patient populations less likely to initiate breastfeeding, such as women who are unmarried, young, have lower income, or have lower education level. All discussions about breastfeeding should focus on the positives of the choice and on ways to make it work for various lifestyles. Mothers who report receiving encouragement from their physicians are more likely to continue breastfeeding.

In the hospital, all attempts to maximize an infant's access to breastfeeding should be encouraged. If a lactation consultant is available, all breastfeeding mothers should have access to this service. The pediatrician needs to reinforce the importance of early, frequent, untimed feeds and of good maternal nutrition and hydration. Mothers should be encouraged to stay inpatient until the newborn is at least 48 hours of age and longer if there are any difficulties. As vitamin D concentrations are low and not readily available in human milk, infants should be started on 400 U vitamin D daily, starting from birth. Supplementation with formula is discouraged unless the infant has greater than 10% weight loss, hypoglycemia, or significant hyperbilirubinemia or if mother is medically unable to breastfeed.

At the first post-hospital office visit, the pediatrician should ask the mother about specifics on breastfeeding, including any hindrances that may occur (Box 9-2). Ideally, infants should be feeding 8 to 12 times in 24 hours and having 3 to 4 voids and 3 to 4 bowel movements by the fourth day of life. The LATCH score can be used as a systematic method for gathering information about an individual breastfeeding session (Box 9-3). The system assigns a numerical score of 0, 1, or 2 to each letter of the acronym LATCH with a maximum score of 10. *L* is for how well the infant latches onto the breast. *A* is for the amount of audible swallowing noted. *T* is for the mother's nipple type. *C* is for the mother's level of comfort. *H* is for the amount of help the mother needs to hold her infant to the breast. Consistent good LATCH scores do have some predictive ability for prolonged successful breastfeeding, but individual subjective questions about mother's perception should also be asked (Evidence Level II-2).

All infants should be plotted on the World Health Organization Growth charts, as they establish breastfed infants as the biological norm. Infants should be followed closely until mother is comfortable with breastfeeding and birth weight is regained at which time infants should be scheduled for regular well-child checks, with reaffirmation of breastfeeding at each visit.

Supporting Return to Work

For working mothers, return to work often occurs at 6 to 8 weeks postpartum, and recommending pumping as soon as breastfeeding is established will help build up supply. Electric pumps are widely available commercially and often for rent through hospitals or health departments. When mothers are separated from their infants, they should pump both breasts at least every 4 to 6 hours, each time allowing for however long it takes to have 2 full let-downs of milk, easily recognized by the mother as a sudden increase in milk flow velocity and volume. The federal Fair Labor Standards Act requires employers to provide reasonable break time for an employee to express human milk for her nursing child for one year after the child's birth, although the employer is not required to compensate her for any work time spent for such purpose. Having a caregiver other than the mother introduce a bottle at least 2 weeks before mother's return to work can greatly improve infant's success at feeding with a synthetic nipple.

Box 9-2. Breastfeeding Questions

- How do you feel breastfeeding is going, and what concerns to you have about it?
- How many wet and soiled diapers is your baby making in 24 hours?
- Do you feel like your breasts are full before, and lighter after, a feed?
- Does it hurt to nurse?
- Do you see milk in the baby's mouth when he is drinking?
- Do you hear your baby swallowing?
- Does your other breast leak when your baby is feeding?
- Do you feel a tingling feeling 2 times during nursing (known as let-down)?
- Does your baby fall asleep after a feed and stay asleep for several hours until the next feed?
- How long and how frequently does your baby feed on each breast?

Box 9-3. LATCH Scoring System

	0	1	2
LATCH	Sleepy or reluctant No latch or suck	Repeated attempts Must hold nipple in mouth Must stimulate to suck	Grasps breast Tongue down Lips flanged Rhythmic suckling
AUDIBLE SWALLOW	None	A few with stimulation	Spontaneous, intermittent (if less than 24 hours old) or Spontaneous, frequent (if greater than 24 hours old)
TYPE OF NIPPLE	Inverted	Flat	Everted (after stimulation)
COMFORT (of breast/nipple)	Engorged breast Cracked, bleeding, large blisters or bruises Severe discomfort	Filling breast Small blisters or bruises Mild to moderate discomfort	Soft Non-tender Intact nipples (no damage)
HOLD (positioning)	Full assist (Staff holds infant at breast.)	Minimal assist Staff teaches one side, mother does other or takes over feed.	No assist from staff Mother able to independently position/hold infant.

Common Problems

Several common problems for maternal-infant breastfeeding dyads are possible, and the pediatrician should be skilled in diagnosing and treating many of them. Care must be given to anticipatory guidance so that mothers understand that the goal of therapy is to relieve the acute issue and persist in breastfeeding.

Jaundice

Jaundice is present in 60% of all infants but may be more common in breastfed infants. In the first 2 to 3 days of life, physiologic jaundice occurs; over the next week, as a mother's milk production increases and the infant's liver clears bilirubin, this jaundice resolves. Breast milk jaundice usually presents at 1 to 2 weeks of age, and pediatricians should not counsel mothers to interrupt breastfeeding as a diagnostic procedure because of its low specificity and the risk to disregarding the detection of a potentially dangerous disease. If an infant is clinically jaundiced, checking an initial total and direct bilirubin to rule out liver disease is recommended; checking other liver functions or obtaining a complete blood count are not routinely necessary in every patient, as they rarely change the patient's course. If the infant is gaining weight well and the clinical picture is consistent with breast milk jaundice, the pediatrician should only recheck total bilirubin until the value decreases or plateaus. It may take up to 3 months for the clinical jaundice to resolve, and parents should be educated that jaundice has no long-term consequences.

Inadequate Weight Gain

Excessive weight loss, defined as greater than 10% of birth weight, is relatively common in the first week of life in the breastfed infant. Several causes are possible, many of which are related to proper technique, maternal medications, and maternal nutrition. The pediatrician should witness a feeding ensuring proper latch and positioning with the infant's lips flanged out and all of the mother's nipple and part of her areola in the infant's mouth. Depending on parental comfort, severity of weight loss, and outpatient resources, admission may be necessary; however, if weight loss is around 10%, outpatient therapy and counseling is often adequate. Mothers should put infants to breast at least every 2 hours and supplement with pumped human milk or formula after feeds, with a weight recheck daily. Volume of supplementation varies, but a general rule is 5 to 15 mL after each feed at 24 to 48 hours of age, 15 to 30 mL after each feed at 48 to 72 hours of age, and 30 to 60 mL after each feed at older than 72 hours. As there is contradicting evidence on nipple confusion when using synthetic nipples, various methods of supplementation such as the Supplemental Nursing System, cup feeding, or syringe feeding should be attempted before synthetic nipples are given.

Mothers need good hydration and nutrition; a practical way to explain this is that mothers should consume 8 ounces of non-caffeinated, nonalcoholic fluid every time the infant goes to breast and eat an extra small meal of approximately 500 kcal a day.

Maternal Breast Pain

Breast pain is a common concern in the breastfeeding mother, and the pediatric clinician should have a plan for diagnosis and management. First-line evaluation for any pain in a lactating woman is history and ensuring adequate latch. Treatments for cracked nipples include keeping nipples dry and clean, breast shells plus lanolin ointment or cream, hydrogel dressings, and peppermint water (Evidence Level II-2). If candidiasis is diagnosed, both infant and mother should be treated simultaneously; for infant, first-line treatment is nystatin suspension. For mother, topical miconazole or clotrimazole is recommended; if concomitant nipple fissures are present, treatment with topical antibiotic is also recommended because of high coinfection with *Staphylococcus aureus.* Refractory candidiasis can be treated with oral fluconazole for mother and infant. Mother should continue to breastfeed throughout the course to prevent milk stasis and ductal candidiasis; the latter is suspected when recurrent nipple candidiasis or persistent breast pain after adequate treatment of nipple candidiasis is present. A dearth of clinical trials assesses efficacy and safety of treatment for ductal candidiasis. If level of suspicion for infection is high, treatment should be with fluconazole for 14 to 21 days. Mothers are recommended to continue treatment for at least 1 week after symptom resolution and should be informed of possible adverse effects of fluconazole. If the pediatrician is unsure or uncomfortable treating the mother, consultation with a breastfeeding-friendly and knowledgeable physician who cares for adults is necessary.

Plugged ducts and engorgement both can occur when the human milk is not emptying fully or frequently enough. Both occur often as infants feed less frequently. Milk often will not flow easily, but warm compresses and frequent pumping will resolve it.

Mastitis refers to a painful, acute inflammation of the breast tissue associated with fever and influenza-like symptoms. Frequently caused by *S aureus,* mastitis can occur after engorgement or nipple cracking and, unlike a plugged duct or engorgement, symptoms do not improve after 24 hours of effective breast emptying. Continued breastfeeding using both breasts is safe and encouraged during mastitis except in mothers with human immunodeficiency infections. Emptying the breast at least every 6 hours may shorten duration of mastitis and improve rates of expected lactation. If the infant refuses to drink on the infected breast, mother should pump and store or discard the milk to maintain her supply and relieve pain.

Suggested Reading

Academy of Breastfeeding. Educational objectives and skills for the physician with respect to breastfeeding. *Breastfeed Med.* 2011;6(2):99–105

Academy of Breastfeeding Medicine Protocol Committee. ABM clinical protocol #3: hospital guidelines for the use of supplementary feedings in the healthy term breastfed neonate. *Breastfeed Med.* 2009;4(3):175–182

Academy of Breastfeeding Medicine Protocol Committee. ABM clinical protocol #8: human milk storage information for home use for full-term infants (original protocol March 2004; revision #1 March 2010). *Breastfeed Med.* 2010;5(3):127–130

Academy of Breastfeeding Medicine Protocol Committee. ABM clinical protocol #9: use of galactogogues in initiating or augmenting the rate of maternal milk secretion (first revision January 2011). *Breastfeed Med.* 2009;6(1):41–49

American Academy of Pediatrics Section on Breastfeeding. Breastfeeding and the use of human milk. *Pediatrics.* 2012;129(3):e827–e841

Lauer B, Spector N. Hyperbilirubinemia in the newborn. *Pediatr Rev.* 2011;32(8):341–349

Lawrence R, Lawrence R. Breastfeeding: more than just good nutrition. *Pediatr Rev.* 2011;132(7):267–280

Wiener S. Diagnosis and management of Candida of the nipple and breast. *J Midwifery Womens Health.* 2006;51(2):125–128

CHAPTER 10

Bronchiolitis

April Wazeka, MD

Key Points

- Acute bronchiolitis is the most common cause of lower respiratory tract infection in the first year of life.
- It is generally a self-limiting condition and is most commonly associated with respiratory syncytial virus.
- Routine laboratory and radiographic studies are not indicated.
- Supportive care remains the mainstay of treatment, including fluid replacement, oxygen therapy, and respiratory support, if indicated.

Overview

Bronchiolitis is a clinical condition characterized by a wheezing illness associated with a viral lower respiratory tract infection (LRTI). It is characterized by a virally induced bronchiolar inflammation, usually affecting children younger than 2 years, with a peak in infants aged 3 to 6 months. Acute bronchiolitis is the most common cause of LRTI in the first year of life and accounts for the majority of hospitalizations in the United States for this age period. It is generally a self-limiting condition and most commonly associated with respiratory syncytial virus (RSV), with late fall and wintertime epidemics occurring in temperate climates.

Respiratory syncytial virus is the most common cause of bronchiolitis, the virus most often detected as the sole pathogen. It is common to be infected more than once, even in the same RSV season, but subsequent infections are usually milder. However, other respiratory viruses have been implicated in causing bronchiolitis (Box 10-1).

Box 10-1. Respiratory Virus Causes of Bronchiolitis

▪ Respiratory syncytial virus	▪ Coronavirus
▪ Rhinovirus	▪ Influenza virus
▪ Adenovirus	▪ Human metapneumovirus
▪ Parainfluenza virus	▪ Human bocavirus

Differential Diagnoses

The differential diagnosis of bronchiolitis is broad (Box 10-2), and includes other viral and bacterial infectious causes, as well as underlying chronic pulmonary and cardiac conditions and anatomic or structural causes. It is important to keep these in mind, particularly if the clinical course of the child's disease does not seem to be following the normal pattern.

Clinical Features

Because bronchiolitis primarily affects young infants, clinical manifestations are initially subtle. Infants may become increasingly fussy and have difficulty feeding during the 2- to 5-day incubation period. A low-grade fever, usually temperature below 101.5°F, and increasing coryza and congestion usually follow the incubation period. In older children and adults, as well as in up to 60% of infants, RSV infection is generally confined to the upper airway and does not progress further.

Over a period of 2 to 5 days, RSV infection progresses from the upper to the lower respiratory tract, and this progression leads to the development of cough, dyspnea, wheezing, and feeding difficulties. When the patient is brought to medical attention, the fever has usually resolved. Newborns younger than 1 month may present as hypothermic. Severe cases progress to respiratory distress with tachypnea, nasal flaring, retractions, irritability, and possibly apnea and cyanosis (Box 10-3). Hypoxia is a predictor of severe illness and correlates best with the degree of tachypnea (>50 breaths/min). First-time infections are usually most severe; subsequent attacks are generally milder, particularly in older children. Apnea occurs early in the course of the disease and may be the presenting symptom.

Evaluation

The diagnosis is made primarily on presenting signs and symptoms, patient age, and seasonal occurrence. Common findings are tachypnea, the presence of profuse coryza, and fine crackles, wheezes, or both on auscultation of the lungs. Laboratory and radiologic studies should not be ordered routinely to make the diagnosis (Evidence Level II-1). Radiographs may be helpful when a hospitalized patient is not improving at the expected rate or if another diagnosis is expected. Laboratory testing of nasopharyngeal aspirates for RSV and other viruses rarely alters management decisions but may be helpful in hospitalized patients for cohorts and surveillance.

Box 10-2. Differential Diagnoses of Bronchiolitis

PULMONARY

Infectious

- Bacterial pneumonia
- *Chlamydophila pneumoniae*
- *Mycoplasma pneumoniae*
- Pertussis
- Croup

Noninfectious

- Aspiration pneumonia
- Aspiration syndromes
- Asthma
- Cystic fibrosis
- Foreign body ingestion
- Pneumothorax
- Chronic obstructive pulmonary disease

ANATOMIC/STRUCTURAL

- Bronchomalacia
- Congenital lobar emphysema
- Congenital structural airway anomalies
- Constrictive bronchiolitis
- Vascular ring

CARDIAC

- Congenital heart disease

GASTROINTESTINAL

- Gastroesophageal reflux disease

Box 10-3. Risk Factors for Respiratory Syncytial Virus

RISK FACTORS FOR SEVERE RESPIRATORY SYNCYTIAL VIRUS

- Prematurity (gestational age <37 weeks)
- Low birth weight
- Younger than 6 to 12 weeks
- Chronic pulmonary disease (bronchopulmonary dysplasia, cystic fibrosis, congenital anomaly)
- Hemodynamically significant congenital heart disease (eg, moderate to severe pulmonary hypertension, cyanotic heart disease, congenital heart disease that requires medication to control heart failure)
- Immunodeficiency
- Neurologic disease
- Congenital or anatomic defects of the airways

ENVIRONMENTAL AND OTHER RISK FACTORS

- Having older siblings
- Concurrent birth siblings
- Native American heritage
- Passive smoke
- Household crowding
- Child care attendance
- High altitude

Management

Because no definitive treatment for the specific virus exists, therapy is directed toward supportive care, symptomatic relief, and maintenance of hydration and oxygenation. Medical therapies used to treat bronchiolitis in infants and young children are controversial. Although numerous medications and interventions have been used to treat bronchiolitis, at present, only oxygen appreciably improves the condition of young children with bronchiolitis (Table 10-1). Bronchodilator therapy to relax bronchial smooth muscle, though common, is not supported as routine practice by convincing evidence (Evidence Level I). Beta agonists and ipratropium bromide, an aerosolized anticholinergic agent, have not shown effectiveness in the management of infants with bronchiolitis. If bronchodilator therapy is started, it may be continued in patients who demonstrate clinical improvement.

Despite the prominent role that inflammation plays in the pathogenesis of airway obstruction, inhaled and systemic corticosteroids have not proved beneficial in improving the clinical status of patients with bronchiolitis (Evidence Level I). Recently, nebulized epinephrine in combination with oral dexamethasone has been shown to potentially decrease the need for hospitalization. However, there is still insufficient evidence on such therapy at this time; additional studies are needed.

Infants who are hospitalized with bronchiolitis require careful fluid monitoring and provision of nasogastric or intravenous fluids when hyperpnea precludes safe oral feeding. Antibiotics are not indicated unless bacterial infection is suggested. Concomitant otitis media is common and may be treated with oral antibiotics.

Oxygen therapy to maintain saturations greater or equal to 90% is indicated in a previously healthy infant if oxyhemoglobin saturation (SpO_2) falls persistently below 90%. Infants with a known history of hemodynamically significant heart or lung disease and who were premature require close cardiorespiratory monitoring.

Long-term Monitoring

Most previously healthy children with bronchiolitis recover with few complications, but the resolution of symptoms may take weeks. Among those with severe disease, a few may develop respiratory failure and experience a protracted hospital course. Some patients will require supplemental home oxygen therapy at the time of discharge. On follow-up, these patients should be evaluated to document resolution of the need for oxygen therapy. An association between RSV-positive bronchiolitis and subsequent wheezing and asthma has been noted, but proof of causality is lacking at present.

Table 10-1. Treatment of Bronchiolitis

Therapy	Comment	Evidence Level
Bronchodilators	Should not be used routinely	Level I
	A carefully monitored trial of a beta-adrenergic medication is an option, but bronchodilators should be continued only if there is a documented positive clinical response using an objective means of evaluation.	Level I
Corticosteroids	Should not be used routinely	Level I
Nebulized epinephrine	Should not be used routinely	Level II-1
	May decrease admission rates from the emergency department	Level II-2
Ribavirin	Should not be used routinely	Level II-1
Antibiotics	Should be used only in children who have specific indications of the coexistence of a bacterial infection	Level II-1
Fluid and hydration therapy	Recommended if risk of dehydration; should be determined clinically	Level III
Chest physiotherapy	Should not be used routinely	Level II-1
Oxygen	Supplemental oxygen recommended if the oxyhemoglobin saturation (Sp_{O2}) is below 90% in previously healthy infants	Level III
Cardiorespiratory monitoring	Infants with a known history of hemodynamically significant heart disease, lung disease, or prematurity require close monitoring as oxygen is being weaned.	Level II-2
Hand washing	Recommended to prevent nosocomial spread of respiratory syncytial virus	Level II-2

Suggested Reading
· · · · · · · · · · · · · · · · · · · ·

American Academy of Pediatrics Subcommittee on Diagnosis and Management of Bronchiolitis. Diagnosis and management of bronchiolitis. *Pediatrics.* 2006;118(4):1774–1793

Corneli HM, Zorc JJ, Mahajan P, et al. A multicenter, randomized, controlled trial of dexamethasone for bronchiolitis. *N Engl J Med.* 2007;357(4):331–339

Fernandes RM, Bialy LM, Vandermeer B, et al. Glucocorticoids for acute viral bronchiolitis in infants and young children. *Cochrane Database Syst Rev.* 2013;6:CD004878

Nagakumar P, Doull I. Current therapy for bronchiolitis. *Arch Dis Child.* 2012;97(9):827–830

Plint AC, Johnson DW, Patel H, et al. Epinephrine and dexamethasone in children with bronchiolitis. *N Engl J Med.* 2009;360(20):2079–2089

CHAPTER 11

Chest Pain

Nicole Sutton, MD; Lacy C. Hobgood, MD; and Christine A. Walsh, MD

Key Points

- Although chest pain is a frequent concern in children and adolescents, it seldom results from cardiac pathology.

- The most important tools in evaluating chest pain in children are a thorough personal and family history and physical examination, which should guide any further testing and management.

- The electrocardiogram should be analyzed for rhythm, atrioventricular block, delta waves (WPW), ventricular hypertrophy, ST–T wave changes, low voltage, prolonged QTc, and a Brugada syndrome pattern.

Overview

Chest pain is a relatively common presenting concern in children and adolescents, occurring in 6 in 1,000 urban pediatric emergency department visits. It occurs equally in girls and boys, with the mean age being about 12 to 13 years. The most important tools in evaluating chest pain in children are a thorough history and physical examination, which should guide any testing and management. Family history is helpful in identifying conditions that have a genetic predisposition. Children younger than 12 years are more likely to have a cardio-respiratory cause, while children older than 12 years are more likely to have a psychogenic cause. Chest pain may become chronic in 45% to 69% of cases, with symptoms lasting for up to 3 years in 19% of patients (Evidence Level II-3).

Causes

Although chest pain is a frequent complaint in children and adolescents, it seldom results from cardiac pathology. Studies have examined the rate of cardiac chest pain in pediatric patients who presented to emergency rooms; a recent study of more than 4,000 visits to pediatric emergency departments, of children younger than 19 years without known cardiac disease, found a cardiac etiology of the chest pain in 24 or 0.6% of the patients. In addition, one study reviewed the National Death Index and the Social Security Index to make sure that no patient discharged from cardiology care after chest pain evaluation died from cardiac causes. Research has shown that the most common cause of chest pain in children is musculoskeletal, with an increased frequency of the diagnosis of non-cardiac chest pain in children with psychiatric disorders, especially anxiety disorder, and in patients with a history of abuse (Evidence Level II-2).

Cardiac Causes of Chest Pain (Box 11-1)

Box 11-1. Cardiac Causes of Chest Pain

Coronary artery disorders
▪ Kawasaki disease
▪ Anomalous coronary artery/ALCAPA
▪ Coronary fistulas
▪ Williams syndrome
▪ Coronary ischemia from ingestion (eg, cocaine)
Cardiomyopathy
▪ Hypertrophic cardiomyopathy
▪ Dilated cardiomyopathy
▪ Acute myocarditis
Pericarditis
Aortic stenosis
Aortic dissection
Arrhythmia

Abbreviation: ALCAPA, anomalous left coronary artery from the pulmonary artery.

Coronary Artery Disorders

The most common parental concern when their child expresses concerns of chest pain is that the child is having a "heart attack." The incidence of coronary ischemia in children is very low, as coronary artery disease is extremely rare in children. Some children are at risk for coronary ischemia, though. Kawasaki disease can lead to coronary aneurysm formation, which has been reported in as many as 20% to 25% of children not treated with intravenous immunoglobin, and in 2% to 4% of treated children.

Patients with an anomalous coronary artery arising from an abnormal location can also have ischemic chest pain. Another type of coronary artery anomaly, anomalous left coronary artery from the pulmonary artery, very rarely presents out of the newborn period but has been reported in older children and even adults who experience chest pain with exercise. Coronary fistulas have been reported to present with chest pain, although this is rare and they are more likely to present with a continuous murmur as blood flows from the high-pressure aorta to the low-pressure pulmonary artery or atrium.

Patients with Williams syndrome are at risk for developing spontaneous coronary vasospasm with resultant chest pain from myocardial ischemia. This is most likely to occur during induction of or waking up from general anesthesia, but it can happen at any time. In addition, patients with Williams syndrome are at increased risk of coronary artery stenosis. Cocaine use is associated with emergency department visits for chest pain and myocardial infarction.

Cocaine causes hypertension, tachycardia, and vasoconstriction. It increases contractility, myocardial oxygen demand, and platelet activation and also accelerates atherosclerosis. This combination leads to myocardial ischemia and infarction. This can occur in patients with normal coronary anatomy and without any prior coronary artery disease, although the risk appears to be higher in patients with preexisting coronary artery disease (Evidence Level II-3).

Cardiomyopathy

Cardiomyopathy is a disease of the myocardium. Both dilated cardiomyopathy and hypertrophic cardiomyopathy can be associated with chest pain resulting from myocardial demand being greater than cardiac output. In general, acute myocarditis is only associated with chest pain when it is accompanied by pericarditis.

Pericardial Disease

Acute inflammation of the pericardium, otherwise known as pericarditis, may lead to severe chest pain. The chest pain is thought to be the result of the apposition of the inflamed visceral pericardium and parietal pericardium. The pain is generally relieved when the patient sits up and worsens when the patient lies flat. Pericarditis can be viral, bacterial, autoimmune, oncologic, or related to surgery when the pericardium is entered.

Aortic Stenosis

Severe valvar aortic stenosis or sub-valvar aortic stenosis can lead to chest pain during exercise. The increased demand for cardiac output by the hypertrophied left ventricle during exercise cannot be supplied and this leads to the development of anginal chest pain. It may also lead to syncope, similar to hypertrophic cardiomyopathy.

Aortic Dissection

Aortic dissection is rare in children and adolescents unless they have Marfan syndrome, Ehlers-Danlos syndrome, Turner syndrome, or other familial aneurysmal diseases. This pain is severe, generally has sudden onset, and radiates to the back. It is diagnosed by computed tomography or magnetic resonance imaging, although a chest radiograph that shows a widened mediastinum can be consistent with aortic root dilation.

Arrhythmia

Children with supraventricular tachycardia can present with the concern of chest pain or "chest discomfort." Key in assessing for arrhythmia is the history of palpitations. For these patients, the most useful test is an outpatient event monitor so that the electrocardiogram (ECG) can be recorded during episodes of palpitations or chest pain when they occur. The ECG should be scrutinized in patients with chest pain for a delta wave of WPW and for a prolonged QT interval. Ventricular tachycardia is more likely to present in patients with a history of congenital heart disease.

Non-cardiac Causes of Chest Pain (Box 11-2)

Box 11-2. Non-cardiac Causes of Chest Pain

Musculoskeletal
- Chest wall strain/overuse injury
- Direct trauma/contusion
- Rib fracture
- Costochondritis
- Tietze syndrome
- Cervical ribs
- Precordial catch syndrome
- Osteomyelitis
- Myositis
- Thoracic outlet obstruction
- Transverse myelitis

Pulmonary
- Severe or chronic cough
- Asthma/reactive airway disease
- Pneumonia (viral, bacterial, fungal, or parasitic)
- Pneumothorax or pneumomediastinum
- Pulmonary embolism
- Pleural effusion (as seen in collagen vascular disease)
- Pleurodynia (as seen in coxsackievirus)
- Foreign body aspiration
- Cystic adenomatoid malformation
- Primary or secondary adenoma or carcinoma

Psychiatric
- Stress-related pain
- Somatoform disorder
- Hyperventilation syndrome
- Panic attacks
- Bulimia nervosa
- Munchausen syndrome

Box 11-2 *(cont)*

Gastrointestinal
- Reflux esophagitis
- Esophageal spasm
- Esophageal diverticulum
- Esophageal foreign body
- Esophageal rupture/Boerhaave syndrome
- Mallory-Weiss tear
- Achalasia
- Subdiaphragmatic abscess
- Cholecystitis
- Pancreatitis
- Fitz-Hugh-Curtis syndrome (perihepatitis)

Hematologic
- Sickle cell pain crisis/acute chest syndrome
- Hypercoagulation syndromes
- Antiphospholipid syndrome
- Factor V Leiden
- Protein C or protein S deficiency
- Antithrombin III deficiency
- Prothrombin gene mutation
- Elevated lipoprotein (a) level
- Elevated homocysteine level

Oncologic
- Hodgkin disease
- T-cell lymphoma
- Thymoma

Infectious Disease
- Shingles

Other
- Breast tenderness
- Pregnancy, gynecomastia, mastitis, fibrocystic disease
- Ingestion (of cocaine, tobacco, methamphetamine, sympathomimetic stimulants)
- Child abuse

Adapted from Kocis KC. Chest pain in pediatrics. *Pediatr Clin North Am.* 1999;46(2):189–203 and Selbst SM. Chest pain in children. *Pediatr Rev.* 1997;18(5):169–173.

Musculoskeletal

Musculoskeletal causes of chest pain reflect about 15% to 31% of pediatric cases of chest pain. Inspection or palpation may reveal signs of direct trauma. Palpation of the chest wall or of a specific muscle group may reproduce the pain. A preceding upper respiratory tract infection suggests the possibility of costochondritis. Palpation or deep breathing could exacerbate the pain. Tietze syndrome can be thought of as a severe form of costochondritis that is confined to the costal cartilages. A palpable abnormality may suggest rib fracture. Precordial catch is a sharp pain lasting only a few seconds, thought to be caused by a pinched nerve. It seems to be associated with a slouched posture. Most musculoskeletal cases can be treated with rest, nonsteroidal anti-inflammatory drugs, and reassurance.

Pulmonary

The overall prevalence of chest pain due to pulmonary causes is 2% to 11%, especially in children younger than 12 years. Reactive airway disease, asthma, and pneumonia may be diagnosed by auscultation. Chest radiography and pulmonary function testing are used when appropriate for confirmation. A prospective study of 88 children referred to a pediatric cardiology office for chest pain found that 73% had evidence of exercise-induced asthma on pulmonary function testing following a treadmill exercise test. Inhaled albuterol led to objective improvement in 70% and subjective improvement in 97% of identified cases (Evidence Level II-2).

Absence of breath sounds or deviation of the airway suggests pneumothorax. Dullness to percussion suggests pleural effusion. Pleurodynia is the sudden onset of sharp or stabbing chest pain in conjunction with a pleural friction rub, fever, and headache. It is most commonly caused by coxsackievirus infection but can also be caused by other enteroviruses.

Pulmonary embolism is rare in children but must be considered in female adolescents who smoke and are using hormonal contraception or in children with hypercoagulability. When considering foreign body aspiration, obtaining inspiratory and expiratory chest radiographs may be helpful. Bronchoscopy may be both diagnostic and therapeutic.

Psychiatric

Psychiatric causes of pediatric chest pain account for 5% to 17% of cases and are common in children older than 12 years. Life stressors such as family discord, peer pressure/bullying, and poor school performance may be disclosed during a careful history. A heightened emotional state or panic attack may lead to hyperventilation, which can directly cause chest pain due to hypocapnic alkalosis, which in turn can lead to coronary artery vasoconstriction. Other psychiatric conditions such as bulimia could lead to repeated bouts of vomiting, increasing the risk of esophageal tear or rupture.

Gastrointestinal

Gastrointestinal causes of pediatric chest pain account for 4% to 7% of cases. The most common diagnosis is gastroesophageal reflux and may be worse when the child is reclining, especially shortly after meals. Diffuse esophageal spasm and achalasia were the most commonly identified motility disorders.

More worrisome findings on history include hematemesis, hematochezia, melena, and altered vital signs, which may be seen with esophageal tear or rupture. Foreign bodies could be suggested by history and confirmed by plain radiography. In general, they pass spontaneously. Notable exceptions include evidence of esophageal obstruction, foreign body lodged in the esophagus for more than 24 hours, or if the object is a disc battery or an object that is especially long and sharp.

Cholecystitis generally causes focal right upper quadrant pain, generally worse after eating a high-fat, high-protein meal. Ultrasound is usually diagnostic. Pancreatitis should be considered in children with growth failure or malabsorption, a family history of pancreatitis, or recurrent abdominal pain with or without vomiting.

Fitz-Hugh-Curtis syndrome, or perihepatitis, is a cause of right upper quadrant pain seen in 10% of young women with pelvic inflammatory disease due to chlamydia or gonorrhea.

Hematologic

Acute chest syndrome is the second most common reason (after acute vaso-occulusive pain crisis) for the hospitalization of children with sickle cell disease. It can be seen in children with asthma, pneumonia, postoperative atelectasis, or other conditions that affect oxygenation. Diagnosis requires a new pulmonary infiltrate on chest x-ray that involves at least one lung segment and the development of chest pain, fever, increased work of breathing, or hypoxemia. The hypercoagulation syndromes could lead to thrombus formation and development of either pulmonary embolism or myocardial infarction.

Oncologic

Hodgkin lymphoma typically presents as low cervical or supraclavicular lymphadenopathy, nonspecific systemic symptoms (eg, fever, night sweats, weight loss, fatigue, anorexia), and discovery of a mediastinal mass on chest radiograph. Bulky mediastinal disease may cause stridor, dysphagia, dyspnea, cough, or the superior vena cava syndrome.

Infectious Disease

Shingles presents with rash and neuritic pain. Acute neuritic pain is the most common symptom, generally described as burning, stabbing, or throbbing (Evidence Level II-2).

Other

Breast pain can be seen in girls with fibrocystic disease or in boys with gynecomastia. Ingestion of stimulants such as cocaine or sympathomimetics can lead to palpitations, coronary artery vasospasm, or myocardial infarction.

Evaluation

The most important part of this evaluation is history of the chest pain because a careful history can determine cause of the chest pain. It is important to obtain history of the chest pain from the patient as well as the parents/caregivers. Start with duration of the chest pain. Most patients will present with weeks or months of chest pain.

A sudden, more acute history may be more suggestive of a cardiac cause of the chest pain. Determine when the pain occurs. Does it occur only at rest, only with exercise, or when the patient is anxious or stressed, such as when a test will be given at school? A thorough history must include a description of the quality of the chest pain (eg, sharp, squeezing, dull, aching, burning, tightness). It is important to avoid giving patients a list of adjectives to choose from, but allow them to use their own words. Key questions include

▶ Does the pain radiate anywhere? Have the patient point with one finger to the spot where the pain is felt and where the pain radiates.

▶ Have patients rate the pain on a scale of 1 to 10, defining the range for them.

▶ Ask about factors that improve or worsen the chest pain. Does the pain get better or worse with a deep breath? Worsening pain with deep inspiration can be consistent with costochondritis. Feeling like something is catching or caught when taking a deep breath is diagnostic of precordial catch syndrome. Does the pain get better with rest or with analgesics? Is the pain related to eating? Ask about changes or stresses at home and school at the time that the pain started or when the pain recurs.

▶ Does anything else occur with the pain such as palpitations, dizziness, syncope, nausea, vomiting, fatigue, cough, shortness of breath, or fever?

▶ What is the frequency of the chest pain? Is it occurring daily? Weekly? Has the pain been getting more or less frequent, and has the severity of the pain changed?

▶ Are you worried about the pain, and, if so, why?

Cardiac chest pain is generally described as crushing pain that is mid-precordial with radiation to the left arm and jaw when it is caused by coronary artery ischemia. Patients with aortic dissection might describe severe crushing pain in the mid-precordium that radiates to the back.

Key points in the past medical history may include any history of a clotting disorder, systemic arthritis or vasculitis, sickle cell disease, Marfan or Ehlers-

Danlos syndrome, or Kawasaki disease. In the family history, are there any first-degree relatives with sudden cardiac death (ie, unexplained sudden death at younger than 35 years), aborted sudden death, cardiomyopathy, or clotting disorder?

On physical examination, the first step is to note the patient's *body habitus*; a tall, thin patient with pectus excavatum or carinatum may have Marfan syndrome. The costochondral joints should be palpated for tenderness. Auscultation of the lungs may reveal wheezing associated with asthma or rales that can be associated with heart failure.

The cardiac examination should be performed with special care when looking for cardiac causes of chest pain. Note the point of maximal impulse; if the heart is enlarged, the patient may have myocarditis. Muffled heart sounds can be seen in patients with pericarditis and pericardial effusions. A friction rub can also be heard with a pericardial effusion, although a very large effusion may not have any rub. A thrill can be felt in patients with left ventricular outflow tract obstruction. A loud harsh systolic ejection murmur along the left and right upper sternal border can represent sub-valvar or valvar aortic stenosis.

With respect to the rest of the physical examination, look for signs of heart failure, such as hepatosplenomegaly, jugular venous distension, and peripheral edema, as well as systemic diseases, such as swollen joints and rashes.

An ECG can be of benefit in the evaluation of chest pain. The ECG should be reviewed for rhythm, atrioventricular block, delta waves (WPW), ventricular hypertrophy (seen in hypertrophic cardiomyopathy), ST–T wave changes (seen with pericarditis or with coronary ischemia), low voltage (seen in pericarditis and myocarditis), prolonged QTc, and a Brugada syndrome pattern. A Standardized Clinical Assessment and Management Plans (SCAMPs) algorithm has been published (Figure 11-1)

Using this strategy, echocardiograms are only performed in patients with positive elements from the personal history (eg, systemic inflammatory disease, malignancy, thrombophilia) or family history (eg, cardiomyopathy, pulmonary hypertension, aborted sudden death, sudden or unexplained death), positive findings on the physical examination (eg, pericardial friction rub, pathologic murmur), or abnormal ECG findings.

Other testing has not been shown to be effective in diagnosing chest pain in children. A recent study was performed looking at the use of troponin assays for pediatric patients. Of the patients with chest pain, only 4% had elevated troponins, 53% of which were diagnosed with myopericarditis. Almost all of the patients with myopericarditis presented with fever and ST changes on ECG (Evidence Level II-2). Exercise stress testing has likewise not been shown to be helpful in the work-up of chest pain, even in patients with exertional chest pain or with palpitations and possible arrhythmias. The evaluation of chest pain associated with palpitations which seem likely due to an arrhythmia is best assessed with an event monitor. An event monitor is unlikely to record an arrhythmia in the setting of chest pain without palpitations and is not recommended (Evidence Level III).

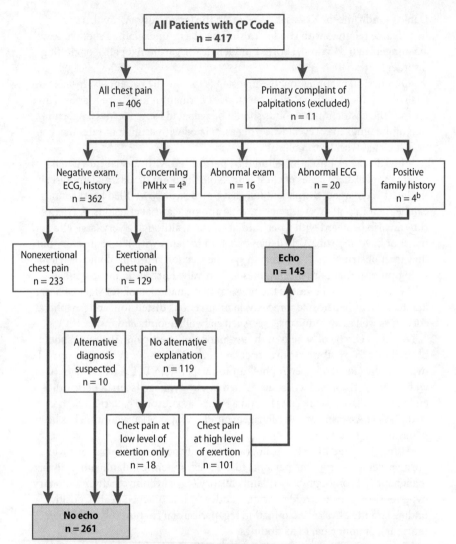

Figure 11-1. Standardized Clinical Assessment and Management Plans algorithm to guide testing in patients with chest pain.
Abbreviations: CP, chest pain; PMHx, past medical history; echo, echocardiogram.
[a] Diagnoses that lead to increased risk of cardiac chest pain (ie, inflammatory disorders, malignancy, thrombophilia).
[b] Family history was considered positive if any of the following were present in a first-degree relative: sudden or unexplained death; aborted sudden death; cardiomyopathy; or pulmonary hypertension. Six patients had an abnormal electrocardiogram result and an abnormal past medical history, family history, or physical examination. Patients with more than 1 abnormality (ie, electrocardiogram, past medical history, family history, and/or physical examination) were counted in only 1 category in this figure.

From Friedman KG, Kane DA, Rathod RH, et al. Management of pedistric chest pain using a standardized assessment and management plan. *Pediatrics.* 2011;128(2):239–245.

Suggested Reading

Anwar S. Pediatric chest pain: findings on exercise stress testing. *Clin Pediatr.* 2012;51(7):659–662

Drossner DM, Hirsch DA, Sturm JJ, et al. Cardiac disease in pediatric patients presenting to a pediatric ED with chest pain. *Am J Emerg Med.* 2011;29(6):632–638

Friedman KG, Kane DA, Rathood RH, et al. Management of pedistric chest pain using a standardized assessment and management plan. *Pediatrics.* 2011;128(2):239–245

Kocis KC. Chest pain in pediatrics. *Pediatr Clin North Am.* 1999;46(2):189–203

Hanson CL, Hokanson JS. Etiology of chest pain referred to cardiologic clinic. *WMJ.* 2011;110(2):58–62

Lipsitz JD, Hsu DT, Apfel HD, et al. Psychiatric disorders in youth with medically unexplained chest pain versus innocent heart murmur. *J Pediatr.* 2012;160(2):320–324

Saleeb SF, Li WY, Warren SZ, Lock JE. Effectiveness of screening for life-threstening chest pain in children. *Pediatrics.* 2011;128(5):e1062–e1068

Takahashi M. Coronary ischemia in pediatric patients. *Pediatr Clin North Am.* 2010;57(6):1261–1280

Verghese GR, Friedman KG, Rathod RH, et al. Resource utilization reduction for evaluation of chest pain in pediatrics using a novel standardized clinical asessment and management plan. *J Am Heart Assoc.* 2012;1(2):jah3-e000349

Weins L, Sabath R, Ewing L, Gowdamarajan R, Portnoy J, Scagliotti D. Chest pain in otherwise healthy children and adolescents is frequently caused by exercise induced asthma. *Pediatrics.* 1992;90(3):350–353

Wyllie R. Foreign bodies in the gastrointestinal tract. *Curr Opin Pediatr.* 2006;18(5):563–564

CHAPTER 12

Colic

Usha Ramkumar, MBBS

Key Points

- Colic is a common problem in infancy.
- Colic is a diagnosis of exclusion. A good history and physical examination is often all that is needed to make the diagnosis.
- Colic resolves spontaneously by 3 to 4 months of age.
- A supportive physician who can understand, educate, and reassure families remains the mainstay of management.
- Some parents may be driven to dysfunctional behavior that may harm the child.

Overview

Colic is a poorly understood condition characterized by excessive crying in the newborn period. It can also be a major source of anxiety and distress for new parents, leading to multiple office visits and frustration for the physician. It is, nonetheless, thought to be benign and self-limiting.

Colic is defined as excessive crying for no apparent reason in the first 3 months of life. A colicky child may cry for more than 3 hours a day, for more than 3 days per week, and for more than 3 weeks (as defined by Wessel et al). The crying usually resolves by 3 to 4 months of age (Box 12-1).

Box 12-1. Characteristics of a Colicky Cry

- Sudden onset often in late afternoon/evening
- Higher intensity, loudness, and pitch than usual crying
- Association with hypertonia
  (eg, clenched fists, knees drawn up, and a pained facies)
- Not related to feedings or environmental stimuli
- Not consolable by the caregiver

Colic is very common and affects up to 40% of newborns. The type of feedings, breast or formula, also does not seem to matter. Most babies will cry when they are hungry, wet, or uncomfortable, and Brazelton TB showed that most babies normally cry for about 2.25 hours in a day for the first 7 weeks of life. Mothers of colicky babies are at risk for postpartum depression, and the babies are at significant risk for abuse. It is therefore important for the physician to understand parental concerns and beliefs and to manage and reassure them adeptly.

Causes

The etiology of colic remains unclear and poorly understood, though it is thought to be multifactorial (Box 12-2).

Box 12-2. Proposed Etiologies of Infantile Colic

GASTROINTESTINAL	NON-GASTROINTESTINAL
Nutritive	**Baby Factors**
■ Aerophagia	■ Hypersensitivity to the environment
■ Colonic fermentation/malabsorption	■ Temperament
■ Excessive intra-intestinal air load	
■ Mode of feeding	**Maternal Factors**
■ Protein allergy/intolerance	■ Family stress
	■ Maternal anxiety
Non-nutritive	■ Maternal smoking
■ Gastroesophageal reflux	
■ Gut hormones	
■ Motility	

Adapted from Gupta SK. Is colic a gastrointestinal disorder? *Curr Opin Pediatr.* 2002;14(5):558–592, with permission.

Gut Factors

Allergy to cow's milk, lactose and fructose intolerance, excessive gas production, and gut hypermotility have been considered and evaluated but not proven as causes for colic. Gastroesophageal reflux and milk-protein allergy may cause excessive crying in babies.

Biological Factors

Baby feeding techniques, such as overfeeding, underfeeding, burping, and air swallowing, have been implicated in the etiology of colic. Motor immaturity of the infant leading to feeding intolerance has been hypothesized.

Psychosocial Factors

A baby's temperament and hypersensitivity to the environment have been considered as factors for causing colic. Parental psychosocial factors including family stress may provoke increased crying in babies.

Clinical Features

A colicky infant presents in the first 2 to 4 weeks of life with sudden onset of prolonged crying, often in the afternoon or evening. Parents describe a "pained" facies with clenched fists and legs drawn up. The infants are often unconsolable and respond poorly to parental soothing, even though they usually are feeding and growing well and have healthy voiding and elimination patterns.

Differential Diagnosis

The differential diagnosis for crying is broad (Box 12-3).

Box 12-3. Common Causes of Crying

IDIOPATHIC COLIC			
Infection	**Gastrointestinal**	**Trauma**	**Other**
■ UTI	■ Constipation	■ Corneal abrasion	■ Overstimulation
■ Meningitis	■ Gas	■ Foreign body in the eye	■ Drug withdrawal
■ Otitis media	■ GE reflux		■ Abuse (eg, fractures, retinal hemorrhage)
	■ Milk protein allergy	■ Hair tourniquet	

Abbreviations: GE, gastrointestinal; UTI, urinary tract infection.

A review of the common organic diseases that may present with colic-like syndrome is helpful (Table 12-1).

Evaluation

Complete dietary history, as well as elimination and sleeping patterns, of the infant need to be assessed. Parents need to be questioned about the nature and duration of crying, its relationship to feedings, and the presence of associated features such as grimacing and straining. Parents' ability to cope with the crying and their thoughts on why the baby is crying also need to be assessed along with any cultural influences that may be present.

The infant's weight and hydration status should be assessed. Growth parameters and vital signs should be reviewed with parents. An extensive head-to-toe physical examination looking for corneal abrasions, retinal hemorrhages, foreign bodies in the eyes, occult fractures, bruises, and hair tourniquets should also to be performed.

Minimal tests needed to make the diagnosis (as directed by the history and physical examination) may have to be considered.

Table 12-1. Organic Diseases Presenting With Colic-Like Syndrome

Disease State	Strength of Evidence in Primary Care Setting	Estimated prevalence
Cow's milk protein intolerance	Strong	<5%
Isolated fructose intolerance	Strong	Rare
Maternal drug effects (ie, Prozac)	Strong	Unknown, changing
Anomalous origin of left coronary artery arising from the pulmonary artery (ALCAPA)	Strong	Very rare
Infantile migraine	Moderate	Rare
Reflux esophagitis	Moderate	Rare
Shaken baby syndrome [Abusive head trauma]	Moderate cause and effect	Difficult to distinguish
Congenital glaucoma	Weak, but suggestive	Rare
Central nervous system abnormalities (ie, Chiari type I malformation)	Weak, but suggestive	Rare
Urinary tract infection	Weak	Probably rare
Lactose intolerance	Very weak	Probably not etiologic

From Walker A, ed. *Pediatric Gastrointestinal Disease.* 4th ed, Hamilton, Ontario: BC Decker Inc; 2004.

Management

Colic is a self-limiting condition, often stopping as mysteriously as it starts, with most infants getting better by 3 to 4 months of age. Despite all the extensive research, safe and effective treatments are not available. Hence, management of colic needs to be individualized to meet the family's needs. Strategies to help the crying as well as improving the parental-child relationship need to be discussed. Reassurance of wellness remains the mainstay of treatment.

Educating families about crying in the newborn period is of utmost importance.

Many hospitals direct parents to The Period of PURPLE Crying Web site or video that is available in many languages. PURPLE is an acronym describing the specific characteristics of an infant's crying (for peak, unexpected, resists soothing, pain-like face, long-lasting, evening). The use of the word *period* is also important, as it tells parents that this kind of crying is a temporary phase that will come to an end. The concept and Web site/video helps educate families about the normalcy of infant crying and the dangers of shaking an infant (Evidence Level 1).

Parental reassurance is an important aspect of management. Listening to families, understanding their beliefs, and addressing their concerns is one of the mainstays of colic management. Acknowledging that the crying behavior is stressful, but reassuring that it is an expected variant that will resolve in time, is the key. Giving parents palliative strategies for managing the crying infant may also be helpful. Rhythmic stimulation with swinging or rocking, soothing music, driving in a car, white noise, and swaddling may be suggested. Encouraging parents to walk away from a crying infant (provided that the infant is in a safe place) may sometimes be necessary. Providing respite for the parent may be beneficial.

Dietary modification remains another mainstay of management. Changing feeding habits, allowing time for the baby to feed without being rushed, and frequent burping during feeds may be suggested. Elimination diets in breastfeeding mothers and formula changes in bottle-fed infants have only shown modest benefits but may be considered. A partially hydrolyzed formula or elimination of cow's milk from the mother's diet while she is breastfeeding may be advised for colic that is refractory to behavioral management (Evidence Level II-2).

Herbal remedies such as teas (Evidence Level II-2), gripe water, and carminatives may be considered. These products may not have significant adverse effects, but studies have not shown them to be helpful. Gripe water has been used in Europe, Asia, and Africa, though many different formulations of gripe water are available and parents need to be warned that some products may contain alcohol and must be avoided.

Medications such as gas drops (eg, simethicone) have some benefit, but most studies show no difference from placebo. Antispasmodics and methylscopolamine are neither safe nor beneficial. Dicyclomine may have some benefits (Evidence Level II-2), but adverse effects like apnea, seizures, and coma outweigh the benefits.

Prognosis/Long-term Effects

Overall, there is considerable evidence for positive outcomes for infants and families with colic. Most available follow-up studies show that infants with colic have good physical and behavioral health.

There may, however, be some negative consequences for the caregivers. Maternal mood may be affected, and family relationships may be difficult for some time. Figure 12-1 represents the worst case scenarios for families.

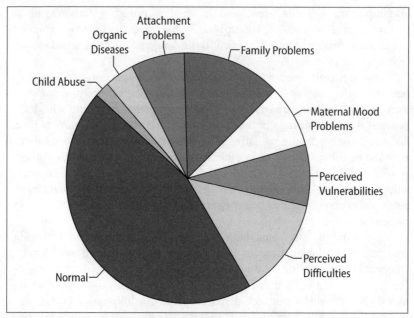

Figure 12-1. Clinical prognostic pie for colic.

Adapted from Lehtonen L, Gormally S, Barr RG. 'Clinical pies' for etiology and outcome in infants presenting with early increased crying. In: Barr RG, Hopkins B, Green JA, eds. *Crying as a Sign, a Symptom, and a Signal.* London, England: Mac Keith Press; 2011, with permission.

Suggested Reading

Barr RG, Hopkins B, Green JA, eds. *Crying as a Sign, a Symptom, and a Signal.* London, England: Mac Keith Press; 2000

Barr RG, Rivara FP, Barr M, Cummings P, Taylor J, et al. Effectiveness of educational materials designed to change knowledge and behaviors regarding crying and shaken baby syndrome in mothers of newborns: a randomized control trial. *Pediatrics.* 2009:123(3):972–980

Brazelton TB. Crying in Infancy. *Pediatrics.* 1962:29(4);579-588

Garrison MM, Christakis DA. A systematic review of treatments for infant colic. *Pediatrics.* 2000;106(1 Pt 2):184–190

National Center on Shaken Baby Syndrome. The Period of Purple Crying Web site. http://www.purplecrying.info. Accessed November 7, 2014

Wessel et al. Paroxysmal fussing in infancy, sometimes call "colic". *Pediatrics.* 1954;14:421-434

CHAPTER 13

Conjunctivitis

Suzette Surratt Caudle, MD

KEY POINTS

- Conjunctivitis is a common pediatric complaint, with acute bacterial conjunctivitis affecting 1 in 8 children each year.

- Most conjunctivitis in childhood is infectious or allergic in etiology. The most common cause is acute bacterial infection, followed by viral infection and allergic conjunctivitis.

- Bacterial cultures are positive in 50% to 80% of children presenting with acute signs and symptoms of conjunctivitis, and nontypable *Haemophilus influenzae* accounts for 50% to 80% of those positive bacterial culture results.

- Cultures for bacterial pathogens can guide treatment but are expensive and slow to return; these are reserved for ophthalmia neonatorum and patients with severe disease or those who have failed empiric topical antibiotic treatment.

- Recent literature supports the use of topical antibiotics for acute bacterial conjunctivitis, based on more rapid resolution of symptoms. The American Academy of Pediatrics (AAP) *Red Book* recommends that children with conjunctivitis who are otherwise well can return to or remain in child care or school as soon as the indicated treatment is initiated (unless their behavior is such that close contact with others is unavoidable).

- Kawasaki disease may manifest with conjunctival injection; Stevens-Johnson syndrome may include significant conjunctival inflammatory changes in association with a severe rash, mucous membrane changes, and other systemic symptoms.

Overview

Conjunctivitis is a common pediatric complaint, with acute bacterial conjunctivitis alone affecting 1 in 8 children each year. Conjunctivitis is defined as inflammation of the conjunctiva. The inflammatory response of the conjunctiva to an inciting agent results in various degrees of injection (often imparting a pink or red hue) and may include some degree of swelling and edema of the conjunctiva (chemosis) or of the eyelid itself. Accompanying secretions may appear to be watery, mucous, or frankly purulent (Figure 13-1). Inflammation of the conjunctiva that lines the eyelids is called palpebral conjunctivitis. Inflammation of the conjunctiva covering the sclera is bulbar conjunctivitis. "Pinkeye" is a nonspecific lay term commonly used to describe conjunctivitis. Conjunctivitis in the first 4 weeks of life is known as ophthalmia neonatorum.

Causes

Many causes of conjunctivitis in childhood are self-limited and benign, but care must be taken to avoid overlooking more significant infections (ie, gonococcal conjunctivitis, human herpesvirus conjunctivitis) that can be vision threatening.

Most conjunctivitis in childhood is infectious or allergic in etiology. The most common cause is acute bacterial infection, followed by viral infection and allergic conjunctivitis (Table 13-1). The remainders of cases result primarily from trauma or irritants or are associated with systemic disease.

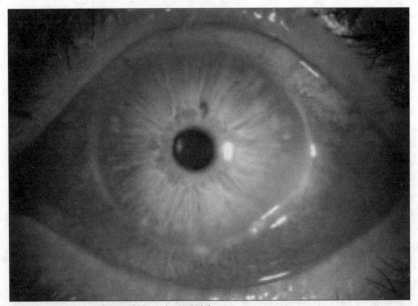

Figure 13-1. Acute bacterial conjunctivitis.

From Richards A, Guzman-Cottrill JA. Conjunctivitis. *Pediatr Rev.* 2010;31(5):196–208. Photograph originally credited to photography department of Casey Eye Institute, Oregon Health and Science University.

Table 13-1. Causes of Conjunctivitis

Category	Specific Etiologies
Infectious	
Bacterial	Nontypable *Haemophilus influenzae, Streptococcus pneumoniae, Moraxella catarrhalis, Staphylococcus aureus, Staphylococcus epidermidis, Pseudomonas, Neisseria gonorrhoeae, Chlamydia trachomatis, Bartonella henselae*
Viral	Adenovirus, coxsackievirus, enterovirus
Allergic	Seasonal allergens, perennial allergens
Irritant/trauma	Chemical conjunctivitis secondary to newborn ophthalmic prophylaxis, smoke, chlorine, trauma, contact lens
Associated with systemic disease	Kawasaki disease, Stevens-Johnson syndrome, ligneous conjunctivitis

Infectious

In studies of conjunctivitis in childhood, bacterial cultures showed positive results in 50% to 80% of cases when children were cultured after presenting with acute signs and symptoms of conjunctivitis.

The most common organism cultured in bacterial conjunctivitis is nontypable *Haemophilus influenzae* (making up approximately 50%–80% of positive bacterial cultures), followed by *Streptococcus pneumoniae* and *Moraxella catarrhalis*. Staphylococcal species, *Streptococcus pyogenes*, *Pseudomonas aeruginosa,* and *Neisseria meningitidis* make up the remainder. Chlamydia and gonorrhea should also be considered as potential pathogens of bacterial conjunctivitis in adolescents through horizontal sexual transmission.

Bacterial causes of ophthalmia neonatorum include *Neisseria gonorrhoeae* and *Chlamydia trachomatis* due to vertical transmission from the maternal genital tract to the neonate (Table 13-2). Other bacterial causes of conjunctivitis are seen in neonates as well, including nontypable *H influenzae, S pneumoniae, Staphylococcus aureus, Staphylococcus epidermidis,* and gram-negative bacilli.

Table 13-2. Major and Minor Etiologies in Ophthalmia Neonatorum

Etiology of Ophthalmia Neonatorum	Proportion of Cases	Incubation Period (d)	Severity of Conjunctivitis[a]	Associated Problems
Chlamydia trachomatis	2%–40%	5–12	+	Pneumonitis 3 wk–3 mo
Neisseria gonorrhoeae	<1%	2–5	+++	Disseminated infection
Other bacterial microbes[b]	30%–50%	5–14	+	Variable
Herpes simplex	<1%	6–14	+	Disseminated infection, meningoencephalitis, keratitis, and ulceration also possible
Chemical	Varies with silver nitrate use	1	+	...

[a] + indicates mild; +++, severe.
[b] Includes skin, respiratory, vaginal, and gastrointestinal tract pathogens such as *Staphylococcus aureus; Streptococcus pneumoniae; Haemophilus influenzae,* nontypeable; group A and B streptococci; *Corynebacterium* species; *Moraxella catarrhalis; Escherichia coli; Klebsiella pneumoniae; Pseudomonas aeruginosa.*

Adapted from American Academy of Pediatrics. Prevention of neonatal ophthalmia. In: *Red Book: 2015 Report of the Committee on Infectious Diseases.* Kimberlin DW, Brady MT, Jackson MA, Long SS, eds. 30th ed. Elk Grove Village, IL: American Academy of Pediatrics; 2015:972–974.

The viral cause of ophthalmia neonatorum is herpes simplex. Viral causes of conjunctivitis beyond the neonatal period include adenovirus, echo-virus, coxsackieviruses, and human herpesviruses. Enteroviruses, influenza, and Epstein-Barr viruses have also been associated with conjunctivitis. Adenovirus is the most frequent viral cause of conjunctivitis.

Allergic

Allergic conjunctivitis may present in childhood. Acute and seasonal allergic conjunctivitis are the result of type 1 (immediate) hypersensitivity reactions mediated by IgE. Acute allergic conjunctivitis is common in children and occurs when antigen is inoculated into the eyes.

Seasonal allergic conjunctivitis occurs more commonly in the late childhood and teen years and is the result of an allergic response to (typically airborne) seasonal allergens such as pollens, grasses, molds, and weeds.

Perennial allergic conjunctivitis is a more chronic form of allergic conjunctivitis and is typically associated with perennial allergens such as dust mites, cockroaches, and animal dander with symptoms of prolonged duration. Seasonal and perennial allergic conjunctivitis make up the vast majority of allergic conjunctival disease and seldom are associated with permanent visual difficulties.

Atopic conjunctivitis occurs in association with eczema and is a severe chronic inflammation of the eyelid skin as well as the conjunctiva, cornea, and even lens. It is typically a disease of the late teen years and adulthood.

Vernal conjunctivitis is a severe form of allergic conjunctivitis associated with the formation of giant papillae on the conjunctiva that result in keratitis secondary to scraping and irritation to the cornea. Papillae can also be seen along the limbus. It is more common in males in warm, temperate climates, particularly India, Africa, and Asia, and in those with personal or family histories of atopy. There is a high concentration of IgE and histamine in secretions, and occurrence is prominent in the warm months of spring and summer, with remission between. It typically lasts 4 to 10 years and ultimately is self-limiting, although ulcerations may occur on the cornea that can threaten vision. This process is best managed in consultation with an ophthalmologist.

Irritant/Traumatic

One form of irritant conjunctivitis is the chemical conjunctivitis resulting from topical ophthalmic prophylactic antibiotics given to neonates to prevent ophthalmia neonatorum. Ocular prophylaxis is indicated for all neonates for the prevention of gonococcal and nongonococcal, non-chlamydial ophthalmia neonatorum. Chemical conjunctivitis in the newborn typically presents within the first 24 hours following antibiotic application. Chemical conjunctivitis, initially described in association with silver nitrate ophthalmologic drops, occurred frequently but is much less frequent with erythromycin and tetracycline ophthalmic ointments. Silver nitrate ophthalmologic drops are no longer available in the United States for this reason. Erythromycin ophthalmic ointment is most commonly used for neonatal ophthalmic prophylaxis as the only option for prophylaxis commercially available in the United States. When chemical conjunctivitis occurs, it is self-limited and resolves after several days.

Smoke and chlorine can induce an irritant conjunctivitis, as can chronic exposure to eye makeup or eye medications or any number of irritants that get into the eyes. Resolution typically occurs with removal of the irritant.

Giant papillary conjunctivitis results from sensitization of the conjunctiva to material on the surface of a contact lens or in contact lens solutions and is associated with prolonged lens wear. Temporary discontinuation of lens wear is necessary in the least, and ophthalmologic consultation is also warranted.

Systemic

Kawasaki disease may manifest with conjunctival injection. Persistent fever and other signs of Kawasaki disease assist with differentiation. Stevens-Johnson syndrome may include significant conjunctival inflammatory changes, also in association with a severe rash, mucous membrane changes, and other systemic symptoms. Ataxia-telangiectasia can include telangiectatic blood vessels on the bulbar conjunctiva. Ligneous conjunctivitis is an unusual conjunctivitis associated with plasminogen deficiency and characterized by chronic pseudomembrane formation on mucous membranes.

Other

In the infant younger than 1 year, nasolacrimal duct obstruction can be confused with conjunctivitis. The infant may be noted to have persistent watery to mucous secretions from the eye or eyes and matting of secretions, but there is generally little inflammation and the problem may persist for months. Gentle massage of the lacrimal sac may result in expression of a small amount of mucous from the puncta. Most cases resolve by approximately 9 months of age. If persistent, referral to an ophthalmologist is necessary.

Other entities in the differential diagnosis for red eye can be found in Chapter 21, Eye Problems.

Evaluation

It can be challenging to distinguish bacterial from viral and even allergic conjunctivitis by physical examination alone. All forms can vary in degree of involvement of the conjunctiva and presence or absence of associated symptoms. However, certain clues can assist in making an accurate diagnosis, and clinical features can help define evaluation strategies. Infection-mediated conjunctivitis is highly contagious, so a history of involved contacts should raise suspicion for an infectious process.

Bacterial

Bacterial conjunctivitis is particularly common in infants, toddlers, and preschoolers. The younger the age at presentation, the more likely the etiology is bacterial. Bacterial conjunctivitis is generally suggested by mucopurulent discharge that may result in matting of the eyelids. Infection is usually bilateral, although early in the course it may present on one side before spreading to the other. Vision should be normal, and although there may be discomfort, there should not be severe pain. Of note is the association between otitis media and acute bacterial conjunctivitis. The presence of acute otitis media has been as high as 30% in acute bacterial conjunctivitis in some studies. The preponderant organism is again nontypable *H influenzae*.

Chlamydial conjunctivitis has onset several days to 2 weeks after birth and is not prevented by neonatal ocular prophylaxis. In addition to inflamed conjunctiva, lid edema and chemosis may occur, unilaterally or bilaterally. Discharge may be watery or mucopurulent. Ocular manifestations of chlamydia infection beyond the neonatal period occur but are rare in children in the United States.

Neisseria gonorrhoeae conjunctivitis usually presents within the first 2 to 5 days after birth and is marked by significant lid swelling, erythema, and copious purulent discharge, typically of abrupt onset. It is rapidly progressive and generally bilateral. Gonococcal infection, untreated, can result in ulceration and perforation of the globe.

Viral

Viral conjunctivitis tends to occur in slightly older children, usually in those of school age. The degree of conjunctival erythema and swelling is highly variable. Discharge is usually watery. While preauricular lymph node enlargement is sometimes described; it is not clear if this is a true association with viral conjunctivitis. Adenoviral conjunctivitis is particularly contagious. Sometimes adenoviral infections are accompanied by pharyngitis and fever (pharyngo-conjunctival fever). Other adenovirus types are associated with epidemic keratoconjunctivitis, a highly contagious form of infection with pseudomembranes, subconjunctival hemorrhages, and corneal infiltrates. Epidemic keratoconjunctivitis is often bilateral and may take weeks to resolve, resulting in visual difficulties and photophobia until the inflammatory cell infiltrates resolve.

Acute hemorrhagic conjunctivitis is more commonly associated with coxsackievirus or echoviruses and results in subconjunctival hemorrhages, acute pain, and sometimes photophobia. It is dramatic and very contagious but self-limiting.

Because herpetic conjunctivitis has potential to lead to keratitis and vision loss, identification is important. Primary herpetic infections can occur in children outside the neonatal period and recurrences are not infrequent but usually occur in adulthood. Eye involvement is typically unilateral. Vesicles may be present on the lid and there may be marked pain as well as swelling of the lid. Dendritic lesions or opacities may be observed on the cornea with fluorescein and close examination. Corticosteroids are contraindicated. Ophthalmologic consultation is indicated. Neonatal herpetic conjunctivitis typically presents within 1 to 2 weeks after birth. Classic vesicular lesions may be on the eyelid, but conjunctivitis may also be the only visible manifestation of neonatal herpes disease.

Allergic

Allergic conjunctivitis is associated with bilateral, watery, itchy eyes with marked injection, significant chemosis, and even bogginess of the conjunctiva and swelling of the lids. There may be an accompanying stringy discharge. Symptoms typically occur within minutes of exposure to the inciting allergen. Allergic conjunctivitis is often accompanied by rhinitis, asthma, or an atopic history. Allergic conjunctivitis tends to have a prolonged course encompassing the period of allergen exposure, although severity may wax and wane.

Perennial allergic conjunctivitis is a more chronic form of seasonal allergic conjunctivitis and may be associated with less itching and more stinging. Perennial allergic conjunctivitis may have seasonal exacerbations.

Signs indicative of more serious etiologies requiring further evaluation include significant pain, photophobia, and vision loss, as well as injection of the limbus. These raise concerns for glaucoma, corneal abrasions, keratitis, uveitis, or iritis. The red reflex and cornea itself should appear normal. Persistent unilateral involvement also raises concern for a foreign body, ulceration, or herpetic keratitis.

Evaluation Strategies

Cultures for bacterial pathogens can guide treatment but are also expensive, and results are usually delayed several days from presentation. Generally, they are reserved for ophthalmia neonatorum and patients with severe disease or those who have failed empiric topical antibiotic treatment. In these cases, Gram stain and culture, including culture for *N gonorrhoeae* as indicated, can be obtained from swabs of the conjunctiva.

Chlamydial conjunctivitis is best tested for with polymerase chain reaction (PCR), enzyme immunoassay, or direct immunofluorescent assay. Nucleic acid amplification tests (NAATs) are generally more sensitive and specific than tissue culture and non-amplified methods. However, there has been only limited study of NAATs for pediatric indications and these tests have not been approved by the US Food and Drug Administration for testing of conjunctival specimens.

Infants suspected to have herpetic conjunctivitis should have human herpesvirus PCR testing of the eye in addition to a more comprehensive assessment for herpetic disease at other sites. Fluorescein and Wood lamp examination, to exclude dendritic lesions, is indicated, as is ophthalmologic consultation and examination of the eye if herpes is suspected or diagnosed. Polymerase chain reaction testing for adenovirus is now available and may become more widely used in the future.

Allergic conjunctivitis may be associated with a high serum IgE level, and conjunctival scrapings may reveal mast cells and eosinophils. Ophthalmologic consultation can offer further diagnostic testing in recalcitrant cases.

Management

Bacterial

Most acute infectious conjunctivitis beyond the neonatal period is self-limited. A previous Cochrane review found that topical antibiotic treatment for acute bacterial conjunctivitis resulted in higher rates of symptom resolution and microbiologic cure at 2 to 5 days and, to a lesser extent, at 6 to 10 days, compared with children who received placebo. After 10 to 14 days, both groups were similar. The most recent Cochrane review (September 2012) continues to support the use of topical antibiotics for acute bacterial conjunctivitis, based on more rapid resolution of symptoms (Evidence Level I). In an effort to minimize costs and risk for resistance associated with unnecessary antibiotic treatment but to maximize appropriate treatment, several investigators have attempted to identify physical findings that make bacterial disease more or less likely. Patel, in a study of 111 patients 2 months to 18 years of age at one institution, found a history of gooey or sticky eyelids or lashes on morning waking and mucoid or purulent discharge on examination were more predictive of bacterial infection. Meltzer prospectively studied 368 children aged 6 months to 17 years presenting with acute conjunctivitis to a pediatric emergency department in one institution and attempted to identify which children were at low risk for bacterial infection. Four features were associated with low risk for bacterial infection: absence of glued eye in the morning, no or watery discharge, age 6 years or older, and presentation in April through November. In the presence of 3 factors, 76% of patients had a negative culture, and in the presence of all 4 factors, 92% of patients had a negative culture.

Initial treatment of presumed bacterial conjunctivitis beyond the neonatal period is with a broad spectrum topical antibiotic that covers gram-negative and gram-positive organisms. Ointments or drops may be used. Ointments may be preferable in children in whom delivery of drops is difficult, but ointments blur vision, making it a less desirable option beyond 1 to 2 years of age.

The choice of topical antibiotic is somewhat controversial. Considerations include time to resolution of symptoms, likelihood of antimicrobial resistance, cost, and likelihood of compliance.

Studies of topical antibiotics in young children are relatively limited and in most cases are drug-to-drug comparisons rather than placebo-controlled trials. Options are shown in Table 13-3.

Polymyxin B–trimethoprim sulfate or newer fluoroquinolones should be the first line of choice for the empiric treatment of presumed bacterial conjunctivitis in children. Proponents for fluoroquinolones argue that these drugs achieve resolution of symptoms faster and that return visits, additional therapies, and additional time out from work and child care for those with polymyxin B–trimethoprim sulfate–resistant cases justifies increased cost of treatment. Proponents for polymyxin B–trimethoprim sulfate argue that clinical rates of improvement are similar and the relatively low rate of overall resistance and decreased cost fully justify its use. Consideration of local resistance patterns and open discussion with families about the pros and cons of different treatment options, with consideration for the specific child and family's situation, appear to offer the most reasonable approach.

Of note, in the case of conjunctivitis-otitis syndrome, oral treatment with a beta-lactamase resistant antibiotic is indicated (amoxicillin-clavulanate, cefdinir, cefixime, cefpodoxime), and topical treatment is then not necessary.

All patients and families should be educated in the usefulness of careful hand washing to minimize spread of disease. While some transmission occurs through large droplets, direct contact through hand-to-eye contamination is a leading method of spread.

Individuals are presumed contagious as long as symptoms persist. The AAP *Red Book* recommends that children with conjunctivitis who are otherwise well can return to or remain in child care or school as soon as the indicated treatment is initiated (unless their behavior is such that close contact with others is likely). Health departments should be notified of outbreaks.

Table 13-3. Topical Antibiotic Treatment Options for Presumed Acute Bacterial Conjunctivitis Beyond the Neonatal Period

Medication	Advantages	Disadvantages
Polymyxin B–trimethoprim sulfate combination	Inexpensive Broad coverage against gram-positive and gram-negative organisms, including MRSA[a] Few side effects	Some *Streptococcus pneumoniae* resistance reported (among some penicillin non-susceptible *S pneumoniae* isolates) Trimethoprim bacteriostatic, associated slower resolution
Newer fluoroquinolones (moxifloxacin, gatifloxacin, besifloxacin)	Broad coverage against gram-negative organisms and enhanced activity gram-positive coverage, including MSSA Cover *Haemophilus influenzae* and *S pneumoniae* and most other bacterial isolates well Moxifloxacin dosed less frequently	Expensive Does not cover MRSA[a]
Older fluoroquinolones (ciprofloxacin, ofloxacin)	Broadly effective but growing resistance Lower cost generics available	Good coverage of *H influenzae;* not as good for *S pneumoniae*
Aminoglycosides (0.3% gentamicin, 0.3% tobramycin)	Good gram-negative organism coverage	Limited gram-positive activity; not active against *S pneumoniae* Associated with chemical conjunctivitis/corneal irritation with extended use
Azithromycin	Dosed less frequently Well tolerated	Bacteriostatic; some *S pneumoniae* resistance reported; weak coverage for *H influenzae*
Erythromycin, 0.5%	Good chlamydia and gram-positive organism coverage Inexpensive	Lacks gram-negative (including *H influenzae*) and staphylococcal coverage Minimal usefulness against childhood acute bacterial conjunctivitis
Sulfacetamide	Inexpensive	Stings the eyes Bacteriostatic, with less coverage of typical pathogens Not recommended

Abbreviations: MRSA, methicillin-resistant *Staphylococcus aureus;* MSSA, methicillin-sensitive *Staphylococcus aureus.*
[a] Studies to date suggest MRSA currently remains an uncommon cause of acute bacterial conjunctivitis in otherwise well children.

Note: Neomycin is generally avoided due to increased likelihood of allergic sensitivity. Unless otherwise noted, antibiotics are typically placed in the eye at least 4 times a day.

Newborns suspected of having *N gonorrhoeae* conjunctivitis should be hospitalized and treated with intravenous (IV) or intramuscular ceftriaxone (single dose unless disseminated disease). Because parenteral treatment is necessary, topical treatment is not necessary for gonococcal conjunctivitis. A full septic work-up to exclude disseminated disease such as arthritis, meningitis, and sepsis should be considered. If Gram stain reveals gram-negative diplococci, urgent ophthalmologic consultation should be considered because of the risk for corneal perforation and permanent vision loss. Lavage of the eye with saline solution may assist in removing inflammatory products until the discharge clears. Maternal and maternal partner treatment should also be insured, and testing for chlamydia in infant and mother should be pursued.

Suspected neonatal chlamydial conjunctivitis is treated with 14 days of oral erythromycin base or ethylsuccinate to eliminate nasal carriage. There are limited data to suggest a shorter course of oral azithromycin may be effective. Mother and partner should also be treated for chlamydia. Topical treatment is not necessary or effective in eradication.

Other bacterial causes of ophthalmic neonatorum can be treated with topical antibiotics, with the exception of *P aeruginosa*. Fortunately, *P aeruginosa* conjunctivitis is rare, but concern is raised when gram-negative rods are found on Gram stain. Infection has been associated with corneal perforation, endophthalmitis, and blindness. There is poor penetration of antibiotics into the anterior chamber, so treatment includes topical and parenteral aminoglycoside therapy.

Of note, uncommonly, *N gonorrhea* and *N meningitidis* cause conjunctival infections beyond the neonatal period. These infections also require parenteral therapy, as the risk of complications is high. Because the organism is typically transmitted through sexual contact, a high level of concern should exist for child abuse if gonococcal conjunctivitis occurs in childhood.

Viral

Viral conjunctivitis is usually self-limited, lasting 1 to 3 weeks. Supportive treatment, including artificial tears and cold compresses, may be helpful for symptomatic relief. The importance of good and frequent hand washing should be stressed to the patient and families, including the use of separate towels by infected and noninfected family members, avoidance of touching eyes, and care with hand-to-hand contact.

Neonatal herpes conjunctivitis requires hospitalization and IV acyclovir for 14 to 21 days (depending on whether ophthalmologic manifestations only whether there is further evidence of disseminated or central nervous system disease), as well as a topical ophthalmic antiviral such as 1% trifluridine, 0.1% iododeoxyuridine, or 3% vidarabine. Beyond the neonatal period, topical antivirals are used, with oral acyclovir for more involved cases.

Corticosteroids are generally avoided in infectious conjunctivitis. They may impede microbial clearance, worsen herpes keratitis, and increase intraocular pressure.

Allergic

Supportive treatment for seasonal allergic conjunctivitis includes lubrication with artificial tears (for ocular mucosal allergen dilution and removal), cold compresses (to assist with itchiness), and avoidance of eye rubbing. Environmental controls should be undertaken to avoid or minimize exposures to triggering allergens. Topical dual antihistamine and mast cell stabilizing therapies (ie, olopatadine, ketotifen, and azelastine) are commonly used options and are the first-line pharmacologic choice for many practitioners. Antihistamine assists with rapid initial symptom improvement, and the mast cell stabilizer confers long-term maintenance benefit. H_1-receptor–specific histamine antagonists (ie, levocabastine, emedastine) can be used for intermittent allergic symptoms, particularly itching, in children 12 years and older. Mast cell stabilizers (ie, lodoxamide, nedocromil, pemirolast) alone can be used for chronic allergic symptoms by decreasing mast cell degranulation when exposed to the allergen.

Perennial allergic conjunctivitis is treated with environmental measures and dual antihistamine–mast cell stabilizer topical treatments. In recalcitrant cases, topical steroids and immunomodulating drugs such as tacrolimus and cyclosporine may be considered to further reduce inflammation, usually in consultation with allergists or ophthalmologists. Steroids may be associated with cataracts, increased intraocular pressure, and corneal irregularities. When used in the setting of herpetic conjunctivitis, they can also cause viral proliferation and scarring of the cornea. Immunotherapy may be considered for persistent symptoms in the face of topical and oral treatments.

Long-term Monitoring and Implications

Most infectious conjunctivitis is not associated with long-standing effects, and permanent visual changes are rare in acute seasonal or perennial allergic conjunctivitis. However, some long-term implications should be considered.

- *Neisseria gonorrhoeae* has the potential to lead to visual loss because of corneal ulceration and perforation.
- If chlamydial neonatal conjunctivitis is left untreated, development of chlamydial pneumonia must be considered.
- Herpetic conjunctivitis or keratitis may recur, with increased risk of scarring and visual problems.

Suggested Readings

American Academy of Pediatrics. *Red Book: 2015 Report of the Committee on Infectious Diseases.* Kimberlin DW, Brady MT, Jackson MA, Long SS, eds. 30th ed. Elk Grove Village, IL: American Academy of Pediatrics; 2015

Block SL. Pediatric acute bacterial conjunctivitis: an update. Healio: Infectious Diseases in Children Web site. http://www.healio.com/pediatrics/eye-care/news/online/%7B364d4d0f-901c-41dc-ad8b-ab2fac10edf0%7D/pediatric-acute-bacterial-conjunctivitis-an-update. Published November 1, 2011. Accessed March 3, 2015

Meltzer JA, Kunkov S, Crain EF. Identifying children at low risk for bacterial conjunctivitis. *Arch Pediatr Adolesc Med.* 2010;164(3):263–267

Patel PB, Diaz MC, Bennett JE, Attia MW. Clinical features of bacterial conjunctivitis in children. *Acad Emerg Med.* 2007;14(1):1–5

Pichichero ME, Wagner RS, Granet DB. Pediatric conjunctivitis: clinical decision-making for optimal treatment. Healio: Infectious Diseases in Children Web site. http://www.healio.com/pediatrics/news/online/%7B6909a6dd-b4ea-40f9-903a-d63158a3f5aa%7D/pediatric-conjunctivitis-clinical-decision-making-for-optimal-treatment. Published June 1, 2011. Accessed March 3, 2015

Richards A, Guzman-Cottrill JA. Conjunctivitis. *Pediatr Rev.* 2010;31(5):196–208

Seth D, Khan FI. Causes and management of red eye in pediatric ophthalmology. *Curr Allergy Asthma Rep.* 2011;11(3):212–219

Sheikh A, Hurwitz B, van Schayck CP, McLean S, Nurmatov U. Antibiotics versus placebo for acute bacterial conjunctivitis. *Cochrane Database of Syst Rev.* 2012;9:CD001211

Wagner RS, Aquino M. Pediatric ocular inflammation. *Immunol Allergy Clin North Am.* 2008;28(1):169–188

Williams L, Malhotra Y, Murante B, et al. A single-blinded randomized clinical trial comparing polymyxin B-trimethoprim and moxifloxacin for treatment of acute conjunctivitis in children. *J Pediatr.* 2013;162(4):857–861

CHAPTER 14

Constipation and Encopresis

Jason E. Dranove, MD

Key Points

- The vast majority of constipation is functional (ie, not due to an underlying organic etiology).

- A thorough history and physical without "red flags" is usually all that is needed to make an accurate diagnosis of functional constipation.

- Fecal impactions must be cleared in order for maintenance treatment to be successful.

- Not all patients with soiling have constipation or a fecal impaction (ie, nonretentive fecal incontinence).

Overview

Up to 3% of visits to general pediatricians and 25% of visits to a pediatric gastro-enterologist concern the issues of constipation and encopresis. Although parents commonly worry about a serious underlying condition, more than 95% of cases are considered "functional" (no identifiable metabolic, neurologic, or anatomic cause) and require no significant work-up. A thorough history and physical examination identifies the diagnosis in most cases (Evidence Level III). Formal definitions have been developed (Box 14-1).

Box 14-1. Definition of Functional Constipation

Two of the following signs/symptoms present for at least 1 month
■ 2 or fewer defecations per week
■ At least 1 episode of incontinence after the acquisition of toileting skills (infants and toddlers) or at least 1 episode of fecal incontinence per week (children 4–18 y)
■ History of excessive stool retention
■ Painful or hard bowel movements
■ Presence of a large fecal mass in the rectum
■ History of large diameter stools that may obstruct the toilet

When constipation progresses to the point of a rectal fecal impaction, encopresis (the involuntary passage of stool) can ensue. A related but pathophysiologically separate condition exists in which the child beyond the toilet-training age (developmental age of at least 4 y) has fecal soiling in the absence of functional fecal retention. This condition is called non-retentive fecal incontinence.

Key facts to assist the practitioner in identifying functional versus organic causes of constipation are as follows (Evidence Level III):

▶ Lack of a meconium bowel movement in the first 48 hours of life warrants mandatory investigation for Hirschsprung disease or anorectal malformations.

▶ Breastfed babies can stool as frequently as every feeding or as infrequently as every 10 to 14 days and still be considered healthy.

▶ Average stool frequency peaks in infancy at roughly 3 times per day and slows to roughly 1 time per day as the child approaches 1 year of age.

▶ Infants often appear to be constipated, strain, and have discomfort when passing stool. Passage of a soft bowel movement relieves the discomfort. This behavior is called infantile dyschezia and typically resolves by 6 months of age.

▶ Functional constipation peaks in onset at 3 particular times: transition from formula or human milk to cow's milk, toilet training, and the commencement of school.

▶ Non-retentive encopresis is often seen in the context of behavioral comorbidities or significant stress.

Causes

Functional constipation is the most common cause of constipation and encopresis in all age groups except the immediate newborn. The most well-accepted cause of constipation is that the child passes a painful or uncomfortable bowel movement and when further urges for defecation occur, the child consciously or unconsciously withholds stool by contracting the gluteal and pelvic muscles. Eventually, the rectum habituates to the stimulus of the enlarging fecal mass, the urge to defecate subsides, and a viscous cycle ensues.

Although children with behavioral and developmental challenges, such as attention-deficit/hyperactivity disorder, sensory integration dysfunction, and autism spectrum disorder, are at higher risk of constipation, they are generally included in the functional category barring other findings. The differential diagnosis is shown in Box 14-2.

Box 14-2. Organic Causes of Constipation

Anatomic malformations	Intestinal muscle/nerve disorders
■ Imperforate anus	■ Hirschsprung disease
■ Anal stenosis	■ Internal anal sphincter achalasia
■ Anteriorly displaced anus	■ Scleroderma
	■ Systemic lupus erythematosus
	■ Generalized hypotonia (eg, Down syndrome, muscular dystrophy)
Metabolic abnormalities	**Drugs**
■ Hypothyroidism	■ Opiates
■ Hypercalcemia	■ Anticholinergics
■ Hypokalemia	■ Phenobarbital
■ Cystic fibrosis	
■ Celiac disease	
Neuropathic	**Other**
■ Myelomeningocele	■ Lead intoxication
■ Spinal cord injury/trauma	■ Botulism
■ Spinal dysraphism	■ Cow's milk protein intolerance
■ Cerebral palsy	■ History of sexual, physical, or emotional abuse

Evaluation

History

Clues to functional constipation include the onset of constipation at common times (eg, transition from formula or human milk to cow's milk, toilet training, or school entrance) and observance of voluntary stool withholding by parents, such as leg straightening, gluteal clenching, standing with legs crossed in a hunched position, and disappearance of the child into another room during times of defecation. The presence of small amounts of bright red blood on the outside of the stool or upon wiping likely indicates an anal fissure. Bright red blood persistently mixed in stool is more concerning for an underlying organic cause. Rectal prolapse can be seen in functional constipation, but recurrent prolapse without obvious constipation should prompt concern for cystic fibrosis. Cow's milk allergy or intolerance is not a proven cause, but if intake is excessive, it could be a possible contributor by an unknown mechanism (Evidence Level III). Patients with fecal impactions frequently have urinary soiling secondary to bladder compression, which can lead to frequent urinary tract infections. Although no direct correlation has been proven, poor clear liquid intake and fiber-poor diets may contribute to constipation (Evidence Level III). The red flags on history which can indicate underlying organic pathology are described in Table 14-1.

Table 14-1. Historical Clues to Etiology of Constipation

Findings on History	Associated Conditions
Delayed passage of meconium	Hirschsprung disease Imperforate anus Small left colon Meconium ileus ·
Poor growth/heat or cold intolerance	Hypothyroidism
FTT, extraintestinal manifestations, abdominal distension, anemia, hypoalbuminemia	Celiac disease
Refractory urinary incontinence/recurrent UTI	Spinal cord abnormality
Acute-onset constipation	Sexual abuse Spinal cord injury/tumor
Recurrent respiratory tract infections and FTT, rectal prolapse	Cystic fibrosis
Honey ingestion in infant	Botulism
Sudden bloody diarrhea in a constipated infant	Hirschsprung enterocolitis
Lower extremity weakness, numbness, tingling	Spinal cord abnormality
Developmental delay/hypotonia	Chromosomal abnormality Muscular dystrophies
Recurrent abdominal distension	Pseudo-obstruction Hirschsprung disease Recurrent sigmoid volvulus
Persistent bright red blood mixed in stool	Large polyp or obstructing mass
Fecal incontinence with no Hx of constipation	Non-retentive encopresis

Abbreviations: FTT, failure to thrive; Hx, history; UTI, urinary tract infection.

Physical Examination

Typical physical examination findings for functional constipation include within–reference range growth parameters, a palpable fecal mass in the suprapubic area, and normal lower extremity deep tendon reflexes, strength, and gait, as well as normal cremasteric reflexes in males. A perianal examination should be performed to assess for anal position, injury, and fissure, as well as gluteal musculature. A digital rectal examination with the fifth finger should be performed in all constipated infants to assess sphincter tone and anal position (Evidence Level III). Rectal examination in older patients is not mandatory if the practitioner is confident in the diagnosis. The lower back should be examined for signs of spinal dysraphism (eg, tuft of hair, deep dimple). The following red flag findings can easily be ascertained on physical examination (Table 14-2).

Table 14-2. Physical Examination Clues to Etiology of Constipation

Examination Finding	Condition Suggested
Short stature, coarse hair, macroglossia	Hypothyroidism
Sacral dimple, sacral tuft, absent DTR	Spina bifida (eg, myelomeningocele) Tethered spinal cord
Explosive stool upon finger withdrawal on rectal examination of infant	Hirschsprung disease
Absent or very small anal opening	Imperforate anus/anorectal malformation
Very tight anal canal of infant	Hirschsprung disease or anal stenosis
FTT, dermatitis herpetiformis, abdominal distension	Celiac disease
Hypotonia	Muscular dystrophy/SMA
Coarse lungs, fingernail clubbing, abdominal distension, rectal prolapse, FTT	Cystic fibrosis

Abbreviations: DTR, deep tendon refleses; FTT, failure to thrive; SMA, spinal muscular atrophy.

Laboratory Studies

Because most cases of functional constipation can be diagnosed based on history and physical examination, no work-up is required (Evidence Level III). If the abdominal examination does not reveal an obvious fecal mass and a rectal examination is not performed, an abdominal radiograph can be helpful (Evidence Level II-2). Work-up is not indicated unless the patient has red flag findings on history or physical examination or has failed aggressive medical management and education. The North American Society for Pediatric Gastroenterology, Hepatology, and Nutrition has published an algorithm to guide practitioners in evaluation of constipation (Figure 14-1).

In children older than 1 year, the only tests recommended for refractory constipation include thyroid studies, a lead level test, serum calcium and potassium concentration tests, a tissue transglutaminase IgA antibody level test, and a total serum IgA count (to rule out celiac disease) (Evidence Level III). A barium enema is not recommended to diagnose Hirschsprung disease, as the diagnosis can be missed by this modality. The only reliable method of diagnosis of Hirschsprung disease is by lack of demonstration of ganglion cells on appropriate depth rectal biopsy or by lack of relaxation of the internal anal sphincter on an anorectal manometry (Evidence Level II-1). Cases truly refractory to medical management may require more in-depth testing (Box 14-3).

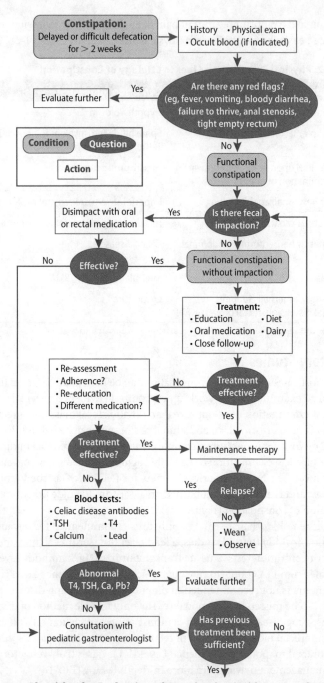

Figure 14-1. Algorithm for Evaluation of Constipation (Evidence Level III).

continued from bottom of previous page

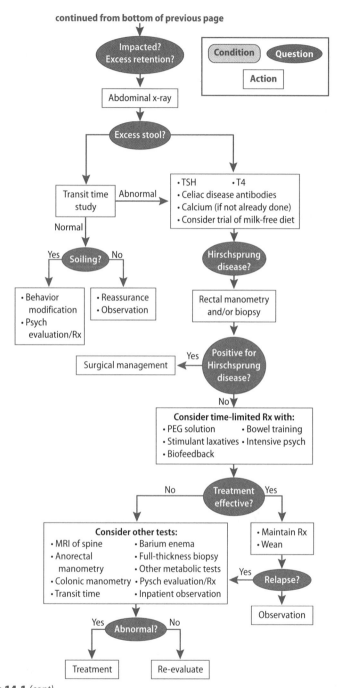

Figure 14-1 *(cont)*

Abbreviations: exam, examination; MRI, magnetic resonance imaging; PEG, polyethylene glycol; psych, psychiatric; T4, anti-thyroxine; Rx, prescription; TSH, thyroid-stimulating hormone.

From Constipation Guideline Committee of the North American Society for Pediatric Gastroenterology, Hepatology, and Nutrition. Evaluation and treatment of constipation in infants and children: recommendations of the North American Society for Pediatric Gastroenterology, Hepatology, and Nutrition. *J Pediatr Gastroenterol Nutr.* 2006;43(3):e1–e13, with permission.

Box 14-3. Additional Testing at Subspecialty Level

Radiography ■ Radiopaque marker transit study ■ Barium enema ■ Lumbosacral spine MRI
Physiologic testing ■ Anorectal manometry ■ Colonic manometry
Tissue sample ■ Rectal suction biopsy ■ Full-thickness rectal wall biopsy

Abbreviation: MRI, magnetic resonance imaging.

Management

Disimpaction

The key to successful management of constipation involves staged therapy with disimpaction followed by maintenance therapy and ongoing educational/behavioral modification. Disimpaction is not necessary in all cases; however, initiating maintenance therapy prior to disimpaction if a fecal impaction is present can lead to soiling, increased patient frustration, and distrust of medications. Clearing a fecal impaction will usually allow the rectum to decompress and regain sensation and tone.

Disimpaction can be accomplished via the oral, rectal, or combined route (Level Evidence II-3). In most cases, an initial trial of oral disimpaction with osmotic and occasionally stimulant laxatives is successful (Evidence Level II-3). Dosing varies by age and practitioner, but most treating clinicians use polyethylene glycol 3350 (PEG 3350), an osmotic laxative, as the main component (Box 14-4).

Maintenance

In children without impaction, or after disimpaction is complete, maintenance treatment is initiated. The goals of treatment are to achieve 1 to 2 soft stools a day (of pudding or mashed potato consistency), resolution of soiling, return of rectal sensation, empowerment of the child, and removing negative emotions associated with the defecation process. Patients with mild cases might respond to simple measures such as increased fiber in the diet, increased clear fluids, and fruit juices with nonabsorbable sugars such as pear, prune, or apple juice (Evidence Level II-3). Polyethylene glycol 3350 is the mainstay of treatment; it is an osmotic laxative that helps soften and lubricate stool. It is safe for use down to 6 months of age (Evidence Level III). No serious adverse effects from PEG 3350 have been reported; the most common adverse effects are diarrhea, bloating, and abdominal cramping, which can usually be managed with titration of dosing. Although PEG 3350 is likely safe for all ages, lactulose is recommended first line for babies younger than 6 months (Evidence Level III). After infancy, stimulant laxatives may be used intermittently for breakthrough constipation or if the symptoms are not adequately responding to osmotic laxatives (Evidence Level II-1) (Table 14-3).

Box 14-4. Levine Children's Hospital One-Day Bowel Cleanout

Age 1-2
PEG 3350, 2 rounded teaspoons mixed in 4 oz of clear liquid hourly until stool clear.

Age 3-5
PEG 3350, 4 capfuls mixed in 24 oz of clear liquid. Give 4 oz q 30 minutes as tolerated; give 1 crushed tablet of Bisacodyl 5 mg prior to and after PEG solution.

Age 6-11
PEG 3350, 6–8 capfuls mixed in 24–48 oz of clear liquid. Give 4 oz q 30 minutes as tolerated; give 1 tablet of Bisacodyl prior to and after PEG solution.

Age 12 and up
PEG 3350, 8–10 capfuls mixed in 32–48 oz of clear liquid. Give 4 oz q 30 minutes as tolerated; give 2 tablets of Bisacodyl prior to and after PEG solution.

Sodium phosphate enema[a] administration (if needed)
Age <2: not routinely recommended
Age 2–4: 33.75 mL
Age 5–11: 67.5 mL
Age 12+: 118 mL
Give one Bisacodyl tablet = 5 mg; give one capful of PEG 3350 = 17 g.

Abbreviation: PEG, polyethylene glycol; q, every.

[a] Sodium phosphate enema = monobasic sodium phosphate monohydrate 19 g and dibasic sodium phosphate heptahydrate 7 g per 118 mL.

Table 14-3. Common Medications for Maintenance Treatment

Medication	Dose	Notes
Osmotic laxatives		
Lactulose	10 g/15 mL liquid 1–3 mL/kg/d in 2 divided doses	Best for age <6 mo Can cause irritability because of flatulence and increased gas
Magnesium hydroxide	400 mg/5 mL 1–3 mL/kg/d	Should be used cautiously in infants
PEG 3350	One capful = 17 g 0.7–1.0 g/kg/d	Widespread use in infants not studied Should be mixed with clear liquid for best palatability
Stimulant laxatives		
Senna	8.8 mg/5 mL 8.6 mg tablet 2–6 y: 2.5–7.5 mL/d ≥6 y: 1–3 tablets per day	Best used intermittently May be used as maintenance therapy in refractory cases
Bisacodyl	5 mg tablet (may be crushed) 3–11 y: 2.5–5 mg/dose >11 y: 5–10 mg/dose	Best used intermittently Use limited by adverse effects of cramping and abdominal pain

Abbreviation: PEG, polyethylene glycol.

Education/Behavioral Modification

When dealing with constipation, education as well as continued reassurance and positive reinforcement are just as important as medications. Attempting bowel movements twice a day, after breakfast and dinner, helps the patient take advantage of the gastrocolic reflex. Other strategies to consider include

▶ Eliminating distractions while in the bathroom (ie, electronic devices and games)

▶ Limiting attempts to 5 to 10 minutes (Longer attempts without successful passage of a bowel movement can increase frustration and defiance.)

▶ Using maneuvers to increase the Valsalva maneuver, such as blowing up a balloon or blowing on the back of the hand

▶ Using a reasonable reward system, focusing on the positives and avoiding negative reinforcement

▶ Increasing intake of clear fluids, fiber, and fruit and vegetables (Although these nourishments are not scientifically proven to help, they are generally viewed as helpful.)

Milk elimination is not routinely recommended, although cutting back on excessive intake is reasonable. In general, if constipation starts during potty training, attempts at weaning therapy prior to successful toileting independence are not advised, as hard or painful stools can impair progress in this endeavor.

Long-term Monitoring

Laboratory or radiographic studies are not recommended routinely during the course of treatment. Poorly controlled constipation over many years can result in quality of life impairment, social isolation, and family stress. In fact, up to 50% of patients relapse within 2 years after an initial successful period (Evidence Level II-3). No official guidelines on length of treatment are available. A large study from Europe showed that up to 70% of patients will be successfully treated 5 years after diagnosis, with most off of laxatives, so overall the prognosis is positive (Evidence Level II-3).

Suggested Reading

Bongers EJ, Tabbers MM, Benninga MA. Functional nonretentive fecal incontinence in children. *J Pediatr Gastroenterol Nutr.* 2007;44(1):5–13

Constipation Guideline Committee of the North American Society for Pediatric Gastroenterology, Hepatology, and Nutrition. Evaluation and treatment of constipation in infants and children: recommendations of the North American Society for Pediatric Gastroenterology, Hepatology, and Nutrition. *J Pediatr Gastroenterol Nutr.* 2006;43(3):e1–e13

Marloes EK, Bongers EJ, Van Wijk MP, Benninga MA. Long-term prognosis for childhood constipation: clinical outcomes in adulthood. *Pediatrics.* 2010;126(1):e156–e162

Kaugars A, Silverman A, Kinservik, et al. Families' perspectives on the effect of constipation and fecal incontinence on quality of life. *J Pediatr Gastroenterol Nutr.* 2010;51(6):747–752

Pashankar DS, Bishop WP. Efficacy and optimal dose of daily polyethylene glycol 3350 for treatment of constipation and encopresis in children. *Pediatrics.* 2001;139(3):428–432

Michail S, Gendy E, Preud'Homme D, Mezoff A. Polyethylene glycol for constipation in children younger than eighteen months old. *J Pediatr Gastroenterol Nutr.* 2004;39(2):197–199

Pashankar DS, Loening-Baucke V, Bisohp WP. Safety of polyethylene glycol 3350 for the treatment of chronic constipation in children. *Arch Pediatr Adolesc Med.* 2003;157(7):661–664

CHAPTER 15

Cough

Erin H. Stubbs, MD

Key Points

- The most common cause of acute cough is viral upper respiratory tract infection.
- Patients with chronic cough warrant further evaluation for a specific cause.
- Use of over-the-counter cough and cold medications is not recommended in children.
- Education and reassurance are essential to alleviate parental anxiety associated with cough.

Overview

Cough is one of the most frequent complaints encountered in pediatric practice. The most common cause of cough is acute viral respiratory tract illness, which is self-limited, although cough may be the presenting symptom for a more serious underlying problem. Cough disrupts sleep, interferes with feeding, may precipitate vomiting, and can affect school performance. During the patient encounter, the pediatrician must identify patients at risk for poorer prognosis or complications and not unnecessarily prescribe antibiotics.

Definitions

The term *cough* refers to a high-velocity expiration, usually against a closed glottis, which makes a characteristic sound.

Acute cough refers to a cough lasting less than 3 weeks. Viral infection of the upper respiratory tract is the most common cause of acute cough. Other causes of acute cough include reactive airway disease, sinusitis, allergy, irritants, and foreign body aspiration. Patients may have recurrent acute cough secondary to repeated acute viral respiratory infections.

Subacute or *prolonged acute cough* is a cough lasting between 3 to 8 weeks. Subacute cough may be secondary to a slowly resolving post viral cough; however, if the cough is progressively worsening during this time frame, further investigation may be warranted.

Chronic cough is defined as a daily cough lasting more than 8 weeks. Chronic cough usually warrants further evaluation or treatment. Conditions associated with chronic cough are listed in Box 15-1.

Box 15-1. Causes of Chronic Cough

- Infection (pertussis, *Chlamydia*, tuberculosis, mycoplasma)
- Asthma
- Sinusitis
- Allergy
- Irritants (tobacco smoke, pollution)
- Occupational exposure
- Foreign body aspiration
- Aspiration
- Gastroesophageal reflux
- Psychogenic cough
- Congenital anomaly
  - Tracheoesophageal fistula
  - Laryngeal cleft
  - Vocal cord paralysis
  - Bronchogenic cyst
  - Aberrant mediastinal vessels
- Tracheobronchomalacia
- Congenital heart disease
- Cystic fibrosis
- Immunodeficiency states
- Primary ciliary dyskinesia
- Mediastinal tumor or other malignancy
- Pulmonary hemosiderosis

A *habit cough* or *psychogenic cough* lasts weeks to months, is not responsive to treatment, and disappears during sleep or with distraction. In many cases, habit cough starts with an upper respiratory tract infection but lingers beyond the expected time frame. Habit cough is often a diagnosis of exclusion.

Evaluation

When taking the history from a patient with concern of cough, it is important to assess the duration of cough as well as the quality, timing, triggers, and any associated symptoms such as fever or postnasal drainage. Distinguishing between acute, subacute, and chronic cough is helpful to aid in diagnosis and management (Figures 15-1 to 15-3). The past medical and family histories may also provide important clues to the etiology of cough. A past history of atopic conditions or a strong family history of asthma may increase suspicion for reactive airway disease, while a history of malabsorption or failure to thrive may suggest cystic fibrosis. The practitioner should inquire about exposure to persons with infections such as tuberculosis or pertussis. For patients with chronic cough, taking an environmental history is also useful to inquire about exposures such as cigarette smoke, mold, dust mites, and pets. Red flags in the history indicating a potentially more serious diagnosis include failure to thrive, weight loss, history of unusual infections, and persistent fever (Table 15-1).

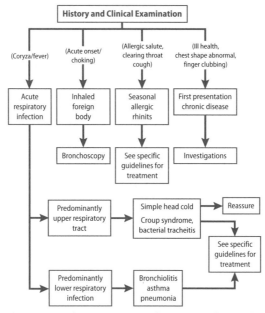

Figure 15-1. Assessment and management of acute cough (<3 wk).

From Shields MD3, Bush A, Everard ML, et al. BTS guidelines: recommendations for the assessment and management of cough in children. *Thorax.* 2008;63:iii1–iii15, with permission.

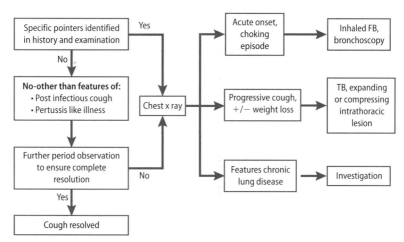

Figure 15-2. Assessment and management of prolonged acute cough (3–8 wk).

Abbreviations: FB, foreign body; TB, tuberculosis.

From Shields MD, Bush A, Everard ML, et al. BTS guidelines: recommendations for the assessment and management of cough in children. *Thorax.* 2008;63:iii1–iii15, with permission.

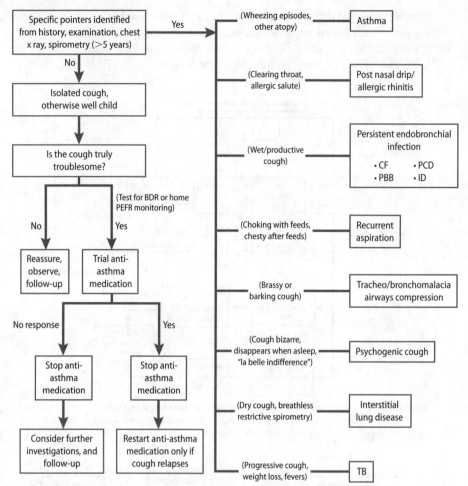

Figure 15-3. Assessment and management of chronic cough (>8 wk).

Abbreviations: BDR, bronchodilator responsiveness; CF, cystic fibrosis; ID, infectious disease; PBB, persistent bacterial bronchitis; PCD, primary ciliary dyskinesia; PEFR, peak expiratory flow rate; TB, tuberculosis.

From Shields MD, Bush A, Everard ML, et al. BTS guidelines: recommendations for the assessment and management of cough in children. *Thorax.* 2008;63:iii1–iii15, with permission.

Table 15-1. Clinical Clues About Cough

Characteristic	Think Of
Staccato, paroxysmal	Pertussis, cystic fibrosis, foreign body, *Chlamydia* spp, *Mycoplasma* spp
Followed by "whoop"	Pertussis
All day, never during sleep	Habit (tic) cough
Barking, brassy	Croup, psychogenic, tracheomalacia, tracheitis, epiglottitis
Hoarseness	Laryngeal involvement (croup, recurrent laryngeal nerve involvement)
Abrupt onset	Foreign body, pulmonary embolism
Follows exercise	Reactive airways disease
Accompanies eating, drinking	Aspiration, gastroesophageal reflux, tracheoesophageal fistula
Throat clearing	Postnasal drip, vocal tic
Productive (sputum)	Infection
Night cough	Sinusitis, reactive airways disease
Seasonal	Allergic rhinitis, reactive airways disease
Immunosuppressed patient	Bacterial pneumonia, *Pneumocystis jiroveci*, *Mycobacterium tuberculosis*, *Mycobacterium avium-intracellulare*, cytomegalovirus
Dyspnea	Hypoxia, hypercarbia
Animal exposure	*Chlamydia psittaci* (birds), *Yersinia pestis* (rodents), *Francisella tularensis* (rabbits), Q fever (sheep, cattle), hantavirus (rodents), histoplasmosis (pigeons)
Geographic	Histoplasmosis (Mississippi, Missouri, Ohio River Valley), coccidioidomycosis (southwest), blastomycosis (north and Midwest)
Workdays with clearing on days off	Occupational exposure

Abbreviation: spp, species.
From Kliegman RM, Greenbaum LA, Lyle PS. *Practical Strategies in Pediatric Diagnosis and Therapy*. 2nd ed. Philadelphia, PA: Saunders; 2004:19, with permission.

The physical examination can help identify the origin of the cough as and is also important to identify signs of a more serious underlying condition. First, the practitioner should note the patient's general appearance, assessing for appropriate growth and development. Then, thorough examination of the upper and lower airway should be completed with the patient's cooperation. Stridor indicates upper airway disease, whereas expiratory wheeze or rhonchi suggest distal airway disease. It is useful to witness the patient's cough for further characterization. The examination should also include evaluation of the nasal mucosa, oropharynx, ears, heart, and extremities (to look for clubbing). For patients with acute cough, fever, tachypnea, and increased work of breathing are all signs of a poorer prognosis. For patients with chronic cough, poor growth, clubbing, heart murmurs, and lymphadenopathy may indicate a more worrisome diagnosis.

Imaging and Laboratory Studies

The diagnostic evaluation should be guided by key features of the patient's history and physical examination. In most cases of acute cough, further evaluation is not necessary. One exception is if foreign body is suspected; urgent bronchoscopy is recommended. For patients with chronic cough, further evaluation is usually warranted with a chest x-ray (CXR). Potential CXR findings include infiltrates (pneumonia), volume loss (foreign body), hyperinflation (asthma), mediastinal nodes (tuberculosis or malignancy), and cardiomegaly (pulmonary edema). Spirometry or trial of a bronchodilator is also useful for evaluation of chronic cough.

Laboratory studies will be guided by the differential diagnosis. A sweat chloride test or CFTR (cystic fibrosis transmembrane conductance regulator) mutation panel should be performed on any patient for whom cystic fibrosis is a concern. A purified protein derivative can be placed to rule out tuberculosis. To diagnose pertussis, polymerase chain reaction is the criterion standard. If gastroesophageal reflux is suspected as the cause of chronic cough, the patient may be started empirically on an acid reducer or may be referred to a gastroenterologist for further testing such as pH probe or a barium swallow. Ultimately, patients with undiagnosed chronic cough may undergo bronchoscopy by a pulmonologist.

Treatment

For treatment of cough, the key is to treat the underlying cause and not just treat cough as a symptom. Parents should be informed that cough associated with a viral upper respiratory tract illness can to last up to 2 to 3 weeks and, in some instances, even longer. Clinicians should avoid overprescribing antibiotics for cough. Antibiotics may also be prescribed when rhinosinusitis is present and not improving after 10 days or for other documented infections such as tuberculosis or pertussis. If reactive airway disease is high on the differential, a trial of a bronchodilator is warranted. Antihistamines and intranasal steroids are beneficial for children with cough due to allergies.

Despite the widespread use of over-the-counter (OTC) cough and cold medicines, their effectiveness has not been proven in children. A recent review found that antitussives, antihistamines, antihistamine decongestants, and antitussive/ bronchodilator combinations were no more effective than placebo at treating cough. Furthermore, the use of OTC cough and cold medicines is associated with medication errors and adverse events; therefore, their use should be strongly discouraged. Similarly, there is no strong evidence for the use of other common remedies, such as humidified air, vitamin C, Echinacea, or zinc. Recent studies have shown honey to be beneficial in improving cough in children with upper respiratory tract infections, and this can be recommended to parents of children 1 year and older.

Suggested Reading

Chang AB. Pediatric cough: children are not miniature adults. *Lung.* 2010;188(Suppl 1):s33–s40

Cohen HA, Rozen J, Kristal H, et al. Effect of honey on nocturnal cough and sleep quality: a double-blind, randomized, placebo-controlled study. *Pediatrics.* 2012;130(3):465–471

Goldman RD. Treating cough and cold: guidance for caregivers of children and youth. *Paediatr Child Health.* 2011;16(9):564–566

Hayward G, Thompson M, Hay AD. What factors influence prognosis in children with acute cough and respiratory tract infection in primary care? *BMJ.* 2012;345:e6212

Marcus MG. Cough. In: McInerny TK, ed. *American Academy of Pediatrics Textbook of Pediatric Care.* Elk Grove Village, IL: American Academy of Pediatrics; 2009;1432–1436

Smith SM, Schroeder K, Fahey T. Over-the-counter (OTC) medications for acute cough in children and adults in ambulatory settings. *Cochrane Database Syst Rev.* 2012;8:CD001831

CHAPTER 16

Croup and Epiglottitis

Kimberly Marohn, MD, and John S. Giuliano, Jr, MD

KEY POINTS

- Croup is one of the most common childhood respiratory illnesses.

- Croup is a clinical diagnosis, and usually no laboratory or radiographic studies are necessary to begin treatment.

- Epiglottitis remains rare but is more commonly diagnosed among school-aged children, and *Streptococcus* is emerging as the predominant pathogen.

- Epiglottitis is a clinical diagnosis confirmed by direct visualization of the epiglottis.

- Establishing an advanced airway prior to the development of total airway obstruction is paramount when managing a patient with epiglottitis.

Croup

Overview

Laryngotracheobronchitis, commonly known as croup, is one of the most common childhood respiratory illnesses. Classically, children present with inspiratory stridor and a characteristic cough that is often described as "barky" or "seal-like." Patients usually present between the ages of 6 months and 3 years, with the highest incidence in the second year of life. The disease is typically benign and self-limiting; however, rare cases can result in significant respiratory distress and failure requiring endotracheal intubation.

The name *croup* has been used to describe a variety of diseases presenting with stridor and cough including viral laryngotracheitis, bacterial tracheitis, epiglottitis, and diphtheria infection. For the purpose of this chapter discussion, the term *croup* will be used to refer to viral laryngotracheitis.

Causes and Differential Diagnosis

Croup is often caused by a virus, parainfluenza type 1 being the most common, but all 3 serotypes have been isolated. Children with parainfluenza type 3 infection are more likely to require hospital admission compared to serotypes 1 and 2. Other viral etiologies include respiratory syncytial virus, influenza, adenovirus, rhinovirus, human coronavirus, and human metapneumovirus. Identification of the specific virus can be helpful when cohorting patients who require hospitalization, but the clinical course and treatment are the same regardless of the underlying viral etiology.

Classically, children with croup wake abruptly in the middle of the night with respiratory distress following a prodrome of cough, coryza, and rhinorrhea. Physical examination findings include inspiratory stridor and a harsh, barky cough in addition to other symptoms of viral upper respiratory infection (URI), including rhinorrhea and nasal congestion. Children with croup may also present with a hoarse voice and fever. Respiratory distress typically occurs 12 to 24 hours following the onset of URI.

Croup is, therefore, a clinical diagnosis, and no laboratory or radiographic studies are necessary to begin treatment. Accurate assessment of the degree of airway obstruction is key to management. The presence of stridor and suprasternal retractions are the most reliable signs of airway obstruction on physical examination. Stridor at rest indicates the presence of fixed airway obstruction, whereas stridor that occurs only when the child is upset indicates dynamic airway obstruction and is less concerning. Children with severe airway obstruction may also present with a prolonged inspiratory phase, decreased breath sounds, retractions, and may appear anxious or air hungry. This may progress to hypoxia and respiratory failure. Signs of impending respiratory failure include fatigue, decreased level of consciousness, cyanosis, poor air entry, and tachycardia out of proportion to what would be expected from fever alone. If there is concern for impending respiratory failure, early intubation is warranted.

Clinical Features

Epiglottitis

Children with bacterial epiglottitis typically present in moderate to severe respiratory distress with high fever (see page 166 for a more detailed account of epiglottitis). On physical examination, they often appear anxious and may sit in a tripod or sniffing position in an attempt to relieve the respiratory distress. Drooling and difficulty swallowing are often present.

Bacterial Tracheitis

Children with bacterial tracheitis also present with a high fever and may appear toxic on examination. This is caused by a bacterial infection within the subglottic level of the trachea. Respiratory distress is the result of airway obstruction from purulent secretions, which may be visible on examination. These children also may have signs of lower airway disease such as crackles or wheeze. Bacterial tracheitis may occur as a primary or secondary infection in the setting of a primary viral process. More of these patients require endotracheal intubation during the acute phase of the disease compared with patients with viral croup.

Spasmodic Croup

Spasmodic croup is often initially difficult to differentiate from viral croup because the presentation is very similar, including barky cough and inspiratory stridor. The hallmark of spasmodic croup is the short duration of symptoms (often resolved by the time the child seeks medical treatment) and the frequent recurrence of symptoms. Children are typically very well appearing between attacks, and the symptoms usually present at night.

Bronchiolitis

Bronchiolitis is a viral infection of the lower airways (see Chapter 10). Children may present with cough, coryza, and fever but typically do not have inspiratory stridor. They usually present with crackles, rhonchi, wheezes, and evidence of decreased air movement on examination consistent with lower airway disease.

Peritonsillar Abscess

Children with peritonsillar abscesses can present with high fevers and toxic appearance in addition to respiratory distress. The classic physical examination finding for a peritonsillar abscess is deviation of the uvula away from the side of the abscess. Children may also present with neck extension, difficulty swallowing, and drooling. The barky cough that is the hallmark of croup is typically absent.

Retropharyngeal Abscess

Children typically present with persistently high fevers and neck extension with retropharyngeal abscesses. These patients usually appear toxic on examination. Lateral neck radiographs will demonstrate thickening of the prevertebral space at the location of the abscess. Barky cough is typically absent. Laboratory studies may show increased white blood cell count as well as other elevated inflammatory markers such as erythrocyte sedimentation rate and C-reactive protein.

Foreign Body Ingestion

If a history of foreign body ingestion is not offered, a high index of suspicion is needed. Many will describe a sudden onset of symptoms in a child who was previously healthy. Inspiratory stridor and barky cough may be present due to upper airway obstruction, but these children will not have fever. Radiopaque objects, such as coins and batteries, may be visible on chest radiographs.

Allergic Reaction/Angioedema/Anaphylaxis

Children with these conditions may have a history of ingesting a substance to which they have a known allergy. Typically, allergic reactions and edema will cause swelling of the face, lips, and tongue that is absent in croup. These children may also have an urticarial rash. Fever and URI symptoms are typically absent.

Upper Airway Injury

Upper airway injury can be caused by blunt trauma to the neck or burns caused by smoke inhalation during a fire. Fever and URI symptoms are generally not present, and these children often will have evidence of other injuries.

Diphtheria

Much less common due to widespread use of immunizations, children with *Corynebacterium diphtheriae* infection will present with high fever and moderate to severe respiratory distress. They generally appear toxic on examination. The hallmark finding of the physical examination is the diphtheritic membrane, which is visible on examination of the oropharynx causing airway obstruction.

Congenital Airway Anomalies

Congenital anomalies such as laryngomalacia, subglottic stenosis, laryngeal webs, airway hemangiomas, and vocal cord paralysis may present as recurrent episodes of severe croup. Underlying narrowing of the airway will make children more susceptible to severe croup in the presence of viral illness. Children with recurrent episodes of croup should prompt an evaluation for congenital airway anomalies.

Evaluation

There are several important questions to be asked when taking a history that will help distinguish croup from other causes of respiratory distress. Fever may be present or absent in viral croup. Persistent high fever is concerning for bacterial infection such as epiglottitis or an abscess. Absence of fever combined with abrupt cessation of symptoms may lead one to consider a diagnosis of spasmodic croup. A hoarse voice and barky cough are characteristic of viral croup but are generally absent in children with epiglottitis or abscess. Additionally, children with croup typically do not present with throat pain, difficulty swallowing, or drooling. The presence of these signs and symptoms is more consistent with more worrisome bacterial infections. Foreign body aspiration may also present similarly but without fever.

Laboratory and radiographic studies are only warranted if the diagnosis of croup is in question. The steeple sign seen on anteroposterior neck radiograph is caused by edema in the proximal trachea and is classically associated with croup. Lateral neck radiographs may also demonstrate subglottic haziness. Children old enough to cooperate with an inspiratory film may demonstrate overdistension of the hypopharynx on lateral neck radiograph. Blood tests are not usually helpful in establishing a diagnosis but may be necessary to rule out other causes of respiratory distress in more severe cases. White blood cell counts may be normal or elevated and can have a lymphocytic or neutrophilic predominance. A significant bandemia on differential may indicate the presence of a more serious bacterial infection. A nasopharyngeal viral direct fluorescent antibody test can be sent to determine the specific viral etiology but will not affect the course of treatment. This may be useful in children who require hospitalization to assist in cohorting.

A number of clinical tools have been developed to assist in assessing the severity of a patient with croup. Some institutions may use croup scoring tools, while others employ croup management algorithms, to drive therapies and patient admission (Figure 16-1), but all available tools focus on stridor at rest and the presence of retractions to assess the degree of respiratory distress. A Westley score of 2 or less is consistent with mild croup; a score of 3 to 7 is consistent with moderate croup; and a score of 8 or more is consistent with severe croup. Prompt identification and treatment of children with severe croup is paramount.

Management

Accurate assessment of the degree of airway obstruction is key to management of croup. Children with severe obstruction and signs of impending respiratory failure may require advanced airway management. The goal of management is to decrease patient agitation and the degree of airway inflammation and swelling to improve respiratory mechanics. Glucocorticoids and nebulized epinephrine are the mainstays of treatment for croup. Most children can be successfully treated as outpatients and few require hospital admission.

Nebulized Epinephrine

Administration of nebulized epinephrine is a very effective way to rapidly reduce airway swelling. Use of racemic epinephrine has been associated with a lower Westley croup score 30 minutes after administration. After 2 hours, this difference is no longer clinically significant; thus, inhaled epinephrine is most effective when used in conjunction with glucocorticoid administration. Children treated with a combination of epinephrine and steroids have decreased duration of hospitalization compared with those treated with steroids alone (Evidence Level I; based on several randomized controlled trials as well as a recent Cochrane review).

Racemic Epinephrine

Racemic epinephrine was initially thought to cause fewer systemic side effects than L-epinephrine alone, but a randomized controlled trial has shown no difference. Either form of inhaled epinephrine is acceptable for use in treating croup. The dose of racemic epinephrine is 0.05 mL/kg/dose. It typically comes as premixed 0.25- and 0.5-mL vials. Children weighing less than 10 kg should receive the 0.25-mL dose. If using L-epinephrine, the dose is always 0.5 mL/kg irrespective of patient weight. The effects can last for 1 to 2 hours and treatments

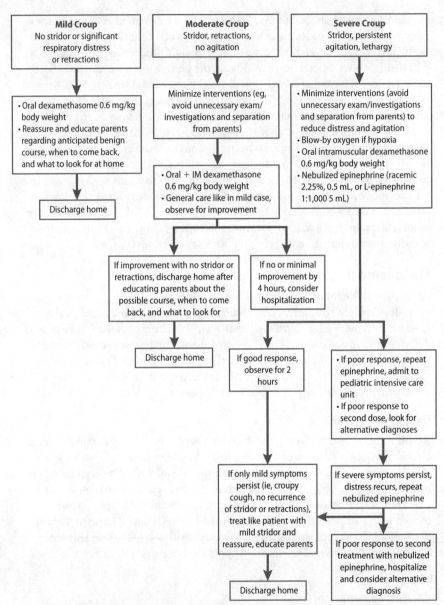

Figure 16-1. Algorithm for the management of croup.

Abbreviations: exam, examination; IM, intramuscular.

From Sharma GD, Conrad C. Croup, epiglottits, and bacterial tracheitis. In: *Pediatric Pulmonology*. Elk Grove Village, IL: American Academy of Pediatrics; 2011.

can be repeated every 15 to 20 minutes, if necessary. Side effects include tachycardia, hypertension, and irritability.

Glucocorticoids

Glucocorticoids are very effective in providing long-term reduction in airway edema and swelling secondary to their anti-inflammatory properties. Typically, improvement in symptoms is seen within 6 hours of administration, meaning that steroids are ineffective as an emergent means to reduce swelling. The use of steroids in the treatment of croup has resulted in decreased length of hospital stay in the emergency department and inpatient settings, decreased unscheduled medical visits, and decreased requirements for racemic epinephrine. Children treated with glucocorticoids also show improvement in Westley scores at 6 hours, although not at 24 hours. Among children with croup who are intubated, steroid administration resulted in decreased length of intubation as well as reduced rate of re-intubation (Evidence Level I; based on several randomized controlled trials as well as a recent Cochrane review).

Dexamethasone

The most commonly used agent to treat croup, dexamethasone, can be administered intramuscularly, intravenously, or orally as a single dose of 0.6 mg/kg. All 3 administration routes have similar pharmacokinetics and bioavailability. It is relatively inexpensive and widely available in most emergency departments. When compared with treatment with prednisolone as a single dose or a 5-day course, children treated with dexamethasone had lower rates of unscheduled return visits and hospital admissions. Prednisolone should only be considered as an option if dexamethasone is not available (Evidence Level I; based on a randomized controlled trial).

Nebulized Budesonide

This therapy may be tolerated better in children with vomiting or severe respiratory distress. It can be mixed with racemic epinephrine to administer medications simultaneously. As a single dose, nebulized budesonide is as effective as a single dose of dexamethasone. It is significantly more expensive than dexamethasone and is not as widely available; therefore, dexamethasone remains the drug of choice in the treatment of croup. There is no good evidence that repeated doses of steroids improve outcomes; in fact, they may be harmful due to the increased risk of side effects. Repeat dosing should only be considered in children with recurrent symptoms or severe croup.

Heliox

Heliox is a mixture of helium and oxygen in percentages ranging from 70% to 80% helium and 20% to 30% oxygen that produces a laminar flow pattern which results in less resistance to gas flow past the airway narrowing. There are no properties inherent to heliox that will decrease the amount of airway edema, but the improved flow may help decrease the agitation associated with hypoxia and air hunger. Heliox is often used in conjunction with racemic epinephrine as a temporizing measure while waiting for glucocorticoids to take effect. A recent review of the use of heliox in conjunction with standard therapies demonstrated a significant reduction in croup scores after 60 minutes compared with children not treated with heliox. Randomized trials comparing the use of heliox to racemic epinephrine and to standard oxygen therapy have not shown significant reduction in croup scores. Heliox should be considered as adjunct to steroids and epinephrine (Evidence Level II-3 because of the lack of any randomized trials).

Humidified Air

Inhalation of warm, moist air may provide some symptomatic relief in children with croup by decreasing dryness of inflamed mucosal membranes. The use of humidified air is currently not recommended in the treatment of croup. However, because it is a cheap and relatively benign therapy, many physicians will use it to provide comfort. It should be discontinued immediately if it causes the child any distress.

Mild croup can be managed in the outpatient setting, but children with moderate or severe disease should be sent to the emergency department. Children who are admitted to the emergency department for croup and treated with nebulized epinephrine and steroids should be observed in the emergency department for at least 4 hours following administration of medications. If they have no recurrence of symptoms, they may be safely discharged home. Children who require more than one dose of nebulized epinephrine should be admitted to the hospital for close observation and monitoring.

Epiglottitis

Overview

Epiglottitis is defined as inflammation and cellulitis of the epiglottis and surrounding supraglottic structures. It is typically a bacterial infection, as opposed to croup, which is more commonly viral. The classic presentation of epiglottitis is a toxic child with high fever, difficulty swallowing, drooling, and respiratory distress. Patients often appear anxious, out of proportion to the degree of respiratory distress manifested on examination, and may position themselves in the tripod or sniffing position in an attempt to relieve respiratory distress. Presently, epiglottitis is more commonly diagnosed among school-aged children; *Streptococcus* is emerging as the predominant pathogen.

Causes and Differential Diagnosis

Epiglottitis is a bacterial infection of the epiglottis. Historically, *Haemophilus influenzae* type b (Hib) was the most common bacterial pathogen; however, the incidence has significantly declined with the development and worldwide implementation of the Hib vaccine. *Streptococcus* and *Staphylococcus aureus* can also cause epiglottitis, and the incidence of these has been increasing as Hib-associated epiglottitis has decreased. Additionally, *Pseudomonas aeruginosa* and *Candida* species have been shown to cause epiglottitis, particularly in adult patients, immunocompromised patients, and patients with long-term hospitalizations. Epiglottitis can also be a rare manifestation of graft-versus-host disease in patients who have undergone bone marrow transplantation. Rare cases of noninfectious inflammation of the epiglottis have been described in patients after neck trauma, foreign body ingestion, thermal injury, or caustic ingestion.

The differential diagnosis of epiglottitis is similar to that of croup; please refer to the previous section in this chapter to review that discussion.

Clinical Presentation

Patients with epiglottitis have rapidly progressive airway edema that quickly leads to complete airway obstruction. The goal of management is to identify patients at risk for epiglottitis quickly and provide advanced airway management before airway obstruction becomes complete. Children typically present with high fever (temperature 38.8°C–40°C), respiratory distress, stridor, and anxiety that often appears out of proportion to the degree of respiratory distress. Older children will often complain of sore throat. Dysphagia and the inability to manage oral secretions manifesting as drooling may be present. The classic 3 Ds presentation of epiglottitis in children includes dysphagia, drooling, and distress. Patients generally appear toxic, especially early in the clinical course. Some children will have a mild viral prodrome, but the characteristic cough associated with croup is typically absent. Speech may be muffled ("hot potato voice") and older children may describe a choking sensation caused by the ball-valve mechanism of their swollen epiglottis. The classic sniffing or tripod position is a sitting position with hyperextension of the neck and the chin thrust forward. This position maximizes airway diameter by aligning the nasal, oral, and tracheal axes and thus relieves some of the distress caused by airway obstruction. Children will often be very reluctant to lie down as they experience increased obstruction and distress in that position.

Evaluation

Epiglottitis is a clinical diagnosis that is confirmed by direct visualization of the epiglottis. If epiglottitis is suspected, the child should immediately be moved to a location where advanced airway management is possible. There have been isolated rare reports of cardiorespiratory arrest associated with attempts to visualize the epiglottis, although most attempts at visualization do not cause arrest. However, it may be prudent not to attempt visualization until advanced airway management is available. In general, children with moderate or severe respiratory distress where epiglottitis is suspected should be kept as calm as possible to avoid worsening of their respiratory distress. This often means delaying further examination until the child has received endotracheal intubation in a controlled environment. Ideally, intubation should take place in the operating room with an experienced anesthesiologist and otolaryngologist, should the need for a surgical airway arise. Laryngoscopy and bronchoscopy can be performed at the same time to provide detailed imaging of airway structures. On physical examination, children with epiglottitis generally have a normal examination of the oropharynx. In some cases, pharyngitis may be noted. The anterior throat may be tender to palpation, particularly at the level of the hyoid bone, and there may be anterior lymphadenopathy. It is generally safe to attempt visualization of the epiglottis in children with only mild to moderate distress using a tongue depressor, although attempts should be discontinued if the child becomes agitated or the epiglottis cannot be seen. Additional imaging or laboratory testing are only helpful if the diagnosis of epiglottitis is in question. Endotracheal intubation should not be delayed in a child with moderate to severe respiratory distress to wait for imaging, but it may be warranted in children with milder respiratory distress. The thumb sign on lateral neck radiographs is pathognomonic for epiglottitis. Lateral neck radiographs may also show loss of the vallecular airspace, thickened aryepiglottic folds, and a distended hypopharynx. Children who are maintaining the sniffing position may show straightening of the cervical spine on lateral neck film. Once intubated, cultures of the trachea and blood should be obtained to help guide antibiotic therapy. White blood cell counts and other inflammatory markers are often elevated but are nonspecific.

Management

Advanced Airway Management

As previously discussed, establishing an advanced airway prior to the development of total airway obstruction is of paramount importance when managing a patient with epiglottitis. Anxiety should be minimized as much as possible and diagnostic testing should be delayed until the airway is secure in patients with moderate to severe distress or signs of impending respiratory failure. Intubation should take place early in a controlled setting with personnel having advanced training in the pediatric airway. Ideally, it should be done in the operating room or sterile environment, should the need for a surgical airway arise. Previously, published data supported the recommendation that all children with epiglottitis be intubated regardless of the degree of respiratory distress on presentation given the relatively small diameter of the pediatric airway and rapid progression of disease (Evidence Level II-2; based on the absence of a randomized controlled trial; however, given the high mortality associated with epiglottitis, it would be impossible to conduct such a study). With the decline of Hib-associated epiglottitis, there is increasing evidence that patients with mild to moderate distress can be managed without intubation if they can be closely observed in a pediatric intensive care unit (ICU). There is some evidence that progression of airway swelling is less rapid with bacterial pathogens other than Hib.

Immediate intubation should be considered if there is a high clinical suspicion of Hib (ie, unimmunized children), in children with epiglottal abscesses, in children younger than 6 years, and in children with known or suspected difficult airway (Evidence Level III; these data primarily come from observational data from a relatively small number of patients).

Antibiotics

Rapid initiation of broad-spectrum antibiotics is the second mainstay treatment for epiglottitis. Empiric therapy should be selected to cover the most common bacterial pathogens, including Hib, *Streptococcus* species, and *Staphylococcus* species. Generally, a combination of a third-generation cephalosporin and coverage for methicillin-resistant *S aureus* is recommended. Vancomycin plus a quinolone antibiotic can be used in patients allergic to cephalosporins. Patients who are immunocompromised or who have had long-term hospitalization should also be covered for *P aeruginosa* infection. Blood and epiglottal cultures should be obtained prior to initiation of antibiotics, if possible, and therapy should be narrowed to target the specific organism when the information becomes available. Typically the length of treatment is 7 to 10 days.

Extubation Criteria

Most patients are monitored, with or without endotracheal intubation, in an ICU for 2 to 3 days. Persistence of epiglottal swelling for longer than this may indicate the presence of an epiglottal abscess. Criteria for extubation include development of air leak around the endotracheal tube, resolution of fever, and the ability to swallow comfortably. Extubation should take place in a controlled setting, usually the operating room, where direct visualization of the epiglottis can be performed to evaluate for decreased swelling.

Glucocorticoids

The efficacy of glucocorticoids in epiglottitis has not been well established. In retrospective case reviews, no clear association between a reduction in length of stay, duration of mechanical ventilation, or duration of ICU stay has been established with the use of glucocorticoids. These medications may be helpful in patients who have failed extubation after several days of appropriate antibiotic therapy.

Complications

Epiglottal Abscess

Epiglottal abscess complication occurs in up to 30% of cases of epiglottitis. Patients may present with more severe symptoms and are at increased risk of airway compromise. Diagnosis is made by direct visualization at the time of endotracheal intubation or by computed tomography scan following intubation. These abscesses require surgical drainage as well as antibiotic therapy. The presence of an epiglottal abscess is an indication for early intubation, with many of these patients remaining intubated for many days until the abscess is properly treated and resolves.

Necrotizing Epiglottitis
Characterized by necrosis of the epiglottis visible on direct examination, necrotizing epiglottitis is a very rare complication of epiglottitis that occurs in immunocompromised patients, most commonly those with HIV.

Secondary Infection
Patients with epiglottitis, especially when caused by *Staphylococcus* or *Streptococcus* species, are at risk for infection at other sites. This can occur as a result of bacteremia or direct extension into local structures. Once an airway has been established, it is important to look for signs of secondary infection to make sure they are properly treated. Patients with concomitant meningitis or osteomyelitis will require longer durations of antibiotic therapy. Patients with abscesses that develop at remote sites may also require surgical drainage.

Suggested Reading

Bjornson C, Russell KF, Vandermeer B, Durec T, Klassen TP, Johnson DW. Nebulized epinephrine for croup in children. *Cochrane Database Syst Rev.* 2011;(2):CD006619

Bjornson CL, Johnson DW. Croup. *Lancet.* 2008;371(9609):329–339

Cherry JD. Clinical practice. Croup. *N Engl J Med.* 2008;358(4):384–391

Choi J, Lee GL. Common pediatric respiratory emergencies. *Emerg Med Clin North Am.* 2012;30(2):529–563

Mayo-Smith MF, Spinale JW, Donskey CJ, Yukawa M, Li RH, Schiffman FJ. Acute epiglottitis. An 18-year experience in Rhode Island. *Chest.* 1995;108(6):1640–1647

Rafei K, Lichenstein R. Airway infectious disease emergencies. *Pediatr Clin North Am.* 2006;53(2):215–242

Russell KF, Liang Y, O'Gorman K, Johnson DW, Klassen TP. Glucocorticoids for croup. *Cochrane Database Syst Rev.* 2011;(1):CD001955

CHAPTER 17

Development:
The Basic Science of Pediatrics

Colleen A. Kraft, MD

Key Points

- Every encounter with a pediatric patient—regardless of whether it is a well-child visit, visit for acute illness, or chronic care management—is an opportunity to assess and promote development.

- Recognize the relationship as a vital sign. The interaction between parent and child is a snapshot of the environment in which the child lives.

- Developmental surveillance and screening are important functions within the medical home. Developing a process within your practice for screening, identification, and referral of children with suspected delay ensures practice success with this function.

- Behavior is communication. Investigate what is being communicated through a child's behavior.

Overview

An understanding of how children acquire motor, language, social-emotional, and cognition skills differentiates pediatrics from all other medical specialties. Pediatricians and pediatric primary health professionals recognize that these foundational skills have a profound impact upon a child's life-course trajectory. As a consequence, pediatricians are in the business of health promotion; they are ideally positioned to counsel families on how to optimize the development of their child as well as monitor for risks and atypical development.

Advances in our understanding of the factors that either promote or undermine early human development reveal the interaction of genetic and environmental factors in building brain architecture. Beginning prenatally, continuing through infancy, and extending into childhood and beyond, development is driven by a cumulative, ongoing, inextricable interaction between biology (genetic predispositions) and ecology (social and physical environment). This dynamic process of brain development sets the life-course trajectory for an individual; in turn, everything from that child's educational achievement to economic stability to healthy behaviors to chronic disease stems from this "dance" between genetics and experience. Given the pivotal role of early childhood experiences in literally sculpting the foundational architecture of the brain, the need for pediatricians to guide families in nurturing the development of their children has never been more clear or critical.

Pediatric visits in the family-centered medical home are occasions for actively building wellness by (a) engaging families in their children's development, (b) promoting wellness by nurturing healthy behaviors, (c) performing developmental surveillance and, when indicated, standardized screenings, and (d) creating therapeutics alliances with families. There remain missed opportunities for developmental promotion and surveillance within our pediatric encounters.

Developmental Disabilities and Behavioral Disorders

Amongst the most common health conditions seen in children in the United States, developmental disabilities and behavioral disorders have an estimated prevalence of 12% to 13% in the pediatric population. Given this, developmental surveillance and screening are important functions of a family-centered medical home (Evidence Level II-2).

Developmental surveillance, a term credited to Dr Paul Dworkin, is the informal assessment of a child's development and behavior at every pediatric encounter. When that encounter is a well-child visit, components include

▶ History
  • Family developmental or behavioral concerns
  • Developmental history with gross motor, fine motor, language, and social-emotional milestones
  • Medical history, family history, and social and environmental risks
  • Identification of child and family protective factors

▶ Developmental observation
  • Gross and fine motor skills
  • Receptive and expressive speech
  • Social and reciprocal interactions
  • Abnormality on physical examination, with focus on neurologic exam

▶ All visits should serve as opportunities for informal assessment of development. Observations of behavior, speech, and social interactions are as important as a targeted physical examination for illnesses.

▶ The reality is that not all children are seen for well-child visits, and an abnormal developmental observation (eg, the 2-year-old with ear pain who is not talking or the 6-year-old who is unable to sit still during a lung examination) should trigger formalized developmental screening.

Developmental screening involves

▶ Use of a standardized test with known reliability, validity, sensitivity, and specificity

▶ Given at key times for the identification of developmental disorders

▶ Interpretation by a pediatric health care professional at the time of the visit

▶ Identification of children at high risk for a developmental disorder

Psychosocial screening can identify risks for developmental and behavioral disorders (Evidence Level II-2). The presence of 4 or more of the following risk factors has been correlated negatively with a child's cognitive ability:

▶ Parental education less than high school

▶ Parental unemployment

▶ Single parent

▶ Three or more children in the house

▶ History of child abuse in the parent

▶ History of parental behavioral health problems

▶ Domestic violence

▶ Frequency of household moves

Anticipatory Guidance

"Immunization" against developmental and behavioral disorders is a primary function of anticipatory guidance to families by pediatric health care professionals. As vaccinations proactively build wellness by protecting children against future infections, social-emotional immunizations proactively build wellness by protecting children from the toxic effects of future adversity. Toxic stress, an inhibitor of healthy brain development and a disruptor of optimal life-course trajectories, occurs when children are unable to "turn off" the physiologic stress response. Efforts to buffer childhood toxic stress might include the following immunizations:

▶ Recognize the relationship as a vital sign.
  • The interaction between parent and child is a window into the ability of the parent to engage with her child and to optimize her child's development.
  • Recognize the difference between the parent who is actively engaged with her child and the parent who is not interacting.
    – An example: One parent is smiling and talking to his infant, whereas a second parent is texting on her phone while the infant is in a car seat.

- – Take the opportunity to reinforce the positive relationship of the first parent and to investigate the lack of interaction with the second parent. Is this caused by a lack of understanding, maternal depression, or distraction due to extreme life stressors?
  - – Education or referral to family support and home-visiting resources may be helpful with the second parent (Evidence Level III).

▶ Participate in Reach Out and Read.
  - An office program in which books are given to young children during well-child visits, Reach Out and Read encourages parents to start reading/interacting with their children, and reading is modeled by an adult in the pediatric waiting room.

▶ Nurture foundational social-emotional skills as they emerge.
  - Note and encourage the infant's social smile, self-regulation, social referencing, use of language skills, and growing emotional awareness.

▶ Collaborate with home-visiting programs.
  - Some evidence-based (Evidence Level II-1) programs such as Healthy Steps or Parents as Teachers can facilitate positive interactions that promote development with vulnerable families.

▶ Provide family support and education.
  - Provide support and education, particularly for those who appear to be struggling, through direct counseling or through community resources.

▶ Promote the 5 Rs.
  - Reading—every day
  - Rhyming—playing and cuddling
  - Routines—so children know what to expect from us, and what is expected of them
  - Rewards—for everyday successes (Praise is a powerful reward!)
  - Relationship—reciprocal and nurturing, the foundation of healthy development

Common Approach to Behavioral Problems

Behavior reflects brain development and is shaped by the child's environment. For typical ages, a child's behavior, despite being appropriate and adaptive, can be problematic to the family. The physician should be aware of different age-related behavior and respond accordingly (Table 17-1).

Table 17-1. Typical Age Behaviors

Age-Related Behavior	Physician Response
Crying in 6-week-old	• This is a developmentally expected occurrence. • Your infant is healthy. • Try holding, rocking, soothing. • Do not become discouraged if your baby does not soothe easily. • Your baby will communicate in other ways when he is a few weeks older.
Temper tantrums in a 15-month old	• This is a developmentally expected occurrence. • Inattention is the best initial parent response. • Comfort and reassure when the tantrum is over. • Teach your child words and signs to communicate. • Your toddler will communicate in other ways as she develops language.
Sleep problems in a 3-year-old	• This is a developmentally expected occurrence. • Keep the sleep environment dark, quiet, and cool. • Keep regular wake-up, nap, and bedtimes. • Keep routines around bedtime; child is fed, sleepy but awake, reading, being soothed, being praised; consistency is key.
School anxiety in a 5-year-old	• This is a developmentally expected occurrence. • Keep a routine around school drop-off and pickup. • Avoid "rescuing" child when anxious at school. • Find a comforting teacher, activity, or object for child when he first arrives at school.
Disrespectful language in a 13-year-old	• This is a developmentally expected occurrence. • Encourage "I feel" communication. • Have a "calm down" activity and place for your teen to go when she is feeling angry or frustrated.

It is important to discuss what behaviors are developmentally typical for a child at a given age. This is most important for younger children, as parents need to understand that this behavior is part of expected development and not defiance on part of the child. Parents need to recognize, for example, that a 12-month-old is not being "bad" but rather is learning by independently exploring the environment. It is the toddler's "job," if you will, to push limits and a parent's job to reinforce limits. This eliminates parental stress and encourages rudimentary but foundation skills as they emerge.

Behavior Management
Behavior management is all about understanding the behavior antecedents and consequences, which can be modified so as to encourage positive behavior and discourage negative behavior.

▶ Parents are encouraged to identify the "purpose" behind repeated behaviors, as these are often done in an attempt to meet an unacknowledged need (eg, "I'm hungry," "I'm tired," "I'm scared," "I want some attention").

▶ Parents should focus not just on how to "stop" the behavior but on how to assist the child in learning more adaptive ways to have these unacknowledged needs met (eg, "use your words," "let's rest a bit," "let's think about something else," "try reading that book while I finish dinner, and then we'll read it together").

Developmental domains include gross motor, fine motor, receptive and expressive language, social/emotional and adaptive, and cognitive/problem-solving.

Developmental quotient is the developmental age/chronologic age × 100 in a specific domain. For example, A 15-month-old child has just started walking alone (developmental quotient = 12/15 × 100, or 80).

Developmental delay is a significant lag in the attainment of developmental milestones. (eg, a 2-year-old who cannot follow a one-step command).

Developmental dissociation is the significant difference in the developmental rates of 2 domains of development (eg, a 2-year-old who can talk in sentences but is not walking independently).

Developmental deviance is non-sequential unevenness in the achievement in developmental milestones (eg, a 2-year-old who identifies all the letters of the alphabet yet does not speak in 2-word phrases and does not make eye contact).

Evaluation of Children with Developmental Disabilities in the Family-Centered Medical Home

The family-centered medical home is an optimal place to serve as the "headquarters" for the evaluation of children who have been identified as having developmental delays. Professionals involved in co-evaluation include

▶ **Developmental pediatricians, child neurologists, and other pediatric subspecialists** who provide medical evaluation and guidance for co-management

▶ **Physical, occupational, and speech therapists** who provide specific treatment to promote development in gross motor skills, fine motor skills, sensory integration, and receptive and expressive language

Behavioral health specialists
- Provide evaluation in specific diagnoses (eg, autism testing)
- Perform cognitive and academic testing
- Apply behavioral interventions (eg, applied behavioral analysis, parent-child interactive therapy)

- ► Early Intervention and local school systems
  - • Referral and ongoing collaboration is essential with the medical home.
  - • Early Intervention provides in-home family support and mentoring in promoting developmental skills.
  - • School systems provide early childhood special education services and therapy directed for educational needs.

Early Intervention

Early Intervention is a federally mandated program authorized under the Individuals with Disabilities Education Act. Available in every community in the United States, Early Intervention identifies and coordinates services for infants and toddlers with disabilities and their families.

- ► Referral can and should be made for any suspected developmental delay, even in the absence of a diagnosis.

- ► Children referred are evaluated by educational specialists and therapists (physical, occupational, and speech), often the same therapists who treat patients in a medical model.

- ► Early Intervention services are mandated to meet the needs of children with demonstrated developmental delays in 1 or more of the following areas:
  - • Physical
  - • Cognitive
  - • Communication
  - • Social and emotional
  - • Adaptive

- ► An Individual Family Services Plan is the child's care plan in Early Intervention.
  - • Early Intervention uses a parent education and mentoring model for therapy.
  - • The medical model of physical, occupational, and speech therapy is more appropriate for some children with known disabilities.
  - • Both methods may be appropriate for the same child at different times.

- ► Early Intervention has been shown to be most successful when
  - • Delays are mild vs severe (before delays in one domain begin to effect other domains).
  - • Children are at environmental vs biological risk for developmental delay (hence the need to change the ecology through education, counseling, and home visits).
  - • Children are at risk for developmental disability vs known disability (Evidence Level II-3) (but funding shortfalls often result in services only for children with demonstrated delays).

Management of Children With Developmental Disabilities in the Family-Centered Medical Home

The family-centered medical home is the optimal place to serve as the "headquarters" for the management of children who have been identified as having developmental delays. Components of management include

▶ Care planning with families of children with developmental disabilities, recognizing the family's expertise and goals for the care of their child

▶ Care plan shared with school, child care, and other personnel who care for the child

▶ Team-based care with practice nurses; care coordinators to help the family/patient access, coordinate, and understand specialty care; educational services; out-of-home care; family support; and other public and private community services

▶ Co-management and communication with pediatric subspecialists

▶ Collaboration with pediatric therapists and behavioral health specialists

Child development is a dynamic and interactive process involving genetics, environment, and education; optimizing cognitive and social-emotional skills; and monitoring for delay, early treatment of delay, and management of children with disabilities. The partnership between families, pediatric medical professionals, and the medical home is crucial in reaching the best developmental outcome for each child.

Suggested Reading

Dubowitz H, Lane WG, Semiatin JN, Magder LS. The SEEK Model of pediatric preventive care: can child abuse be prevented in a low risk population. *Acad Pediatr.* 2012;12(4):259–268

Fine A, Mayer R. *Beyond Referral: Pediatric Care Linkages to Improve Developmental Health.* Commonwealth Fund publication 976. The Commonwealth Fund; 2006

Garner AS, Shonkoff JP; American Academy of Pediatrics Committee on the Psychosocial Aspects of Child and Family Health; Committee on Early Childhood, Adoption, and Dependent Care; Section on Developmental and Behavioral Pediatrics. Early childhood adversity, toxic stress and the role of the pediatrician: translating developmental science into lifelong health. *Pediatrics.* 2010;129(1):e224–e231

Hagan JF, Shaw JS, Duncan PM, eds. *Bright Futures: Guidelines for Health Supervision of Infants, Children, and Adolescents.* 3rd ed. Elk Grove Village, IL; American Academy of Pediatrics; 2008

Jellinek M, Patel BP, Froehele MC, eds. *Bright Futures in Practice: Mental Health Tool Kit.* Vol 2. Arlington, VA: National Center for Education in Maternal and Child Health; 2002

Peacock S, Konrad S, Watson E, Nickel D, Muhajarine N. Effectiveness of home visiting programs on child outcomes: a systematic review. *BMC Public Health.* 2013;13(1):17

Pipan ME, Blum NJ. Basics of child behavior and primary care management of common behavioral problems. In: Voight RG, Macias MM, Myers SM, eds. *Developmental and Behavioral Pediatrics.* Elk Grove Village, IL: American Academy of Pediatrics; 2011:37–57

Shonkoff JP, Garner AS. The lifelong effects of early childhood adversity and toxic stress. *Pediatrics.* 2012;129(12):232–224

CHAPTER 18

Diarrhea

Ricardo A. Caicedo, MD

Key Points

- Acute diarrhea is typically caused by infectious agents, is self-limited, and resolves within 1 to 2 weeks but can lead to dehydration.

- Chronic diarrhea persists beyond 2 weeks, has a broad differential diagnosis, and can adversely impact nutritional status.

- Diagnostic evaluation of diarrhea in infants and children often entails stool studies and laboratory testing, which may prompt further studies.

- Management of acute diarrhea revolves around maintaining hydration, whereas that of chronic diarrhea is aimed at the causative process.

Overview

Diarrhea is an increase in frequency or water content of stools. It results from an imbalance between intestinal water and electrolyte secretion and absorption. Expected stool frequency and volume varies by age (Table 18-1).

Table 18-1. Reference Range of Stool Frequency or Volume by Age Group

Population	Reference Range of Stool Frequency or Volume
Breastfed infants	Once every 7 days, 7 times per day
Infants	5–10 g/kg per day
Children	0–3 stools per day 10 mL/kg per day
Adolescents	0–2 stools per day 200 g per day

With this in mind, a more practical definition of diarrhea (except in breastfed infants) is the passage of liquid stools more than 3 times per day, or as stools that are looser or more liquid than normal for the individual. *Acute diarrhea* in children is usually caused by infectious processes and typically has onset and resolution within 1 to 2 weeks. When it is not self-limited and persists beyond this time frame, it is referred to as *chronic diarrhea*.

Causes and Differential Diagnosis

Most cases of acute diarrhea in infants and children are caused by gastrointestinal (GI) infection. In about two-thirds of cases, the infectious agent is identified. Viral causes are more common (50%–80%) and tend to present with watery diarrhea, and often with concomitant vomiting, as in acute gastroenteritis. Other etiologic categories for acute diarrhea include non-GI infection, toxin/drug, and allergic (Table 18-2).

Table 18-2. Causes of Acute Diarrhea

GI Infection		
Viral	**Bacterial**	**Protozoan**
Rotavirus	Enteroinvasive *Escherichia coli*	*Giardia lamblia*
Norovirus	Enterohemorrhagic *E coli*	*Cryptosporidium parvum*
Enterovirus	Enterotoxigenic *E coli*	*Entamoeba histolytica*
Calicivirus	Enteropathogenic *E coli*	*Isospora belli*
Astrovirus	*Shigella* species	
	Salmonella species	
	Yersinia species	
	Campylobacter species	
	Clostridium difficile species	
	Vibrio cholerae species	
	Aeromonas species	
Non-GI Infection		**Other**
Influenza		Antibiotic associated
Otitis media		Drug adverse effect
Other respiratory tract infection		Food poisoning
Urinary tract infection		Allergic reaction
Meningitis		Acute appendicitis
Sepsis		Intussusception

Abbreviation: GI, gastrointestinal.

The differential diagnosis of prolonged or chronic diarrhea is much broader than that of acute diarrhea. Causes of chronic diarrhea can be categorized by mechanism (Table 18-3). Since many of these conditions appear primarily at specific ages, it is also helpful to stratify them by age of onset (Table 18-4).

In developing countries, chronic diarrhea is more likely to be caused by chronic parasitic (including helminths or worms), bacterial, or mycobacterial infection. Postinfectious villous injury and disaccharidase deficiency is also common. The most common causes of chronic diarrhea in industrialized nations are functional/dietary causes, carbohydrate malabsorption, celiac disease, and inflammatory bowel disease.

Table 18-3. Causes of Chronic Diarrhea

Mechanism	Examples
Infection	Giardiasis, cryptosporidiosis (especially in immunocompromised host) *Entamoeba histolytica*
Villous injury	Celiac disease[a] Post-enteritis enteropathy Secondary lactase/disaccharidase deficiency Allergic enteropathy Milk/soy protein intolerance
Gastrointestinal organ disease	Short bowel syndrome[a] Small intestinal bacterial overgrowth Necrotizing enterocolitis Hirschsprung disease enterocolitis[a] Intestinal lymphangiectasia[a] Intestinal dysmotility or pseudo-obstruction[a] Pancreatic exocrine insufficiency (cystic fibrosis, Shwachman-Diamond syndrome)[a] Liver disease with secondary cholestasis and bile salt deficiency
Maldigestion/ malabsorption	Lactase deficiency (lactose intolerance) Sucrase isomaltase deficiency Glucose-galactose malabsorption[a] Fructose malabsorption
Autoimmune	Inflammatory bowel disease[a] (Crohn disease, ulcerative colitis, indeterminate colitis) Celiac disease[a] Autoimmune enteropathy[a] Lymphocytic colitis
Congenital/inborn error of metabolism	Abetalipoproteinemia[a] Congenital chloride diarrhea[a] Congenital sodium diarrhea[a] Galactosemia[a] Microvillus inclusion disease[a] Tufting enteropathy[a] Syndromatic diarrhea[a] Acrodermatitis enteropathica[a]
Hypersecretory	Neuroblastoma Ganglioneuroma (secretes vasoactive intestinal peptide) Gastrinoma
Hypermotility	Hyperthyroidism[a] Pseudo-obstruction[a] Short bowel syndrome[a]
Dietary/functional	Toddler's diarrhea (chronic nonspecific diarrhea of childhood) Hyperosmolar formula or juice Sorbitol Laxative overuse/abuse Encopresis (retentive fecal soiling) Irritable bowel syndrome

[a] Associated with poor weight gain, malnutrition, or failure to thrive.

Table 18-4. Causes of Chronic Diarrhea by Age of Onset

Infant	Child	Adolescent
Milk/soy protein intolerance	Post-enteritis enteropathy	IBS
Post-enteritis enteropathy	Toddler's diarrhea	Post-enteritis enteropathy
Hyperosmolar formula	IBS	Lactose intolerance
Cystic fibrosis	Lactose intolerance	Inflammatory bowel
Celiac disease	Celiac disease	disease
Short bowel syndrome	Inflammatory bowel disease	Celiac disease
Rare: Congenital/inborn	Cystic fibrosis	*Rare:* Hyperthyroidism,
errors of metabolism,	Encopresis	laxative abuse
autoimmune enteropathy	*Rare:* Pseudo-obstruction,	
	secretory tumor	

Abbreviation: IBS, irritable bowel syndrome.

Clinical Features

Acute diarrhea is often watery and presents as part of acute gastroenteritis. Associated symptoms include nausea, vomiting, anorexia, cramping abdominal pain, and, in some cases, fever, fatigue, and generalized malaise. Blood and mucus in the stools in the acute scenario suggests infectious colitis. The term *dysentery* is often used to describe a syndrome of bloody diarrhea, tenesmus, and abdominal pain. Common infectious agents causing dysentery include *Salmonella, Shigella, Campylobacter,* and *Yersinia* species and enterohemorrhagic *Escherichia coli.*

Dehydration is another important clinical feature of acute diarrhea. The degree of dehydration is determined by stool volume, rapidity of onset, and duration of the diarrheal illness, as well as concomitant losses as with vomiting. Cardinal signs of dehydration include thirst, lack of tears, dry mucous membranes, decreased skin turgor, decreased urine output, and tachycardia.

The clinical picture in chronic diarrhea is more diverse. Stools may be watery, bloody, mucus laden, oily, foamy, or explosive or contain undigested food particles. The consistency and color of the stools are typically observed and reported by parents. Stool colors of red (blood), black (melena), and white (cholestasis) should prompt concern, but other hues including green and yellow can be within the reference range. Chronic diarrhea may lead to dehydration but more commonly affects nutrition and growth. In general terms, osmotic diarrhea (as seen with lactose intolerance) is associated with bloating and flatulence and improves with fasting. Voluminous diarrhea that persists in the fasting state implies a secretory process, as in cholera or a catecholamine-secreting tumor. Table 18-5 lists clinical features that are clues to particular diagnoses in chronic diarrhea.

Evaluation

Initial history should consider the child's age and focus on onset, duration, and associated symptoms. It should be apparent within the first few minutes of the encounter if the case is one of acute or chronic diarrhea. In acute diarrhea, history should center on travel, food exposure, group child care, ill contacts, antibiotic exposure, and community outbreak. Physical examination should assess degree of dehydration. The clinical diagnosis of a viral infection can be made without stool examination or other laboratory tests in many cases. Routine stool testing for bacterial, viral, or protozoan pathogens is not recommended in most cases of acute diarrhea (Evidence Level III). Exceptions include infants younger than 3 months of age, toxic or septic appearance, high fever, bloody stools, history of foreign travel, or community outbreak.

The approach to the child with chronic diarrhea starts with determining the character of the stools and any associated symptoms that may provide diagnostic clues (see Table 18-5). As with other digestive complaints, "red flag" symptoms such as weight loss, nocturnal defecation, abdominal pain, and vomiting should prompt consideration of an underlying organic disease process. Dietary and family history is critically important. Physical examination should start with review of

Table 18-5. Clinical Manifestations in Chronic Diarrhea

Sign or Symptom	Suggested Diagnoses
Bloating/cramping	Lactose intolerance, IBS, giardiasis
Excessive flatus, explosive stools	Carbohydrate malabsorption
Oily/greasy stools (*steatorrhea*)	CF, celiac disease, Shwachman-Diamond syndrome
Bloody/mucous stools	IBD, allergic colitis
Undigested food particles in stool	Toddler's diarrhea (CNSD)
Watery, profuse stools, hypokalemia, alkalosis	Secretory tumor (VIPoma, neuroblastoma)
Nocturnal defecation	IBD
Recurrent abdominal pain	IBD, celiac disease, IBS
Pain relieved with defecation	IBS
Constipation/stool withholding	Encopresis, laxative overuse
Weight loss	Celiac disease, IBD, CF, hyperthyroidism
Growth failure/short stature	Celiac disease, IBD, CF
Normal growth	CNSD, overfeeding, fructose/sorbitol malabsorption
Anemia	IBD, celiac disease
Arthritis	IBD, celiac disease
Recurrent oral ulcers	IBD
Erythema nodosum	IBD
Dermatitis herpetiformis	Celiac disease
Abdominal distention, vomiting	Pseudo-obstruction, dysmotility

Abbreviations: CF, cystic fibrosis; CNSD, chronic nonspecific diarrhea; IBD, irritable bowel disease; IBS, irritable bowel syndrome.

the growth parameters and nutritional status, including the body mass index in children and weight-for-length ratio in infants and young toddlers. Depending on the initial differential diagnosis, several stool and laboratory tests may be useful; these results may prompt further diagnostic investigation (Table 18-6).

Management

Acute Diarrhea

The treatment of acute diarrhea is directed toward maintaining hydration. Most patients will have mild to moderate dehydration, and the first-line recommended treatment is oral rehydration. Glucose-electrolyte oral rehydration solutions enhance intestinal absorption of salt and water and can relatively rapidly (3–4 hours) rehydrate a child. If the child is unable to drink, the solution can be given via nasogastric tube. Intravenous rehydration is indicated if there is excessive vomiting, ongoing losses, or severe dehydration. Once rehydrated, the infant or child should resume an age-appropriate normal diet, which reduces intestinal permeability as well as protein and energy deficits (Evidence Level I). The popular "BRAT" (bananas, rice, applesauce, toast) diet is nutritionally inadequate and thus not recommended. Breastfed infants should continue to breastfeed at all times, including during rehydration. There is no indication for the use of diluted formula and only a limited role for lactose-free formula. This would be in cases of severe diarrhea or if the diarrhea clearly worsens on reintroduction of milk.

Most cases of diarrhea caused by GI infection do not require antimicrobial therapy. In some cases, such as with enterohemorrhagic *E coli,* antibiotics are contraindicated because they may increase the risk of developing hemolytic uremic syndrome. Specific antimicrobial therapy is recommended in the following infectious scenarios:

- *Salmonella typhi*
- *Salmonella* species in young infants, sickle cell disease, immunocompromised (Evidence Level III)
- *Shigella* species (Evidence Level I)
- *Campylobacter* species (for severe cases) (Evidence Level II-3)
- Cholera (Evidence Level I)
- *Clostridium difficile* (metronidazole as first line, with oral vancomycin for recurrent or severe cases) (Evidence Level I)
- *Giardia* species (Evidence Level I), *Cryptosporidium* species, *Entamoeba histolytica*

Table 18-6. Diagnostic Tests in the Evaluation of Chronic Diarrhea

Test	Use/Implication
Stool	
Lactoferrin level/white blood cell count	Colonic inflammation (nonspecific to cause)
Bacterial culture	Infectious enterocolitis
Clostridium difficile toxin assay	*C difficile* infection
Giardia/cryptosporidium antigen level	Specific protozoan infection
Presence of ova and parasites	*Entamoeba histolytica, Cyclospora,* helminths
pH/reducing substances	Carbohydrate malabsorption
Fat stain	Fat malabsorption
72-hour fecal fat collection	Evaluation of steatorrhea
Elastase (pancreatic elastase-1) level	Pancreatic exocrine insufficiency (low)
Alpha$_1$-antitrypsin level	GI protein loss (high)
Osmotic gap [290 − 2 x (Na + K)]	Classification of watery diarrhea (secretory vs osmotic)
Blood	
CBC/differential	Anemia in IBD, celiac disease, thrombocytosis, leukocytosis in IBD
ESR, C-reactive protein concentration	Elevated in IBD
Electrolyte level	Deranged in hypersecretory processes (hypokalemia, hyponatremia)
Albumin level	Low in IBD, protein-losing enteropathy
Total/direct bilirubin level	Cholestasis, CF
Tissue transglutaminase IgA titer	Celiac disease—first-line screening test[a] (Evidence Level I)
Levels of vitamins A, D, E	Fat malabsorption (CF, IBD, celiac disease)
Cholesterol, triglycerides levels	Low in abetalipoproteinemia
Other	
Sweat chloride	CF
Breath hydrogen testing	Carbohydrate malabsorption, small intestinal bacterial overgrowth
Abdominal radiograph	Fecal impaction, encopresis
Small bowel follow-through	Dysmotility, Crohn disease
EGD with biopsies	Celiac disease,[a] IBD,[a] disaccharidase deficiency
Pancreatic enzyme analysis	Pancreatic exocrine insufficiency
Colonoscopy with biopsies	IBD,[a] allergic colitis, lymphocytic colitis
Anorectal manometry/rectal biopsies	Hirschsprung disease

Abbreviations: CBC, complete blood count; CF, cystic fibrosis; CNSD, chronic nonspecific diarrhea; EGD, esophagogastroduodenoscopy; ESR, erythrocyte sedimentation rate; IBD, irritable bowel disease; IBS, irritable bowel syndrome; K, potassium; Na, sodium; vs, versus.

Probiotics, or live active microorganisms with a beneficial effect on the host, may be useful in certain cases of acute diarrhea. These include rotaviral diarrhea, the duration and severity of which can be reduced by using *Lactobacillus* GG (Evidence Level I). Probiotic preparations have also been shown to reduce the severity of antibiotic-associated diarrhea (Evidence Level I). The same effect has not been observed in bacterial infectious diarrhea.

Zinc supplementation is recommended by the World Health Organization for the treatment of diarrhea in children 6 months and older. The mechanism is as yet undetermined, but benefit has been shown for patients in areas having high prevalence of zinc deficiency and malnutrition (Evidence Level I). There is no role for antimotility agents such as loperamide or diphenoxylate in acute diarrhea. Their use may protract an acute infectious process or lead to ileus.

Chronic Diarrhea

Treatment of chronic diarrhea is specific to the underlying cause (Table 18-7). Furthermore, enteral or parenteral nutrition support may be needed in those cases involving undernutrition or failure to thrive.

Table 18-7. Treatment of Chronic Diarrhea by Diagnosis

Diagnosis	Treatment(s)
Allergic enteropathy	Protein hydrolysate or elemental formula
Autoimmune enteropathy	Immunosuppression
Bile acid malabsorption	Cholestyramine
Celiac disease	Gluten-free diet (Evidence Level I)
Chronic nonspecific diarrhea (toddler's diarrhea)	Reduce fructose/carbohydrate intake, liberalize fat, fiber
Congenital/neonatal diarrheas (microvillus inclusion disease, tufting enteropathy, congenital chloride or sodium diarrhea)	Parenteral nutrition, aggressive fluid/electrolyte replacement, intestinal transplantation
Cystic fibrosis	Pancreatic enzyme supplementation, enteral nutrition, fat soluble vitamins
Giardiasis	Metronidazole (Evidence Level I), nitazoxanide
Glucose-galactose malabsorption	Fructose-based formula/diet (Evidence Level II-1)
Hirschsprung disease (enterocolitis)	Antibiotics, surgery
Inflammatory bowel disease	Immunosuppression, immunomodulation (Evidence Level I), enteral nutrition, biologics (Evidence Level I), antibiotics, surgery
Irritable bowel syndrome	Dietary modification, stress reduction, fiber (Evidence Level III), antimotility agents, antispasmodics

Table 18-7 *(cont)*

Diagnosis	Treatment(s)
Lactose/fructose intolerance	Lactose/fructose-limited diet, lactase
Secretory diarrheas	Fluid/electrolyte replacement, parenteral nutrition, octreotide, racecadotril
Short bowel syndrome	Enteral and parenteral nutrition, loperamide, bowel lengthening surgery, intestinal transplantation
Small intestinal bacterial overgrowth	Antibiotics (metronidazole, rifaximin) (Evidence Level II-1)
Sucrase-isomaltase deficiency	Dietary restriction, sacrosidase (Evidence Level I)

Long-term Monitoring

In many cases of chronic diarrhea, identification and treatment of the underlying cause will lead to resolution of symptoms and prevent nutritional deficiencies. Patients on a low lactose diet for lactose intolerance may require alternative sources of calcium to meet recommended targets. Patients with inflammatory bowel disease, celiac disease, cystic fibrosis, and short bowel syndrome should have longitudinal follow up with specialists in gastroenterology and nutrition (Evidence Level III). This also pertains to any infant or child receiving home parenteral nutrition or being evaluated for intestinal transplantation. These children will benefit from careful serial monitoring of weight velocity, linear growth, dietary intake, stooling pattern, blood counts, inflammatory markers (or tissue transglutaminase level in the case of celiac disease), protein status, and micronutrients/vitamins.

Suggested Reading

Armon K, Stephenson T, MacFaul R, et al. An evidence and consensus based guideline for acute diarrhea management. *Arch Dis Child.* 2001;85(2):132–142

Binder HJ. Causes of chronic diarrhea. *N Engl J Med.* 2006;355(3):236–239

Davidson G, Barnes G, Bass D, et al. Infectious diarrhea in children: Working Group Report of First World Congress of Pediatric Gastroenterology, Hepatology and Nutrition. *J Pediatr Gastroenterol Nutr.* 2002;35(Suppl 2):S143–S150

Hempel S, Newberry SJ, Maher AR, et al. Probiotics for the prevention and treatment of antibiotic-associated diarrhea: a systematic review and meta-analysis. *JAMA.* 2012;307(18):1959–1969

Hill ID, Dirks MH, Liptak GS, et al. Guideline for the diagnosis and treatment of celiac disease in children: recommendations of the North American Society for Pediatric Gastroenterology, Hepatology, and Nutrition. *J Pediatr Gastroenterol Nutr.* 2005;40(1):1–19

King CK, Glass R, Bresee JS, Duggan C; Centers for Disease Control and Prevention. Managing acute gastroenteritis among children: oral rehydration, maintenance, and nutritional therapy. *MMWR Recommend Rep.* 2003;52(RR-16):1–16

Lazzerini M, Ronfani L. Oral zinc for treating diarrhea in children. *Cochrane Database Syst Rev.* 2008;3:CD005436

Zella GC, Israel EJ. Chronic diarrhea in children. *Pediatr Rev.* 2012:33(5):207–217

CHAPTER 19

Dysuria

Richard Hobbs, MD, and Richard J. Chung, MD

Key Points

- Although dysuria typically stems from a select few common causes, the differential diagnosis includes a broad spectrum of less common local and systemic etiologies.

- A detailed clinical history and careful physical examination often yield a specific clinical diagnosis without need for further testing.

- Younger children may present with behavioral changes rather than subjective complaints.

- Many causes of dysuria are more common in pregnant females, and pregnancy testing is strongly encouraged in sexually active girls.

Overview

Dysuria is defined as pain or burning associated with urination. As such, it is a symptom and not a diagnosis. Dysuria can present in isolation or as part of a larger constellation of symptoms and can occur at any time from early childhood through adulthood.

Several conditions can cause dysuria. In some instances, however, skin-borne lesions may also cause discomfort during urination.

Clinical Presentation and Initial Examination

In addition to urinary discomfort, it is important to identify other associated symptoms when formulating a differential diagnosis. Such symptoms might include pruritus, urethral or vaginal discharge, abdominal or pelvic symptoms, rash or other skin lesions, conjunctivitis or other mucosal symptoms, and systemic symptoms such as fever. Developmental history, local exposures (eg, bath soaps, detergents, tightly fitting clothes), traumatic injuries, menstrual history for adolescent girls, and sexual activity are also important historical elements.

A detailed history is often sufficient to significantly narrow one's differential diagnosis. However, younger children may be unable to articulate symptoms and may present only with suggestive behavioral changes, including reluctance to urinate, overt urinary retention, and general irritability. In addition, adolescents may not be comfortable divulging private details related to sexual activity, so it is important to provide confidential care, interviewing the adolescent patient alone if possible, while maintaining a low threshold for further questioning if the history remains unclear. Finally, even in the context of a private interview, patients may be hesitant to divulge certain sensitive causes of local trauma, including abuse, masturbation, and unintentional injuries, including retained foreign body. On physical examination, key findings might include fever; rash; ocular or other mucosal involvement; arthritis; abdominal, pelvic, or costovertebral angle tenderness or masses; local lymphadenopathy; and genitourinary tract findings, such as adhesions, urethral meatus abnormalities, mucosal or skin lesions, urethral or vaginal discharge, and lymphadenopathy. For sexually active girls, examination of the clitoral and periurethral areas is particularly important. Additionally, a speculum examination, vaginal and cervical sample collection, and bimanual examination may be indicated in certain situations. For boys, regardless of sexual history, inspection and palpation of the testicles and penis, and retraction of the foreskin if uncircumcised, are important components of the examination.

Differential Diagnosis

The differential diagnosis of dysuria is broad. For younger children, a urinary tract infection (UTI) and mechanical or chemical causes are the most common etiologies (Table 19-1). Most cases in adolescence stem from a select few common causes, most notably UTIs or a sexually transmitted infection (STI) (Table 19-2). UTIs most commonly stem from coliforms and are generally rare in male adolescents without structural abnormalities. Typical presenting symptoms are urinary frequency, hesitancy, nocturia, malodorous urine, and sometimes fever, abdominal/flank pain, nausea, and vomiting, particularly in the setting of pyelonephritis.

Table 19-1. Common Etiologies of Dysuria in Children

Cause	Key Features	Evaluation/Management
Urinary tract infection	Fevers, abdomen/flank pain, frequency	UA, UCx, urinary tract imaging, antibiotics, preventive counseling, phenazopyridine
Irritant vulvovaginitis/urethritis	Urethral or vulvar irritation on examination; odor and blood associated with foreign body, bubble baths/soaps, tight underwear, sand, frequent masturbation, pinworms	Avoidance for most, removal of foreign body, improved toileting skills for newly trained children, sitz baths or bland emollients
Anatomic	Associated findings on physical examination (eg, labial adhesions, phimosis, trauma, prolapse)	Speculum examination, urinary tract imaging, surgical procedures when conservative measures fail
STI	Signs of trauma on examination, discharge, behavioral change	STI testing, pregnancy testing, counseling, antimicrobials, child protective services

Abbreviations: STI, sexually transmitted infection; UA, urinalysis; UCx, urine culture.

Table 19-2. Common Etiologies of Dysuria in Adolescents

Cause	Key Features	Evaluation/Management
Urinary tract Infection	Fevers, abdomen/flank pain, frequency	UA, UCx, antibiotics, preventive counseling, phenazopyridine
Candidal vulvovaginitis	Recent antibiotics, diabetes/impaired immune system, sexually active	Wet prep, antimicrobials
STI	Sexually active, discharge	STI testing, pregnancy testing, counseling, antimicrobials
Irritant vulvovaginitis	Soaps, douches, spermicide, masturbation	Avoidance

Abbreviations: STI, sexually transmitted infection; UA, urinalysis; UCx, urine culture.

Sexually transmitted infection syndromes include urethritis, cervicitis, and pelvic inflammatory disease in girls and urethritis and epididymitis in boys, all of which typically present with discharge. The most common sexually transmitted organisms implicated in dysuria are *Chlamydia trachomatis, Neisseria gonorrhoeae, Trichomonas vaginalis,* and herpes simplex virus. *Ureaplasma urealyticum* and *Mycoplasma genitalium* are other important causes of nongonoccocal urethritis. A history of having had sexual partners with similar symptoms strongly suggests the possibility of an STI.

Conditions localized to the periurethral area can also result in dysuria. In boys, these include balanitis and balanoposthitis. In girls, these include labial adhesions and tears, as well as chemical irritation from cleansers, spermicides, or other agents. In both genders, periurethral conditions may include local trauma such as mucosal abrasions from consensual sexual activity, abuse, or self-manipulation, as well as varicella, herpes simplex virus infection (which can also cause urethritis), and traumatic causes, both unintentional and intentional.

Vaginitis is another potential cause of dysuria among female adolescents and can stem from *Candida albicans,* bacterial vaginosis, allergens, chemical irritation, foreign bodies, and the sexually transmitted causes noted above. In younger patients, group A streptococci and *Shigella* species should also be considered.

Dysuria is also associated with an array of less common etiologies. These include Stevens-Johnson syndrome, which is a life-threatening manifestation of erythema multiforme, which affects a variety of mucosal surfaces including, potentially, the urethra. Other less common etiologies include Behçet syndrome, reactive arthritis, urinary tract stones, nephrolithiasis, hypercalciuria, hyperuricosuria, dysfunctional voiding, urethral stricture, lichen sclerosis, virginal vaginal ulcers (Lipshutz), endourethral syphilitic chancres, *Enterobius vermicularis* infestation, and psychogenic dysuria.

Laboratory Evaluation

Laboratory evaluation of dysuria is often minimal, although urinalysis and urine culture from a cleanly voided midstream sample are often very helpful as a first step toward establishing a diagnosis. Pyuria is evidenced by positive leukocyte esterase or greater than 5 to 10 white blood cells per high powered field on microscopy. A concurrent positive nitrite test typically suggests UTI. If the first 10 milliliters of urine are examined and pyuria is present, this is suggestive of inflammation in the genitourinary tract and may be present with either UTI or STI. Meanwhile, microscopic or gross hematuria, while often associated with UTI, can also suggest other etiologies such as nephrolithiasis or traumatic injury.

Other laboratory tests might include direct fluorescent antibody (DFA) testing and viral culture from lesions suspicious for herpes simplex virus, saline wet prep for bacterial vaginosis and trichomoniasis, 10% potassium hydroxide (KOH) wet prep for *Candida* vaginitis, vaginal pH to distinguish various causes of discharge, gonorrhea and chlamydia testing (typically nucleic-acid amplification testing on urine, urethral, vaginal, or cervical samples), and *Candida* culture if necessary.

In sexually active adolescents, pregnancy should always be considered, as many common causes of dysuria, including UTI, are more common during pregnancy. Vague complaints such as nausea, irregular menses, abdominal pain, and irregular spotting, may suggest pregnancy. A qualitative urine pregnancy test is appropriate for point-of-care testing.

Management

Management of dysuria involves directed treatment of the specific etiology as well as supportive measures targeted at alleviating symptoms. For infectious causes of dysuria, pain tends to improve promptly after initiation of antimicrobial therapy and improvement of local inflammation. For other causes, the course of dysuria after treatment can be variable.

Supportive measures, including oral analgesics such as acetaminophen, nonsteroidal anti-inflammatory medications, and rarely opioids in the case of extreme pain, are important. Locally active agents such as phenazopyridine, flavoxate, and oxybutynin can also be employed depending on the etiology of symptoms, although age restriction apply to their use. Other supportive options include sitz baths and topical barrier ointments if painful lesions are present.

Prevention of recurrent causes of dysuria should focus on treatment of the primary etiology, as in cases of anatomic abnormalities, and on avoidance of precipitating causes, such as mechanical or chemical irritants, poor genitourinary tract hygiene, and improper toileting techniques. Though data is lacking, some clinicians may choose to counsel sexually active female patients with recurrent UTIs to void before intercourse and immediately afterward. Spermicide also increases risk for UTIs. Prophylactic antibiotics may be considered for recurrent UTIs in certain situations, on a daily, postcoital, or patient-initiated basis. Meanwhile, cranberry juice was recently been found to be less efficacious than previously thought.

Suggested Reading

Jepson RG, Williams G, Craig JC. Cranberries for preventing urinary tract infections. *Cochrane Database Syst Rev.* 2012;10:CD001321

Musacchio NS, Gehani S, Garofalo R. Emergency department management of adolescents with urinary complaints: missed opportunities. *J Adol Health.* 2009;44(1):81–83

Shaikh N, Morone NE, Lopez J, et al. Does this child have a urinary tract infection? *JAMA.* 2007;298(24):2895–2904

CHAPTER 20

Ear Pain

Charles Willson, MD, and Suzette Surratt Caudle, MD

Key Points

- Otalgia may be severe and immediate; satisfactory pain relief is indicated.

- Otalgia may be caused by local inflammation of the structures of the ear or referred pain. Because many important structures are in close proximity of the ears, impairment of function of these structures may point to the cause of the pain.

- A red tympanic membrane is not a sufficient finding to diagnose acute otitis media.

- If the aural structures appear to be healthy, consider referred or "phantom" pain.

- Most causes of otalgia may be diagnosed and managed in the outpatient setting.

- Accurate diagnosis and management of otalgia is necessary to maintain auditory function.

Overview

Ear pain, otherwise known as otalgia, is a frequent presenting concern. Causes of ear pain range from the entirely benign to far more serious, but fortunately less common, disorders. Many parents struggle with trying to decide if the 6-month-old pulling on her ear has a painful condition or is merely exploring the sensations of her new body. Some older children learn that when they tell their parent that their ear hurts, they will get immediate attention (phantom ear pain).

Over the years, greater than 50% of acute otitis media (AOM) cases do not require antibiotic therapy and will resolve with comfort therapy and time. Rarely, however, a bacterial acute otitis media will cause the tympanic membrane to rupture or even progress to acute mastoiditis or osteomyelitis with extension into the cranium. An inadequately treated acute otitis media may become chronically infected with formation of a cholesteatoma. Hearing loss may occur with recurrent bacterial otitis media, but this, too, is rare. However, these complications take time to develop, and a vigilant parent need not worry that she will miss the signs of these serious complications.

Differential Diagnosis (Table 20-1)

Table 20-1. Differential Diagnosis of Otalgia

Primary Ear Pain	Referred Ear Pain
External ear/ear canal • Trauma • Rash • Cellulitis • Otitis externa • Furuncle • Infection of the pinna • Foreign body • Cerumen impaction • Perichondritis **Middle ear/eustachian tube** • Acute otitis media • Eustachian tube dysfunction or blockage • Myringitis • Skull fracture leading to hemotympanum • Cholesteatoma **Inner ear** • Labyrinthitis	• Lymphadenitis • Parotitis • Ramsey-Hunt syndrome • Pharyngitis/tonsillitis/retropharyngeal abscess • Brain abscess • Brain tumor, acoustic neuroma • Cervical spine injury, dislocation, tumor • Behavioral—exploration, attention seeking • Sinusitis • Dental disease • Neural syndromes—Bell palsy, trigeminal neuralgia, migraines • Skull fracture • Temporomandibular arthralgia/arthritis • Thyroiditis **Behavioral** • "Phantom" ear pain

Evaluation

The ear may be the primary site of pain, or pain may be referred from another site. Pain due to pathology in a nearby but anatomically distinct location may present as ear pain. Therefore, an evaluation of a patient with otalgia should include a search for causes of both primary and referred pain. A thorough examination of the structures of the head and neck should be performed on all patients with otalgia (Table 20-2).

Pain directly attributable to the ear may indicate pathology of the external ear and canal, the middle ear and eustachian tube, or the inner ear.

The External Ear and Canal

The external ear may be the site of trauma, a painful rash, or cellulitis. Cellulitis of the ear lobe has become more frequent with the cultural practice of piercings. Without good daily care, a piercing may embed the distal end of the "earring" in the ear lobe and require minor surgery for removal.

With otitis externa, the ear canal becomes swollen and extremely painful because of irritation of the periosteum of the base of the skull. Simple manipulation of the pinna will produce a marked painful response, confirming the diagnosis. A parent can easily be taught how to apply traction to the pinna to

Table 20-2. Clues and Considerations in Evaluation of Otalgia

Chief Concern of Otalgia	Thorough History for Symptoms Suggestive of Primary or Referred pain	Complete Physical Examination of Entire Head and Neck Area
Primary and referred sources of pain	Fever: infections including AOM, mastoiditis, sinusitis, pharyngitis, oral/pharyngeal abscesses, intracranial infections	**Ear** • Erythema, lesions • Pain on pinna movement • Obstruction (including foreign body) or debris in ear canal • Abnormal tympanic membrane: effusion, hemotympanum, vesicles, tumor/masses • Postauricular swelling/tenderness
	Ear drainage: AOM w/ perforation or otitis externa	**Oropharynx** • Oral lesions
	History of trauma/possible trauma to head, neck	• Erythema/tenderness of mouth • Erythema, swelling, lesions
	Pain w/ eating: dental etiology	• Throat or tonsils
	Spitting, other symptoms of gastroesophageal reflux	**Face** • Tenderness over sinuses • Nasal drainage
	Headaches/family history of migraines	• TM joint abnormality • Parotid swelling
	Dizziness/balance concerns: labyrinthitis	**Neck** • Lymphadenopathy • Tenderness/enlargement thyroid
	Hearing problems	**Skull** • Tenderness, bruising
		General status • Alert, oriented • Ill appearing
		Neurologic examination focusing head, neck, and upper extremities • Cranial nerve examination • Tenderness or trauma of cervical spine

Abbreviations: AOM, acute otitis media; TM, tympanic membrane; w/, with.

distinguish between the otalgia of an acute otitis externa versus an otitis media. An otitis externa may proceed to a cellulitis at the base of the pinna. When the base of the pinna becomes swollen and painful, a "malignant" otitis externa may be present that will require parenteral antibiotics rather than the usual antibiotic eardrops that resolve a simple otitis externa. An otitis externa may also become chronic with persistent purulent drainage from the ear canal, especially if the tympanic membrane (TM) is perforated.

A furuncle is a purulent infection of a hair root, which may occur within the ear canal or adjacent to the pinna and may mimic an acute otitis externa. Inflammation of the perichondrium, known as perichondritis, may occur on the pinna or inside the ear canal.

Ear pain may also develop acutely when a toddler decides to insert a foreign body into the external auditory canal. Foreign bodies in the ear canal should be removed as soon as possible to prevent damage to the ear canal or tympanic membrane. If the pediatrician is hesitant to remove the foreign body or the child is uncooperative in holding still during the quick procedure, otolaryngologists are equipped to remove the foreign body safely with local analgesia, using an operating microscope.

The Middle Ear and Eustachian Tube

Pain associated with an acute otitis media is caused by stretching of the highly innervated TM by the rapid development of pus behind the membrane. Once the TM is fully stretched (usually over a couple of hours), the pain subsides. Sometimes the TM will rupture, bringing immediate relief from the pain. A parent should understand that providing an oral or topical analgesic is an acceptable approach to managing this phase of acute otitis media. If the TM ruptures, it will quickly repair itself when the infection is controlled. Examining the child during regular office hours will confirm the suspected AOM. Purulent fluid will be visible behind the now opaque TM. Pneumatic otoscopy or tympanometry will confirm the presence of an effusion (Figure 20-1). In contrast, when air is present in the middle ear space, the TM will move as air pressure in the external canal is increased and then decreased. In AOM, the TM will be bulging and red with inflammation, and often yellow or white pus may be seen within the middle ear cleft. When an acute otitis media does not respond to appropriate antibiotic therapy, a tympanocentesis using a 22-gauge lumbar puncture needle through an operating otoscope may release the pressure of the abscess-like infection and provide a positive culture of the organism to assess antibacterial sensitivities. Eustachian canal dysfunction or blockage can lead to negative pressure behind the TM, causing retraction of the membrane. Positive air pressure transmitted through an open eustachian canal may be caused by screaming, diving, or air travel, resulting in acute pain. Gastroesophageal reflux can result in a swollen proximal end of the eustachian tube with subsequent disruption of function.

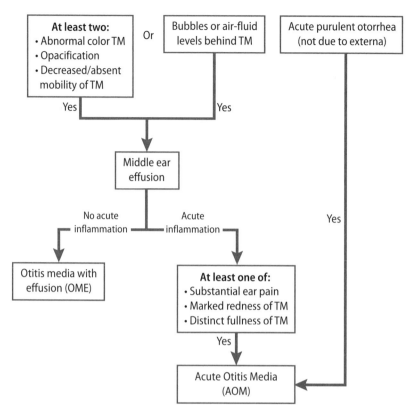

Figure 20-1. Algorithm for distinguishing between acute otitis media (AOM) and otitis media with effusion (OME).

Abbreviation: TM, tympanic membrane.

From Kerschner JE. Otitis media. In: Kliegman RM, Stanton BF, St. Geme JW, Schor NF, Behrman RE, eds. *Nelson's Textbook of Pediatrics.* 19th ed. Philadelphia, PA: Saunders; 2011:2203, with permission.

Referred Pain

Lymphadenitis. Swelling of the preauricular and postauricular lymph nodes may extend to the base of the ear and cause pain. Rubella often causes postauricular lymph node enlargement. With a solitary node enlargement, tuberculosis or cat-scratch disease should be considered.

Parotitis. Swelling of the parotid gland with fever may be viral or bacterial in origin. Differentiation between parotid swelling and acute lymphadenitis is important. Fortunately, immunization against mumps virus has made viral parotitis much less common.

Dental disease. A dental abscess or exposed dental nerve may cause pain referred to the ear. Management includes penicillin, pain medications, and referral to a dentist.

Pharyngitis. Inflammation of the posterior oropharynx may cause a feeling of fullness and even pain in one or both ears. Viral syndromes such as herpangina due to Coxsackie A virus may present with otalgia as part of the symptom complex. On careful examination, the presence of vesicles and erythema of the posterior oropharynx confirms the diagnosis.

Tonsillitis/tonsillar disease. Severe swelling and inflammation of the tonsils will suggest this diagnosis. With swelling superiorly and medially to the tonsil, an abscess must be considered. High-dose penicillin will often be sufficient treatment, but if airway compromise is suspected, an urgent referral to an otolaryngologist should be made.

Retropharyngeal cellulitis/abscess. Painful swallowing, high fever, and systemic toxicity are the usual presenting concerns of a patient with retropharyngeal abscess. Only imaging may differentiate between a cellulitis or an abscess. Hospitalization with otolaryngologist consultation is required until any possibility of airway compromise is alleviated.

Sinusitis. Infection in the maxillary and even ethmoid sinuses has been known to cause unilateral otalgia. Local tenderness and swelling of the surrounding structures will suggest the diagnosis.

Brain abscess/tumor. An abscess may arise in the mastoid air cells with extension into the cranium or vice versa. A meningeal tumor or acoustic neuroma (eg, schwanoma) may erode into the inner ear structures or mastoid region. Careful assessment of cranial nerve function may suggest this possibility.

Neural syndromes including migraine. Otalgia may accompany Bell palsy, trigeminal neuralgia, and rarely migraine headaches. A family history of migraine headaches is an important clue.

Cervical spine injury, dislocation, tumor. A history of major trauma with cervical nerve root involvement will help guide the diagnosis. Presentation of tumors in the region are more subtle, with appropriate imaging showing mass effects.

Skull fracture. A history of trauma and the presence of blood behind the TM will suggest a basilar skull fracture.

Temporomandibular arthralgia/arthritis. Confirm the diagnosis by palpation of the joint as the patient opens and closes her mouth. Anti-inflammatory agents, especially nonsteroidal agents, are the mainstay of therapy. If bruxism is causing trauma to the TM joint, dental appliances may be used to lessen the pressure on the joint and damage to the teeth. In patients with idiopathic juvenile arthritis, the TM joint may be involved and managed as part of that syndrome. A normal examination of the ear structures will confirm that the pain is referred.

Thyroiditis. Rarely, a viral or bacterial infection will cause thyroiditis with pain referred to the ears. Autoimmune thyroiditis is heralded by the presence of a goiter.

Management

Because of the extreme sensitivity of the innervation of the ear, pain medications are often appropriate. Acetaminophen, ibuprofen, and even opiates may be required to bring relief while waiting for curative therapy to become effective. The pain associated with stretching of the eardrum with acute otitis media or air with barotrauma will be self-limited, as the pain usually subsides within an hour or two as the stretch receptors accommodate. If the tympanic membrane is intact, a topical benzocaine may be safely instilled to bring immediate relief. Worsening of the swelling of the canal after using the drops may indicate an allergy to benzocaine.

Irritation may develop beneath impacted cerumen, so when seen as an incidental finding, cerumen should be gently removed.

Trauma

Parents and patients should be advised to never insert anything into the ear canal. When trauma has caused swelling and pain, it may be managed as an acute otitis externa with care to rule out trauma to the tympanic membrane and possible damage to the ossicles.

Otitis Externa

Antibiotic drops are the mainstay of therapy for otitis externa. An antibiotic suspension rather than a solution is preferred. Neomycin-Polymyxin B-cortisone is a popular combination eardrop but must be used cautiously because of the ototoxicity of neomycin and the tendency to develop allergy to neomycin. Ciprofloxacin drops do not have these disadvantages but are considerably more expensive. Prior to instilling the drops, all debris in the ear canal should be gently removed or rinsed out. A wick may be inserted into the canal to hold the suspension against the ear canal. As the swelling of the ear canal lessens, the wick will fall out. Usually instilling the drops 4 times a day for 5 days will suffice.

For patients that get recurrent otitis externa due to swimming, a 1:1 mixture of vinegar and isopropyl alcohol may be instilled into the child's ear at bedtime and immediately allowed to drain out to prevent the development of an otitis externa.

Otitis Media

In younger children, viral upper respiratory tract infections cause swelling of the lining of the eustachian tube, leading to a negative pressure behind the eardrum. Serous fluid develops in the middle ear space (ie, otitis media with effusion), and a bacterial infection may develop (ie, acute otitis media). Viral pathogens that predispose to otitis media include parainfluenza, influenza, and adenovirus. Bacterial pathogens originate in back of the nasal passage at the base of the eustachian tube. Pneumococcal infection, *Hemophilus influenzae, Moraxella* species infection, and group A streptococcal infection should be considered. With a perforated eardrum, *Staphylococcus aureus* and pseudomonas may enter the middle ear space, leading to chronic otitis media.

When a decision has been made to treat the child with antibiotics, and the child has not received amoxicillin in the past 30 days, does not have concurrent purulent conjunctivitis, or is not allergic to penicillin, amoxicillin at 80 to 90 mg/kg/day divided 3 times a day remains the mainstay treatment for AOM. A 10-day course is typical, especially in infants, but in older children, a 5-day course may be sufficient. If antibacterial resistance to penicillin develops, especially when the AOM has recurred within 30 days of a previous course of amoxicillin, or there is a history of recurrent AOM unresponsive to amoxicillin, amoxicillin-clavulanate (β-lactamase coverage) should be considered. In a patient with vomiting or unusual toxicity, an intramuscular dose of ceftriaxone may be given and repeated over the next 2 days. For children with penicillin allergy, alternate second- or third-generation cephalosporin such as cefuroxime, cefdinir, or cefixime may be used, with the caution that a 10% cross-reactivity between penicillin and cephlosporin antibiotics is possible.

Extension of AOM into the mastoid sinus requires parenteral antibiotics.

A cholesteotoma is a benign tumor of the middle ear usually precipitated by chronic infection. Surgical removal is required to prevent destruction of the ossicles.

For a child with otalgia, purulent effusion, and an inflamed TM, management with analgesics and antipyretics is acceptable because up to 40% of patients with this presentation will recover without antibacterial therapy. Some clinicians faced with this presentation will educate the parent about the natural course of otitis media and give the parent a prescription for an antibiotic to fill should the ear pain worsen and fever develop.

Bacterial infection of the inner ear is rare, but viruses may cause labyrinthitis with tinnitus and vertigo. Management is supportive.

Referred Pain

Management of the source of the pain is crucial.

Conclusion

Otalgia is a common presenting concern in a busy primary care office and a frequent cause of referral to an otolaryngologist. Attention to the anatomic location of the painful structure with an understanding of the conditions that may lead to direct or referred pain to the ear is crucial in making an accurate diagnosis and beginning specific management. Maintenance of hearing acuity is a prime consideration requiring accurate and timely diagnosis and treatment. Fortunately, most cases of otalgia will resolve with appropriate management.

Suggested Reading

Kerschner JE. Otitis media. In: *Nelson's Textbook of Pediatrics*. 19 ed. Philadelphia, PA: Saunders; 2011:2636–2646

Leung A, Fong J, Leong A. Otalgia in children. *J Natl Med Assoc*. 2000;92(5):254–260

Lieberthal AS, Carroll AE, Chonmaitree T, et al; American Academy of Pediatrics Subcommittee on Diagnosis and Management of Acute Otitis Media. Clinical practice guideline: the diagnosis and management of acute otitis media. *Pediatrics*. 2013;131(3):e964–e999

Neilan RE, Roland RS. Otalgia. *Med Clin North Am*. 2010;94(5):961–971

Venekamp RP, Sanders S, Glaziou P, Del Mar CB, Rovers MM. Antibiotics for acute otitis media in children. *Cochrane Database Syst Rev*. 2013;1:CD000219

Wood DN, Nikos N, Gregory CW. Clinical trials in assessing ototopical agents in the treatment of pain associated with acute otitis media in children. *Int J Pediatr Otorhinolaryngol*. 2012;76(9):1229–1235

CHAPTER 21

Eye Problems: Red Eye and Swelling

Suzette Surratt Caudle, MD

Key Points

- Tearing, a large eye or cornea, or a dull red reflex in a neonate raise concern for congenital glaucoma and should prompt rapid referral to a pediatric ophthalmologist.

- A red eye with ciliary flush or an irregular pupil should raise concern for uveitis.

- In the setting of periorbital or orbital cellulitis, ophthalmoplegia, pain on extraocular movement, and proptosis warrant urgent thin slice computed tomography of the orbit and sinuses, but failure to improve, a difficult physical examination, marked edema, or other factors may also indicate the need to proceed with imaging.

- Multidisciplinary management of orbital cellulitis, with pediatrics, otolaryngology, or ophthalmology, is essential to determine if and when surgical intervention may be indicated to avoid vision loss and other morbidity.

Overview

Red eye is a common presenting symptom in pediatric practice. Causes can range from benign to life-threatening illnesses, a common cause being conjunctivitis.

Like red eye, eye and eyelid swelling can also be associated with relatively benign etiologies or more serious systemic or local pathology.

Causes

Causes of the red or swollen eye include keratitis, corneal abrasion, conjunctivitis, blepharitis, other disorders of the eyelid, iritis, glaucoma, and infections of the eye and orbital soft tissues (eg, periorbital or preseptal cellulitis, orbital cellulitis, and orbital abscesses). This chapter will focus on preseptal and orbital cellulitis, after a brief review of other eye problems resulting in the red or swollen eye.

Blepharitis

Blepharitis is inflammation of the eyelid margin. Onset is generally 6 to 7 years of age, but it may persist for months before it is diagnosed. It is usually caused by a staphylococcal infection, and scaling, crusting, and redness along the eyelid margin, especially in the morning, are hallmarks. Tearing, photophobia, and swollen eyelids are also telltale signs. There is minimal to no discharge, but lids may crust shut overnight. The eyelid may be chronically inflamed with acute exacerbations, with the lid margins red, thickened, and vascularized. In some instances, there is breakage, misdirection, or loss of eyelashes. Secondary conjunctival and corneal involvement may include punctuate erosions, keratitis, ulceration, and even corneal scarring and revascularization. Treatment of blepharitis includes keeping the eyelids clean and free of crusts, using warm compresses and gentle scrubbing of the eyelid with a cotton swab dipped in a baby-shampoo/water mix. This treatment needs to be continued over a long period of time as a preventive measure and as some degree of symptoms may persist. Staphylococcal infection can be treated using topical antibiotics, such as erythromycin or bacitracin, on the eyelids for approximately one week, with exact duration being guided by severity. For severe cases, topical steroids may be required. As meibomian gland dysfunction can lead to drying of the eye and tear deficiency, lubricants, such as artificial tears, can be useful adjunct treatments. Blepharitis may also be complicated by hordeola and chalazia.

Hordeolum

A hordeolum is an acute infection of either Zeis glands (eg, external hordeolum or stye) or of a meibomian gland (ie, internal hordeolum). Infection is usually caused by *Staphylococcus epidermidis* or *Staphylococcus aureus*. Spread to neighboring issue can cause preseptal cellulitis, and a persistent hordeolum can lead to chronic inflammation resulting in a chalazion. Hordeola are treated with warm compresses 4 times daily. Topical antibiotics do not help with earlier resolution but may help prevent spread.

If severe and not improving, surgical drainage may be necessary.

Chalazion

A chalazion is a focal inflammatory lesion eyelid from obstruction of a meibomian gland (ie, internal hordeolum) and is a sterile inflammation. Seborrhea, acne, and blepharitis can predispose to the development of chalazia. The role of *S aureus* in chalazia is not clear. Pain is absent or mild; however, continued inflammation can lead to disfigurement of the eyelid, pyogenic granuloma, and preseptal cellulitis. Most chalazia can be managed conservatively with warm compresses 4 times daily and topical antibiotic ointment if there are signs of infection.

Intralesional steroids can help accelerate healing but can cause hypo-pigmentation of the overlying skin. Large persistent lesions may require surgical drainage and curettage.

Contact Dermatitis

Contact dermatitis is the most common cause of eyelid skin inflammation. Eyelid involvement may be the only or the initial presenting site for contact dermatitis. Contact dermatitis may be allergic or irritant in etiology. Irritant dermatitis is caused by the direct toxic effect of the irritant, and allergic dermatitis is a type IV hypersensitivity. Contact dermatitis presents as erythema, edema, and vesiculation when acute, with scaling and desquamation in more long-standing cases. Treatment is avoidance of causative agents and low-dose topical steroids to the lids for 5 to 10 days.

Atopic Dermatitis

Atopic dermatitis involving the eyelid is marked by red, thickened, and macerated eye lids. Atopic dermatitis of the eyelids is often associated with chronic staphylococcal blepharitis and hyperemic and boggy conjunctiva. Atopic dermatitis is treated with oral antihistamines and systemic or topical steroids during flares.

Dacryocystitis

Dacryocystitis is bacterial infection of the lacrimal sac that usually occurs as a result of bacterial superinfection after a viral upper respiratory tract infection (URTI). Fever, redness, swelling, and tenderness are noted in the area lateral to and below the medial canthus. When pressure is applied to the region, pus may be exuded from the sac. In neonates, *Streptococcus pnuemoniae* is a common pathogen, while *S aureus* and *S epidermidis* are more common in older children. Patients who are toxic appearing need intravenous antibiotics such as nafcillin or clindamycin.

Dacryoadenitis is infection of the lacrimal gland and manifests as sudden redness and swelling of the outer end of the upper eyelid. It is most often caused by viruses (mumps, Epstein Barr virus, cytomegalovirus, enteric cytopathic human orphan [ECHO] virus, varicella) and bacteria (staphylococci, *S pyogenes,* chlamydia, and *Neisseria gonorrhea*). Treatment is typically oral antibiotics, but occasionally intravenous antibiotics are required.

Congenital Glaucoma

Congenital glaucoma is an increase of intraocular pressure shortly after birth. Clinical signs include tearing, photophobia, blepharospasm, a large cornea, corneal clouding, and sometimes red eye. Disease is bilateral approximately 70% of the time. In some cases, physical signs are minimal. The red reflex may look dull. Intraocular pressure must be reduced to avoid damage to the optic nerve. Medications (such as beta-adrenergic inhibitors and carbonic anhydrase inhibitors) and sometimes surgery (ie, opening outflow channels of trabecular network) are necessary. Congenital glaucoma can be associated with systemic and genetic abnormalities including Sturge-Weber syndrome, neurofibromatosis I, and Marfan syndrome.

Uveitis

Uveitis is inflammation of any part of the uveal tract (ie, iris, choroids, ciliary body, or retina), and can result in blindness. Uveitis is associated with multiple systemic disorders such as juvenile arthritis. Iridocyclitis (ie, inflammation of the iris and ciliary structures) is marked by the sudden onset of redness, pain, photophobia, tearing, and mild decreases in visual acuity. The conjunctiva and sclera may appear congested (a ciliary flush) and the pupil may appear small and irregular. Diagnosis is made with a slit lamp, demonstrating cells and protein within the aqueous chamber. Early treatment improves prognosis and includes topical corticosteroids, nonsteroidal anti-inflammatory agents, and cycloplegic-mydriatic agents. Many vision-threatening complications can occur for which prompt recognition and immediate referral to ophthalmologic care may help to mitigate.

Infections of the Eye

Infections involving the eyelid, its surrounding structures, and the orbit itself typically present as a red, swollen eye. Preseptal or periorbital cellulitis is infection restricted to the areas (eyelid and adnexa) anterior to the septum. Orbital cellulitis involves tissues behind the septum and can further include subperiosteal abscesses and orbital abscesses.

Periorbital Cellulitis

Periorbital cellulitis is approximately 3 times more common than orbital cellulitis and is largely a disease of childhood. It occurs mostly in children younger than 5 years. It is often caused by direct inoculation of the organism into the eye by a complicated URTI, by disruption of skin integrity (either through an insect bite or minor trauma that gets secondarily infected), or through impetigo, eczema or acne, direct extension from a hordeolum or lacrimal infection, or a dental abscess. Prior to effective immunization against *Haemophilus influenzae* type b, and to some extent *Streptococcus pneumoniae,* hematogenous spread was a significant factor. It plays a lesser role at this time.

Orbital Cellulitis

Orbital cellulitis occurs when infection involves the structures posterior to the orbital septum. Infection may spread to the orbit through the bone from the paranasal sinuses surrounding the orbit on 3 of 4 sides. The most common predisposing factor for pediatric orbital cellulitis is rhinosinusitis, especially ethmoiditis. In addition, the orbital veins are valveless with anastomosing fibers and allow passage of infection in either a retrograde or antegrade fashion via hematogenous spread. Penetrating trauma and foreign bodies can also result in orbital cellulitis. Uncommonly, orbital cellulitis may represent spread of a periorbital cellulitis through the septum.

Orbital cellulitis occurs in all ages but is more common in childhood. Most cases are unilateral. Orbital cellulitis is more common in winter because of its association with sinus and upper respiratory tract infections.

The most common organisms cultured from patients with periorbital infections are *S aureus, S epidermidis,* and *Streptococcus pyogenes.* Of cases cultured, these organisms accounted for 75% of pediatric periorbital infections. Staphylococcal and streptococcal organisms are the most common organisms in orbital cellulitis as well. Community-acquired MRSA is gaining in prominence and is estimated to account for as many as two-thirds or even three-fourths of *S aureus* isolates from patients with orbital cellulitis. Other streptococci, nontypeable *H influenzae, Moraxella catarrhalis,* and anaerobes have also been identified. Polymicrobial infections are sometimes seen in orbital cellulitis, especially in older pediatric patients, and can include anaerobes. Polymicrobial infections may follow dental infections as well as sinusitis. Rare fungal infections have been described.

Other Causes

Other causes of swollen eyelids include allergic reactions and edema secondary to hypoproteinemia. Allergic responses typically respond to an antihistamine. Hypoproteinemia would be expected to present as bilateral involvement, typically with other systemic signs, and is typically worse upon arising in the morning but improves over the course of the day.

Clinical Features

Virtually all of the recommendations for diagnosis, evaluation, and management of periorbital and orbital disease are based on Evidence Level II-3 or III.

Both disorders usually involve unilateral redness, swelling and induration, and tenderness and pain of the eyelid. Fever is common, and onset is usually rather abrupt. General malaise may be present. Erythema may extend over the superior orbital rim into the brow.

Particularly in young children, ill appearance and preceding URTI symptoms raise concern for hematogenous seeding. A history of recent URTI and possible sinus symptoms, trauma, and recent dental issues should be elicited.

Visual changes and decreased visual acuity, ophthalmoplegia, proptosis, and chemosis signal orbital involvement. Pain is also typically present. Patients may appear ill and even toxic.

Evaluation

Periorbital cellulitis can often be diagnosed on clinical features. A complete blood count, while not necessary in most cases, will typically reveal an elevated white blood cell count. If hematogenous spread is a concern or systemic symptoms are present, blood cultures should be considered. Overall yield of blood cultures is low, although somewhat higher in children than adults. Culture of eye drainage or the conjunctival sac may be of use. In cases requiring surgical management, wound (orbital abscess or sinus fluid) cultures offer high yield.

Thin sagittal, coronal, and axial slices of a computed tomography (CT) scan of the sinuses and orbits with contrast enhancement will differentiate periorbital from orbital cellulitis and delineate the degree of orbital involvement. It is most critical to differentiate patients who have orbital or intracranial abscesses early because early identification benefits these patients most at risk for vision and even life-threatening complications, as well as identifying them for closer follow-up. Computed tomography is classically indicated in the presence of proptosis, neurologic involvement (eg, lethargy or other altered mental status, seizures, focal deficits), ongoing loss of vision, or impaired extraocular movements, or if the diagnosis is unclear or complete examination unobtainable. Proptosis, oph-thalmoplegia, and pain on extraocular movements as indications for CT, do identify a group at high risk for intraorbital and intracerebral complications, but using those criteria alone missed about half of cases with complications. Other predictors of having orbital abscess on CT are an absolute neutrophil count greater than 10,000, with moderate to severe edema extending beyond the peri-orbital area, and previous antibiotic use (Evidence Level II-3). Computed tomog-raphy imaging will not only identify orbital involvement such as diffuse fat infiltration, subperiosteal involvement, and orbital abscess but also potentially identify foreign bodies, as well as far less common causes of proptosis, such as orbital pseudotumor, sarcoidosis, Wegener granulomatosis, and malignancies.

Management

Uncomplicated periorbital cellulitis is treated with oral or parenteral antibiotics to cover staphylococci and streptococci. Local patterns of methicillin-resistant *S aureus* (MRSA) prevalence and sensitivity should be considered in treatment choices. There is no evidence that parenteral therapy offers faster resolution or decreases complications from the disease compared to oral therapy in patients with simple periorbital cellulitis. Treatment decisions regarding route of therapy should be made based on the clinical appearance of the child and the disease progression, the ability to successfully take oral medications and compliance concerns, and the assurance of close follow-up. Oral therapy may include amoxi-cillin-clavulanate or a cephalosporin to cover beta-lactamase producers as well as clindamycin. Preseptal cellulitis in neonates is treated with hospitalization and parenteral therapy. When suspicion for hematogenous spread is present, parenteral therapy to empirically cover gram positive and gram negative organisms, including those associated with rhinosinusitis, should be undertaken. Typically oral therapy lasts 7 to 10 days. Parenteral therapy can be transitioned to oral therapy when clear improvement and resolution of systemic symptoms is noted, for a 10- to 14-day total course of therapy.

Indications for inpatient admission and intravenous antibiotics include (1) ill-appearing patients or who have signs of central nervous system involvement such as lethargy, seizures, focal neurologic deficits, headache, or vomiting; (2) patients with diplopia, decreased visual acuity, proptosis, abnormal extraocular movements, or abnormal light reflexes; and (3) patients in whom a complete clinical eye examination is not possible because of marked swelling or age/ability to cooperate. Coverage for orbital cellulitis includes coverage for *S aureus*, *S pyogenes*, sinus pathogens such as *S pneumoniae* and non-typeable *H influenzae*, and anaerobes. Coverage for MRSA should be strongly considered as well. A second- or third-generation cephalosporin or ampicillin-sulbactam, with clindamycin, is an appropriate initial response. Vancomycin may be used in the ill-appearing child. In all cases, improvement should be evident within 2 days of initiating therapy. Some sources advocate 21 days of therapy in cases secondary to complications of sinusitis, but most recommend shorter courses with adjustment based on monitoring of clinical response to therapy.

Consultation with ophthalmologic or otolaryngological colleagues for possible surgical intervention should be undertaken in the case of orbital cellulitis, particularly complicated orbital cellulitis. While many cases are managed medically, including cases with subperiosteal abscesses, surgical intervention may be needed for drainage of large abscesses, release of pressure on orbital contents, and to obtain cultures. Any deterioration of vision or signs of progression generally prompt surgical management. Various studies have described situations in which medical management is less likely to be successful, including abscesses greater than 10 mm, the presence of non-medial subperiosteal abscesses or intracranial disease, increasing age (older than 9 years), proptosis, gas in the orbit, and in the setting of a dental infection. Sinus surgery, orbital surgery, and at times neurosurgery may be indicated. Ophthalmoplegia, abscess, acuity worse than 20/60, blindness, progression of orbital signs, and lack of improvement after 48 hours of aggressive medical management are indications to strongly consider surgical management.

Long-term Monitoring and Implications

Orbital cellulitis can extend to the venous sinus, resulting in cavernous sinus thrombosis. Initial symptoms are similar to those of orbital cellulitis, and may progress to loss of vision and meningismus.

Further intracranial complications of orbital cellulitis include subdural empyemas, extradural abscesses, intracranial abscesses, and meningitis.

Vision loss and even blindness may occur secondary to retinal artery occlusion, compression, or inflammation of the optic nerve or corneal ulceration. When intracranial complications, including cavernous sinus thrombosis, are suspected magnetic resonance imaging is indicated.

Suggested Reading

Baring DE, Hilmi OJ. An evidence based review of periorbital cellulitis. *Clin Otolaryngol.* 2011;36(1):57–64

Bedwell J, Bauman NM. Management of pediatric orbital cellulitis and abscess. *Curr Opin Otolaryngol Head Neck Surg.* 2011;19(6):467–473

Hauser A, Fogarsi S. Periorbital and orbital cellulitis. *Pediatr Rev.* 2010;31(6):242–249

Rudloe TF, Harper MB, Prabhu SP, Rahbar R, VanderVeen D, Kimia AA. Acute periorbital infections: who needs emergent imaging? *Pediatrics.* 2010;125(4):e719–e726

Sethuraman U, Kamat D. The red eye: evaluation and management. *Clin Pediatr.* 2009;48(6):588–600

Wong IB, Nischal KK. Managing a child with an external ocular disease. *J AAPOS.* 2010;14(1):68–77

CHAPTER 22

Failure to Thrive

Melinda A. Williams-Willingham, MD, and Patricia D. Morgan, MD

Key Points

- It is important to obtain accurate measurements and use appropriate growth charts.
- A thorough history, complete physical examination, and ancillary evaluation are essential.
- Be sure to look for psychosocial factors that may play a role in growth failure in infants and children.

Overview

Failure to thrive (FTT), or growth failure, is one of the most common problems in pediatrics and may be seen in any age group, though especially significant during the first 3 years when critical growth and development occur. Failure to thrive accounts for 1% to 5% of pediatric hospital admissions for children younger than 2 years in the United States. A systematic approach is necessary to determine the cause, which often involves multiple factors that lead to FTT.

Definition

There is no consensus on the definition for FTT. Interchangeable terms such as *growth failure* and *poor weight gain* are appropriate, while terms such as *organic* and *non-organic* are no longer used.

Failure to thrive in infants and children is a symptom that usually results from (a) inadequate caloric intake or undernutrition; (b) poor utilization; or (c) increase in metabolic demand, which prevents them from maintaining adequate physical growth and development compared to recognized references for age and gender. A traditional approach toward the diagnosis for FTT includes a combination of anthropometric criteria rather than one criterion which will lead to a more accurate identification for children at risk for failure to thrive (Box 22-1) (Evidence Level III).

Box 22-1. Common Anthropometric Criteria for Diagnosing Failure to Thrive

- Weight for age below the 3rd or 5th percentile on more than one occasion
- Weight for length less than the 5th percentile
- Shift of greater than or equal to 2 major growth percentiles downward in a standardized growth grid using the 90th, 75th, 50th, 25th, 10th, and 5th percentiles as the major percentiles during a 6-month period
- Length for age below the 5th percentile
- Weight less than 70% of ideal weight for age, which may require prompt attention (Evidence Level III)

Causes

A variety of medical and nonmedical causes may contribute to FTT; however, the immediate factor is commonly caused by inadequate nutrition. Pediatricians must, therefore, consider possible secondary causes in addition to the primary contributing factor. The cause is often multifactorial and includes biological, psychosocial, and environmental contributions, making the evaluation complex.

Failure to thrive can be seen in cases of child neglect, and a social history is an important aspect in identifying social factors as a cause of growth failure. Failure to thrive as a consequence of child maltreatment must be considered in families with profiles indicating a high risk of abuse or neglect, ones that consistently fail to adhere to the recommended interventions or are unable to maintain a safe environment for their child. Child neglect or physical abuse must be considered in children with FTT because children with FTT are 4 times more likely to be abused than children without growth failure.

Poverty is the greatest single factor for FTT in developed and developing countries. Family factors can contribute at any age and may include inadequate nutritional knowledge and inadequate finances. Although only about 20% of children with FTT have an underlying medical condition as a cause for their growth failure, it is still important to exclude significant medical problems related to inadequate caloric intake, inadequate caloric absorption, or excessive caloric expenditures (Table 22-1) (Evidence Level III).

In many instances, the infant or child may simply not being fed enough. This may be because the infant or child is not being offered enough formula, human milk, or other foods.

Inadequate caloric absorption may be seen with persistent losses, as with malabsorption and persistent emesis. Malabsorption may be seen with chronic diarrhea, excess juice intake, protein-losing enteropathy, celiac disease, certain food sensitivities, and pancreatic insufficiency.

Persistent vomiting due to gastroesophageal reflux, medications, anatomic abnormalities, metabolic conditions, and food sensitivities may also be the cause.

Excessive caloric use may be seen in conditions such as immunologic problems and recurrent infections, hyperthyroidism, congenital heart disease, pulmonary disease, malignancy, other chronic diseases such as diabetes, and renal disease such as renal tubular acidosis.

Table 22-1. Differential Diagnosis of FTT

Inadequate Caloric Intake	Inadequate Caloric Absorption	Increased Calorie Requirements
Lack of Appetite • Anemia • Psychosocial problems • CNS pathology • Chronic infection **Difficulty With Ingestion** • Psychosocial problems (apathy and rumination) • CNS disorder • Craniofacial anomalies • Dyspnea • Feeding disorder • Generalized muscle weakness/pathology • Tracheoesophageal fistula • Genetic syndrome • Congenital syndrome **Unavailability of Food** • Inappropriate feeding technique • Insufficient/inadequate volume of food • Inappropriate food for age • Withholding of food (abuse, neglect) **Vomiting** • CNS pathology • Intestinal tract obstruction • Gastroesophageal reflux • Drugs	**Malabsorption** • Biliary atresia • Celiac disease • Cystic fibrosis • Enzymatic deficiencies • Food (protein) sensitivity/intolerance • Immunologic deficiency • Inflammatory bowel disease • NEC/short gut **Diarrhea** • Bacterial gastroenteritis • Parasitic infection • Starvation diarrhea **Hepatitis** **Hirschsprung Disease** **Psychosocial Problems** • Refeeding diarrhea	**Increased Metabolism/Increased Use of Calories** • Chronic/recurrent infection • Chronic respiratory insufficiency • Congenital heart disease/acquired heart disease • Malignancy • Chronic anemia • Toxins (lead) • Drugs • Endocrine disorders **Defective Use of Calories** • Metabolic disorders • Renal tubular acidosis • Chronic hyopxemia

Abbreviations: CNS, central nervous system; NEC, necrotizing enterocolitis.
Adapted from Zenel JA. Failure to thrive: a general pediatrician's perspective. *Pediatr Rev.* 1997;18(11):371–378.

Clinical Features

Poor growth is the most common clinical presentation of FTT and is based on the appropriate use of standardized growth charts. Often the key to recognition of FTT is to accurately measure and plot a child's weight, length/height, and head circumference over a period of time and then assess the growth trend.

Evaluation

The evaluation of a child who has FTT will require a thorough review of the growth chart (specifically, identifying the time or age of the change in growth), complete history including feeding and dietary history, review of systems, thorough head-to-toe physical examination, and diagnostic work-up as indicated.

Expected monthly weight gain for infants is listed in Table 22-2 (Evidence Level III). The expected gain in length during the first year of life is 25 cm/y (25 cm/y), during the second year is 12.5 cm/y (4.5 in/y), and beyond 3 years of age to puberty is 5 to 6 cm/y (2 in/y). The average head circumference at birth is 35 cm (13.5 in) and increases to approximately 47 cm (18.5 in) by 1 year of age. By 6 years of age, the rate of head circumference growth decreases to an average of 55 cm (21.5 in) by 6 years of age.

Table 22-2. Average Monthly Weight Gain

Age, mo	Pounds, lb/mo	Kilograms, kg/mo
0–3	2.2	1
3–6	1.1	$\frac{1}{2}$
6–9	$\frac{3}{4}$	$\frac{1}{3}$
9–12	$\frac{1}{2}$	$\frac{1}{4}$

Growth Charts

The basis for the approach to differential diagnosis of FTT utilizes the appropriate validated growth chart. It is very important to obtain accurate serial measurements of the weight, length or height, and head circumference of the child over time.

Keep in mind that properly assessing the patient's growth may require contacting previous medical providers for the infant or child to accurately assess the trend of growth over time. Recently, the Centers for Disease Control and Prevention (CDC) recommended the adoption of the World Health Organization (WHO) growth charts in the United States replacing the previous recommendations to use the growth chart form the CDC. For children 2 years and younger, the CDC WHO growth charts should be used. Based on these changes, the clinician will notice the following differences:

- Breastfed infant will no longer appear to grow too rapidly the first 6 months nor look like he is failing to grow sufficiently during the second 6 months.
- Non-breastfed infants may now appear to grow at a lower percentile during the first 6 months and more rapidly during the second 6 months of life.
- Overall, WHO growth charts will result in increased rates of children classified as underweight during the first 6 months of life.

The use of modified growth charts for premature infants, infants with genetic syndromes, such as trisomy 21 syndrome and Turner syndrome, and other special populations should prevent an inaccurate diagnosis of FTT.

In many cases of FTT, the weight loss or poor weight gain will precede any decrease in length/height. The head circumference is usually the last parameter to be affected. Cases in which all 3 growth parameters are low initially or decrease simultaneously usually indicate an underlying medical problem. In addition, decreased weight for height is an index to identify the child at acute risk and who needs nutritional treatment immediately, perhaps on an inpatient basis.

History

The most important investigative technique is an accurate, detailed account of the child's eating habits, caloric intake, and parent-child interaction. A careful history should include the assessment of diet and feeding or eating behaviors and past and current medical, social, and family history.

Dietary history should include breastfeeding problems, such as problems with latching on; poor milk supply; number of feedings; type and volume of formula; formula preparation; juice quantity; and specific diets, such as vegan. A dietary recall of amount of breastfeeding, amount of formula (specifically, volume and number per day), and meals, snacks, and fluid intake for children is useful on subsequent visits in the evaluation of FTT.

The developmental status at the time of FTT is also important because children with FTT have a higher incidence of developmental delays than the general population.

Ideally, observing the parent-child interaction during feedings in the office, hospital, or home setting via home visits provides invaluable information. Situations such as when and where the child eats, what happens with food refusal, or distractions during feedings or meals are important in the assessment.

In evaluating the time of growth failure, it is important to ask about certain stressors in the family, such as job loss, divorce, births, or deaths. A review of systems should determine if the following signs are present: appetite changes, food allergies, fever, abdominal pain, vomiting, bowel pattern, diarrhea, urinary abnormalities, or fatigue.

Physical Examination

The physical examination requires that the child be undressed for a thorough examination. The first consideration in examining the child with presumed FTT is ensuring the measurements are accurate (Table 22-3) (Evidence Level III). The examiner needs to focus on a few main goals, which include the following:

- Detection of underlying disease that may impair growth
- Identification of any dysmorphic features suggestive of a genetic disorder impeding growth
- Assessment for signs of possible child abuse or neglect
- Assessment of severity and possible effects of malnutrition

Table 22-3. Failure to Thrive Physical Examination

Approach to FTT	Physical Examination
Vital signs	Blood pressure, temperature, pulse, respirations, anthropometry
General appearance	Activity, affect, posture, dysmorphic features
Skin	Hygiene, rashes, neurocutaneous markings, signs of trauma, signs of vitamin deficiency
Head	Hair whorls, quality of hair, alopecia, fontanel size, frontal bossing, sutures, shape, dysmorphisms, philtrum
Eyes	Ptosis, strabismus, palpebral fissures, conjunctival pallor, fundoscopic examination
Ears	External form, rotation, tympanic membrane
Mouth, nose, throat	Thinness of lip, hydration, dental health, glossitis, chelosis, gum bleeding, unusual odor of breath
Neck	Hairline, masses, lymphadenopathy
Chest	Breath sounds, cardiac examination for murmurs, cardiomegaly or arrhythmias
Abdomen	Protuberance, hepatosplenomegaly, masses
Genitalia	Malformations, hygiene, trauma
Rectum	Fissures, trauma, hemorrhoids
Extremities	Edema, dysmorphisms, rachitic changes, nails
Neurologic	Cranial nerves, reflexes, tone, retention of primitive reflexes, voluntary movement

Abbreviation: FTT, failure to thrive.
Adapted from Failure to thrive. In: Kleinman RE, ed. *Pediatric Nutrition Handbook*. 6th ed. Elk Grove Village, IL: American Academy of Pediatrics; 2009:601–636.

Laboratory Investigation

Any laboratory investigation should be guided by information obtained by history and physical examination findings. Routine laboratory testing identifies a cause of FTT in less than 1% of children and is generally not recommended.

If it is indicated to rule out a medical etiology, the following are initial studies: complete blood count, basic metabolic profile, thyroid function tests, and urinalysis (UA). Additional work-up based on evaluation may include stool fat, erythrocyte sedimentation rate (ESR), and screening for lead and cystic fibrosis (Figure 22-1).

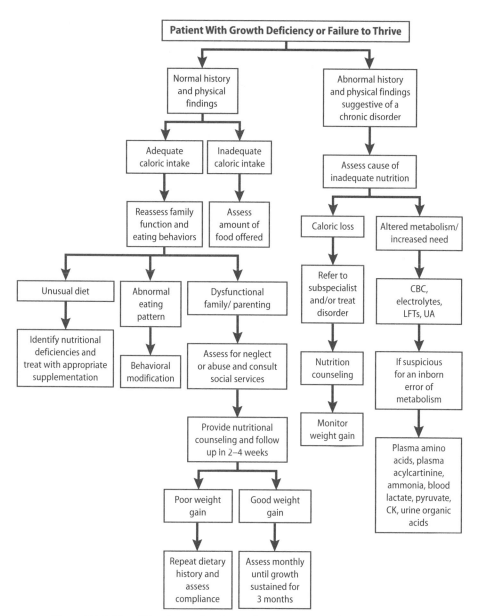

Figure 22-1. Algorithm for evaluation and management of FTT.

Abbreviations: CBC, complete blood count; CK, creatine kinase; LFT, liver function test; UA, urinalysis.

Adapted from Weston JA. Growth deficiency/failure to thrive. In: Bajaj L, Hambridge SJ, Kerby G, Nyquist AC, eds. *Berman's Pediatric Decision Making.* 5th ed. Philadelphia, PA: Mosby; 2011:302–307.

Management

The goals of management of FTT are provision of adequate calories, protein, and other nutrients; nutritional counseling; monitoring of growth and nutritional status; specific treatment of disorders, complications, or deficiencies; long-term monitoring or follow-up; supportive economic assistance if needed; and education of family.

Of the stated goals, an important goal of management involves appropriate nutritional goals and catch-up growth. Age appropriate nutritional counseling should be provided to parents of children with FTT to help ensure catch-up growth. Minimal catch-up growth should generally be 2 to 3 times the average weight gain for corrected age.

Approximately 20% to 30% more energy along with increased protein may be required to achieve catch-up growth in children. Catch-up in linear growth may lag several months behind that of weight.

There should be an assessment of the FTT based on weight for length/height as follows: mild (80%–90%), moderate (70%–80%), or severe (<70%). Treatment should be geared toward severity of the growth failure. Mild to moderate FTT may be managed by the health care professional on an outpatient basis. Increase caloric intake by ensuring the appropriate amount of calories and formula, and possibly increase the amount of calories per ounce of human milk or formula to make 22 kcal/oz, 24 kcal/oz, or 27 kcal/oz. These options should only be done under the guidance and monitoring of the primary care physician or dietitian. For outpatient management for children, it is helpful to limit 100% fruit juice to less than 6 to 8 oz/day; increase calories by adding foods such as margarine, peanut butter, and cheeses; avoid liquids until after meals; and offer healthy snacks.

Other behavioral tips for caregivers may be needed to ensure a healthy, relaxed feeding/mealtime, such as eating together, allowing a long time for the child to eat, offering meals or snacks every 2 to 3 hours, and positively reinforcing good eating habits versus threatening, punishing, forcing, or bribing a child to eat. Failure to thrive often requires a consistent multidisciplinary group of health care professionals.

Hospital Admission

Indications for hospitalization should be considered in certain circumstances such as moderate to severe FTT in which a child is less than 70% of her predicted weight for length or severe impairment of the caregiver or non-compliance is evident. The following situations should prompt admission for further evaluation and management:

- Dehydration or electrolyte abnormalities
- Concerns for abuse or neglect
- Failed outpatient management
- Non-compliance with outpatient management

During an admission, patients will typically undergo strict calorie count, daily naked weights, social work consultation, additional ancillary evaluation, and possible involvement of speech therapists and pediatric subspecialists, including a gastroenterologist. Other potential management includes zinc supplementation and, depending on severity of the growth failure, may include a nasogastric tube or gastrostomy tube.

Long-term Implications and Monitoring

Children with FTT are at risk for adverse outcomes. Maximal postnatal brain growth occurs in the first 6 months of life; therefore, FTT in the first year of life can be ominous. Failure to thrive is a common problem with long-term risks of growth, developmental, and behavioral problems in children.

Cognitive and school outcomes of children who have had FTT are worse than those of children who have not experienced undernutrition. Although many children with FTT experience growth and recovery by school age, they continue to be at risk for poor growth, low academic achievement, and poor academic work habits, which is likely to undermine future performance.

Multidisciplinary interventions, including home nursing visits, should be considered to improve weight gain, parent-child relations, and cognitive development of children with FTT. The multidisciplinary team can include the pediatrician, a nurse, a dietitian, a nurse practitioner, a social worker, a gastroenterologist, and speech or occupational therapists.

Several studies indicate that early home intervention mitigated many of the negative effects of FTT. Particular attention should be paid to these children's growth, nutritional intake, parent-child interaction, and appropriate access to early intervention resources such as food stamps and WIC (Supplemental Nutrition for Women, Infants, and Children), Social Security Income (SSI), and subspecialty care if necessary.

Parental guidance and education are essential to ensure that adequate nutrition and calories are being provided, as well as addressing behavioral and psychosocial factors that may play a role. Given the evidence of long-term problems, the primary care physician must closely monitor the ongoing growth and development of all children who have been diagnosed with FTT.

Suggested Reading
· · · · · · · · · · · · · · · · · ·

Block RW, Krebs NF. Failure to thrive as a manifestation of child neglect. *Pediatrics.* 2005;116(5):1234–1237

Cole S, Lanham JS. Failure to thrive: an update. *Am Fam Physician.* 2011;83(7):829–833

Foote JM, Brady LH, Burke AL, et al. *Evidence-based Clinical Practice Guideline on Linear Growth Measurement of Children.* Rockville, MD: Agency for Healthcare Research and Quality; 2009. http://www.ahrq.gov. AHRQ Guideline Summary NGC-7631. Accessed October 20, 2012

Gahagan S. Failure to thrive: a consequence of undernutrition. *Pediatr Rev.* 2006;27(1):e1–e11

KidsGrowth. Tables for normal growth. KidsGrowth Web site. www.kidsgrowth.com /resources/articledetail.cfm?id=811. Accessed November 9, 2014

Mei Z, Grumer-Strawn LM. Comparison of changes in growth percentiles of US children on CDC 2000 growth charts with corresponding changes on WHO 2006 growth charts. *Clin Pediatr.* 2011;50(5):402–407

Zenel JA Jr. Failure to thrive: a general pediatrician's perspective. *Pediatr Rev.* 1997;18(11):371–378

CHAPTER 23

Febrile Seizures

Russell C. Bailey, MD

Key Points

- Febrile seizures are the most common seizures of childhood and are generally benign events with a very low risk of injury or associated comorbidities.

- Febrile seizures are categorized as simple or complex based on several specific clinical features. Simple febrile seizures are brief (lasting less than 10 to 15 minutes), generalized without focality, and isolated, occurring once within a single 24-hour period or single febrile illness. Complex febrile seizures may last longer than 10 to 15 minutes, often are associated with focal features during the seizure or following the seizure (eg, Todd paralysis), or occur more than once within a single 24-hour period or febrile illness.

- Evaluation of a child with a febrile seizure should focus on identifying the underlying etiology to the febrile illness. Evidence-based guidelines help define appropriate evaluation principles.

- In most cases, children who experience febrile seizures do not develop epilepsy in the future; the risk appears to be in the range of 2% to 7% in previously non-epileptic children with a first febrile seizure.

- Most children who experience febrile seizures do not require treatment beyond general education and reassurance; abortive therapy measures may be employed in the event of prolonged or recurrent febrile seizures.

Overview

Febrile seizures are the most common form of seizures in childhood, with 2% to 5% of children experiencing a febrile seizure. The International League Against Epilepsy defines a febrile seizure as a seizure "associated with a febrile illness not caused by an infection of the central nervous system, without previous neonatal seizures or a previous unprovoked seizure, and not meeting criteria for other acute symptomatic seizures." Defined further, febrile seizures occur (1) in association with a febrile illness, (2) in the absence of a central nervous system infection or acute electrolyte abnormality, (3) in the absence of prior afebrile seizures, including neonatal seizures, and (4) in patients older than 1 month. Clinically, febrile seizures are divided into simple febrile seizures and complex febrile seizures, with the latter category including febrile status epilepticus.

There is no consensus opinion on the age range in which febrile seizures occur, with studies employing lower age limits ranging from 1 to 6 months of age and upper age limits often unspecified. However, most febrile seizures occur between 6 and 60 months of age, which is in accordance with often-cited age ranges for typical febrile seizures. The peak age for febrile seizures is between 18 to 24 months, with onset rare after 7 years of age.

While the exact pathophysiology of febrile seizures is unknown, there is a clear genetic predisposition that can be defined in some patients. However, such a genetic predisposition is not seen in all children. Febrile seizures represent age-dependent seizures that occur during a period in which all children, regardless of genetic influences, are susceptible to fever-induced seizures. In contrast to previous thought, the rate of temperature rise of the fever is not the catalyst for febrile seizures; instead, the peak temperature appears to be most important with a required temperature greater than 38.4°C (101.12°F). However, the temperature may not be evident at the time of the seizure, as approximately 21% of children experience a febrile seizure prior to or within 1 hour of onset of fever.

Causes

Any febrile illness, regardless of etiology, can produce a febrile seizure. While often the underlying infectious etiology remains unidentified, viral infections, otitis media, pneumonia, gastrointestinal illness, and urinary tract infections are frequently implicated in febrile seizures. Identifying the underlying etiology of the febrile illness is of utmost importance to guide treatment and exclude potentially life-threatening infections such as meningitis or other intracranial infections.

The incidence of meningitis in patients presenting with febrile seizures is approximately 2% to 5%. In 2011, Batra and coworkers investigated the prevalence and clinical predictors of bacterial meningitis among 497 children aged 6 to 18 months with a first febrile seizure. They reported the overall prevalence of meningitis to be 2.4% among patients with a first febrile seizure, 0.86% among those who experienced a simple febrile seizure, and 4.8% among patients who experienced a complex febrile seizure. Furthermore, they identified clinical predictors of meningitis among patients experiencing a first febrile seizures and found seizure duration greater than 30 minutes, postictal drowsiness, and persistent neurologic deficit as the most consistent clinical predictors of bacterial meningitis.

Clinical Features

Febrile seizures are divided into simple and complex based on several clinical features. Simple febrile seizures are brief (lasting less than 10 to 15 minutes), generalized without focality, and isolated, occurring once within a single 24-hour period or single febrile illness. In contrast, complex febrile seizures may last longer than 10 to 15 minutes, are often associated with focal features during or following the seizure (eg, Todd paralysis), or occur more than once within a single 24-hour period or febrile illness. Approximately 35% of febrile seizures are complex. A child's prior neurologic history does not influence classification of a febrile seizure. Included within the category of complex febrile seizures is febrile status epilepticus, defined as a single febrile seizure lasting longer than 30 minutes or a series of discrete febrile seizures with no return to baseline between seizures.

Evaluation

Diagnostic evaluation in the setting of a febrile seizure should focus on identifying the underlying etiology of the febrile illness. As discussed previously, there are a multitude of potential etiologies, and identification of an underlying etiology helps guide treatment and exclude underlying meningitis or other intracranial infections. While recommendations on the routine evaluation of patients with simple febrile seizures exist, ultimately the specifics of each child dictate neurodiagnostic decision-making.

In 1996, the American Academy of Pediatrics (AAP) published a practice parameter addressing neurodiagnostic evaluation of the child with a first simple febrile seizure. In 2011, the AAP updated this practice parameter and published a clinical practice guideline that once again addressed neurodiagnostic evaluation of a child with a simple febrile seizure (Evidence Level III). Both of these guidelines addressed the evaluation of a child 6 to 60 months of age in the setting of a simple febrile seizure and explicitly state that guidelines are not intended for patients who have experienced a complex febrile seizure, a history of afebrile seizure, or preexisting neurologic abnormalities.

Routine analysis of blood chemistries, including basic electrolytes and glucose, and complete blood cell counts are not recommended in the setting of simple febrile seizures unless clinically indicated, as in the case of persistent vomiting or diarrhea (Evidence Level II-1). Likewise, blood cultures are not routinely indicated and are considered of low yield given the relative low incidence of occult bacteremia in children with febrile seizures. However, basic diagnostic evaluation again should be directed at identifying the underlying etiology. In line with this fact, consideration of diagnostic tests for treatable conditions, such as rapid tests for influenza, chest radiographs for pneumonia, and urinalysis with urine culture for urinary tract infections, all of which require specific treatment, should be considered when clinically indicated.

Given the morbidity and mortality associated with meningitis, the decision whether to perform a lumbar puncture for cerebrospinal fluid analysis has garnered substantial attention. For this reason, numerous studies provide recommendations on the performance of lumbar punctures in the setting of febrile seizures. First, in accordance with AAP guidelines, any child with a history of febrile seizure and signs or symptoms of meningitis or intracranial infection should undergo a lumbar puncture (Evidence Level III). The revised AAP guidelines differ from those published in 1996, which recommended that a lumbar puncture be strongly considered in all patients younger than 12 months given the subtlety of the signs and symptoms of meningitis in this age group. Addressing this change and in light of widespread vaccination against the most common causes of bacterial meningitis in children, in 2004 the AAP wrote, "Current data no longer support routine lumbar puncture in well-appearing, fully immunized children who present with a simple febrile seizure" (Evidence Level III). However, it is highly recommended that any infant younger than 6 months undergo a lumbar puncture. Second, lumbar puncture is a consideration in infants 6 to 12 months of age who are considered deficient with regard to immunizations, specifically *Haemophilus influenzae* type b and *Streptococcus pneumoniae* immunizations. Third, a lumbar puncture is a consideration in children pretreated with antibiotics prior to presenting with a febrile seizure, as prior antibiotic use potentially can mask signs and symptoms of meningitis. Unfortunately, no agreed-on definition of *pretreated* exists.

Electroencephalography (EEG) is of limited value and low yield and should not be included in routine evaluation of simple febrile seizures (Evidence Level III). Electroencephalograms do not alter the outcome, influence the treatment decision for febrile seizures, or predict future febrile seizure recurrence or development of epilepsy. Electroencephalograms are occasionally abnormal in the setting of febrile seizures, but such findings are of unclear significance and are not predictive of recurrence or future epilepsy.

Routine neuroimaging is also not indicated in the routine evaluation of a simple febrile seizure (Evidence Level III). The risk of radiation exposure associated with computed tomography (CT) scans and sedation required for magnetic resonance imaging (MRI) scans offset the low likelihood of benefit from such imaging. However, such decisions should be made within the context of clinical presentation, particularly with regard to CT scans, which should be pursued when concern for trauma, intracranial hemorrhage, or increased intracranial pressure exists.

Finally, neurodiagnostic evaluation of complex febrile seizures warrants independent discussion. Unfortunately, no clinical guidelines exist and data are lacking with regard to routine evaluation of a patient who experiences a complex febrile seizure including febrile status epilepticus. Still, a number of studies address this important question. First, as in the case of simple febrile seizures, one should focus on identifying the underlying etiology of the febrile illness, including evaluation for and exclusion of meningitis or other intracranial infection. One should consider performing a lumbar puncture in the setting of a complex febrile seizure, particularly following the first complex febrile seizure. Second, while there is not enough evidence to support routine use of neuroimaging, one should consider it to assess for underlying structural abnormality in the setting of a complex febrile seizure, again particularly following an initial complex febrile seizure. Outside the setting of the concern for trauma, intracranial hemorrhage, or increased intracranial pressure, an MRI is the preferred neuroimaging modality. Finally, in the setting of complex febrile seizures, the routine use of EEG generally remains of limited value for reasons discussed earlier. However, the EEG may be useful in specific scenarios given its high diagnostic value for certain causes of viral encephalitis, specifically herpes encephalitis. Additionally, an EEG is helpful in the evaluation of possible ongoing subclinical seizures or nonconvulsive status epilepticus when clinically indicated.

Management

Approaches to the treatment of febrile seizures essentially fall into 2 categories: acute treatments and preventive or prophylactic treatments. In terms of the acute treatment of febrile seizures, focus must be on treating the underlying infection and the acute seizure, if necessary. Should evaluation of the patient identify a treatable infection, appropriate treatment of that underlying infection is imperative. For acute or abortive seizure treatment, use of benzodiazepines is effective and recommended in an effort to abort ongoing seizures. In the home setting, abortive treatment primarily involves the use of rectal diazepam, although intranasal and buccal forms of midazolam exist. In the hospital setting, a variety of benzodiazepines and modes of delivery are available. The goal of this treatment approach is not to prevent febrile seizure recurrence, but to abort an ongoing seizure and prevent prolonged febrile seizures, given the concerning association between prolonged febrile seizures and future risk of epilepsy. While no consensus exists on when to administer abortive therapy, the author's practice is to administer abortive therapy for a febrile seizure lasting 5 minutes or longer.

Various approaches to the prevention of febrile seizure recurrences exist, including the use of antiepileptic medications, on a chronic or intermittent basis, and antipyretics, primarily acetaminophen and ibuprofen. However, given the expense of treatment, adverse effects associated with the medications, low risk associated with febrile seizures, uncertainty of febrile seizure recurrence, low association with future development of epilepsy, and lack of evidence that prophylactic treatment in any form prevents development of epilepsy, prophylactic treatment of febrile seizures is not recommended in most cases (Evidence Level II-2).

No studies demonstrate that the intermittent use of antipyretics effectively prevents febrile seizure recurrence (Evidence Level II-1 and Evidence Level II-2). Furthermore, potential adverse effects associated with regular use of such medications, including hepatotoxicity, respiratory failure, metabolic acidosis, renal failure, and coma, argue against their use in this manner. Antiepileptic medications, however, are effective in preventing febrile seizure recurrences.

Continuous, daily use of some antiepileptic medications effectively reduces the risk of febrile seizure recurrence (Evidence Level II-2). Phenobarbital, primidone, and valproic acid are antiepileptic medications considered effective in preventing such recurrences, but adverse effects of these medications, including sedation, irritability, hyperactivity, weight gain, thrombocytopenia, hepatotoxicity, and pancreatitis, limit their use in the setting of febrile seizures. Furthermore, no data suggest that prophylactic use of antiepileptic medications in a continuous manner reduces future risk of epilepsy. Therefore, continuous use of antiepileptic medications is not recommended as preventive treatment of febrile seizures (Evidence Level II-2).

Intermittent use of antiepileptic medications, primarily oral diazepam given at the onset of a febrile illness, also has proved effective in preventing febrile seizure recurrences. However, once again, this method of treatment is limited by the adverse effects frequently experienced, including sedation, irritability, ataxia, dizziness, and possibly respiratory suppression. Additionally, because febrile seizures occasionally occur simultaneously with onset of fever, this approach commonly fails to prevent recurrence. Furthermore, the use of benzodiazepines in this manner could complicate the clinical picture of the sick child. Benzodiazepines frequently produce sedation in children, creating an encephalopathic picture, which in turn could mask or mimic an evolving central nervous system infection and exceedingly complicate the clinical decision-making of the treating physician. Given these shortcomings, intermittent use of antiepileptic medications at onset of a febrile illness in an effort to prevent febrile seizure recurrence is not recommended.

Finally, a necessary part of the management of febrile seizures involves educating and reassuring the family. Families benefit greatly from education on the incidence and natural course of febrile seizures, risk of febrile seizure recurrence and subsequent epilepsy, and reassurance of the benign nature of febrile seizures. Families should receive instruction on appropriate management of a seizure (Box 23-1). Finally, instruction in general seizure precautions is necessary to educate the family on activities that possibly place a child at risk of injury in the event of a seizure (see Box 23-1).

Box 23-1. Home Management of Febrile Seizures

In the event of a seizure, families should be instructed to
- Remain calm.
- Place the child in the lateral decubitus position to avoid aspiration.
- Never place anything in the child's mouth or give the child anything by mouth, including medications.
- Loosen tight clothing.
- Not restrain the child.
- If possible, place a soft pillow or object under the child's head.
- Time the seizure.
- Administer abortive medications as directed.
- Notify emergency services in the event of respiratory distress, a prolonged seizure, recurrent seizures, or a prolonged postictal state.

Families should also pursue general seizure precautions for the child (to minimize risk of injury in event of seizure).
- Avoid unnecessary heights and trampolines due to the risk of falls.
- Maintain constant supervision when in or around water due to risk of drowning, including the bathtub.
- Maintain constant supervision around sources of heat or fire, such as campfires or stoves, or boiling water due to risk of burning or scalding oneself.
- When appropriate, do not operate machinery or drive, and never bike without a helmet.

Prognosis

Morbidity/Mortality

Febrile seizures are considered benign events with no long-term adverse effects and a very low associated risk of morbidity and mortality. With all seizures, there is the risk of injury during the seizure itself, such as falls or drowning. However, there is no evidence of neurocognitive decline, lasting behavioral abnormalities, or permanent motor dysfunction as a result of febrile seizures. Studies have reported no deaths from febrile seizures and an extremely low mortality rate associated with febrile status epilepticus.

Risk of Recurrent Febrile Seizures

Following the initial febrile seizure, approximately one-third of patients experience a recurrent febrile seizure and approximately 10% experience 3 or more recurrences. Family history of febrile seizures and younger age are the most consistent predictors of recurrence. In fact, some studies report a 50%

recurrence risk among children who experience their initial febrile seizure at younger than 12 months. Low peak temperature refers to the peak temperature during the febrile illness, with a lower peak temperature increasing risk of recurrence. The duration of recognized fever refers to the time between onset of fever and the febrile seizure, with a shorter time between fever onset and febrile seizure increasing likelihood of recurrence.

Risk of Epilepsy

Studies investigating the risk of developing epilepsy following a febrile seizure vary, with reports ranging from 2% to 7% compared with the general population risk of approximately 1%. Neligan and coworkers performed a prospective follow-up study among 181 patients from onset of febrile seizures for a median duration of 24 years with the goal to establish the long-term risk of developing epilepsy and found that 7% experienced a single afebrile seizure and 6% developed epilepsy, as defined as 2 or more afebrile seizures. A family history of epilepsy, history of prior neurologic abnormality, complex febrile seizures including prolonged febrile seizures and febrile status epilepticus, and short duration between recognized fever and febrile seizure are 4 factors increasing the risk of future epilepsy. Clearly, an association exists between febrile seizures and epilepsy, but the nature of this association remains poorly understood. The most pressing question is whether febrile seizures themselves, particularly prolonged febrile seizures, produce alterations in the brain that then contribute to an epileptogenic process, a question currently under investigation.

Suggested Reading

American Academy of Pediatrics Provisional Committee on Quality Improvement, Subcommittee on Febrile Seizures. Practice parameter: the neurodiagnostic evaluation of the child with a first simple febrile seizure. *Pediatrics*. 1996;97(5):769–772

American Academy of Pediatrics Steering Committee on Quality Improvement and Management, Subcommittee on Febrile Seizures. Febrile seizures: clinical practice guideline for the long-term management of the child with simple febrile seizures. *Pediatrics*. 2008;121(6):1281–1286

American Academy of Pediatrics Subcommittee on Febrile Seizures. Febrile seizures: guideline for the neurodiagnostic evaluation of the child with a simple febrile seizure. *Pediatrics*. 2011;127(2):389–394

Batra P, Gupta S, Gomber S, Saha A. Predictors of meningitis in children presenting with first febrile seizures. *Pediatr Neurol*. 2011;44(1):35–39

Capovilla G, Mastrangelo M, Romeo A, Vigevano F. Recommendations for the management of "febrile seizures": ad hoc Task Force of LICE Guidelines Commission. *Epilepsia*. 2009;50(Suppl 1):2–6

Guidelines for epidemiologic studies on epilepsy. Commission on Epidemiology and Prognosis, International League Against Epilepsy. *Epilepsia*. 1993;34(4):592–596

Neligan A, Bell GS, Giavasi C, et al. Long-term risk of developing epilepsy after febrile seizures: a prospective cohort study. *Neurology*. 2012;78(15):1166–1170

Oluwabusi T, Sood SK. Update on the management of simple febrile seizures: emphasis on minimal intervention. *Curr Opin Pediatr*. 2012;24(2):259–265

Shinnar S, Glauser TA. Febrile seizures. In: Pellock JM, Bourgeois BFD, Dodson WE, eds. *Pediatric Epilepsy: Diagnosis and Therapy*. 3rd ed. New York, New York: Demos Medical Publishing; 2008:293–302

Shinnar S, O'Dell C. Febrile seizures. *Pediatr Ann*. 2004;33(6):394–401

CHAPTER 24

Fever

Carl J. Seashore, MD; Andrew Z. Heling, MD; and Jacob A. Lohr, MD

Key Points

- It is rarely necessary to specifically treat a fever, as a fever in the setting of an infectious source is a beneficial response mechanism in the host. Instead, the underlying cause of the fever should be identified and treated when possible.

- Rectal measurement is the standard method to measure body temperature and is the preferred method for children younger than 6 months unless contraindicated.

- Acetaminophen and ibuprofen (for those 6 months or older) are both acceptable antipyretics to judiciously administer when patient discomfort or comorbidities outweigh the benefits of a fever. Alternating or co-administering both antipyretics, though a common practice, should be discouraged in routine settings.

- The evaluation and management of the underlying cause of a fever depends on multiple factors, including the patient's clinical status, age, comorbidities, and duration of fever.

- Consider a broad differential diagnosis in children with recurrent fevers or with fever of unknown origin. Consultation with a local specialist is reasonable for these children.

Overview

A fever is defined as an abnormal elevation in core body temperature for a given age via a central nervous system–mediated process. A widely accepted threshold level for all ages is a rectal temperature of greater than or at 38.0°C (100.4°F).

A fever is not a primary pathology but rather the body's secondary response to a variety of pathologic processes, including infections, inflammatory disorders, and malignancy, among others. The most common cause of fever is a self-limited viral illness. Although the differential diagnosis for the underlying source of fever is broad, frequently the primary source of a fever can be elicited through a thorough history and physical examination, as fever is rarely the sole presenting sign or symptom. The extent of the work-up depends on multiple factors, including the patient's clinical status, age, comorbidities, and duration of fever.

Management should focus on the underlying cause of the fever and not on the fever itself, as a fever in the presence of an infection is a natural and beneficial defense mechanism in the host. No evidence shows that fevers result in long-term neurologic sequelae. However, certain patients have comorbidities that may be exacerbated by fevers, and for some patients the subjective discomfort of their fever outweighs its beneficial effects. In such patients, the judicious use of antipyretics is warranted.

Clinical Documentation of Fever

Body temperature can be measured in multiple ways, including via a thermometer placed in the axilla (axillary), mouth (oral), or rectum (rectal); infrared analysis of the ear canal; and skin temperature strips placed on the forehead. Rectal measurement is the most accurate method and is the criterion standard, though both patient and physician acceptance of this approach decrease with increasing patient age, as does the necessity for such precise measurements beyond infancy (Table 24-1). In addition, rectal measurement is contraindicated in certain conditions, including neutropenia.

Table 24-1. Fever Definition and Preferred Method of Measurement Based on Age

Age	<6 mo	6 mo–3 y	≥4 y
Preferred method to objectively measure temperature	Rectal unless contraindicated	Axillary if patient tolerates; otherwise, rectal unless contraindicated	Oral if patient tolerates, otherwise, axillary
Definition of fever	≥38.0°C (100.4°F)	≥38.0°C (100.4°F)	≥38.0°C (100.4°F)

A normal rectal temperature is variable and ranges from 36.6°C to 37.9°C (97.9°F–100.3°F). It is important to note that daily variations of up to 0.5°C (0.9°F) occur regardless of the method used to assess temperature, with lowest average temperatures occurring in the early morning and highest average temperatures occurring in the afternoon. Age, circulating hormones, and external factors (including ambient temperature, recent ingestion of food or drinks, and degree of clothing or swaddling) can all affect patient temperature recordings depending on the method of assessment utilized.

Initial Diagnostic Assessment of Fever

Patients with a fever may subjectively show concern for malaise and anorexia and have tachycardia on physical examination. If patients' temperatures have not yet reached a new elevated thermal set point (ie, their internal temperature is still rising), they may subjectively feel cold or complain of chills and on physical examination may shiver or have pallor. Conversely, if patients' temperatures have exceeded their new thermal set point (ie, their internal temperature is falling), they may subjectively feel hot and on physical examination may be diaphoretic or flushed.

While the most common source of fever in all age groups is an acute, self-limited viral illness, it is imperative to identify and treat more severe causes of fever, including serious bacterial infections. Obtaining a thorough history and physical examination is key to identifying an underlying cause of fever. Warning signs that are of particular concern and that necessitate emergent work-up include, but are not limited to, those found in Box 24-1. A thorough physical examination must also be performed. All clinically unstable patients must be identified, worked up, and managed, including, but not limited to, those found in Box 24-2.

Box 24-1. Warning Signs Obtained via the History Examination That Necessitate Emergent Work-up

- Altered mental status, including behavioral changes, unresponsiveness, and lethargy
- Seizures or other abnormal movements beyond simple febrile seizures
- Severe localized pain, including that of the head, abdomen, joints, or extremities
- Inability to bear weight, walk, or otherwise use extremities
- Difficulty breathing or productive cough
- Bloody diarrhea
- Major comorbidities (such as immune-deficient states, including AIDS, sickle cell disease, and malignancy)

Box 24-2: Warning Signs Obtained via the Physical Examination That Necessitate Emergent Work-up

- Vital sign instability, including hypotension, significant tachycardia, tachypnea, and hypoxemia
- Altered mental status, including lethargy, irritability, and inconsolability
- Meningeal signs, including Kernig and Brudzinski maneuvers in older children, and poor tone or bulging fontanelle in infants
- Hyperventilation or hypoventilation, respiratory distress, or increased work of breathing
- Swollen, tender joints; abnormal gait; or inability to use joint or bear weight
- Petechial rash, cyanosis, or mucous membrane abnormalities, including dry cracked lips and strawberry tongue
- Ill appearance

Clinical Subtypes of Fever

Fever with source is defined as the presence of a fever in the setting of a suspected source, obtained either via history, physical examination, or diagnostic testing. *Fever without source* is defined as the presence of a fever for fewer than 10 days when no source is identified via history, physical examination, or diagnostic testing. *Fever of unknown origin* has had various historic definitions but in this chapter is defined as a fever without source occurring for all or most of 10 or more days. *Periodic fever syndromes* are conditions in which fevers are secondary to innate immune system disorders and have a pattern of recurrence over time.

Fever With Source

The definition of fever with source includes the presence of a fever with an obvious source obtained either via history examination, physical examination, or selected diagnostic testing. The evaluation and management of fever with source is straightforward and depends on the illness that is suspected. In low-risk populations, including those older than 28 days who are otherwise well without major comorbidities, evaluation is complete when obvious sources of fever are identified either via a thorough history and physical examination alone or in conjunction with limited laboratory or radiographic testing. Management is then tailored to treat the inciting source of the fever, if indicated. High-risk populations, including immunocompromised patients, newborns 28 days or younger, and those with significant comorbidities or who are clinically unstable, warrant a more thorough work-up. For these high-risk patients, management should err on aggressive and early initiation of broad antimicrobial coverage.

Fever Without Source

The evaluation and management of pediatric patients with a fever without source is largely based on age and clinical status. The specific age stratification, as set forth in the next sections, while partly arbitrary, reflects changes in both infectious organism frequency and immune responses with increasing age, as well as historic data from multiple clinical studies that were based on specific age ranges.

Younger Than 3 Months

The rate of serious bacterial infections is highest in this age group, particularly among those 28 days or younger, because of immature defense mechanisms and insufficient vaccination. Therefore, the evaluation and management of a fever in this patient population must be more urgent and more conservative to identify and treat potentially devastating bacterial infections (Figure 24-1).

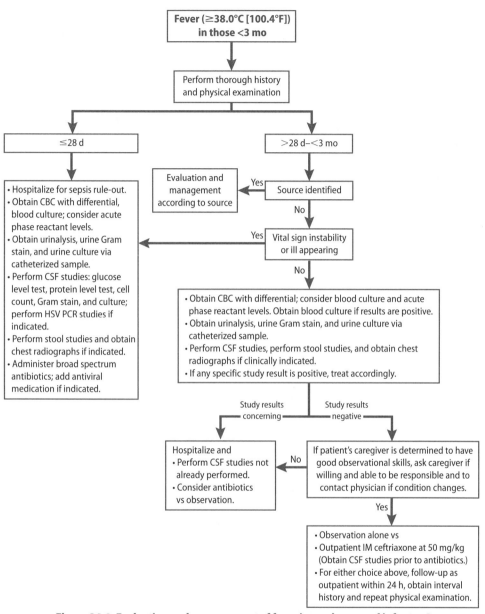

Figure 24-1. Evaluation and management of fever in newborns and infants <3 mo.
Abbreviation: CBC, complete blood count; CSF, cerebral spinal fluid; HSV, herpes simplex virus; PCR, polymerase chain reaction; IM, intramuscular; IV, intravenous; vs, versus; WBC, white blood cell.
[a] The presence of comorbid conditions such as inflammatory conditions, oncologic disease, or hardware alter fever evaluation. Recognition of fever pattern is essential and would change clinical decision-making if a specific pattern arises.

Younger Than or at 28 Days

Newborns younger than or at 28 days with a fever constitute a medical emergency, as this patient population is at particular risk of serious bacterial infections and their associated adverse sequelae due to limited immune system functioning (Table 24-2). For this patient population, even if a source is identified, a complete sepsis work-up should be performed, including a blood culture, urinalysis with Gram stain, and urine culture obtained via catheterization or suprapubic aspiration, as well as a lumbar puncture with cerebrospinal fluid (CSF) evaluation, including protein and glucose level analysis, complete cell count and differential, Gram stain, and culture. In addition, herpes simplex virus (HSV) polymerase chain reaction (PCR) should be obtained if the patient's clinical course, an objective examination including CSF analysis, maternal and delivery history, or a combination thereof warrants it. Recent evidence suggests enterovirus PCR should be considered in large part to identify low-risk patients and facilitate shorter hospital stay and antibiotic exposure. A complete blood count (CBC) with white blood cell (WBC) count with differential is frequently obtained and can be used to trend values over time. Chest radiographs, including both anterior-posterior and lateral projections, are indicated if the patient presents with at least one clinical sign of pulmonary disease (ie, tachypnea, oxygen desaturation, cough, coryza, rales, rhonchi, wheezing, stridor, or increased work of breathing, including grunting, retractions, or nasal flaring). Stool WBC count and culture should be obtained in the presence of hematochezia or diarrhea.

Newborns with a fever must be admitted to a hospital for empiric parenteral antibiotic medication as well as antiviral medication if HSV infection is suspected. If the patient is clinically well, antibiotic medication may be discontinued after at least 36 hours if all bacterial cultures (ie, blood, urine, and CSF) are continuously monitored and are found to be negative at that time, and antiviral medication may be discontinued once HSV PCR returns negative. All obtained cultures should be followed until they are finalized as negative. A longer antibiotic course is required if cultures are positive or if the patient does not clinically improve after admission.

Older Than 28 Days to Younger Than 3 Months

For patients who are older than 28 days to younger than 3 months, a full sepsis work-up is not required if a source of an infection can be identified by history or physical examination and if the newborn or infant is otherwise well appearing. However, if no source is identified, a partial work-up is indicated, even for well-appearing patients. For this age range, prudent laboratory evaluation includes a CBC with differential with or without both a blood culture and acute phase reactant test such as for C-reactive protein or procalcitonin level, as well as a urinalysis, Gram stain, and urine culture obtained via catheterization or suprapubic aspiration. A blood culture should be obtained if any of the above laboratory values are suspicious for an infection, and it is frequently drawn and sent to the laboratory at the same time as other blood tests to limit the number of blood draws required. The presence of hematochezia or diarrhea warrants stool studies, while respiratory signs or symptoms, including oxygen desaturation, tachypnea, or respiratory distress, warrant chest radiographs.

Table 24-2: Evaluation and Management for a Newborn ≤28 d With a Fever, Including a Sepsis Rule-Out and Parenteral Antimicrobials

Fever in Newborn ≤28 d, Regardless of Clinical Appearance (Evidence Level II)	
Evaluation	
Blood	Culture, CBC with differential
Urine	Urinalysis, Gram stain, culture (via catheterized specimen or suprapubic aspiration)
CSF	Protein and glucose level test, complete blood cell count with differential, Gram stain, culture; HSV PCR if indicated by history and physical examination or CSF findings, enterovirus PCR to be considered
Radiographs	Chest radiographs in presence of respiratory signs or symptoms
Stool	Culture and WBC count in presence of gastrointestinal signs or symptoms
Management	
Antibiotics	Inpatient admission with broad spectrum, parenteral antibiotics to be continued until blood, urine, and CSF bacterial cultures are negative after at least 36 h of culturing and if patient is clinically well; a longer treatment course required if bacterial cultures are positive or if patient has not returned to clinical baseline Example empiric antibiotic regimens for infants born at term include both • IV ampicillin at 100 mg/kg/dose every 12 h and IV gentamicin at 4 mg/kg/dose every 24 h (preferred regimen) OR • IV ampicillin at 100 mg/kg/dose every 12 h and IV cefotaxime at 50 mg/kg/dose with frequency dependent on postnatal age Antibiotic regimens and doses to be tailored based on suspicion for meningitis, the organism being treated, and gestational age
Antivirals	IV acyclovir at 20 mg/kg/dose every 8 h if concerned for HSV; HSV PCR assay should be obtained if treating; can discontinue treatment with negative PCR assay

Abbreviation: CBC, complete blood count; CSF, cerebral spinal fluid; HSV, herpes simplex virus; PCR, polymerase chain reaction; UTI, urinary tract infection; IV, intravenous; WBC, white blood cell.

For well-appearing patients, positive findings via the above laboratory or radiographic tests warrant admission for inpatient management. If tests are negative but outpatient follow-up is unlikely to occur for a well-appearing patient, inpatient management is also recommended.

Conversely, for well-appearing infants in whom the history and physical examination findings are unrevealing as to the source of fever, the laboratory test findings are negative, and reliable follow-up is available within 24 hours, the patient can be managed on an outpatient basis, as the likelihood for a serious bacterial infection is low. Follow-up must occur within 24 hours, and urine and blood cultures must be monitored in a timely manner. It is acceptable to treat such patients with observation alone or with empiric outpatient antibiotic treatment using a third-generation cephalosporin (such as IM ceftriaxone at 50 mg/kg/dose daily with a maximum of 1 g per day) until urine and blood cultures are negative for at least 36 hours if cultures are continually monitored. However, prior to empiric antibiotic administration, CSF analysis and culture should be obtained via a lumbar puncture. Regardless of treatment choice, patients should be reassessed within 24 hours.

In the case of a patient who is clinically unstable or ill appearing, a full sepsis work-up is indicated (Table 24-3). Such patients must be admitted to a hospital for parenteral antibiotic medication as well as antiviral medication if HSV infection is suspected. Patients must remain inpatient until cultures are negative for at least 36 hours, if cultures are continuously monitored, and, if viral illness is suspected, PCR is negative. Positive bacterial cultures or viral PCR necessitate a longer hospitalization for continued antimicrobials, as does the infant with negative culture results who does not clinically return to a baseline state of health.

Table 24-3. Evaluation and Management for Children >28 d–<3 mo With Fever

Fever, Well Appearing and Source Identified (Evidence Level III)	
Evaluation	
Specific to identified source; patient not considered to have fever without source	
Management	
Treatment related to source; patient not considered to have fever without source	

Fever, Well Appearing and Source Not Identified (Evidence Level II)	
Evaluation	
Blood	Obtain CBC with differential; consider blood culture and acute phase reactant test such as for CRP or procalcitonin level. (Obtain blood culture if CBC with differential is abnormal or you are planning to administer antibiotics.)
Urine	Urinalysis, Gram stain, culture (via catheterized specimen or suprapubic aspiration)
CSF	Prior to initiating antibiotics, obtain protein and glucose level, cell count with differential, Gram stain, and culture. Consider HSV and enterovirus PCRs depending on history and physical examinations and CSF findings.
Radiographs	Chest radiographs in presence of respiratory signs or symptoms
Stool	Culture and WBC count in presence of gastrointestinal signs or symptoms

Table 24-3 *(cont)*

Fever, Well Appearing and Source Not Identified (Evidence Level II)	
Management	

- If initial study findings test negative, you may consider observation alone vs outpatient IM ceftriaxone at 50 mg/kg/dose once daily up to 2 days while cultures and studies are pending (perform CSF analysis, including CSF culture and blood culture, prior to initiating antibiotics); either management option requires close follow-up within 24 hours.
- If CBC with differential reveals an abnormal WBC count (ie, <5,000 cells/mm³ or >15,000 cells/mm³), elevated absolute neutrophil count (>10,000 cells/mm³), or elevated band count (>1,500 cells/mm³), obtain blood culture and perform CSF analysis if you have not already done so; it requires inpatient admission for management with broad antibiotic coverage until cultures are negative for at least 36 hours. An example antibiotic regimen includes IV ampicillin at 50 mg/kg/dose every 6 h and IV ceftriaxone at 50 mg/kg/dose daily with maximum of 1 g per day. If treating for meningitis, administer meningitic dosing of antibiotics and add IV vancomycin at 20 mg/kg/dose and adjust doses according to serum levels.

Fever and Ill Appearing (Evidence Level III)	
Evaluation	
Blood	CBC with differential, blood culture
Urine	Urinalysis, Gram stain, culture (via catheterized specimen or suprapubic aspiration)
CSF	Protein and glucose level, cell count with differential, Gram stain, culture. Consider HSV and enterovirus PCRs depending on history and physical examinations and CSF findings.
Radiographs	Chest radiographs in presence of respiratory signs or symptoms
Stool	Cultures and studies in presence of gastrointestinal signs or symptoms
Management	

Inpatient admission with broad spectrum, parenteral antimicrobials until cultures are negative for at least 36 h. An example antibiotic regimen includes IV ampicillin at 75 mg/kg/dose every 6 h and IV ceftriaxone at 100 mg/kg/dose daily with maximum of 2 g/dose if treating for a severe infection. If treating meningitis, ensure you are administering meningitic dosing of antibiotics and add IV vancomycin at 20 mg/kg/dose and adjust doses according to serum levels.

Abbreviation: CBC, complete blood count; CRP, C-reactive protein; CSF, cerebral spinal fluid; PCR, polymerase chain reaction; UTI, urinary tract infection; WBC, white blood cell.

3 Months to 3 Years of Age

Of patients 3 months to 3 years of age with a fever, approximately 20% have no identifiable source on history or physical examination. Just as for all other age ranges, acute self-resolving viral illnesses remain the number one source of fevers in this patient population. The advent of *Haemophilus influenzae* type b and *Streptococcus pneumoniae* vaccines has markedly reduced the rate of bacteremia. Accordingly, global testing for bacteremia in this age range via blood culture and CBC with differential is no longer recommended, though these tests may be obtained if clinical suspicion is high and should be obtained for patients who are not immunized.

For patients in this age range who are otherwise well appearing and without vital sign instability, have no significant comorbidities, and are fully immunized for their age, evaluation for a fever without localizing a source can consist of watchful waiting without antibiotics and with close follow-up by a health care professional. Blood and urine tests may be obtained if clinician suspicion is high, though it is not necessary to do so and empiric antibiotics should not be prescribed.

Additional evaluation is indicated for certain patient populations. For those with a temperature greater than or at 39°C (103°F) and who are girls younger than 2 years, uncircumcised boys younger than 2 years, or circumcised boys younger than 6 months, a urinalysis, urine Gram stain, and urine culture should be obtained via catheterization or suprapubic analysis because in these population subsets, a urinary tract infection is a likely source of high fever. Blood work is not required unless the patient is unimmunized and therefore at higher risk of a serious bacterial illness, which would then warrant an evaluation and more conservative management.

For patients who are clinically unstable, including those with vital sign instability, altered mental status, or who are otherwise ill appearing, urgent evaluation and management are warranted and a full sepsis work-up is required (Table 24-4). Such patients should receive a third-generation cephalosporin antibiotic parentally and be transferred to an inpatient setting for further evaluation and management until stabilization occurs.

3 Years of Age

In this patient population, a thorough history and physical examination will most often identify a cause of the fever, as rarely in this age range do patients with a fever present without additional signs or symptoms. Evaluation and management for those older than 3 years with a fever and without an identified source, who are otherwise well and without significant comorbidities, can be managed more conservatively on an outpatient basis with observation and close follow-up. Conversely, ill-appearing patients and those with significant comorbidities should be more aggressively worked up and managed with broad-spectrum antibiotics as determined clinically at the discretion of the physician. Clinical discretion should be used for situations that fall in between.

Table 24-4. Evaluation and Management for Patients 3 mo–3 y With a Fever

Fever, Well Appearing and Source Identified (Evidence Level III)
Evaluation
Specific to identified source; patient not considered to have fever without localizing signs
Management
Treatment related to source; patient not considered to have fever without localizing signs

Table 24-4 *(cont)*

Fever <39°C (103°F); Otherwise, Well Appearing and Source Not Identified (Evidence Level II)	
Evaluation	
Consider blood and urine work-up if clinically suspicious or has had prior urinary tract infection.	
Management	
Watchful waiting with close observation within 48 h	

Fever ≥39°C (103°F); Otherwise, Well Appearing, Fully Vaccinated for Age, and Source Not Identified (Evidence Level II)	
Evaluation	
Blood	No studies required; is also acceptable to obtain CBC with differential and obtain a blood culture if leukocytosis is observed
Urine	For girls <24 mo, uncircumcised boys <24 mo, circumcised boys <6 mo, or patients with prior history of UTI: urinalysis, urine Gram stain, and urine culture
Radiographs	Chest radiographs in presence of respiratory signs or symptoms
Stool	Cultures and studies in presence of gastrointestinal signs or symptoms
Management	
Watchful waiting acceptable if patient has arranged follow-up within 24–48 h. If still febrile at 24–48 h, may elect to provide IM ceftriaxone at 50 mg/kg/dose once; prior to administering antibiotics, CSF analysis should be performed in addition to obtaining CBC with differential, blood culture, and urine studies if not previously done.	

Fever and ill-appearing (Evidence Level III)	
Evaluation	
Blood	CBC with differential, blood culture
Urine	Urinalysis, Gram stain, culture (via catheterized specimen or suprapubic aspiration)
CSF	If concerned for meningitis: protein and glucose level tests, cell count with differential, culture; consider HSV and enterovirus PCR
Radiographs	Chest radiographs in presence of respiratory signs or symptoms
Stool	Cultures and studies in presence of gastrointestinal signs or symptoms
Management	
Inpatient admission with broad spectrum, parenteral antimicrobials until cultures are negative for at least 36 h. An example antibiotic regimen includes IV ceftriaxone at 100 mg/kg/dose daily with maximum of 2 g/dose if treating for a severe infection. If treating meningitis, ensure you are administering meningitic dosing of antibiotics, add vancomycin at 20 mg/kg/dose and adjust vancomycin dosing according to serum levels.	

Abbreviation: CBC, complete blood count; CSF, cerebral spinal fluid; HSV, herpes simplex virus; IM, intramuscular; IV, intravenous; PCR, polymerase chain reaction; UTI, urinary tract infection.

Patients With Comorbidities

Many children with chronic illnesses require collaboration with treating specialists to aid in evaluation and management of fever in these special populations (Table 24-5). Developing a proactive plan for how to respond to fever can be helpful in minimizing unnecessary hospitalization or quickly identifying a patient with more urgent needs.

Table 24-5. Comorbidities Affecting Fever Evaluation and Management

Inflammatory Conditions	Oncologic Disease	Presence of Hardware
Inflammatory bowel disease Juvenile idiopathic arthritis Lupus Hemophagocytic lymphohistiocytosis	Any cancer diagnosis Any chemotherapy treatment Fever with neutropenia	Central venous lines Gastric feeding tubes Tracheostomy Orthopedic hardware Cardiac hardware Ventriculoperitoneal shunt

Fever of Unknown Origin

Fever of unknown origin in the pediatric population is defined as a documented fever that persists for all or most of 10 or more days without a known source despite repeated examination by a provider and selected laboratory or radiographic testing. Similar to fevers without source, fevers of unknown origin can be secondary to a broad range of pathologies, including infections, inflammatory disorders, malignancy, and drug fever, among others. Frequently the cause of fever is secondary to a common disorder presenting with an atypical course, but often the source of fever of unknown origin is never identified.

A detailed history and physical examination should be obtained about the fever, including its timing, duration, frequency, severity, and associated symptoms, both at the onset of the fever as well as on subsequent days. In addition, emphasis must be placed on the patient's past medical history, including growth curves, a comprehensive review of systems, medications currently and recently taken, allergies, immunizations received, social history (including recent and past travel history), sick contacts, pet and animal exposures, and family history focusing on genetic disorders and ethnic background. It is imperative to perform serial physical examinations, ideally by the same physician, though additional insight may be gained when a fresh set of eyes intermittently examines the patient. Subtle findings on examination can sometimes lead to the source of fever.

If the history and physical examination findings do not yield clues as to possible etiologies, reasonable laboratory and radiographic studies to obtain include a CBC with differential, examination of peripheral smear, erythrocyte sedimentation rate, C-reactive protein level, blood culture (preferably at time of febrile illness), and urine studies, including urinalysis, Gram stain, and culture. Additional laboratory and radiographic testing should ideally be performed sequentially and only if supported by the history and physical examination findings. Studies to consider include serum electrolytes including liver enzymes, lactate dehydrogenase, and uric acid; rheumatologic studies; stool guaiac; and human immunodeficiency virus testing. A tuberculosis skin test with a control or interferon-gamma release assay; stool studies, including cultures, WBC count, and ova and parasite examination; ferritin level; specific testing for infectious diseases that are common causes of fever of unknown origin; and radiographic studies of the chest, mastoids, or sinuses may also be reasonable if supported by the history and physical examination findings.

If the presenting patient is clinically stable other than the continued presence of a fever, it is reasonable to continue with outpatient management with serial examinations and stepwise, focused laboratory and possibly radiographic assessment while either a cause is elucidated or the fever abates. However, if the patient clinically deteriorates, admission for inpatient management should occur.

Periodic Fever Syndromes

Periodic fever syndromes must be considered in the patient who presents with a recurring fever. This category of fever is secondary to an innate immune system disorder in which inflammatory pathways are activated, resulting in a fever. Examples of such periodic fever syndromes include: familial Mediterranean fever; periodic fever, aphthous stomatitis, pharyngitis, adenitis syndrome (PFAPA); familial cold autoinflammatory syndrome; hyperimmunoglobulin D syndrome; TNF-receptor–associated periodic syndrome; Muckle-Wells syndrome; and neonatal-onset multisystem inflammatory disease. Of these, familial Mediterranean fever is the most common. An overview of selected periodic fever syndromes can be found in Table 24-6.

Table 24-6. Selected Examples of Periodic Fever Syndromes

Condition	Typical Age at Onset	Fever Duration	Fever Frequency	Common Findings (in Addition to Fever)
Familial Mediterranean fever	<10 y	1–3 d	4–8 wk	Mediterranean or Middle Eastern descent; pain (abdomen, arthralgias, myalgias)
Periodic fever, aphthous stomatitis, pharyngitis, and adenitis	<5 y	3–5 d	4–6 wk	Aphthous stomatitis, pharyngitis, and cervical adenitis; rash, abdominal pain, diarrhea
Hyperimmunoglobin D syndrome	<1 y	4–7 d	4–6 wk	Abdominal pain, diarrhea, maculopapular rash, lymphadenopathy
TNF-receptor–associated syndrome	<5 y	Days to weeks	Irregular intervals	Abdominal pain, arthralgias, myalgias with overlying erythema, eye abnormalities

Derived from Seashore CJ, Lohr JA. Fever of unknown origin in children. *Pediatr Ann.* 2011;40(1):26–30.

A common feature amongst all subtypes listed above is a cyclical pattern of fevers, for which the fever persists for a typical amount of time before abating for a longer period of time, with the cycle then repeating. Additional findings depend on the condition, though abdominal concerns, rashes, arthralgias, and mucocutaneous findings are common signs for many of the periodic fever syndromes.

Management

Fevers in otherwise healthy patients rarely need to be managed with antipyretics. In the setting of an infection, fevers are primarily beneficial to the patient and result in decreased microbial replication and enhanced immune functioning. In addition, no data show long-term harm associated with the presence of fevers, including a lack of long-term neurologic sequelae, nor does antipyretic use result in a shortened course of illness.

However, there are certain circumstances in which fevers should be managed with antipyretics. Fevers can be uncomfortable to patients, and higher temperatures can result in increased discomfort and insensible fluid loss. In certain populations, fevers should be treated more aggressively, including those who have epileptic disorders or who are younger than 6 years with a prior febrile seizure, those with a decreased oxygen-carrying capacity at baseline (including those with cardiopulmonary disorders or chronic anemia), and those with metabolic instability (including those with inborn errors of metabolism). In such patients, antipyretic use prevents exacerbation of underlying conditions. In addition, fever management is warranted if the source of fever is known to be noninfectious in etiology.

Appropriate antipyretics to reduce temperatures in those with a fever include ibuprofen for children older than 6 months and acetaminophen for all children. Ibuprofen is at least as effective of an antipyretic as acetaminophen (Evidence Level I). Aspirin should be avoided because of concern for Reye syndrome.

Alternating between ibuprofen and acetaminophen increases the overall frequency of antipyretic administration and decreases patient temperature, though using this method has not been shown to improve overall outcomes. Alternating between medications places patients at increased risk for caregiver confusion and for subsequent medication overdose (Table 24-7). In general, patients should be advised to adhere to dosing recommendations based on age and weight and should not exceed 48 hours of maximal use without consulting with a health care professional.

Table 24-7. Overview of Antipyretics (Evidence Level I)

Antipyretic	Age	Dosage	Frequency	Maximum Dosage	Cautions
Acetaminophen	All ages	10–15 mg/kg/dose PO/PR/IV	Every 4–6 h	**Per dose:** Maximum of 650 mg/dose if given every 4 h **Per day:** Maximum of 90 mg/kg/d (not to exceed 4 g/d)	Hepatic disorders, OTC medicines containing acetaminophen
Ibuprofen	≥6 mo	10 mg/kg/dose PO	Every 6 h	**Per dose:** Maximum of 600 mg/dose **Per day:** Maximum of 40 mg/kg/d (not to exceed 2.4 g/d)	Gastrointestinal or renal disorders, dehydration, concomitant use of additional nephrotoxic medications
Aspirin	Should not be used in children because of concern for Reye syndrome				

Abbreviations: IV, intravenous; OTC, over the counter; PO, by mouth; PR, programed release.

Suggested Reading

American Academy of Pediatrics Section on Clinical Pharmacology and Therapeutics, Committee on Drugs, Sullivan JE, Farrar HC. Fever and antipyretic use in children. *Pediatrics.* 2011;127(3):580–587

American College of Emergency Physicians Clinical Policies Committee, Clinical Policies Subcommittee on Pediatric Fever. Clinical policy for children younger than three years presenting to the emergency department with fever. *Ann Emerg Med.* 2003;42(4):530–545

Avner JR. Acute fever. *Pediatr Rev.* 2009;30(1):5–13

Baraff LJ. Management of infants and young children with fever without source. *Pediatr Ann.* 2008;37(10):673–679

Cincinnati Children's Hospital Medical Center. *Evidence-based Care Guideline for Fever of Uncertain Source in Infants 60 Days or Less.* Cincinnati, OH: Cincinnati Children's Hospital Medical Center; 2010

Goldsmith DP. Periodic fever syndromes, *Pediatr Rev.* 2009;30(5):e34–e41

Nield LS, Kamat D. Fever. In: Kliegman RM, Stanton BMD, Geme JS, Schor N, Behrman RE, eds. *Nelson Textbook of Pediatrics.* 19th ed. Philadelphia, PA: Elsevier; 2011:896e.8–896e.11

Nield LS, Kamat D. Fever without a focus. In: Kliegman RM, Stanton BMD, Geme JS, Schor N, Behrman RE, eds. *Nelson Textbook of Pediatrics.* 19th ed. Philadelphia, PA: Elsevier; 2011:896–902

Seashore CJ, Lohr JA. Fever of unknown origin in children. *Pediatr Ann.* 2011;40(1):26–30

Sur DK, Bukont EL. Evaluating fever of unidentifiable source in young children. *Am Fam Physician.* 2007;75(12):1805–1811

CHAPTER 25

Fluids and Electrolytes

Suresh Nagappan, MD, MSPH; Nicole L. Chandler, MD;
and Kenneth B. Roberts, MD

Key Points

- For dehydrated children, 4 phases of fluid and electrolyte therapy should be considered separately: initial fluid resuscitation, replacement of fluid deficit, provision of maintenance, and replacement of ongoing losses.

- Oral rehydration is the method of choice to replace fluid and electrolytes in mild to moderately dehydrated children.

- Children with clinical signs of severe hypovolemia should receive intravenous isotonic fluid replacement in the form of rapidly administered fluid boluses.

- After 1 or 2 fluid boluses, moderate to severely dehydrated children still need additional fluid and electrolytes to replace their deficit.

Overview

The ability to replace fluid and electrolytes lost during illness and to maintain homeostasis during fasting and thirsting was a major advance in the care of infants and children in the past century. The key distinction in determining the amount, rate, and electrolyte composition of fluid is whether the child (a) is severely dehydrated (hypotensive); (b) has a mild-moderate fluid deficit, or (c) has no deficit but simply needs to maintain homeostasis. Children with hypovolemia or a fluid deficit require a higher concentration of solute than children who only have to meet the needs of basal metabolism. It is useful to consider the following 4 phases of fluid and electrolyte therapy:

1. Resuscitation phase (reserved for those with clinical signs of hypovolemia, such as tachycardia)
2. Deficit phase (to replace losses from processes such as diarrhea)
3. Maintenance phase
4. Replacement of ongoing losses

Normal saline (NS) or lactated Ringer (LR) solution are best suited for quickly restoring intravascular volume during the resuscitation phase (Table 25-1). Dextrose, 5%, in ½ NS (D5½NS) has a sodium (Na) concentration similar to the composition of fluid lost in common pediatric illnesses and, with added potassium (K), is suitable for replacement of the deficit once clinical signs of hypovolemia are no longer present. Finally, dextrose, 5%, in ¼ NS (D$_5$¼NS), with added K, most closely resembles the fluid and electrolyte needs for maintenance of homeostasis. If the patient is able to tolerate small amounts of oral intake, World Health Organization oral rehydration solution should be used rather than intravenous therapy.

Table 25-1. Commercially Available Electrolyte Solutions for Parental Use

Common Name	Chemical Name	Na and Cl	Notes
Normal saline	0.9% NS	154 mEq/L of each	With or without 5% dextrose
Lactated Ringer		130 mEq/L of Na, 109 mEq/L of Cl	K 4 mEq/L, Ca 2.7 mEq/L, lactate 28 mEq/L; with or without 5% dextrose
½ normal saline	0.45% NS	77 mEq/L	With or without 5% dextrose
¼ normal saline	0.225% NS	38 mEq/L	With 5% dextrose

Abbreviations: Ca, calcium; Cl, chloride; Na, sodium; NS, normal saline.

Evaluation

Resuscitation Phase (Severe Hypovolemia)

Patients with hypotension need rapid intravascular volume replacement that is best be provided with boluses (20 mL/kg) of fluids that have sodium concentrations similar to intravascular fluid: NS or LR. Children in uncompensated shock (15% dehydration) typically need at least three 20 mL/kg (2%) boluses: the first bolus brings the child from 15% to 13% reduction in body weight, supporting the blood pressure but not improving heart rate; by the end of the second bolus, blood pressure should be normal; the third bolus brings the child to a 9% deficit, with beneficial effect on the heart rate. Note that simply starting maintenance fluids in a child who is still moderately dehydrated is not sufficient to rehydrate the child successfully, nor is giving an increased rate of maintenance intravenous fluids.

Deficit Phase

The classic example of a child who has incurred a deficit is one who has diarrheal losses from acute gastroenteritis. A common and dangerous mistake is simply using fluid composition appropriate for maintenance (D$_5$¼NS) and increasing the fluid rate (for example, "1.5 times maintenance") without determining the actual water and electrolyte of the deficit. This can lead to hyponatremia and serious injury.

Assessing the Severity of Dehydration

The first step is to determine the severity of dehydration, most accurately done by calculating the difference between the pre-illness weight and current weight. Pre-illness weight, however, is not always available and often clinical estimates of dehydration must be used (Table 25-2).

Table 25-2. Estimating the Severity of Dehydration

Clinical Data	Hemodynamic Changes	Severity of Dehydration	Infant Est fluid loss	Adolescent Est fluid loss	Problems in Assessment
• Dry mucous membranes • Decreased urine output • Absent tears	Normal	Mild	5% (50 mL/kg)	3% (30 mL/kg)	Oral mucosa may be dry in chronic mouth breathers. Frequency and amount of urination may be difficult to assess during diarrhea, especially in infant girls.
• Poor skin turgor • Sunken fontanel • Sunken eyes • Abnormal respirations • Tachycardia (heart rate >150 beats/min) • Mental status (fatigued or irritable)	Tachycardia	Moderate	10% (100 mL/kg)	6% (60 mL/kg)	Turgor affected by serum $[Na^+]$[a] Heart rate affected by fever, $[Na^+]$,[a] underlying disease
• Hypotension • Poor perfusion (CR >2 sec)	Hypotension, poor perfusion	Severe	15% (150 mL/kg)	9% (90 mL/kg)	Both possibly affected by $[Na^+]$,[a] underlying disease

Abbreviations: CR, capillary refill; est, estimated.
[a] $[Na^+]$ >150 mEq/L gives falsely low estimate of severity; $[Na^+]$ <130 mEq/L exaggerates clinical estimate of severity.

Estimates are based on dry mucous membranes, decreased urine output, absent tears, skin turgor, sunken fontanel, sunken eyes, abnormal respirations, tachycardia, mental status, hypotension, and poor perfusion. The absence of dry mucous membranes is the most sensitive sign for ruling out dehydration (negative likelihood ratio of 0.41). Children with moist mucous membranes are unlikely to be dehydrated. The most specific signs for ruling in dehydration, according to a meta-analysis, are skin turgor, abnormal respirations, and delayed capillary refill (likelihood ratios between 2 and 4). In contrast, decreased urine output is nonspecific (likelihood ratio of only 1.3). Depending on which signs are present, one can estimate the percentage of body weight that has been lost. Clinical signs are typically apparent by the time the child has lost 3% to 5% of body weight (eg, "is 3%–5% dehydrated"). Laboratory tests are no better at determining the extent of dehydration than clinical signs.

It needs to be clear that all guidelines regarding fluids and electrolytes are approximations that in no way can replace careful monitoring of the patient. Furthermore, no single, simple sign or test infallibly reflects fluid and electrolyte balance. The following measures are listed in decreasing order of practical value in monitoring: physical signs of dehydration; body weight; urine volume and specific gravity; input and output measurements with direct measurements of all losses; serum urea nitrogen concentration; hematocrit; concurrent serum and urine osmolalities; and serum electrolyte concentrations (which, by themselves, say little about the state of hydration). The frequency of monitoring must be individualized, depending on the present severity of the disorder and the potential rate of change. Once daily is not sufficient in a child whose dehydration is severe enough to warrant hospitalization.

Amount of Deficit

As noted above, estimates of the percentage of body weight lost can be converted to milliliters of fluid by recognizing that 1% of body weight lost = 1% dehydration = 10 mL/kg water. Therefore, a patient who weighs 5 kg and is "5% dehydrated" (5% weight loss) has lost 250 mL; if "10% dehydrated" (10% weight loss), has lost 500 mL; and if "15% dehydrated" (15% weight loss), has lost 750 mL.

Composition of Deficit

The composition of deficit fluids is dependent on 3 factors: the time period of fluid lost, the source of fluid lost (Table 25-3), and the patient's current electrolytes.

1. *Time period of fluids lost.* Hyperacute loss of fluids occurring over hours is most often from the extracellular space and most closely resembles the sodium concentration of NS or LR. In acute loss over days (eg, gastroenteritis), the body has a chance to equilibrate and fluid loss contains less Na and more K. Chronic loss over weeks (eg, pyloric stenosis), contains even less Na and more K.
2. *Source of fluids lost.* Common sources of fluid loss (ie, diarrhea, vomiting, diabetic ketoacidosis) during illness are similar in sodium concentration to ½ NS.

3. *Current electrolytes.* Hyponatremia and hypernatremia both affect the clinical signs of dehydration as noted in Table 25-2. They should be considered as special situations and are discussed later in the chapter.

Table 25-3. Electrolyte Loss From Various Sources

Fluid	Sodium (mEq/L)	Potassium (mEq/L)	Chloride (mEq/L)
Gastric	20–80	5–20	100–150
Bile	120–140	5–15	80–120
Ileostomy	45–135	3–15	20–115
Diarrheal	10–90	10–80	10–110
Sweat: normal	10–30	3–10	10–35
Sweat: cystic fibrosis	50–130	5–25	50–110
Burns	140	5	110

Maintenance Phase

Maintenance requirements are distinctly different from deficits and should be calculated separately. Normally, fluid and electrolyte maintenance is achieved orally, but if the patient is unable to tolerate oral intake, maintenance needs can be provided parenterally. Maintenance fluid and electrolyte needs result from basal metabolism, which creates 2 by-products: heat and solute (Figure 25-1). *Heat* is lost from the body mainly by evaporating water from the skin and water vapor from the upper respiratory tract. These water losses are often referred to as "insensible losses," which also includes a minimal amount of secretions from the gastrointestinal tract. Sweating is an active process, not an insensible loss, and does not apply to homeostasis in a thermoneutral environment. Several methods have been described to estimate maintenance fluid and electrolyte needs, but the Holliday-Segar method is the most frequently used because it is simple and easy to remember.

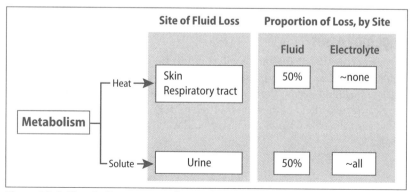

Figure 25-1. Metabolism creates 2 by-products: heat and solute.

Amount of Maintenance

Using the Holliday-Segar method, for every 100 kcal expended, 50 mL of water are lost insensibly (to dissipate heat) and approximately 50 mL of water are excreted in urine (to dispose of solute), for a total of 100 mL, thereby equating kcal and mL. The "4-2-1" rule adapted from the work of Holliday and Segar (Table 25-4) quickly estimates maintenance fluid needs in milliliters per hour and reflects decreasing metabolic rate with age.

Table 25-4. Fluid Requirements Formula Using the Holliday-Segar Method for the Average Hospitalized Patient at Maintenance

Weight (kg)	Kcal or mL	Kcal or mL
0–10 kg	100/kg per day	4/kg per hour
11–20 kg	1,000 + (50/kg/d for each kilogram between 10 and 20)	40 + (2/kg/h for each kilogram between 10 and 20)
>20 kg	1,500 + (20/kg/d for each kilogram over 20)	60 + (1/kg/h for each kilogram over 20)

Derived from Holliday MA, Segar WE. The maintenance need for water in parenteral fluid therapy. *Pediatrics.* 1957;19(5):823–832.

Composition of Maintenance Fluids

As just described, water losses can be divided into "insensible" losses and urinary losses. The water lost insensibly (from the skin and the respiratory tract) contains minimal electrolytes because it is due to evaporation. Thus, urinary output is the primary factor in determining electrolyte composition of maintenance fluids. The commercially available solution $D_5\frac{1}{4}NS$ with the addition of 20 mEq/L of K acetate is the universal maintenance fluid that best matches physiologic requirements. Other fluid types (such as NS) provide an excess of sodium compared with basal requirements and no potassium.

Ongoing Losses

Many patients with dehydration will continue to have ongoing losses after initiation of therapy. When possible, measuring the ongoing losses is helpful in determining fluid needs. The origin of the losses can also help with determining the electrolyte content of the fluid (see Table 25-3). A simple rule to remember is that gastrointestinal losses can be replaced with $D_5\frac{1}{2}NS$ and transudates with NS or LR.

Summary

Summarizing the concepts of fluid and electrolyte physiology, one can generalize the fluid composition most appropriate for specific situations.

1. NS or LR to begin deficit replacement until normalization of vital signs.

2. $D_5\frac{1}{2}NS$ with 20 mEq/L K acetate to replace the remaining deficit in most patients. Oral rehydration with oral rehydration solutions (ORS) is preferable for those able to drink. Simply increasing the rate of maintenance fluid to replace a deficit never makes physiologic sense.

3. $D_5\frac{1}{4}NS$ with 20 mEq/L K acetate for maintenance once deficit is replaced if child is still not drinking. Oral hydration is once again preferable.

4. Ongoing losses (eg, from continued diarrhea) should be replaced with deficit fluid (see summary point 2) if significant.

Management

Oral Rehydration

Case Example 1

A 10 kg 1-year-old boy has a 3-day history of vomiting and diarrhea. Based on clinical signs of dry mucous membranes, delayed skin turgor, decreased wet diapers, and tachycardia, but normal blood pressure and capillary refill, you estimate that he is 10% dehydrated. His Na is 137 mEq/L. Based on the discussion in this chapter, he needs both replacement of this deficit as well as provision of maintenance needs.

The most appropriate method of replacement is oral rehydration whenever possible. Multiple studies have shown that patients rehydrated orally compared to those rehydrated parenterally have equivalent resolution of moderate dehydration, production of urine, absence of severe emesis, and rate of return to care. Notably, orally rehydrated patients have a lower hospitalization rate and shorter time spent in the emergency department. These studies specifically looked at children with moderate rehydration, thus dispelling the idea that oral rehydration is appropriate only for children with mild dehydration. Oral rehydration should not be used in children who are severely dehydrated, in uncompensated shock, or have a suspected intra-abdominal pathology. Children who have high volume diarrheal loss (eg, cholera) or who have derangements in Na can still receive oral rehydration, however. In our case, the patient has 10% weight loss secondary to dehydration.

Since 1% of body weight = 10 mL/kg water, 10% = 100 mL/kg water;
100 mL/kg x 10 kg = 1,000 mL = 1 L deficit fluid loss.

This can be provided orally over 6 hours with 150 mL each hour or approximately 1 tbsp (15 mL) every 5 to 10 minutes. The fluid choice to replace this must account for the electrolyte losses described in the Composition of Maintenance Fluids section.

As seen in Table 25-5, beverages such as apple juice and soda provide too little Na and too much glucose (they are the equivalent of dextrose, 12%, in water). Absorption occurs via a Na-glucose co-transporter, so absorption of salt (and water) is aided by a small amount of glucose; exceeding this amount can lead to an osmotic diarrhea from the unabsorbed glucose molecules that remain in the lumen
of the gastrointestinal tract (eg, excess sugar in juice). In patients with nausea and emesis, a ketogenic state exists and can lead to further emesis and inability to tolerate oral liquids. The glucose component of ORS halts the production of ketones and allows for clinical improvement of anorexia, nausea, and emesis and increased ability to tolerate oral rehydration. The World Health Organization solution and other commercially available drinks have a favourable glucose to Na ratio (the equivalent of dextrose, 1.35%, to dextrose, 2.5%, in ¼ to ½ NS).

Parenteral Rehydration (Isotonic Dehydration)

Case Example 2

A 10 kg 1-year-old girl has acute gastroenteritis with 3 days of diarrhea and decreased oral intake. You estimate approximately 10% weight loss from dehydration based on physical examination findings of dry mucous membranes, poor skin turgor, decreased urine output, tachycardia, and normal blood pressure. Her Na is 140 mEq/L. Your first approach would be oral rehydration, but this patient is unable to tolerate oral liquids at this time.

1. *Resuscitation phase.* The patient is tachycardic with a stable blood pressure. This child could be rehydrated successfully with ORS, but because she is not tolerating oral fluids, even in small amounts, parenteral access is needed. Fluid composition appropriate for resuscitation (NS or LR) should be used to quickly restore intravascular volume. LR is preferable to NS because it can begin to replace some of the bicarbonate (HCO_3^-) lost in diarrheal stool. A standard approach would be to give the child a bolus of approximately 20 mL/kg of LR and repeat the bolus as needed to normalize her heart rate.

2. *Deficit phase.* Deficit needs must be calculated and replaced. Providing maintenance-type fluid composition (ie, D_5¼NS) to a patient that is dehydrated can be dangerous. As just described, deficit fluid needs are distinctly different.

   Recall that 1% of body weight = 10 mL/kg water, 10% = 100 mL/kg water. In this case, 100 mL/kg x 10 kg = 1,000 mL = 1 L deficit fluid loss.

Table 25-5. Composition of Commercial Oral Rehydration Solutions and Commonly Consumed Beverages

Solution	Carbohydrate (gm/L)	Sodium (mmol/L)	Potassium (mmol/L)	Chloride (mmol/L)	Base[a] (mmol/L)	Osmolarity (mOsm/L)
Oral Rehydration Solution						
World Health Organization (WHO) (2002)	13.5	75	20	65	30	245
WHO (1975)	20	90	20	80	30	311
European Society of Paediatric Gastroenterology, Hepatology and Nutrition	16	60	20	60	30	240
Enfalyte®[b]	30	50	25	45	34	200
Pedialyte®[c]	25	45	20	35	30	250
Rehydralyte®[d]	25	75	20	65	30	305
CeraLyte®[e]	40	50–90	20	NA	30	220
Commonly used beverages (not appropriate for diarrhea treatment)						
Apple juice[f]	120	0.4	44	45	NA	730
Coca-Cola[g]	112	1.6	NA	NA	13.4	650

[a] Actual or potential bicarbonate (eg, lactate, citrate, or acetate).
[b] Mead-Johnson Laboratories, Princeton, New Jersey.
[c] Ross Laboratories (Abbott Laboratories), Columbus, Ohio. Data regarding Flavored and Freezer Pop Pedialyte are identical.
[d] Ross Laboratories (Abbott Laboratories), Columbus, Ohio.
[e] Cera Products, LLC, Jessup, Maryland.
[f] Meeting US Department of Agriculture minimum requirements.
[g] Coca-Cola Corporation, Atlanta, Georgia. Figures do not include electrolytes that might be present in local water used for bottling. Base = phosphate.
From Centers for Disease Control and Prevention. Managing acute gastroenteritis among children: oral rehydration, maintenance, and nutritional therapy. *MMWR Recommen Rep.* 2003;52(RR-16):12.

If patient was given one fluid bolus (20 mL/kg), 200 mL deficit was replaced.

Total deficit = 1,000 mL – 200 mL = 800 mL (8%) deficit remaining.

Once circulation has been stabilized, the remaining deficit can be provided based on source of loss. In this case, the source is diarrheal, which most closely resembles ½ NS with 20 mEq K acetate per liter (see Table 20-3). One approach is to give the remainder of the deficit over 6 to 8 hours.

Deficit remainder = 800 mL D$_5$½NS over 8 hours = 100 mL/hour. Note that because 8% of the deficit was given over 8 hours, this is equivalent to 1%/hour or 10 mL/kg/hour.

3. *Maintenance phase.* As just described, maintenance fluid needs to reflect basal metabolism and should be addressed after the deficit has been replaced and continued until the child is drinking sufficiently well to sustain herself orally and no longer needs parenteral fluids. The addition of dextrose to the deficit fluids will help to halt the nausea and anorexia caused by ketosis and improve oral intake. Using the Holliday-Segar method,

Total water need calculation: (100 mL/kg/day x 10 kg) = 1,000 mL/day = 1 L/day. Maintenance fluid: D$_5$¼NS + 20 mEq/L K acetate at 40 mL/hour.

However, in this example, we have used 8 hours to replace the deficit and have not provided any maintenance fluid during this time. Maintenance fluid could be administered simultaneously with the fluid used to replace the deficit, but the fluids have different composition, so administering them sequentially keeps the calculations simpler. To complete the day on which the deficit was replaced and make up for the 8 hours without maintenance fluids, maintenance fluid for that day could be given over 16 hours rather than 24 as follows:

Maintenance fluid: 1,000 mL/16 hours = D$_5$¼NS + 20 mEq/L K acetate at 63 mL/hour for 16 hours.

4. *Ongoing losses.* These can be replaced, if significant, using the same composition as the deficit fluid just described.

Special Situations: Parenteral Rehydration (Hypotonic Dehydration)

Case Example 3

A 10 kg 1-year-old girl has acute gastroenteritis with 3 days of diarrhea and decreased oral intake. The parents have been giving her only apple juice at home in amounts insufficient to replace her diarrheal losses. Her serum sodium is 125 mEq/L. Her weight at a clinic visit 3 days ago was 11 kg. Based on the weight change, you estimate approximately 10% weight loss from dehydration.

Her physical examination findings can lead one to overestimate the degree of dehydration because of fluid shifts due to hyponatremia.

1. *Resuscitation phase.* This phase is the same as for isotonic dehydration. After one 20 mL/kg (2%) bolus of NS or LR, the patient's vital signs stabilize.

2. *Deficit phase.* In the prior example, we already determined the patient's fluid deficit to be 1 L. The sodium deficit with 1 L of fluid deficit would be 1 L (total fluid deficit) x 0.6 x 145 mEq/L = 87 mEq.

   However, this patient has an additional Na deficit as indicated by her serum sodium of 125. The additional Na deficit can be calculated with the following equation:

   Excess Na deficit = (Goal Na – Actual Na) x 0.6 (proportion from extracellular fluid) x weight = 135 – 125 mEq/L x 0.6 x 10 kg = 60 mEq Na.
   Total sodium deficit = 87 mEq + 60 mEq = 147 mEq Na.

   Because this patient has received 1 bolus already (200 mL of NS = 31 mEq Na), there is a remainder of 147 − 31 mEq Na = 116 mEq Na and 800 mL of fluid.

   116 mEq Na ÷ 800 mL water = 145 mEq/L.

   Therefore, NS would best reflect this patient's remaining deficit needs. K acetate can be added (20 mEq/L) given that 10 to 80 mEq K is lost in 1 L of diarrheal stool output (see Table 25-3). Care must be taken to avoid correcting the sodium too quickly due to the risk of developing central pontine myelinolysis (especially if the patient had an initial serum sodium less than 115 mEq/L). The sodium should be monitored closely to ensure an increase in sodium no greater than 12 mEq/L in 24 hours.

3. *Maintenance phase.* Once the deficit is replaced, maintenance fluid requirements will remain the same as in the prior example. This can be done orally (if the child is tolerating liquids) or parenterally.

4. *Ongoing losses.* These can be replaced, if significant, using the same composition as the deficit fluid above.

Special Situations: Parenteral Rehydration (Hypertonic Dehydration)

Case Example 4

A 10 kg 1-year-old girl has acute gastroenteritis with 3 days of diarrhea and decreased oral intake. Her serum sodium is 155 mEq/L. Her weight at a clinic visit 3 days ago was 11 kg. Based on the weight change, you estimate approximately 10% weight loss from dehydration. Her physical examination findings can lead one to underestimate the degree of dehydration because of fluid shifts due to hypernatremia.

1. *Resuscitation phase.* NS or LR can still be used initially for fluid resuscitation, but care must be taken to not further exacerbate the hypernatremia. Bolus fluid should be given only until clinical signs such as hypotension resolve.

2. *Deficit phase.* In this scenario, the total fluid loss remains the same, 1,000 mL fluid, but the amount of sodium differs as the patient has a free water deficit as reflected in the high serum sodium. The most important concept in treating hypernatremic dehydration is to slowly correct the serum sodium. The correction should be done over approximately 48 hours with care to not correct the sodium more than 12 mEq in 24 hours. In this case, the deficit fluid should initially be replaced with NS, as the sodium concentration of NS is close enough to the patient's serum sodium to avoid over-rapid correction. $D_5\frac{1}{2}NS$ with 20 mEq K acetate per liter can be added (y-in) in addition to the NS to provide dextrose, slightly lower Na concentration (aiming for a Na concentration in intravenously administered fluids no more than 15 mEq/L less than the patient's serum Na) and K needs. The patient's serum sodium should be monitored regularly to ensure that the sodium is not falling too quickly.

3. *Maintenance phase.* Again, the maintenance needs do not change and are similar to the examples above.

On the Forefront: Hypertonic Approach Versus Physiologic Approach to Maintenance Fluid Management

The physiologic approach championed by Holliday and Segar in 1956 has been challenged in recent years by a collection of studies looking at the risk of hyponatremia when providing intravenous fluids. The studies focus on 3 different patient populations: general pediatric inpatients, postoperative patients, and intensive care patients.

For general pediatric inpatients, the literature at first glance suggests that hypotonic fluids can lead to clinically significant hyponatremia. However, there are several limitations. In a randomized control trial in children who had gastroenteritis, children who received hypotonic fluids did have lower sodiums than those who received hypertonic fluids. But the lowest Na in either group was 131 mEq/L. It is unlikely that a sodium in this range (130–134 mEq/L) would cause clinical harm. It is possible, however, that a large drop in sodium, regardless of the final level, could be problematic, but the average sodium drop was only 2 mEq/L in this study. Some studies also conflated maintenance and deficit fluids. If a child received large amounts of hypotonic fluid in which the maintenance rate is simply doubled (instead of calculating maintenance and deficit separately and giving appropriate fluid types for each), hyponatremia may well ensue. The 38 mEq/L of sodium in $D_5\frac{1}{4}NS$ replaces maintenance needs but is inadequate to replace losses from diarrhea or emesis. Finally, some studies randomized children who were initially hyponatremic to receive $D_5\frac{1}{4}NS$, as noted in the "hypotonic" example, this would not be appropriate treatment and reflects lack of calculation. Thus, if one approaches dehydrated patients as described, with an initial isotonic bolus, followed by deficit replacement and then provision of maintenance, there is no evidence that dangerous clinical sequelae of hyponatremia will occur. While no studies have shown hypernatremia caused by using isotonic maintenance fluids, there is a risk of hyperchloremic metabolic acidosis.

Intensive care and postoperative patients need to be considered separately, mainly because anesthesia, pain, and central nervous system injury all stimulate the release of antidiuretic hormone (ADH). Providing hypotonic fluids in the setting of increased levels of ADH without first restoring the circulation with isotonic fluids can lead to hyponatremia. Appropriately addressing hypovolemia and understanding the potential for increased ADH in these patients should prompt the provider to utilize isotonic fluids for restoration of circulatory volume before beginning maintenance intravenous fluids.

Suggested Reading

Gorelick M, Shaw KN, Murphy KO. Validity and reliability of clinical signs in the diagnosis of dehydration in children. *Pediatrics.* 1997;99(5):E6

Holliday MA, Segar WE. The maintenance need for water in parental fluid therapy. *Pediatrics.* 1957;19(5):823–832

King CK, Glass R, Bresee JS, Duggan C; Centers for Disease Control and Prevention. Managing acute gastroenteritis among children: oral rehydration, maintenance, and nutritional therapy. *MMWR Recomm Rep.* 2003;52(RR-16):1–16

Neville KA, Verge CF, Rosenberg AR, O'Meara MW, Walker JL. Isotonic is better than hypotonic saline for IV rehydration of children with gastroenteritis. *Arch Dis Child.* 2006;91(3):226–232

Roberts KB. Fluid and electrolytes: parental fluid therapy. *Pediatr Rev.* 2001;22(11): 380–387

Spandorfer PR, Alessandrini EA, Joffe MD, Localio R, Shaw KN. Oral versus intravenous rehydration of moderately dehydrated children: a randomized, controlled trial. *Pediatrics.* 2005;115(2):295–301

Steiner MJ, DeWalt DA, Byerley J. Is this child dehydrated? *JAMA.* 2004;291(22): 2746–2754

CHAPTER 26

Gastrointestinal Bleeding

Lay Har Cheng, MD, MSPH, and Victor M. Piñeiro, MD

Key Points

- Upper gastrointestinal bleeding is usually self-limited in children, but children with ongoing bleeding warrant urgent evaluation.

- Heart rate and orthostatic vital signs can help determine the presence of significant gastrointestinal bleeding.

- Initial hemoglobin and hematocrit may falsely underestimate the degree of gastrointestinal bleeding.

- Gastroccult test can be used to assess for blood in gastric contents. Hemoccult (stool guaiac) test can be used to detect blood in stool.

- Extra-intestinal sources of bleeding should always be considered and ruled out quickly if possible.

Overview

Gastrointestinal (GI) bleeding is an anxiety-producing experience for both parents and children. Fortunately, most common causes of GI bleeding are minor and self-limited. However, though most children with GI bleeding are clinically stable, rarely GI bleeding can be massive and life threatening. Rapid assessment of the child's hemodynamic status should be made and if necessary hemodynamic stabilization should take priority over further diagnostic evaluation. For a child with hemodynamic instability and ongoing GI bleeding, early gastroenterology and surgical consultation is imperative for possible emergency endoscopic or surgical therapy.

In the stable patient, a detailed history and physical examination is necessary to help discern whether the source of the bleeding is gastrointestinal as well as to identify children at greatest risk of GI bleeding. Upper gastrointestinal (UGI) bleeding, defined as bleeding proximal to the ligament of Treitz, may present as vomiting of gross blood (hematemesis) or coffee-ground vomiting caused by degradation of the heme by gastric acid. Massive UGI bleeding can present with melena (black tarry stools), with or without the presence of hematemesis, or with hematochezia (red bloody stools) in the setting of rapid transit due to the cathartic effects of blood. Lower gastrointestinal (LGI) bleeding, or bleeding distal to the ligament of Treitz, may present with bright red blood on the toilet tissue paper after passing a bowel movement, small clots of blood mixed with the stool, bloody diarrhea, or hematochezia. The clinical presentation for occult GI bleeding may be unexplained fatigue, pallor, or iron deficiency anemia.

Causes

The primary causes of GI bleeding vary by age of the patient, clinical presentation, associated symptoms, and clinical appearance of the child. Upper gastrointestinal bleeding may present as a small volume bright blood or coffee-ground emesis in a well-appearing child or as massive hematemesis or melena (Table 26-1). Occasionally, a child will be initially asymptomatic, only to develop signs and symptoms of cardiovascular collapse with ongoing severe GI bleeding. As in UGI bleeding, the primary causes of LGI bleeding also vary by age of patient, associated symptoms, and appearance of the child (Table 26-2). Very often melena is caused by a UGI source (see Table 26-1).

Table 26-1. Main Causes of Upper Gastrointestinal Bleeding[a] (By Age and Appearance of the Patient)

Age	Well-appearing child	Ill-appearing child
Newborn/ infant	Swallowed maternal blood Vitamin K deficiency Reflux esophagitis Reactive gastritis Milk-protein sensitivity Vomiting-induced hematemesis (prolapse gastropathy syndrome) Gastrointestinal duplications	Stress gastritis or ulcer Coagulopathy (DIC) Mallory-Weiss tear Duodenal/gastric web Bowel obstruction
Preschool (2–5 y)	Vomiting-induced hematemesis (prolapse gastropathy syndrome) Acid-peptic disease Mallory-Weiss tear	Esophageal varices (liver disease) Hemorrhagic gastritis Stress gastritis or ulcer Caustic ingestion Bowel obstruction
Older child/ adolescent	Vomiting-induced hematemesis (prolapse gastropathy syndrome) Mallory-Weiss tear Reflux esophagitis Reactive gastritis	Esophageal varices (liver disease) Hemorrhagic gastritis Stress gastritis ors ulcer Bowel obstruction Dieulafoy lesion

Abbreviation: DIC, disseminated intravascular coagulation.
[a] Rare causes of upper gastrointestinal bleeding: vascular malformation, hemobilia, intestinal duplication, vasculitis, aortoenteric fistulae.

Table 26-2. Main Causes of Lower Gastrointestinal Bleeding[a]
(By Age and Appearance of the Patient)

Age	Well-appearing child	Ill-appearing child
Newborn/infant	Allergic proctocolitis Anal fissure Nodular lymphoid hyperplasia Intestinal duplication Infectious colitis Hemorrhagic disease of the newborn Meckel diverticulum	Necrotizing enterocolitis Malrotation with volvulus Infectious colitis Hirschsprung disease enterocolitis Intussusception
Preschool (2–5 y)	Anal fissure Juvenile polyp Perianal streptococcal cellulitis Rectal prolapse Meckel diverticulum Nodular lymphoid hyperplasia Inflammatory bowel disease	Infectious colitis Intussusception Malrotation with volvulus Henoch-Schönlein purpura Hemolytic uremic syndrome Ulcerative colitis
Older child/adolescent	Anal fissure Infectious colitis Hemorrhoid Polyp Inflammatory bowel disease Meckel diverticulum	Infectious colitis Ulcerative colitis Henoch-Schönlein purpura

[a] Rare causes of bleeding: vascular malformation, hemobilia, intestinal duplication, intestinal ischemia.

Initial Presentation and Assessment

Based on the answers to specific questions, the physician can approximate the severity, source, and duration of bleeding and where the patient needs to be sent (Box 26-1). Large-volume bleeding or ill appearance would prompt emergent transport to a local emergency department. A directed social and family history may direct the physician to specific conditions that could be presenting for the first time. In addition, various foods and medications can cause stools or emesis to falsely appear to contain blood (eg, candies, fruit juices, beets, blueberries, iron, bismuth).

Upper Gastrointestinal Bleeding

Initial Evaluation

The presence of blood in gastric contents is best confirmed using the Gastroccult test if a specimen can be obtained. Epistaxis, oropharyngeal bleeding, and hemoptysis should be considered and ruled out in cases of suspected UGI bleeding. For newborns or for breastfeeding infants, swallowed maternal blood must be considered, and the Apt-Downey test can be used to distinguish the presence of fetal hemoglobin from adult hemoglobin A. Initial evaluation of children with UGI bleeding should include a targeted physical examination (Box 26-2) and laboratory evaluation (Box 26-3).

A careful individualized approach depending on associated symptoms, signs, and severity of bleeding is needed. An initial hemoglobin and hematocrit is critical but may underestimate the degree of bleeding. A normal saline gastric lavage is useful to confirm the presence of esophageal or gastric bleeding, as well as to identify active bleeding. Note that duodenal bleeding may be missed on gastric lavage since it is transpyloric. Upper gastrointestinal bleeding is usually self-limited in children. However, children with ongoing bleeding warrant urgent evaluation.

Box 26-1. Historical Information

OPEN-ENDED QUESTIONS

- Describe the location, quantity, and appearance of the bleeding.
- What are the physical appearance and vital signs of the patient (if available)?
- What medical conditions does the child have (eg, liver disease, inflammatory bowel disease, etc)?
- What medication is the child on (eg, anticoagulants, nonsteroidal anti-inflammatory drugs)?

HISTORY .

- Description of onset, location, duration, occurrence
- Exposure to raw food, reptiles, travel, or toxins
- Foreign body ingestion
- Exposure to others with similar symptoms
- Ingestion of specific foods or medications
- Other associated symptoms (ie, mouth sores, pain, rashes, vomiting, swelling, headaches, neck pain, chest pain, diarrhea, fevers, bruising, and infections)
- Medications (ie, nonsteroidal anti-inflammatory drugs, warfarin, hepatotoxins, antibiotic use)

REVIEW OF SYSTEMS

- Gastrointestinal disorders
- Liver disease
- Bleeding diatheses
- Anesthesia reactions

FAMILY HISTORY

- Gastrointestinal disorders (eg, polyps, ulcers, colitis)
- Liver disease
- Bleeding diatheses
- Anesthesia reactions

From Wyllie R, Hyams JS, Kay M, eds. *Pediatric Gastrointestinal and Liver Disease.* 4th ed. Philadelphia, PA: Saunders Elsevier; 2011, with permission.

Box 26-2. Targeted Physical Examination

Vital signs: orthostasis, pulse pressure, instability, urine output

General: appearance (well or ill), fever, mental status

Head, eyes, ears, nose, and throat: trauma, scleral injection, petechiae, lip and buccal pigmentation, epistaxis, erythema or burns to posterior pharynx, bleeding

Chest/cardiovascular: tachycardia, murmur, capillary refill

Abdomen: tenderness, splenomegaly, hepatomegaly, caput medusa, distention, ascites

Genitourinary: fistula, swelling

Rectal: gross blood, melena, tags, tenderness, fissure, fistula, swelling, inflammation

Dermatological: pallor, jaundice, rash, arteriovenous malformation, bruising, petechiae

From Wyllie R, Hyams JS, Kay M, eds. *Pediatric Gastrointestinal and Liver Disease.* 4th ed. Philadelphia, PA: Saunders Elsevier; 2011, with permission.

Box 26-3. Possible Laboratory Studies

- Complete blood count
- Prothrombin time/international normalized ratio/partial thromboplastin time
- Complete metabolic profile (electrolytes, liver function tests)
- Type and screen
- If significant loss: type and cross, fibrinogen level
- Stool culture including assay for *Escherichia coli* O157:H7, *Shigella, Salmonella, Yersinia, Campylobacter; Clostridium difficile* toxins A and B; *Cryptosporidium* and *Giardia* assays; and ova and parasite smear if indicated by history
- Erythrocyte sedimentation rate, C-reactive protein, γ-glutamyl transpeptidase (GGT) if indicated by history
- Hemoccult and Gastroccult testing

From Wyllie R, Hyams JS, Kay M, eds. *Pediatric Gastrointestinal and Liver Disease.* 4th ed. Philadelphia, PA: Saunders Elsevier; 2011, with permission.

Additional Evaluations

Diagnostic studies that may be useful to further evaluate the child with UGI bleeding include radiographic and endoscopic studies (Table 26-3). Esophago-gastroduodenoscopy (EGD) is the preferred method to confirm the diagnosis and possibly treat the bleeding lesion when necessary (see Therapy section). If the patient presents with hematemesis or has a positive nasogastric lavage, radiographic testing is rarely indicated unless the EGD is negative. However, radiographic studies may be useful in certain clinical scenarios. Plain abdominal radiographic studies can be used to identify an esophageal or bowel perforation, or a bowel obstruction. Abdominal ultrasound can identify portal hypertension responsible for esophageal or gastric varices. In the setting of brisk bleeding (ie, ≥0.5 mL/min), angiography allows for identification of the bleed as well as for therapy by embolization through placement of coils.

Table 26-3. Imaging Studies and Associated Indications

Test	Indication
Abdominal x-ray	Constipation Foreign body Vomiting
Upper gastrointestinal series	Dysphagia Odynophagia Drooling Obstruction Vomiting
Barium enema	Suspected stricture Intussusception Hirschsprung disease (late)
Ultrasound (Doppler recommended for liver disease)	Portal hypertension Intussusception Possible inflammatory bowel disease
Meckel scan	Meckel diverticulum
Tagged RBC scan	Obscure gastrointestinal bleeding
MRI/CT	Obstruction Suspected inflammatory bowel disease Obscure gastrointestinal bleeding
Angiography	Suspected arteriovenous malformation

Abbreviations: CT, computed tomography; RBC, red blood cell.
Adapted from Wyllie R, Hyams JS, Kay M, eds. *Pediatric Gastrointestinal and Liver Disease.* 4th ed. Philadelphia, PA: Saunders Elsevier; 2011, with permission.

Therapy

Initial fluid resuscitation and stabilization are the first priority for both UGI and LGI bleeding. Options for medical treatment of UGI bleeding include acid reduction, vasoconstriction, and cytoprotection (Box 26-4). Antacids, H_2-receptor antagonists, and proton pump inhibitors are useful to treat suspected acid-peptic disease, as well as to aid in reducing continued acid injury to an existing mucosal defect. Octreotide is useful to reduce splanchnic blood flow, particularly in the setting of portal hypertension. Sucralfate is activated in an acidic environment (pH <4) to form a buffer and an insoluble barrier that binds to proteins on the surface of ulcers. Use of sucralfate should be avoided in patients with chronic renal failure because of its aluminum content.

Box 26-4. Therapy of GI Bleeding

SUPPORTIVE CARE

- IV fluids
- Blood products (packed red blood cells, fresh frozen plasma)
- Pressors (dopamine, etc)

SPECIFIC CARE

- Proton pump inhibitors (omeprazole, lansoprazole, pantoprazole)
- Somatostatin analogue (octreotide)

ENDOSCOPIC THERAPY

- Injection (sclerosant, epinephrine, normal saline, hypertonic saline)
- Coagulation (bipolar, monopolar, heater probe, laser, argon plasma)
- Variceal injection and ligation
- Band ligation
- Polypectomy
- Endoscopic clip
- Endoscopic loop

From Wyllie R, Hyams JS, Kay M, eds. *Pediatric Gastrointestinal and Liver Disease.* 4th ed. Philadelphia, PA: Saunders Elsevier; 2011, with permission.

Endoscopic therapy includes electrocoagulation, laser photocoagulation, argon plasma coagulation, injection of epinephrine and sclerosants, band ligation, and mechanical clipping. Use of these modalities comes with the risk of intestinal necrosis and perforation but can be critical to stop ongoing bleeding.

Early surgical consultation should be obtained prior to any endoscopic intervention in which the risk of severe bleeding is high. Surgical intervention should be reserved for patients in whom hemodynamic stability is tenuous or in whom there is uncontrolled bleeding. Exploratory laparotomy may be necessary in children with a GI perforation or an obstruction.

Lower Gastrointestinal Bleeding

History and Physical

A detailed history and physical can help the clinician narrow down the list of potential causes of LGI bleeding. Family history of a first-degree relative with allergy, inflammatory bowel disease, familial adenomatous polyposis, hereditary hemorrhagic telangiectasia, Ehlers-Danlos syndrome, or bleeding disorder raises the possibility of the same disorder in the patient. Personal history of neonatal sepsis, omphalitis, umbilical catheterization, abdominal surgery, previous GI bleeding, hematologic abnormalities, or liver disease can further direct the clinician towards the most likely source of the LGI bleeding. Risk factors such as day care attendance and recent use of antibiotics raise the possibility of bacterial or viral GI infection.

The clinical characteristics can also elucidate the most likely causes of the LGI bleeding (Tables 26-4 and 26-5).

Table 26-4. Principal-Associated Gastrointestinal Symptoms in Relation to the Underlying Cause(s) of Lower Gastrointestinal Bleeding

Amount of Blood Loss	Appearance of Bleeding	Characteristics of Stools	Pain	Underlying Disease
Small	Red	Hard	Yes (anorectal)	Anal fissure
Small to moderate	Red	Loose	Variable (abdominal)	Allergic proctocolitis, infectious colitis, hemolytic uremic syndrome, inflammatory bowel disease
Small to moderate	Red	Normal, coated with blood	No	Polyp
Moderate	Red to tarry	Normal	Yes (abdominal)	Henoch-Schönlein purpura
Moderate	Red to tarry, currant jelly	Normal	Yes (abdominal)	Intussusception
Moderate	Red to tarry	Loose	Yes (abdominal)	Hirschsprung disease enterocolitis
Large	Red to tarry	Normal	No	Meckel diverticulum, angiodysplasia

From Turck D, Michaud L. Lower gastrointestinal bleeding. In: Walker WA, Goulet O, Kleinman R, et al, eds. *Pediatric Gastrointestinal Disease.* 4th ed. Ontario, Canada: BC Decker; 2004:268.

Table 26-5. Principal Physical Findings in Relation to the Underlying Cause(s) of Lower Gastrointestinal Bleeding

Location	Physical Finding	Underlying Disease
Abdomen	Hepatosplenomegaly, ascites, dilated venous channels on the abdomen, caput medusa	Portal hypertension
	Abdominal mass	Intussusception, IBD, intestinal duplication
Perineal area	Anal fissure	Constipation, Crohn disease
	Skin tag, fistula, abscess	Crohn disease, chronic granulomatous disease, immunodeficiency syndromes
	Hemorrhoids, rectal varicosities	Portal hypertension, constipation (adolescent)
	Rectal mass at digital rectal examination	Polyp

Table 26-5 *(cont)*

Location	Physical Finding	Underlying Disease
Skin and mucous membranes	Eczema	Food allergy
	Purpura	Henoch-Schönlein purpura, hemorrhagic disease, hemolytic uremic syndrome
	Jaundice, palmar erythema, spider angioma	Liver cirrhosis
	Digital clubbing	Liver cirrhosis, IBD
	Pyoderma gangrenosum	Ulcerative colitis
	Erythema nodosum	Crohn disease
	Telangiectasia	Hereditary hemorrhagic telangiectasia
	Soft tissue tumor (skull, mandible)	Gardner syndrome
	Café au lait spots	Turcot syndrome
	Pigmentation of the lips, buccal mucosa, face	Peutz-Jeghers syndrome
	Alopecia, onychodystrophy, hyperpigmentation	Cronkhite-Canada syndrome
	Breast hypertrophy	Cowden disease
	Bluish soft nodules	Blue rubber bleb nevus syndrome
	Soft tissue hypertrophy	Klippel-Trénaunay syndrome
Eye	Iritis	IBD
Joint	Arthritis	Henoch-Schönlein purpura, IBD
Growth	Failure to thrive	IBD, Hirschsprung disease
	Very short stature, webbed neck, widespread nipples	Turner syndrome

Abbreviation: IBD, inflammatory bowel disease.
From Turck D, Michaud L. Lower gastrointestinal bleeding. In: Walker WA, Goulet O, Kleinman R, et al, eds. *Pediatric Gastrointestinal Disease.* 4th ed. Ontario, Canada: BC Decker; 2004:269.

Initial Evaluation

Fecal occult blood testing, or guaiac test, can be used to confirm the presence of blood in the stool. Rarely, false-positives can potentially result from consumption of myoglobin or hemoglobin in meat or ascorbic acid in uncooked fruits and vegetables. Epistaxis, oropharyngeal bleeding, hemoptysis, hematuria, and menses should be considered and ruled out in cases of suspected LGI bleeding. For newborns or for breastfeeding infants, swallowed maternal blood must be considered, and the Apt-Downey test can be used to distinguish the presence of fetal hemoglobin from adult hemoglobin A. Upper gastrointestinal bleeding must also be considered, as it may also present with melena, hematochezia, and anemia.

Initial evaluation of children with LGI bleeding should include a targeted physical examination (see Box 26-1) and laboratory evaluation (see Box 26-2). A normal saline gastric lavage is useful to confirm the presence of UGI bleeding in the presence of large volume melena or hematochezia.

Additional Evaluations

Radiographic studies are often performed and are especially useful when trying to exclude a surgical emergency (see Table 26-3). Plain upright and supine abdominal radiographs should be obtained in patients suspected of having an obstruction, ischemia, or perforation. Barium enema should be avoided as part of an initial evaluation, as it will lead to delays in endoscopic and scintigraphic evaluation. Abdominal ultrasound can evaluate an abdominal mass or suspected intussusception. If findings are suspicious for intussusceptions, air contrast enema with a pediatric surgeon present is the next step for diagnostic confirmation and treatment.

Endoscopic evaluation is colonoscopy. Small bowel enteroscopy, available at certain centers only, allows for visualization and sampling of the small bowel between the ligament of Treitz and the ileocecal valve. Video capsule endoscopy can be used to evaluate the small bowel for bleeding and ulceration. It should be avoided in those with potential partial obstruction that may prevent safe and successful passage of the camera.

Abdominal scintigraphy with technetium (Tc) 99m pertechnetate, also known as a Meckel scan, can be used to identify the heterotopic gastric mucosa found in a Meckel diverticulum or intestinal duplication. A radioisotope-tagged red blood cell scan performed with a sample of the patient's own red blood cells tagged with Tc 99m can identify sources of bleeding when the rate of blood loss is at least 0.5 mL/min. Angiography, also used when the bleeding rate exceeds 0.5 mL/min, has the added benefit of allowing for intra-procedure embolization or local infusion of vasopressin but comes at the risk of serious complications including arterial spasm, arterial thrombosis, contrast reaction, and acute renal failure.

Therapy

Many of the medical or surgical treatment options of LGI bleeding are similar to the treatment of UGI bleeding just discussed and listed in Box 26-4. Once colonic preparation (ie, cleanout) is complete, colonoscopy can often identify the bleeding lesion. Other specific medical and surgical treatment options are tailored to the underlying cause of the bleeding and are beyond the scope of this chapter.

Suggested Reading

Boyle JT. Gastrointestinal bleeding in infants and children. *Pediatr Rev.* 2008;29(2):39–52

Fox VL. Gastrointestinal bleeding in infancy and childhood. *Gastroenterol Clin North Am.* 2000;29(1):37–66

Walker WA, Goulet OJ, Kleinman RE, Sherman PM, Shneider BL, Sanderson IR, eds. *Pediatric Gastrointestinal Disease.* 4th ed. Ontario, Canada: BC Decker; 2004

Wyllie R, Hyams JS, Kay M, eds. *Pediatric Gastrointestinal and Liver Disease.* 4th ed. Philadelphia, PA: Saunders Elsevier; 2011

CHAPTER 27

Headaches and Migraines

Marcelo E. Bigal, MD, PhD, and Marco A. Arruda, MD, PhD

Key Points

- Migraine is common in the pediatric population. It may affect performance at school and even disrupt social and family life.

- Diagnosing migraine requires a systematic yet simple approach: look for red flags and investigate further only when they are present or when therapeutic response is below expectations.

- In the absence of red flags, children with headaches disabling enough to require medical consultation are considered to have migraine until proven otherwise.

- Migraine requires no single criterion to diagnose but rather a combination of criteria.

- The hallmark of migraine is headache with associated symptoms.

- Treatment of migraine needs to be conducted systematically. Stratify acute therapies as a function of migraine characteristics. One size does not fit all.

- Some children will also require preventive therapies. Drug choice should be based on comorbidities or clinical symptoms that could also benefit from that specific drug.

Overview

Although migraine is common at all ages, the effects of age on migraine prevalence and clinical features are dramatic. The age influence on migraine is best studied for prevalence and gender distribution. Before puberty, migraine prevalence is slightly higher in boys than in girls; as adolescence approaches, incidence and prevalence increase more rapidly in girls than in boys. The prevalence continues to increase throughout childhood and early adult life.

Nonetheless, the influence of age on migraine goes far beyond determining its prevalence by also influencing clinical presentation, differential diagnosis, and therapeutic outcomes. Indeed, diagnosis and treatment of migraine in children and adolescents resemble a kaleidoscope with many facets and striking peculiarities with only some resemblance to migraine at adulthood. Among the resemblances, we emphasize that migraine is the most common diagnosis among children seeking care for headache in primary care and, as in adults, it imposes a significant burden to children by affecting quality of life, school attendance and performance, and sometimes the extended family and family life.

Migraine in children often lacks its most distinguishing feature seen in adults, the headaches (as in the periodic syndromes of childhood), or else is characterized by headaches of shorter duration and a different phenotype. Furthermore, secondary headaches are more common in the pediatric population relative to adult, although migraine is by far the most common diagnosis in children with headaches. Finally, not all migraine medications available to the adult population are approved for pediatric use, creating therapeutic challenges. Improper migraine treatment is a risk factor for progression from episodic to chronic migraine, a condition characterized by headaches on more days than not, and an outcome to be aggressively avoided.

Accordingly, proper diagnosis and care of migraine in childhood require a systematic approach and meticulous follow-up. A structured process for the clinician to comfortably navigate diagnosis and treatment of migraine in childhood is key to care of these children.

Clinical Features and Evaluation

Distinguishing Primary From Secondary Headaches

An important first step in headache diagnosis for all ages is to distinguish primary from secondary headaches. In secondary headaches, there is an underlying cause that may be ominous (eg, brain tumor, meningitis). In primary headaches (eg, migraine, tension-type headaches), there is not an underlying cause. Distinguishing primary from secondary headaches require 3 steps: 1) obtaining a good history and detailed physical and neurologic examination; 2) looking for red flags; and 3) investigating properly as guided by the red flags or assigning a primary headache diagnosis in the absence of red flags.

Step 1: Obtain a Good Medical History and Detailed Physical and Neurologic Examination

The second edition of the *International Classification of Headache Disorders* (*ICHD-II*) describes 14 headache categories subdivided into a total of 196 possible headache diagnoses, of which 113 have been described in the pediatric population. Most of these headaches are rare, and indeed, few medical disorders can be so accurately diagnosed on clinical grounds as headache disorders. Without being reductionists, we affirm that the vast majority of children with headaches without red flags who seek medical care have migraines. In those children who do not seek health care, tension-type headaches are the most common. Other headaches exist but are much rarer and will appear very different to the primary care physician. Children with these headaches should be referred to a pediatric neurologist or a headache specialist for diagnosis and care.

History

Accordingly, history for children with headaches focuses on trying to spot the atypical red flags. It also focuses on defining severity as a prelude to treatment. Important elements of history include

▶ Age of onset and temporal pattern (ie, acute, chronic, progressive, non-progressive). Look for very early onset (eg, younger than 5 years), non-remitting headaches, or chronic or progressive headaches.

▶ Pain quality when the pain is at its peak of intensity. All "mild" headaches look the same (eg, dull, non-characteristic). It is important to ask about the quality of the headache when it is at its worst. Features to look for include throbbing pain (a migraine feature) versus other forms (eg, dull, stabbing, pressure).

▶ Pain severity and duration of pain with and without treatment. Sometimes pain severity needs to be inferred by behavior. With mild pain, children typically complain but continue with their activities; with moderate pain, children become quiet and lay down; with severe pain, they often go to bed or cry.

▶ Location of pain when it is at its worst. Is it bilateral with both sides hurting the same? Bilateral with one side hurting more than the other? Unilateral fixed versus alternating (from attack to attack)? Migraine attacks are bilateral or unilateral alternating. Totally side-locked headaches (all attacks are in the same side) should be assessed carefully.

▶ Associated symptoms with an emphasis on nausea (do you get sick to your stomach or can you eat when you have the headaches?), photophobia (does light bother you more when experiencing the headache than when you don't have pain?), and phonophobia (does sound bother you more when experiencing the headache than when you don't have pain?).

▶ Symptoms suggestive of aura (see Migraine With Aura section), including scintillating scotomata, hemisensory disturbance, hemiparesis, dysphasia, and vertigo.

▶ Headache triggers (eg, emotions, foods, exertion, odors, excessive light, sleep deprivation).

▶ Relieving and worsening factors during headache attacks. Migraines are typically relieved by compression of the superficial temporal artery, cold compresses on the temples, rest in a dark and silent room, sleep, and vomiting. Migraine is typically worsened by physical activities, but secondary headaches are typically worsened as well; therefore, this finding should be interpreted in context.

▶ A detailed history of medications used and all examinations performed in the past, as well as the degree of functional impact, which may be helpful as a gauge of severity, duration, and frequency of the headaches.

As diagnosis is often based on the first encounter with a patient, use of a headache diary may contribute considerably to an accurate diagnosis (Figure 27-1). Headache diaries can also be very useful to assess outcomes with treatment.

Month: Year:

Days	1	2	3	4	5	6	7	8	9	10	11	12	13	14	15	16	17	18	19	20	21	22	23	24	25	26	27	28	29	30	31	HI
Dawn (0-6)																																
Morning (6-12)																																
Afternoon (12-18)																																
Night (18-24)																																
Unilateral																																
Bilateral																																
Pressure/tightning																																
Throbbing/pulsating																																
Worsening by exercise																																
Nausea																																
Vomiting																																
Photophobia																																
Phonophobia																																
Aura																																
Medication																																
Relief (++ / + / –)																																
Menstruation																																
Trigger factor																																

HI =

Pain intensity: 1 = low, the child continues to play; 2 = moderate, the child stops physical activities but does not lies down; 3 = severe, the child lies down and may cry. HI (headache index): monthly sum of headache intensity.

Fill according to the pain intensity — Fill with an X — Fill according to the pain relief in response to medication (+,–)

Figure 27-1. Pediatric headache diary.

Physical Examination

The general physical examination is of particular importance in children with headaches. It should include examination of the skull, including bruits over the temples, mastoids, and orbits. Hemotympanum may be found in head trauma. Examination should include measurement of head circumference, palpation and percussion of sinuses and mastoids, and attention to the neck (including carotid thrills and bruits, meningismus), abdomen (palpate for visceromegaly, which can indicate presence of storage diseases), spine (look for scoliosis and any sacral anomalies), and skin (look for stigmata of the neurocutaneous syndromes, such as café au lait spot and port-wine stain). Particular attention must be given to the measurement of arterial blood pressure.

Neurologic Examination

Neurologic examination should look for potential signs of ominous disorders. The primary care pediatrician should focus on mental state (ie, level of consciousness), cranial nerves (eg, funduscopic examination, pupils and conjugated eye movements), focal weaknesses, deep tendon reflexes, coordination, tremors (eg, rapid alternating movements, finger to nose), and gait (eg, regular, toe, heel, tandem, running, turning).

Step 2: Look for Red Flags

At this point, physicians should have easily spotted red flags, if any exist. The authors have developed the mnemonic SAFETIPS to help physicians remember what to explore.

▶ **S**udden-onset headache: when a very severe headache reaches its peak in only a few seconds or minutes (versus the more gradual onset of migraine headaches).

▶ **A**ssociated with seizures, unexplained behavior changes, or important decline in school achievement.

▶ **F**ocal neurologic signs or symptoms other than typical visual or sensory aura: papilledema (intracranial hypertension), sensory or motor deficits, incoordination, and cranial nerves deficits (eg, hearing loss, monocular blindness, visual field deficits, diplopia, strabismus, nystagmus, turning of head).

▶ **E**xertion-triggered headaches (or **e**xplosive headaches) starting during exercise, coughing, or Valsalva maneuver. Note that what defines this red flag is the intense, rapid onset of a headache in close association with these activities. Migraine is often triggered by exercises, but its onset is gradual and its presentation is typical.

▶ **T**emporal pattern: Worsening pattern, important changes in the quality of pain, its location, or frequency of headaches are red flags. Furthermore, clinicians should also fear when the complaint is about "the worst headache of the person's life."

▶ **I**nfection signs or symptoms: fever, coryza, sore throat, impaired peripheral circulation, petechiae, meningeal irritation (ie, neck stiffness, Kernig sign, Brudzinski sign, or bulging fontanelle in infants younger than 1 year).

▶ **P**rominent vomiting, especially if it does not relieve headaches (which often is the case with migraine) or is delinked from headaches.

▶ **S**leep disruption by headache: Children with migraine are often capable of sleeping during the attack and feel relieved by it. Headaches that often wake children in the middle of the night should be investigated.

In the presence of red flags, the physician must conduct the proper work-up or refer the patient to a neurologist (Table 27-1). In the absence of red flags, the pediatrician is expected to diagnose and treat the primary headache. Lack of

Table 27-1. Red Flags in Diagnosis of Headache in Children and Adolescents: The SAFETIPS Mnemonic and Suggested Investigation

Red Flags	Consider	Possible Investigation(s)
Sudden onset	Subarachnoid hemorrhage, bleeding into a mass, arteriovenous malformation, or aneurysm	Neuroimaging and lumbar puncture (after neuroimaging)
Associated with • Seizures • Recent behavior changes • Declining in school achievement	Intracranial hypertension, intracranial mass lesions, and psychiatric comorbidity	Neuroimaging Psychiatric evaluation
Focal neurologic signs/symptoms	Intracranial hypertension, intracranial mass lesions	Neuroimaging
Exertion triggered (or **e**xplosive)	Subarachnoid hemorrhage, bleeding into a mass, arteriovenous malformation, or aneurysm	Neuroimaging
Temporal pattern • Time from onset <6 mo • Worsening pattern • Change of headache pattern • Worst headache in life	Intracranial hypertension, intracranial mass lesions, arteriovenous malformation, or aneurysm	Neuroimaging
Infection signs/symptoms	Acute sinusitis, meningitis, encephalitis, Lyme disease, systemic infection, collagen vascular disease, arteritis	Paranasal sinuses CT, lumbar puncture, blood tests
Prominent vomiting	Intracranial hypertension, intracranial mass lesions	Neuroimaging
Sleep disruption by headache	Migraine, cluster headache, hypnic headache,[a] and intracranial hypertension	Neuroimaging

Abbreviation: CT, computed tomography.

[a] Hypnic headache is a primary headache characterized by attacks of dull headache that always awaken the patient from sleep. It is extremely uncommon in the pediatric population.

expected improvement or worsening after proper treatment with proper doses for proper times is a red flag.

We emphasize that obtaining neuroimaging studies in children without red flags is not recommended. According to practice parameters of the American Academy of Neurology, neuroimaging should be considered in children with an abnormal neurologic examination such as focal findings, signs of increased intracranial pressure, significant alteration of consciousness, and coexistent seizures. In addition, there may be historical features in the individual to suggest recent onset of severe headache, change in the type of headache, or associated features that suggest neurologic dysfunction (Evidence Level II-2).

The SAFETIPS approach provides good guidance as to when neuroimaging or other forms of testing should be requested (see Table 27-1).

Step 3: Diagnose the Primary Headache (Figure 27-2)

In the absence of red flags, children with headaches that are significant enough to require medical consultation are considered to have migraine until proven otherwise.

Migraine is a chronic, relapsing, remitting disorder with a strong genetic component. It typically aggregates in the family and is associated with primary dysfunction in inhibitory brain systems accountable for the sensitive-sensorial process (thus, hypersensitivity to light, sounds, and odors). Pain is often but not always present and is not the only symptom. Migraine is subdivided in several categories; the 2 most common forms are migraine with and without aura. In young children, migraine sometimes occurs without headache. This subtype was formerly known as acephalgic migraine but is now referred to as childhood periodic syndromes that are commonly precursors of migraine. These 3 migraine subtypes are detailed herein.

Migraine Without Aura

Criteria for migraine without aura, according to *ICHD-II,* are described in Box 27-1. Migraine without aura is characterized by reoccurring attacks of headache lasting from 1 to 72 hours each (attacks typically last less than 24 hours). The headache must have 2 of the following characteristics: 1) unilateral location (or more severe in one side than on the other); 2) throbbing nature (when pain is most severe); 3) moderate to severe pain intensity at some point of the attack; or 4) exacerbation of headache by routine physical activity. During headache attacks, at least one of the following should also be present: nausea and/or vomiting, photophobia and/or phonophobia.

In children, attacks are usually shorter than in adults and last less than 4 hours or even less than 1 hour. Because young children may not be able to verbalize some of these characteristics, it is important to ask about their behavior during the attack (eg, seeking bed rest, turning off the television).

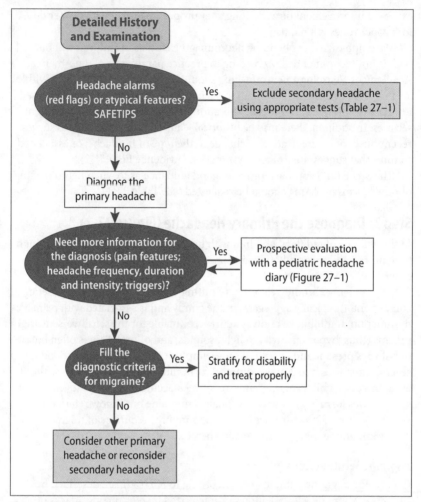

Figure 27-2. Algorithm for the diagnosis of migraine in children.

Understanding that migraine requires a combination of criteria and that no single criterion need be present is key to diagnosis. Bilateral headache that is non-throbbing and not associated with photophobia or phonophobia but is severe, worsened by physical activities, and accompanied by nausea fulfills the criteria for migraine as well as more typical presentations. Indeed, the hallmark of migraine is not the headache but the associated symptoms.

When the syndrome fulfills all but one criterion for migraine, diagnosis is probable migraine. The diagnosis of probable migraine in children very often evolves to a definitive diagnosis of migraine with or without aura. Treatment approaches are the same.

Box 27-1. Diagnostic Criteria of Migraine With and Without Aura According to the Second Edition of the *International Classification of Headache Disorders*

Migraine Without Aura	Migraine With Aura

A: At least 5 attacks fulfilling criteria B–D
 	
B: Headache attacks lasting 1–72 h
 	
C: Headache has at least 2 of the following characteristics:
  1: Unilateral location
  2: Pulsating quality
  3: Moderate or severe pain intensity
  4: Aggravation by or causing avoidance of routine physical activity (eg, walking, climbing stairs)
 	
D: During headache, at least one of the following symptoms:
  1: Nausea or vomiting
  2: Photophobia and phonophobia
 	
E: Not attributed to another disorder[a]
	A: At least 2 attacks fulfilling criteria B–D
	
	B: Aura consisting of at least one of the following symptoms but no motor weakness:
	  1: Fully reversible visual symptoms including positive features (eg, flickering lights, spots, or lines) or negative features (ie, loss of vision)
	  2: Fully reversible sensory symptoms including positive features (ie, pins and needles) or negative features (ie, numbness)
	  3: Fully reversible dysphasic speech disturbance
	
	C: At least 2 of the following symptoms:
	  1: Homonymous visual symptoms or unilateral sensory symptoms.
	  2: At least one aura symptom develops gradually over ≥5 min or different aura symptoms occur in succession over ≥5 min.
	  3: Each symptom lasts ≥5 and ≤60 min.
	
	D: Headache fulfilling criteria B–D for migraine without aura. Migraine without aura begins during the aura or follows aura within 60 minutes.
	
	E: Not attributed to another disorder[a]

[a] History and physical and neurologic examinations do not suggest any secondary headache; history or physical or neurologic examinations do suggest such a disorder but it is ruled out by appropriate investigations; or such a disorder is present but attacks do not occur for the first time in close temporal relation to the disorder.

Migraine With Aura

Migraine with aura (see Box 27-1 for criteria) accounts for approximately 25% of migraine cases. Very often, children have some attacks with and others without aura. Aura is defined as fully reversible focal neurologic symptoms, which usually precede or sometimes accompany the headache. Symptoms develop gradually over 5 to 20 minutes and last for less than 60 minutes. Visual aura is the most common form, characterized by positive (eg, flickering lights, spots, or lines) or negative features (ie, loss of vision). Positive (ie, pins and needles) or negative sensory features (ie, numbness) and dysphasic speech may occur. Headache with the features of migraine without aura usually follows aura symptoms.

Most of the time, aura is typical and its diagnosis does not impose a challenge. When visual aura is atypical, the most important differential diagnosis is epilepsy. The key features to differentiate these conditions are

▶ The positive and negative visual manifestations of epilepsy affect the central visual field, while in aura they are more peripheral.

▶ Symptoms in epilepsy typically last less than 1 minute.

▶ Other epileptic manifestations occur in immediate relationship to visual disturbance in children with epilepsy (eg, automatisms, altered consciousness, olfactory symptoms, aphasia, déjà vu).

Hemiplegic migraine (HM) is a rare form of migraine with aura, characterized by fully reversible attacks of motor weakness with or without other aura symptoms. It is subdivided into familial or sporadic. In familial HM, there is at least one first- or second-degree relative with migraine aura including motor weakness. In sporadic HM, there is no family history. Hemiparesis or single limb paresis must be present; bilateral paresis provides evidence against the diagnosis. In the course of HM, common symptoms include severe and prolonged attacks of hemiplegia, fever, seizure, confusion, and sometimes even coma. Therefore, we emphasize that, for the most symptomatic cases (when the diagnosis has not been previously described or when cognitive symptoms occur), a diagnosis of HM can only be made after exclusion of secondary conditions. Differential diagnosis of HM in children and adolescents includes basilar migraine, stroke (mainly ischemic transient attacks), Todd paralysis (when temporary paresis or paralysis follows a seizure), epilepsy, and the syndrome of transient headache and neurologic deficits with cerebrospinal fluid lymphocytosis.

Basilar-type migraine is a common subtype of migraine with aura. Diagnosis requires at least 2 of the following fully reversible aura symptoms: dysarthria, vertigo, tinnitus, hypacusia, diplopia, visual symptoms simultaneously in temporal and nasal fields, ataxia, decreased level of consciousness, and simultaneously bilateral paresthesias. Basilar-type migraine is not an ominous form of migraine and treatment is similar to other migraine subtypes.

Childhood Periodic Syndromes That Are Commonly Precursors of Migraine

Childhood periodic syndromes refer to recurrent, transient, and otherwise unexplained signs and symptoms that seem to be precursors of migraine. Among them, more robust evidence exists for cyclic vomiting, abdominal migraine, and benign paroxysmal vertigo of childhood.

Cyclic vomiting syndrome is defined as recurrent and episodic stereotypical attacks of severe nausea, vomiting, pallor, and lethargy lasting from 1 hour to 5 days with complete resolution of symptoms between attacks, which are not attributed to another disorder. History and physical examination do not show signs of gastrointestinal disease. Family history of migraine is often present.

Abdominal migraine, in turn, is an idiopathic disorder characterized by recurrent attacks of abdominal pain lasting from 1 to 72 hours (untreated or unsuccessfully treated). Pain is referred to as dull or "just sore" in quality, of moderate to severe intensity, and located in the midline or periumbilical area or poorly localized. During attacks of abdominal pain, at least 2 of the following symptoms are present: anorexia, nausea, vomiting, or pallor. History and physical examination do not show signs of gastrointestinal or renal disease, or such disease has been ruled out by appropriate investigations.

Benign paroxysmal vertigo in childhood is characterized by recurrent attacks of severe vertigo resolving spontaneously after minutes to hours in otherwise healthy children. During attacks, nystagmus, vomiting, and unilateral throbbing headache may occur. The neurologic examination, audiometric and vestibular functions, and electroencephalogram are normal between attacks.

Management

The same structured approach required to diagnose migraine is also required for proper treatment because one size does not fit all. As for adults, treatment choices for children should follow a stratified approach, in which the medication is prescribed as appropriate for the burden of disease. Clinicians should avoid step-care strategies, in which all children are treated with nonspecific medications first, which are subsequently switched to other classes of medication in cases of failure (eg, acetaminophen switched to nonsteroidal anti-inflammatory drugs [NSAIDs], then to ergotamine compounds, and then to triptans).

Step 1: Define Reasons for Consultation and Disability

Children with headaches are often brought to the doctor because parents fear ominous causes, such as a brain tumor or an aneurysm. In these cases, after being reassured, they may not accept the recommended treatment. If children are disabled by migraines (see Step 2: Define the Effect of Migraine), management approach includes having an open discussion on the benefits of treatment, consequences of migraine, and potentially evolving nature of the disease if improperly treated (Evidence Level III). If children are indeed not disabled, we see no problem in allowing families to manage the problem with over-the-counter analgesics, emphasizing situations (eg, increase of frequency, lack of response) that would suggest a return visit for additional evaluation (Evidence Level III).

Step 2: Define the Effect of Migraine

The burden of migraine may vary substantially from individual to individual. Assessing the effect of migraine is mandatory because it will guide therapeutic decisions (eg, initiation of preventive therapies) (Evidence Level I in adults; Evidence Level III in children).

Effect should be measured in terms of school attendance and performance, leisure and physical activities, social life, and family. Several tools can assist physicians in this regard. The authors favor the Pediatric Migraine Disability Assessment (PedMIDAS) (www.cincinnatichildrens.org/service /h/headache-center/pedmidas), which evaluates the effect of headaches on school, home, play, and social activities for the past 90 days using only 6 questions. The PedMIDAS uses a total score grading scale of no (0–10), mild (11–30), moderate (31–50), and severe (>50) effect and has been shown to be sensitive to intervention effects (Evidence Level I in adults; Evidence Level II-2 in children).

Step 3: Take Advantage of Non-pharmacologic Measures

Non-pharmacologic approaches should always be used. Eventually they may even become mainstream therapy (Evidence Level III). Among the strategies in use, the author recommend the following measures:

Encourage a Structured Daily Routine (Evidence Level III)

Migraine is a neurologic disorder characterized by sensory dysmodulation, with attacks often triggered by internal or external stimuli. Most adult migraineurs are well aware that any change in routine habits often triggers attacks. Thus, frequent changes in hours of sleep (ie, sleeping less or more than usual) or meals (eg, skipping meals) should be avoided. When possible, parents should establish a routine for children to sleep, eat, play, and study.

Educate Parents and Children About Avoidable Triggers (Evidence Level II-3)

Life happens and children shouldn't fear life. As such, the authors do not advocate major behavior changes in children with migraine. Nonetheless, most parents come to recognize migraine triggers such as specific foods, fasting, odors (eg, perfume, paint, gasoline), irregular sleep habits, prolonged exposure to light, negative or positive emotions, school events, excessive extracurricular activities, excessive noise, and menstruation.

Food triggers include specific cheeses (tyramine), chocolate (theobromine and phenylethylamine), citrus (phenolic amines and octopamine), sausages (nitrite, nitric oxide donors), dairy products (allergenic proteins), fried foods (oleic and linoleic acids), flavor enhancers commonly used in some Asian cuisines (monosodium glutamate [Chinese restaurant syndrome]), preservatives and additives (tartrazine and sulfites), artificial sweeteners (aspartame), wine and beer (histamine, tyramine, sulfites, and alcohol), and tea, coffee, and soda (caffeine).

When triggers are suspected, they should be documented in the headache diary (see Figure 27-1 and the following section) to rule out misperceptions. True triggers should be avoided. It is important to document the trigger rather than empirically recommending trigger avoidance (Evidence Level III). Categorically banning foods and activities the child might find pleasurable is not the proper way to treat migraine.

Encourage Use of Headache Diary (Evidence Level III)

The headache diary (see Figure 27-1) is an essential tool for monitoring patients with headaches. When possible, it is particularly important to initiate its use before starting preventive therapies. A physician's initial impression is often modified by the information provided by the headache diary. Headache diaries are of particular importance for monitoring treatment outcomes. Sometimes benefit may only be perceived by the patient when change in headache frequency is documented by the headache diary.

In addition to the strategies listed previously, others are added in specific circumstances, including parents not wanting pharmacologic treatment, pharmacologic treatment only being partially effective, and absolute contraindications for the use of prophylactic drugs. In this context, cognitive and behavioral therapies are emerging as effective interventions to help children and adolescents manage chronic and recurrent pain. Behavioral strategies include biofeedback, relaxation training, and behavioral management programs to reinforce adaptive behaviors. Cognitive strategies include stress management, guided imagery, and cognitive coping skills. Cognitive and behavioral programs incorporate both strategies.

The utility of relaxation training and biofeedback is well supported by evidence, and these measures seem to work better in children as compared with adults (Evidence Level I). Describing these methods is beyond the scope of this chapter. While holistic approaches to the child with migraine can be useful, multidisciplinary interventions (with involvement of psychologists and other professionals) for refractory or complicated cases are usually employed (Evidence Level III).

Step 3: Use Pharmacologic Treatment Stratified by Needs

Overview of Drug Therapy

Pharmacotherapy is usually divided into 2 categories: drugs that are acutely taken to treat attacks (acute treatment) and drugs that are taken whether or not headache is present to reduce frequency and severity of attacks (preventive therapy). Acute treatment is subdivided into nonspecific pharmacologic treatments, which are useful for a range of pain disorders (eg, aspirin, acetaminophen, NSAIDs, opiates, combination analgesics) and migraine-specific treatments (eg, ergotamine, dihydroergotamine, triptans).

While virtually every patient benefits from acute treatment, preventive therapies are reserved for selected migraine sufferers (Evidence Level I).

Acute Treatment

Figure 27-3 displays an algorithm for the acute treatment of migraine attacks in children and adolescents. Table 27-2 summarizes doses, side effects, and evidence levels of these symptomatic medications.

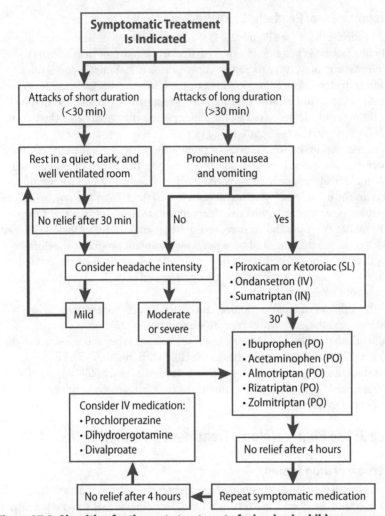

Figure 27-3. Algorithm for the acute treatment of migraine in children.
Abbreviations: IN, intranasal; IV, intravenous; min, minutes; PO, per os (by mouth, orally); SL, sublingual.

Table 27-2. Drugs for the Acute Treatment of Migraine in Children

Drug	Dose	Age (y)	Side Effects	Level of Evidence[a]
Acetaminophen[b]	15 mg/kg; PO	4–16	No or minor side effects Nausea, vomiting, urticaria, skin rashes, and hepatotoxicity (All are rare.)	I[c]
Ibuprofen[b]	10 mg/kg; PO	4–16	No or minor side effects Dizziness, headache, dyspepsia, nausea, vomiting, diarrhea, abdominal pain, and flatulence	I[c]
Almotriptan[b]	6.25–12.5 mg; PO	12–17	No or minor side effects Nausea, vomiting, upper abdominal pain, transient mild stiffness, and somnolence	I[c]
Rizatriptan[b]	5–10 mg; PO	12–17	No or minor side effects Asthenia, dizziness, and dry mouth	I[c]
Sumatriptan	10–20 mg; IN	6–17	Taste disturbance	I
Zolmitriptan	2.5–5 mg; PO	6–18	No or minor side effects Dizziness, drowsiness, and weakness	I
Piroxicam	20 mg; SL	12–18	Mouth ulceration, nausea, epigastric distress, abdominal pain, constipation, diarrhea, flatulence, and dizziness	II-1
Ketorolac	0.5–1 mg/kg; SL (single dose)	4–18	Diarrhea, headache, nausea, heartburn, dizziness, and drowsiness	III
Prochlorperazine[d]	0.15 mg/kg; IV	5–18	No or minor side effects Akathisia	I

Table 27-2 *(cont)*

Drug	Dose	Age (y)	Side Effects	Level of Evidence[a]
Dihydroergotamine[d]	Initial IV dose 0.1–0.15 mg (6–9 y) 0.2 mg (9–12 y) 0.25 mg (12–16 y) Repeat every 8 h until headache-free (max of 20 doses).	6–16	Nausea, vomiting, anxiety, chest tightness, urticaria, face flushed, and elevated blood pressure	II-3
Divalproex sodium[d]	15–20 mg (over 5 min); IV (max of 1 g)	13–17	Cold sensation, dizziness, nausea, paraesthesia, and tachycardia	II-3
Ondansetron[d]	0.1 mg/kg (<12 y or <40 kg) 4 mg single dose (>12 y or >40 kg); IV (over 2–5 min)	3–18	No or minor side effects Headache, drowsiness/sedation, malaise/fatigue, and extrapyramidal symptoms (All are rare.)	I

Abbreviations: IN, intranasal; IV, intravenous; max, maximum; PO, per os (by mouth, orally); SL, sublingual.

[a] Level I: Evidence obtained from at least one properly designed randomized controlled trial. Level II-1: Evidence obtained from well-designed controlled trials without randomization. Level II-2: Evidence obtained from well-designed cohort or case-control analytic studies, preferably from more than one center or research group. Level II-3: Evidence obtained from multiple time series with or without the intervention. Dramatic results in uncontrolled trials might also be regarded as this type of evidence. Level III: Opinions of respected authorities, based on clinical experience, descriptive studies, or reports of expert committees.

[b] US Food and Drug Administration approved.

[c] See Figure 27-3 for medication frequency.

[d] Drugs indicated for IV use.

Important principles for physicians to follow in acute treatment of migraine include the selection of proper medication using stratified care, rapid return to normal activity without relapse as the goal of treatment, strong consideration of preventive therapy if children need to use acute medications more than twice per week, use of appropriate and tailored dosages for children, and treatment of attacks as soon as possible. Evidence suggests that delayed treatment is associated with sensitization of neurons involved in the pathophysiology of the attack and decreased therapeutic response (Evidence Level II-2). Accordingly, acute treatment should not be delayed.

In children whose migraine attacks are typically short (less than 30 minutes), it may be enough to recommend rest in a quiet, dark, and well-ventilated room. Such conditions will alleviate photophobia and phonophobia and facilitate sleep. Many children with short-duration attacks do not require symptomatic medication given the brevity of symptoms. However, if the attacks are usually prolonged, non-pharmacologic approaches are always useful starting points, but a symptomatic medication is necessary.

Medications approved for use in the pediatric population are nonspecific (ibuprofen and acetaminophen) and specific (almotriptan and rizatriptan) (Evidence Level I). Regardless of the medication, parents can be asked to try a medication for at least 3 attacks. A "good response" can be considered if improvement was significant for all attacks. The trial can be repeated if there was improvement in 2 out of 3 attacks and will continue or change as per the satisfaction of the child and parents. Medication can be changed if there was improvement in fewer than 2 attacks (Evidence Level III).

For mild to moderate headaches that typically are not associated with nausea, paracetamol or ibuprofen are good choices. When headaches are mild to moderate and nausea is present, NSAIDs with antiemetic medications can be used. Ketorolac tromethamine sublingually (Evidence Level I) is a good choice, given its rapid absorption, fast onset of action, efficacy, and safety. In case of pronounced nausea and vomiting, ondansetron can be used instead. Metoclopramide is a very effective migraine medication for nausea and pain, but its use should be reserved because of the potential for dramatic but fully reversible extrapyramidal side effects (eg, dystonia, akathisia).

For children with more debilitating headaches, triptans are usually the drugs of choice. Triptans can be given to children with less debilitating headaches who have not responded to nonspecific medications. Although all triptans seem to be effective in children, only almotriptan and rizatriptan have been approved by the US Food and Drug Administration for use in adolescents.

If the first dose of the common analgesic, NSAID, or triptan does not work after 4 hours, a second dose is recommended. If a second dose does not work, consider hospitalization and use of the following drugs intravenously: prochlorperazine (Evidence Level I), dihydroergotamine (Evidence Level II-3), and divalproex sodium (Evidence Level II-3).

Although effective, there is general agreement that compounds with caffeine, barbiturates, and narcotics should be avoided in primary care treatment of migraine (Evidence Level III).

Preventive Therapy

Figure 27-4 displays an algorithm addressing preventive therapy for migraine in children and adolescents. Table 27-3 contains a summarization of the doses, therapeutic opportunities, side effects, and evidence level of prophylactic medications.

When to Start and When to Stop

There are no formal recommendations as to when to start preventive therapy. Expert consensus recommends that the decision should be based on frequency of headaches (certainly for 6 or more days of headache per month, potentially for those with 4–5 and for less frequent but very disabling cases), burden of attacks (due to duration, lack of response to acute therapies, or associated symptoms), presence of debilitating associated symptoms (eg, prolonged aura, hemiparesis), and response to acute medications.

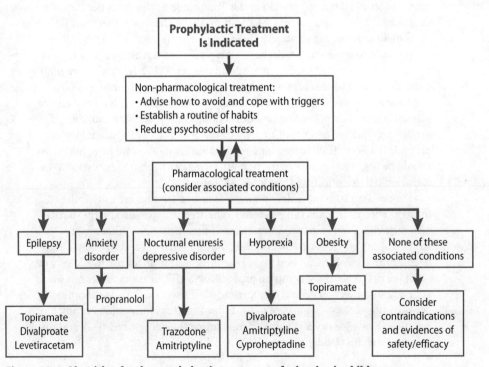

Figure 27-4. Algorithm for the prophylactic treatment of migraine in children.

Table 27-3. Drugs for the Prophylactic Treatment of Migraine in Children

Drug[a]	Dose	Age (y)	Therapeutic Opportunities (Associated Conditions)	Side Effects	Evidence Level[b]
Topiramate	3–9 mg/kg/d; bid[c]	8–15	Epilepsy, obesity, and bipolar disorder	Poor appetite, weight loss, paresthesias, drowsiness, fatigue, dizziness, and oligohidrosis Attention or memory difficulties are less frequent than in adults.	I
Trazodone[d]	1 mg/kg/d; ode	7–18	Depressive disorder	Increase in suicidal thoughts, worsened symptoms of depression	I
Propranolol	2–3 mg/kg/d; bid–tid	7–16	Anxiety and symptomatic mitral valve prolapse	No or minor side effects Fatigue, sleep disturbance, bronchospasm, and asthma exacerbation	II-1
Divalproate	15–45 mg/kg/d; bid	7–16	Epilepsy Bipolar disorder	Gastrointestinal upset, weight gain, somnolence, dizziness, and tremor	II-3
Levetiracetam	250–500 mg/d; tid	3–17	Epilepsy	Somnolence, dizziness, and irritability	II-3
Amitriptyline	0.25 mg/kg/d; e	3–17	Depressive disorder	Somnolence, increased appetite, weight gain, dry mouth, constipation	II-3
Cyproheptadine	4–8 mg/d; e	3–17	Respiratory allergy, hyperoxia	Somnolence, increased appetite, and weight gain	III

Abbreviations: bid, twice a day; tid, 3 times a day.

[a] Flunarizine (Evidence Level I) was not included in the list because it is unavailable in the United States.

[b] Level I: Evidence obtained from at least one properly designed randomized controlled trial. Level II-1: Evidence obtained from well-designed controlled trials without randomization. Level II-2: Evidence obtained from well-designed cohort or case-control analytic studies, preferably from more than one center or research group. Level II-3: Evidence obtained from multiple time series with or without the intervention. Dramatic results in uncontrolled trials might also be regarded as this type of evidence. Level III: Opinions of respected authorities, based on clinical experience, descriptive studies, or reports of expert committees.

[c] It is recommended that therapy be initiated at 25 to 50 mg/day followed by titration to an effective dose in increments of 25 to 50 mg/day every week.

[d] The US Food and Drug Administration warns about increased risks of suicidal thinking and behavior, known as suicidality, in children, adolescents, and young adults aged 18 to 24 years during initial treatment with antidepressants (generally the first 1–2 months).

[e] At bedtime.

Preventive medication should also be considered when excessive acute medication is being taken as well as for associated periodic syndromes.

To reiterate, one size does not fit all. A child with monthly headache attacks that consistently cause him or her to miss school despite acute treatment qualifies as much for preventive therapy as a child with daily headaches.

Once a decision to start preventive medication is made, consideration should be given to the duration of treatment. After the proper dose is established and clinical control is considered satisfactory (no more than 2 days of headache per month that are not severe and responding well to acute medication are worthy goals), the child can remain on preventive medication for 6 months to 1 year (Evidence Level III). Discontinuation should be as gradual as the introduction of medication. Good principles to follow are to start with a low dose, go slow (titrate properly to avoid adverse events), do not rush discontinuation, and taper gradually over a few weeks (Evidence Level III).

Which Medication?

There are a few well-designed studies on prophylaxis of migraine in childhood and adolescence; level I evidence exists only for flunarizine (unavailable in the United States), topiramate, and trazodone. In adults, there is level I evidence for some beta-blockers (propranolol and nadolol), tricyclic antidepressants (amitriptyline, nortriptyline), calcium channel blockers (verapamil), divalproex and other antiepileptic drugs, and nutraceuticals. Pizotifen and cyproheptadine are also often used in children (see Table 27-3 and Figure 27-4).

The efficacy of all preventive medications is similar in adults and in children (Evidence Level III). The choice is largely based on contraindications for use (eg, beta-blockers in children with asthma) and potential to use the drug profile to address comorbid conditions.

In Figure 27-4, the principle of selecting preventive medications while using their "adverse profiles" to address comorbidities is illustrated. We highlight the use of beta-blockers for children who are anxious or dysautonomic (eg, cold extremities, excessive sweating, tachycardia); topiramate (which causes weight loss) for children with obesity; topiramate, divalproate, or levetiracetam for children with epilepsy; divalproate, amitriptyline, pizotifen, or cyproheptadine for children with hyperoxia; and amitriptyline, imipramine, or trazodone for children with depressive disorder or nocturnal enuresis.

Concerning prophylactic treatment, it is important to recognize that lack of evidence for efficacy is not the same as evidence of lack of efficacy. Failure to appreciate this may limit the efficacy of management of children with migraine. To the extent that it is possible, the physician should keep in mind the incredible burden of migraine on affected children; always treat within label, giving preference to approved drugs when possible; and select a drug based on plausibility or proven efficacy in studies with adults and proven safety in children when evidence is not available or first-line therapies have failed.

Long-term Implications

Preventing Development of Chronic Migraine

As mentioned, the goal of migraine treatment is to avoid current debilitation and prevent future poor outcomes. Migraine is a chronic, recurrent disorder that progresses in some individuals. Chronic migraine—when individuals evolve to a state where they have headaches on more days than not—is the result of this progression.

Risk factors for migraine progression have been identified and are traditionally divided into 2 categories: modifiable and non-modifiable by health interventions. Among non-modifiable risk factors are earlier ages of migraine onset, female gender, low family income, and prenatal exposures to nicotine and alcohol. For these children, more aggressive treatment may become necessary (Evidence Level III).

Modifiable, robust risk factors for progression include frequency of migraine attacks (pain causes pain), obesity, excessive use of acute migraine medication (more than 8 days per month), excessive caffeine consumption, and comorbidities such as depression, anxiety, and sleep disorders. Physicians should aspire to not just relieve current pain and disability but to also avoid migraine progression. Reducing attack frequency, avoiding medication overuse, practicing appropriate use of preventive drugs and behavioral therapies, and encouraging weight loss, if appropriate, should be part of migraine therapy to improve patients' lives today and prevent progression in the future.

Conclusion

Proper treatment of migraine requires a structured yet easy-to-follow approach. By obtaining a good medical history, conducting detailed physical and neurologic examinations, and searching for red flags, physicians can clinically diagnose migraine confidently.

Selection of an antimigraine (acute or preventive) drug for a patient depends on the stratification of the patient's migraine attack by peak intensity, time to peak intensity, level of associated symptoms, time to associated symptoms, comorbid diseases, and concomitant treatments that might cause drug-drug interactions. Physicians have in their armamentariums an ever-expanding variety of medications, available in multiple formulations and dosages, with good safety and tolerability profiles. Continued clinical use will yield familiarity with the various drugs and it may become possible to match individual patient needs with the specific characteristics of a drug, optimizing therapeutic benefits.

Suggested Reading
• • • • • • • • • • • • • • • • • •

Abu-Arafeh I, Razak S, Sivaraman B, Graham C. Prevalence of headache and migraine in children and adolescents: a systematic review of population-based studies. *Dev Med Child Neurol.* 2010;52(12):1088–1097

Arruda MA, Albuquerque RC, Bigal ME. Uncommon headache syndromes in the pediatric population. *Curr Pain Headache Rep.* 2011;15(4):280–288

Arruda MA, Bigal ME. Behavioral and emotional symptoms and primary headaches in children: a population-based study. *Cephalalgia.* 2012;32(15):1093–1100

Arruda MA, Bigal ME. Migraine and migraine subtypes in preadolescent children: association with school performance. *Neurology.* 2012;79(18):1881–1888

Bigal ME, Liberman JN, Lipton RB. Age-dependent prevalence and clinical features of migraine. *Neurology.* 2006;67(2):246–251

Hershey AD, Powers SW, Vockell AL, LeCates S, Kabbouche MA, Maynard MK. PedMIDAS: development of a questionnaire to assess disability of migraines in children. *Neurology.* 2001;57(11):2034–2039

Lewis D, Ashwal S, Hershey A, et al. Practice parameter: pharmacological treatment of migraine headache in children and adolescents: report of the American Academy of Neurology Quality Standards Subcommittee and the Practice Committee of the Child Neurology Society. *Neurology.* 2004;63(12):2215–2224

Lewis DW, Ashwal S, Dahl G, et al. Practice parameter: evaluation of children and adolescents with recurrent headaches: report of the Quality Standards Subcommittee of the American Academy of Neurology and the Practice Committee of the Child Neurology Society. *Neurology.* 2002;59(4):490–498

Olesen J. The International Classification of Headache Disorders. 2nd edition (ICHD-II). *Rev Neurol (Paris).* 2005;161(6–7):689–691

Termine C, Ozge A, Antonaci F, et al. Overview of diagnosis and management of paediatric headache. Part II: therapeutic management. *J Headache Pain.* 2011;12(1):25–34

CHAPTER 28

Hematuria: Macroscopic and Microscopic

Leonard G. Feld, MD, PhD, MMM

Key Points

- Microscopic hematuria is a medical (nonsurgical) disease. Most cases only require limited biochemical evaluation and maybe a renal sonogram. For patients with persistent microscopic hematuria, minimal evaluation is usually necessary, although periodic monitoring for the development of hypertension or proteinuria is required. Isolated microscopic hematuria is not a presentation of urinary malignancy.

- Patients with hematuria with proteinuria require an extensive work-up to delineate the cause in order to initiate appropriate treatment and because of the risk of chronic kidney disease.

- Gross hematuria does require imaging of the urinary tract. Most common glomerular diseases are poststreptococcal glomerulonephritis, IgA, and Alport syndrome. Patients with recurrent gross hematuria with persistent microscopic hematuria should be evaluated for Alport syndrome (use of skin biopsy, family history) and IgA nephropathy (recurrence is associated with respiratory infection; consider a renal biopsy).

- Cystoscopy is rarely required for the evaluation of hematuria in children.

Overview

Primary care practitioners frequently discover microscopic hematuria as an incidental finding in children during routine well-child examinations (eg, preschool, pre-camp, pre-sports), coincident to an evaluation of an acute illness or with the onset of urinary tract symptoms. On the other hand, gross hematuria is relatively uncommon and implications are generally more concerning than microscopic hematuria. The differential diagnosis for microscopic and macroscopic (ie, gross) hematuria is extensive; the causes and extent of the evaluation will be based on whether the hematuria is asymptomatic or symptomatic. As a general rule, hematuria is a medical rather than urologic problem.

Definition
· · · · · · · · · ·

Hematuria is defined as a positive urine reagent strip (ie, dipstick) reaction with the presence of 5 or more red blood cells (RBCs) per high-power field (HPF) in 3 consecutive freshly centrifuged specimens or greater than 6 RBCs per HPF on an un-centrifuged specimen obtained at least 1 week apart (Evidence Level II-2). Confirmation of hematuria is critical. A false-positive urine reagent strip reaction for hematuria can result from myoglobinuria or hemoglobinuria, in which the urine has no RBCs on microscopy. If no RBCs are noted on microscopic evaluation, measurement of urinary myoglobin (possible rhabdomyolysis) or the presence of hemolysis on serum or blood smear analysis will redirect the evaluation and management. Drugs, foods, and other substances can cause discoloration of the urine, although the urine dipstick reaction will be negative for blood (Table 28-1).

Table 28-1. Discoloration of Urine Due to Medications, Foods, Chemicals, Toxins, Infections, and Other Causes (Selected)

Medications	Foods or Other Causes
Black or brown urine	
Chloroquine	Alkaptonuria
Ferrous salts/iron dextran	Aloe
Levodopa	Copper or phenol poisoning
Methyldopa	Porphyria
Metronidazole	Povidone-iodine (Betadine) contamination
Nitrates	Rhubarb, fava beans[a]
Nirtofurantoin	Tyrosinosis
Quinine[a]	Viral hepatitis (acute) or cirrhosis
Sorbitol	
Sulfonamides[a]	
Blue, blue-green, or green urine	
Amitripyyline	Artificial colors from foods
Cimetidine	Bilirubin
Doxorubicin	Familial hypercalcemia (blue diaper
Indigo carmine	syndrome)
Indomethacin	Indicanuria
Methylene blue	Pseudomonas urinary tract infection
Phenergan	
Propofol	
Triamterene	
Multivitamins (some)	

Table 28-1 *(cont)*

Medications	Foods or Other Causes
Dark yellow or orange urine	
B complex and C vitamins Carotene Heparin Laxatives Phenazopyridine (Pyridium) Phenacetin Rifampin Sulfasalazine Warfarin	Carrots Uric acid crystals
Pink or red urine	
Compazine Daunorubicin/doxorubicin Deferoxamine Heparin Ibuprofen Methyldopa Phenothiazines Phenytoin Rifampin Salicylates	Beets Blackberries Lead poisoning Porphyria Renal causes—cystitis, Wilms tumor, hemolytic anemia,[a] glomerulonephritis (usually brown)
Discoloration of urine with hemoglobinuria	
Aspidium Betanaphthol Carbolic acid Carbolic acid Carbon monoxide Chloroform Fava beans Mushrooms Naphthalene Pamaquine Phenylhydrzine Potassium chlorate Quinine Snake venom Sulfonamides Turpentine	Blood transfusions Cardiovascular bypass Fresh-water drowning Hemolytic anemias Sepsis—typhoid, yellow fever, scarlet fever, diphtheria, malaria, syphilis Paroxysmal nocturnal hemoglobinuria

[a] Discoloration of urine with microscopic hematuria.

From Drugdex—Drug Consults, Micromedex, vol 62, Rocky Mountain Drug Consultation Center, Denver CO.

Diagnosis and Evaluation

Localization of the Hematuria

During the evaluation of hematuria, the differentiation of glomerular bleeding versus non-glomerular/extraglomerular/lower urinary tract causes is critical (Table 28-2). It is essential to assess the duration of gross hematuria and whether persistent microscopic hematuria follows episodes of gross hematuria or whether both resolve completely. If phase-contrast microscopy is available to assess urinary RBC morphology, the differentiation of dysmorphic (ie, glomerular bleeding) versus eumorphic (ie, normal or non-glomerular bleeding) RBCs can be useful (Evidence Level III). The presence of RBC casts is associated with glomerular hematuria, whereas blood clots or sediment (ie, visible stone fragments) suggest lower tract involvement.

Table 28-2. Distinguishing Glomerular From Non-glomerular Sources of Hematuria (Evidence Level III)

Test	Glomerular	Non-glomerular
Urinalysis		
Dysmorphic RBCs	+	−
Cellular casts	+	−
Brown or tea colored	+ +	+
Bright red	−	+ +
Clots	−	+
Crystals	−	+
Protein	+	−
History		
Family history of kidney failure	+	−
Systemic disease	+	−
Nephrolithiasis or hypercalciuria	−	+
Trauma	−	+
Symptomatic voiding	−	+
Physical examination		
Systemic signs	+	−
Hypertension	+ +	+
Edema	+	−
Abdominal mass	−	+
Genital bruising	−	+

Abbreviation: RBC, red blood cell.
From Feld LG, Waz, WR, Perez LM, Joseph DB. Hematuria: an integrated medical and surgical approach. *Pediatr Clin North Am.* 1997;44(5):1191–1210, with permission.

The presentation of urinary tract symptoms (such as frequency, urgency, dysuria, blood clots, blood not persistent throughout the urinary stream, flank or abdominal pain) associated with hematuria is consistent with extra-glomerular hematuria. Glomerular bleeding presenting with oliguria, hypertension, proteinuria, impaired kidney function, or symptoms of systemic diseases (eg, arthritis/arthralgias, rash, mouth ulcers, cough, hemoptysis, pericardial rub) suggest primary or secondary glomerular disease. In children, trauma, foreign bodies, and child maltreatment should also be considered.

A family history of renal diseases such as nephrolithiasis, chronic kidney disease, hereditary nephritis (ie, family members with high-frequency neuro-sensory hearing loss), and urinary tract abnormalities may guide additional investigations (Table 28-3). As indicated previously, the physical examination may suggest renal manifestations of systemic diseases (such as systemic lupus erythematosus, granulomatosis with polyangiitis, Henoch-Schönlein purpura, Goodpasture syndrome, hepatitis, sickle cell disease, diabetes mellitus) or signs of trauma, child maltreatment, uveitis, edema, hypertension, or abdominal masses. Linear growth, growth velocity, weight, and body mass index may suggest chronic kidney disease or systemic disease. Hematuria has 6 general categories or patterns (Table 28-4).

Table 28-3. Useful Information in History and Physical Examination for the Diagnosis of Hematuria

History	Physical Examination
Review of systems/medications	
• Category of hematuria (See Table 28-4.) • Medication and food history (See Table 28-1.) • Recent illness (throat or skin infections, exercise, or trauma [includes child maltreatment]) • Menstrual history if appropriate • Systemic symptoms—headaches, weight loss or gain, fatigue, alopecia, fever, rash, visual problems (possible uveitis), mouth ulcers, cough, hemoptysis, arthralgias, arthritis, abdominal or flank pain, gastrointestinal or urinary symptoms (dysuria, urgency, frequency, polyuria, urine discoloration), constipation, hematochezia, localized or generalized swelling, hearing loss	• Linear height, growth velocity, and weight • Elevated blood pressure • Hair loss • Periorbital/pretibial or other areas of edema • Eye examination/acuity • Skin lesions or rashes (malar, petechia, or purpura) • Heart sounds—murmurs, pericardial rub, gallops • Lung—decreased breath sounds • Abdominal/flank pain or masses or ascites (Glomerular bleeding is painless.) • Genitourinary tract—trauma • Joint examination
Past medical and family history, including travel	
• Neonatal problems • Hemoglobinopathies such as sickle cell trait or disease • Polycystic kidney disease • Hematuria, hearing loss, or both • Hypercalciuria or renal stones • Chronic kidney disease • Collagen vascular disease • Urinary tract infections • Prior surgeries	

Table 28-4. Categories of Hematuria

Category of Hematuria	Typical Causes
Persistent microscopic	Familial hematuria (thin basement membrane nephropathy), idiopathic or benign familial nephritis (Alport syndrome), IgA nephropathy, hypercalciuria, hydronephrosis, or secondary to prior diseases such as postinfectious glomerulonephritis, polycystic kidney disease, sickle cell hemoglobinopathy, Henoch-Schönlein purpura, renal tuberculosis, congenital urologic diseases (multicystic renal disease, ADPKD), nutcracker syndrome
Persistent microscopic with proteinuria	Primary or secondary glomerulonephritis, interstitial nephritis, advanced autosomal dominant polycystic kidney disease, vasculitides (Henoch-Schönlein purpura) (See Chapter 42 on proteinuria.)
Intermittent microscopic	Fever, exercise, loin pain hematuria, nutcracker syndrome
Persistent microscopic and persistent or intermittent macroscopic	Vasculitides (Henoch-Schönlein purpura), IgA nephropathy, familial nephritis, recurrence of acute glomerulonephritis
Persistent macroscopic	Familial nephritis, coagulopathies, acute glomerulonephritis, rhabdomyosarcoma, Wilms tumor, AV malformation, sickle cell hemoglobinopathy, renal vein thrombosis, renal tuberculosis, urinary tract infection associated with ADPKD, trauma, urinary tract infections
Intermittent macroscopic	Exercise, sickle cell hemoglobinopathy (trait > disease), loin pain hematuria, urethrorrhagia, nutcracker syndrome

Abbreviations: AV, arteriovenous; ADPKD, autosomal dominant polycystic kidney disease.
From Feld LG, Waz, WR, Perez LM, Joseph DB. Hematuria: an integrated medical and surgical approach. *Pediatr Clin North Am.* 1997;44(5):1191–1210, with permission.

History and Physical Examination

For both microscopic and macroscopic hematuria, key information can direct the evaluation and management (see Table 28-3).

Specific Causes and Selected Evaluation of Hematuria (Figures 28-1 and 28-2)

The differential diagnosis of hematuria can be divided based on anatomic location, parenchymal origin (glomerular or interstitial), hematology/oncology, or miscellaneous/fictitious causes. A mnemonic **A–I** of causes of hematuria created by Richard Neiberger may guide the evaluation of patients (**A**natomy, **B**oulders, **C**ancer, **D**rugs, **E**xercise, **F**oreign body/trauma, **F**amilial, **G**lomerulonephritis, **H**ematology, **I**nfection).

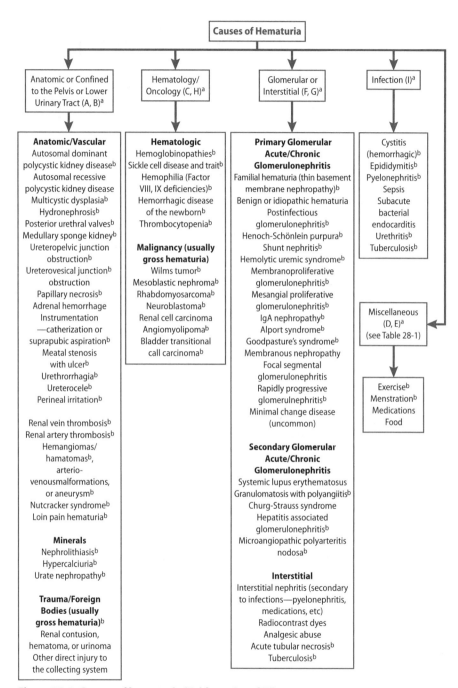

Figure 28-1. Causes of hematuria (Evidence Level III).

*May present with macroscopic hematuria with or without microscopic hematuria.

[a] Letters from mnemonic (see text).

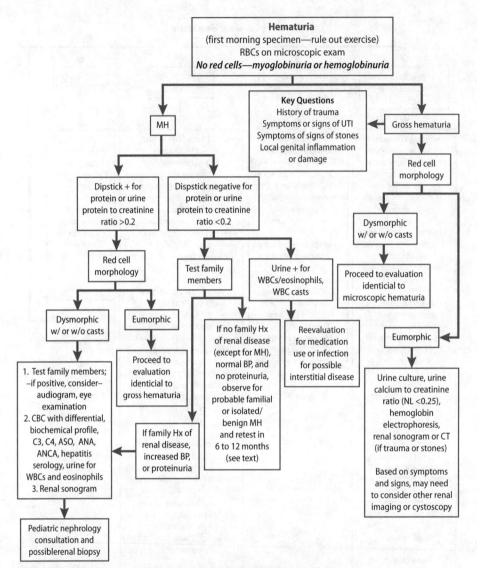

Figure 28-2. Evaluation of hematuria (Evidence Level II-2 and III).

Abbreviations: +, positive; ANA, antinuclear antigen; ANCA, antineutrophil cytoplasmic antibody; ASO, anti-streptolysin O; BP, blood pressure; CBC, complete blood count; CT, computed tomography; exam, examination; Hx, history; MH, microscopic hematuria; NL, normal; RBC, red blood cell; UTI, urinary tract infection; WBC, white blood cell; w/, with; w/o, without.

Modified from Feld LG, Waz, WR, Perez LM, Joseph DB. Hematuria: an integrated medical and surgical approach. *Pediatr Clin North Am.* 1997;44(5):1191–1210, with permission.

Anatomic or Confined to the Pelvis or Lower Urinary Tract

Anatomic Vascular

Most anatomic and vascular etiologies present with macroscopic hematuria. For most children who present to the physician's office, urgent care center, or emergency department with gross hematuria, the hematuria has an identifiable cause. Prenatal sonogram may suggest congenital anomalies such as posterior urethral valves, ureteropelvic junction obstruction, multicystic dysplasia, autosomal dominant, or recessive polycystic kidney disease. During the evaluation of urinary tract symptoms or infection, vesicoureteral reflux, posterior urethral valves, ureterocele, ureteropelvic junction, or ureterovesical junction obstruction may be discovered.

Other causes include nutcracker syndrome, which is the compression of the left renal vein between the aorta and superior mesenteric artery with the development of collateral veins. It is usually diagnosed by Doppler renal ultrasound. Patients present with left flank pain and hematuria. Other anatomic causes include hypercalciuria (Table 28-5). Renal stones usually present with hematuria along with severe pain (known as renal colic) referable to the urinary tract. A family history of nephrolithiasis is an important clue to the diagnosis, especially in the southeast United States (sometimes referred to as the "stone belt"). Urethrorrhagia presents in prepubertal boys (ie, ≈10 y) with bloody spots in the underwear. It is painless, and almost 50% of all cases will resolve in 6 months; greater than 90%, in 1 year, although it may persist for 2 years. The approach is watchful waiting in most cases.

Table 28-5. Normal Values for Urinary Calcium and Uric Acid Excretion (Evidence Level II-2)

Urinary calcium to urinary creatinine ratio in mg: mg based on years of age (95th percentile)		24-hour urinary calcium excretion
0.5–1 years	<0.81	<4 mg/kg/day
1–2 years	<0.56	
2–3 years	<0.5	
3–5 years	<0.41	
5–7 years	<0.3	
7–17 years	<0.25	
Uric acid excretion per glomerular filtration rate (GFR) in mg/dL GFR		**24-hour urinary uric acid excretion**
0.1–1 years	<2.38	<814 mg/1.73 m²/day
1–2 years	<2.08	
2–3 years	<1.93	
3–5 years	<1.64	
5–7 years	<1.19	
7–10 years	<0.83	
10–17 years	<0.59	

Modified from Feld LG. Nephrology. In: Feld LG, Meltzer AJ, eds. *Fast Facts in Pediatrics*. Philadelphia, PA: Saunders; 2007:454, with permission.

Most causes of renal injury represent blunt abdominal trauma. As described in Table 28-6, computed tomography of the abdomen and pelvis with contrast is the imaging modality of choice. Children with more than 50 RBCs per HPF have an increased association for significant renal damage whether the hematuria is microscopic or macroscopic. Blood in the urethral meatus after trauma suggests injury in the pelvic region where urethral injury is possible. Retrograde urography should be performed before bladder catheter placement.

Box 28-1. Preferred Tests for Various Patterns of Hematuria (Evidence Level II-2 to III)

Isolated microscopic hemauria
Kidney/bladder ultrasound Voiding cystourethrogram, if abnormal findings on ultrasound
Painful hematuria (nontraumatic)
CT abdomen/pelvis without contrast Kidney/bladder ultrasound (alternative)
Macroscopic or microscopic hematuria (traumatic)
CT abdomen/pelvis with contrast

Abbreviation: CT, computed tomography.

Renal venous thrombosis is most common in the first year of life and presents with hematuria, thrombocytopenia, and a flank mass.

As a general rule, painful gross hematuria is usually associated with infection, calculi, or urologic problems, whereas glomerular causes of hematuria are painless. Microscopic hematuria is an extremely rare presentation of a renal or abdominal tumor.

The kidney and bladder sonogram are the best initial radiographic evaluations for hematuria based on availability and cost. They will exclude renal cystic disease, hydronephrosis, and masses. However, genitourinary imaging should be tailored to specific clinical entities. Cystoscopy is rarely indicated for microscopic hematuria.

Hematology/Oncology

Sickle cell disease and trait are the most common hematologic diseases presenting with hematuria. Microscopic hematuria is more common than macroscopic hematuria with sickle cell disease. Sickle cell trait may present with unilateral, painless macroscopic hematuria most often from the left kidney. A renal sonogram may show early papillary necrosis. Wilms tumor may present with macroscopic hematuria (with a red or deep cherry color) and a detectable abdominal mass. It is rare for Wilms tumor and rhabdomyosarcoma (associated with the bladder) to present with microscopic hematuria.

Glomerular or Interstitial Disease

Primary Glomerular Disease

Familial hematuria, thin basement membrane glomerulopathy, and idiopathic/ benign hematuria present at any age with the incidental finding of persistent microscopic hematuria. Macroscopic hematuria, hypertension, impaired renal function, and proteinuria are not characteristic of this disorder in children. In most cases, a renal biopsy is not necessary. These forms of hematuria have no biochemical abnormalities and only hematuria reaction on dipstick without proteinuria. A renal sonogram is the only imaging study considered, and a renal biopsy is not necessary.

IgA nephropathy, postinfectious/poststreptococcal glomerulonephritis (PIAGN/PSAGN), familial nephritis (ie, Alport syndrome), Henoch-Schönlein purpura, mesangiocapillary glomerulonephritis, and hemolytic uremic syndrome can present with macroscopic or microscopic hematuria. The work-up is a biochemical and urinary evaluation without imaging studies. Based on the work-up, a percutaneous renal biopsy may be necessary to make the diagnosis and assist in the decision for pharmacologic therapy. The laboratory studies include a complete blood count with differential and smear analysis to assess hemolysis and thrombocytopenia (ie, hemolytic uremic syndrome), urinary protein measurement (see Chapter 42 on proteinuria) and an antistreptolysin titer to detect prior streptococcal infection. Poststreptococcal glomerulonephritis occurs most often in children aged 2 to 12 years. It develops most frequently after an acute throat or skin infection with a nephritogenic strain of group A beta-hemolytic streptococci with M types 47, 49, and 57 in skin infections and M types 1, 2, 4, and 12 frequently seen in upper respiratory tract infections. Antistreptolysin is elevated following pharyngeal streptococcal infections, whereas antihyaluronidase and antinicotinamide adenine dinucleotidase titers are increased in most patients with streptococcal skin infections. Complement studies (C3 and C4) will be decreased in primary and secondary glomerular disease. Usually, C3 and CH50 are decreased more than C4 in PIAGN/PSAGN and return to normal in 8 to 12 weeks. If C3 levels are depressed for more than 8 to 12 weeks, membranoproliferative glomerulonephritis or lupus nephritis should be considered and a renal biopsy should be performed for diagnosis. In contrast, there is a proportionate reduction in both C3 and C4 is systemic lupus erythematosis (SLE) and cryoglobulinemia. Levels of C3 are not depressed in Henoch-Schönlein purpura, hemolytic uremic syndrome, IgA nephropathy, benign/idiopathic hematuria, or Alport syndrome.

IgA nephropathy presents with recurrent episodes of gross hematuria coincident with a nonspecific upper respiratory tract infection and typically with persistence of microscopic hematuria between episodes. Although the prognosis is generally excellent, some patients develop hypertension, proteinuria, and chronic kidney disease. Alport syndrome presents similar to IgA without a respiratory tract illness. The diagnosis can be made by the absence of epidermal staining for collagen type IV chain on skin biopsy (used instead of a kidney biopsy); by history of family members with proteinuria, progressive renal disease, and high-frequency sensorineural hearing loss or anterior lenticonus (or both); or by a combination thereof.

The most common secondary glomerular diseases are SLE, granulomatosis with polyangiitis (formally Wegener granulomatosis), and hepatitis (B or C) associated glomerulonephritis. As indicated previously, C3 and C4 levels may be depressed with elevated antinuclear antibodies and anti-DNA antibodies in SLE. Antineutrophil cytoplasmic antibodies may be present in granulomatosis with polyangiitis and Churg-Strauss syndrome. If these diseases are considered, a renal biopsy is needed to make the diagnosis or assess the type of renal involvement in the case of SLE.

Interstitial Disease

The most common forms are related to medications such as antibiotics (eg, penicillins, cephalosporins, sulfa drugs, quinolones), nonsteroidal antiinflammatory drugs, proton pump inhibitors, and phenytoin; infections (viruses such as cytomegalovirus and human immunodeficiency virus, bacteria, and fungi); obstructive uropathy; hypercalcemia; lead nephropathy; or tubulointerstitial nephritis with uveitis. The presentations include macroscopic or microscopic hematuria, fatigue, anemia, white blood cells/eosinophils on urine microscopy, eosinophilia, and sometimes depressed renal function. In many cases, diagnosis is made by exclusion or by biopsy. The differential diagnosis includes acute glomerulonephritis and urinary tract infection.

Infection

Lower urinary tract inflammation can result in both macroscopic and microscopic hematuria. However, bacterial urinary tract infections are uncommon as a cause of gross hematuria. Both subacute bacterial endocarditis and shunt nephritis present similar to other forms of acute glomerulonephritis and have hypocomplementemia (low C3) in greater than 90% of patients. In shunt nephritis (uncommon), patients have recurrent fever, hepatosplenomegaly, anemia, and central nervous system symptoms.

Miscellaneous/Factitious

As shown in Table 28-1, many medications, foods, chemicals, toxins, and infections can discolor the urine. When it is difficult to differentiate menstruation versus hematuria, urinary catheterization should be performed. Many children have macroscopic or microscopic hematuria following exercise. By limiting physical activity for 24 to 48 hours and obtaining a first-morning sample, exercise-induced hematuria will be differentiated from other causes of hematuria. This test is important to allow participation in sports or entry into the military.

Selected Management of Hematuria

Figure 28-3 provides a brief description of the management of hematuria. For patients with persistent microscopic hematuria, minimal evaluation is usually necessary, although periodic monitoring for the development of hypertension,

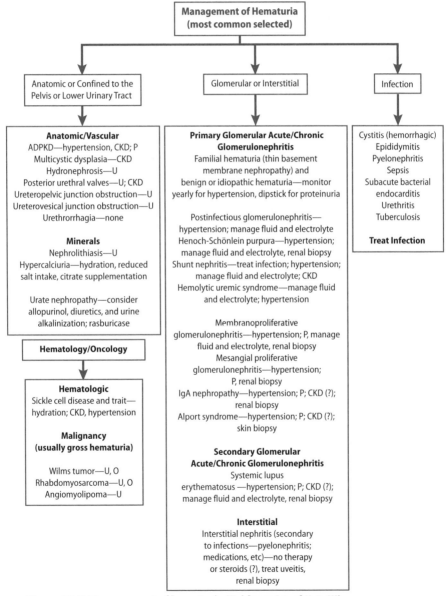

Figure 28-3. Management of hematuria (Evidence Level II-2–III).

Abbreviations: ADPKD, autosomal dominant polycystic kidney disease; CKD, chronic kidney disease; O, oncology consultation; P, proteinuria (manage with angiotensin-converting enzyme); U, urologic or surgical intervention.

proteinuria, or both is required. Because of the large number of causes of hematuria, individual evaluation and management are appropriate.

Suggested Reading

American College of Radiology. ACR Appropriateness Criteria® Hematuria—Child. http://www.acr.org/~/media/ACR/Documents/AppCriteria/Diagnostic /HematuriaChild.pdf. Accessed June 25, 2015.

Bergstein J, Leiser J, Andreoli S. The clinical significance of asymptomatic gross and microscopic hematuria in children. *Arch Pediatr Adolesc Med.* 2005;159(4):353–355

Boineau FG, Lewy JE. Evaluation of hematuria in children and adolescents. *Pediatr Rev.* 1989;11(4):101–107

Diven SC, Travis LB. A practical care approach in hematuria in children. *Pediatr Nephrol.* 2000;14(1):65–72

Feld LG, Waz WR, Perez LM, Joseph DB. Hematuria: an integrated medical and surgical approach. *Pediatr Clin North Am.* 1997;44(5):1191–1210

Feld LG, Meyers KEC, Kaplan MB, Stapleton FB. Limited evaluation of microscopic hematuria in pediatrics. *Pediatrics.* 1998;102(4):1–5

Fitzwater DS, Wyatt RJ. Hematuria. *Pediatr Rev.* 1994;15(3):102–107

Greenfield SP, Williot P, Kaplan D. Gross hematuria in children: a ten-year review. *Urology.* 2007;69(1):166–169

Massengill S. Hematuria. *Pediatr Rev.* 2008;29(10):342–348

Pan CG. Evaluation of gross hematuria. *Pediatr Clin North Am.* 2006;53(3):401–412

Patel HP, Bissler JJ. Hematuria in children. *Pediatric Clin North Am.* 2001;48(6): 1519–1537

Stapleton FB. Morphology of urinary red blood cells: a simple guide in localizing the site of hematuria. *Pediatr Clin North Am.* 1987;34(3):561–570

Youn T, Trachtman H, Gauthier B. Clinical spectrum of gross hematuria in pediatric patients. *Clin Pediatr.* 2006;45(2):135–141

CHAPTER 29

Hypertension

Donald J. Weaver, Jr, MD, PhD

Key Points

- The prevalence of hypertension is increasing in the pediatric population.

- The diagnosis of hypertension requires confirmation of elevated blood pressure readings obtained at 3 separate office visits using an appropriate cuff.

- The more severe the elevation in blood pressure and the younger the patient, the more likely a secondary cause of hypertension will be identified.

- All patients with confirmed hypertension should undergo laboratory and radiologic evaluation.

- Lifestyle changes are the primary tool for initial management of hypertension.

Overview

Because of the increased rate of obesity in youth, the prevalence of hypertension is increasing in the pediatric population. *The Fourth Report on the Diagnosis, Evaluation, and Treatment of High Blood Pressure in Children and Adolescents* (4th Report) defines systolic and diastolic blood pressure levels according to the 50th, 90th, 95th, and 99th percentiles based on the patient's age, height percentiles, and gender (Evidence Level III). Blood pressure measurements below the 90th percentile are within reference range (Table 29-1). Because of the dependence of blood pressure on age and height in the pediatric patient, several authors have developed novel tools to facilitate recognition of elevated blood pressures (Figure 29-1).

Table 29-1. Classification of Hypertension in Children

Classification	SBP or DBP Percentile	Follow-up
Prehypertension	90th to <95th or if BP exceeds 120/80 to <95th percentile	Recheck in 6 mo, and consider school or home BP monitoring.
Stage 1 hypertension	95th to 99th plus 5 mm Hg	Evaluate within 1 mo.
Stage 2 hypertension	>99th plus 5 mm Hg	Evaluate with 1 wk or immediately if symptomatic.
White-coat hypertension	BP >95th in the medical setting but within reference range outside the medical setting	Consider ABPM as well as school or home BP monitoring.
Masked hypertension	BP <95th in the medical setting but >95th outside the medical setting	Consider ABPM in high-risk populations (ie, chronic kidney disease and diabetes).

Abbreviations: ABPM, ambulatory blood pressure monitoring; BP, blood pressure; DBP, diastolic blood pressure; SBP, systolic blood pressure.

Modified from National High Blood Pressure Educational Program Working Group on High Blood Pressure in Children and Adolescents. The Fourth Report on the Diagnosis, Evaluation, and Treatment of High Blood Pressure in Children and Adolescents. *Pediatrics*. 2004;114:555–576.

The 4th Report suggests that all children older than 3 years seen in the medical setting should have their blood pressure measured during office visits (Evidence Level III). In addition, select patients with specific medical conditions younger than 3 should also have their blood pressure measured (Evidence Level III) (Box 29-1). Although oscillometric devices are convenient, auscultation is the preferred method for determining blood pressure except in infants in whom Korotkoff sounds may be difficult to hear and in the intensive care setting, in which blood pressures must be monitored frequently (Evidence Level II-2). The 4th Report suggests that the average of several measurements taken by an oscillometric device can be used for comparison with the blood pressure tables (Evidence Level III). In addition, blood pressures measured by oscillometric devices exceeding the 90th percentile should be repeated using auscultation (Evidence Level III). Finally, correct assessment of blood pressure in children also depends on the selection of a cuff that is appropriate for the size of the child's arm (Evidence Level II-2).

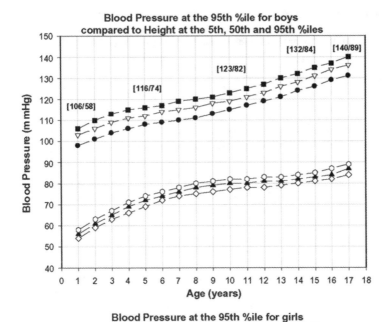

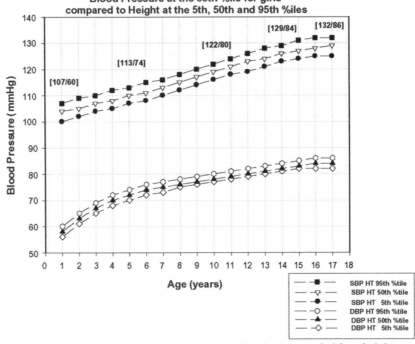

Figure 29-1. Blood pressure at the 95th percentiles for boys and girls at height percentiles.

From Feld LG, Corey H. Hypertension in childhood. *Pediatr Rev.* 2007;28(8):283–298.

Box 29-1. Children <3 y Who Should Have Blood Pressure Assessed

- History of prematurity or very low birth weight
- Congenital heart disease
- Known renal or urologic malformations
- Solid-organ transplant
- Malignancy or bone marrow transplant
- Treatment with medications known to raise blood pressure
- Systemic illnesses associated with increased blood pressure (ie, tuberous sclerosis)

Modified from National High Blood Pressure Educational Program Working Group on High Blood Pressure in Children and Adolescents. The Fourth Report on the Diagnosis, Evaluation, and Treatment of High Blood Pressure in Children and Adolescents. *Pediatrics.* 2004;114:555–576.

The diagnosis of hypertension requires confirmation of elevated readings at 3 or more separate office visits, and the appropriate timing of those visits is listed in Table 29-2 based on the staging of the blood pressures (see Table 29-1) (Evidence Level III). The term *white-coat hypertension* is applied to patients who demonstrate within-range blood pressure readings outside the medical setting, but office-based blood pressures are consistently above the 95th percentile (see Table 29-1).

Table 29-2. Common Causes of Pediatric Hypertension

Age Group	Etiology
Neonates	Renal artery or venous thrombosis Renal artery stenosis Congenital renal abnormalities Coarctation of the aorta Bronchopulmonary dysplasia Iatrogenic
30 d–1 y	Renal artery stenosis Renal parenchymal disease Coarctation of the aorta Iatrogenic
1–6 y	Renal parenchymal disease Renal artery stenosis Coarctation of the aorta Endocrinopathies Iatrogenic
6–12 y	Renal parenchymal disease Renovascular disease Primary hypertension Coarctation of the aorta Endocrinopathies Iatrogenic
12–18 y	Primary hypertension Iatrogenic Renal parenchymal disease Endocrinopathies Renal artery stenosis

Causes and Differential Diagnosis

The causes of hypertension based on age are listed in Table 29-2. Hypertension in the neonatal period deserves special consideration. As in older children, renovascular and renal parenchymal diseases are important causes of hypertension in neonates. In addition to renal artery stenosis, renovascular causes specific to the neonatal period include the development of arterial thrombi associated with placement of umbilical artery catheters with a prevalence of 25% to 80%. A second cause of renovascular hypertension specific to the neonatal period is renal vein thrombosis, which typically presents with hypertension, gross hematuria, and thrombocytopenia. Infants of diabetic mothers are at higher risk for developing renal vein thrombosis. Coarctation of the aorta is also an important cause of vascular hypertension early in life, accounting for 30% of hypertension in the first year of life. Congenital renal parenchymal diseases are the next most common group of causes in the neonatal period, specifically autosomal recessive polycystic kidney disease and renal obstruction. Hypertension associated with bronchopulmonary dysplasia is an important consideration in the premature infant. Finally, iatrogenic causes are another category of diagnoses, including medications such as dexamethasone, caffeine, and other adrenergic agents.

The increasing prevalence of increased body weight and obesity has been associated with an increase in the prevalence of primary or essential hypertension in children and adolescents. Dietary and lifestyle factors such as increased body mass index, carbohydrate intake, and sedentary behavior have all been associated with the development of primary hypertension in children. More important, primary hypertension remains a diagnosis of exclusion in children.

Clinical Features

The 4th Report emphasizes that evaluation of hypertension should begin with a history and physical examination (Evidence Level II-3) (Table 29-3). On physical examination, 4 extremity blood pressures and pulses should be assessed in all patients to evaluate for coarctation of the aorta. Skin examination can reveal evidence of systemic disease including systemic lupus erythematosus, neurofibromatosis, or tuberous sclerosis. Detection of an abdominal mass may suggest hydronephrosis, Wilms tumor, or polycystic kidney disease. An abdominal bruit provides evidence of renovascular disease.

Table 29-3. Pertinent Findings on History, Physical Examination, and Relevant Studies in Pediatric Patients With Hypertension

Etiology	History	Physical Examination	Studies
Renal parenchymal disease	Swelling Gross hematuria Urinary tract infections Polyuria Nocturia History of oligohydramnios Failure to thrive Muscle weakness Family history of renal disease	Edema Short stature Palpable mass Pallor	CBC Serum creatinine BUN Electrolytes Urinalysis Renal ultrasound Consider genetic testing for monogenetic forms of hypertension
Renovascular disease	Neonatal history of a UAC	Carotid or abdominal bruit Abdominal mass Café au lait spots Adenoma sebaceum Ash leaf spots Neurofibromas	Renal ultrasound with Doppler Serum renin Serum aldosterone CTA, MRA Angiography
Endocrinopathies	Weight loss Flushing Tremor Heat intolerance Muscle weakness	Acne Moon facies Striae Tachycardia Goiter Hirsutism Virilization	Free T4, TSH Serum renin Serum aldosterone Cortisol ACTH Adrenal imaging Plasma and urine steroids
Primary hypertension	Smoking Family history of cardiovascular disease Sedentary behavior Weight gain Daytime fatigue Snoring	Elevated BMI Acanthosis nigricans	Hemoglobin A1$_c$ Fasting lipids Polysomnography
Iatrogenic	Prior medical history Decongestants Stimulants Immunosuppressants Contraceptive pills		Drug screening

Table 29-3 (cont)

Etiology	History	Physical Examination	Studies
Cardiac	History of congenital cardiac disease Shortness of breath	Decreased pulses in lower extremity Leg BP 10 mm Hg lower than arm BP	Echocardiogram

Abbreviations: ACTH, adrenocorticotropic hormone; BMI, body mass index; BP, blood pressure; BUN, blood urea nitrogen; CBC, complete blood count; CTA, computed tomographic angiography; Free T4, free thyroxine; MRA, magnetic resonance angiography; TSH, thyroid stimulating hormone; UAC, umbilical arterial catheter.

Evaluation

The 4th Report recommends that the evaluation of all patients with persistent blood pressure above the 95th percentile include a complete blood count, urinalysis, serum blood urea nitrogen level test, serum creatinine level test, electrolytes level test, urine culture, and renal ultrasound because renal disorders are common causes of secondary hypertension (Evidence Level III). All hypertensive patients as well as obese patients with prehypertension should have a fasting lipid panel and a fasting blood glucose (Evidence Level III).

Plasma renin can be used to assess for monogenetic forms of hypertension, including Liddle syndrome, glucocorticoid-remediable aldosteronism, and apparent mineralocorticoid excess in which salt retention and volume expansion often lead to suppression of plasma renin activity. Hypokalemia and metabolic alkalosis are a result of secondary hyperaldosteronism. A high plasma renin activity is a specific but not sensitive measure of renovascular disease, as up to 20% of patients with renovascular disease will have a within-range renin level.

If an endocrinopathy is suspected, thyroid stimulating hormone, free T4, serum aldosterone, and plasma steroid concentrations are indicated (Evidence Level III). In cases of a pheochromocytoma, 24-hour urine measurement of fractionated metanephrine, epinephrine, norepinephrine, or spot urine samples may also be considered (Evidence Level III). In fact, plasma-free metanephrine (performed in recumbency) have a very high sensitivity of 99% for detection of catecholamine-secreting tumors.

Urine drug screening and polysomnography for obstructive sleep apnea are also useful in targeted populations based on information obtained during the history (Evidence Level III).

In terms of imaging, intra-arterial digital subtraction angiography and renal vein renin measurements are the gold standard for evaluation of the renal vasculature (Evidence Level II-2). Other imaging techniques have limitations, and no consensus is available on alternative approaches to angiography. Renal ultrasonography with Doppler, magnetic resonance angiography, radionuclide renal scans, and computed tomographic angiography have been used as screening tests for renovascular disease but may not detect stenosis in the segmental renal arteries.

Ambulatory blood pressure monitoring (Evidence Level III) allows for determination of mean blood pressure over 24 hours, over waking hours, and while asleep. This technique is helpful in assessing patients with white-coat hypertension as well as assessing the response to antihypertensive therapy. It is also recognized that high-risk populations including patients with diabetes and chronic kidney disease may have within-range office-based blood pressures but demonstrate significant elevations outside of the office. Termed *masked hypertension,* these elevations are associated with development of end-organ damage.

Finally, evaluation of hypertension also includes assessment of end-organ changes (Evidence Level III). Left ventricular hypertrophy (LVH) is associated with increased risk of cardiovascular morbidity and mortality in adult patients with hypertension. The presence of LVH is an indication for initiation of antihypertensive therapy in patients with borderline blood pressures or for intensification of antihypertensive therapy in patients currently on therapy. If LVH is present, echocardiograms should be performed every 6 to 12 months to assess for progression. Retinal vascular narrowing has also been associated with hypertension and may be a prognosticator for cardiovascular risk. Proper examination requires referral to an experienced ophthalmologist on a yearly basis. Hypertensive retinopathy is graded from I to IV. No specific treatment is recommended, but grades I and II are generally reversible in children upon lowering of blood pressure.

Management

Non-pharmacologic Therapy

Healthy lifestyle changes are the primary treatment tool for initial management of prehypertension and hypertension (Evidence Level II-2). Specific behaviors that need to be addressed include dietary modifications, enhanced physical activity, minimized sedentary behavior, and smoking cessation. Recommendations include reducing sodium intake to 2 to 3 g per day, reducing cholesterol intake, and reducing intake of sweetened drinks and other high sugar/carbohydrate foods. Using a family-based approach, patients should be instructed to limit portion sizes, to reduce high caloric snacks, and to eliminate skipping meals. Although sodium restriction is difficult in children, families should be advised to avoid processed foods, refrain from adding additional salt to foods, and follow the sodium content on food labels.

Physical activity should be encouraged (Evidence Level II-3). A meta-analysis involving children and adolescents demonstrated a 1% reduction in systolic blood pressure and a 3% reduction in diastolic blood pressure with exercise. Both resistance training and aerobic activity are recommended for the treatment of hypertension in youth. However, patients with uncontrolled stage 2 hypertension should be restricted from participation in competitive sports. A history of exercise-associated chest pain or trouble breathing as well as a family history of sudden death may warrant additional investigation before an exercise regimen is initiated. Once in place, 60 minutes of daily physical activity with a reduction in sedentary behavior to 2 hours daily is recommended.

Pharmacologic Therapy (Table 29-4)

The timing for initiation of pharmacologic therapy is based on the following concepts:

- Pharmacologic therapy should be started immediately in patients with confirmed hypertension and evidence of end-organ damage, diabetes, chronic kidney disease, significant symptoms, and secondary hypertension.
- In patients with persistent hypertension despite implementation of non-pharmacologic therapy, initiation of pharmacologic therapy depends on the severity of the blood pressure elevations.
- In patients with asymptomatic stage 2 hypertension, pharmacologic therapy should be initiated early in the hopes of preventing the development of end-organ changes (Evidence Level III).

Figure 29-2 summarizes the evaluation and treatment of hypertension.

Table 29-4. Pharmacologic Agents in Pediatric Hypertension

Class	Agent	Dose
Angiotensin-converting enzyme inhibitor	Captopril	Initial: 0.3–0.5 mg/kg/dose (3–4 times a day) Maximum: 6 mg/kg/day
	Enalapril	Initial: 0.08 mg/kg/day (1–2 times a day) Maximum: 0.6 mg/kg/day–40 mg/day
	Lisinopril (in children >6 y)	Initial: 0.07 mg/kg/day (once daily) Maximum: 0.6 mg/kg/day–40 mg/day
Angiotensin receptor blocker	Irbesartan	Children 6–12 y: 75–150 mg/day
	Losartan	Initial: 0.7 mg/kg/day Maximum: 1.4 mg/kg/day–100 mg/day

Table 29-4 *(cont)*

Class	Agent	Dose
Calcium channel blocker	Amlodipine	Children 6–17 y: 2.5–5 mg once daily
	Felodipine	Initial: 2.5 mg/day Maximum: 10 mg/day
	Isradipine	Initial: 0.15–0.2 mg/kg/day (3–4 times a day) Maximum: 0.8 mg/kg/day up to 20 mg/day
	Nifedipine XR	Initial: 0.25–0.5 mg/kg/day (1–2 times a day) Maximum: 3 mg/kg/day up to 120 mg/day
Beta blocker	Atenolol	Initial: 0.5–1 mg/kg/dose (1–2 times a day) Maximum: 2 mg/kg/day up to 100 mg/day
	Metoprolol	Initial: 1–2 mg/kg/day (2 twice daily) Maximum: 6 mg/kg/day–200 mg/day
	Propranolol	Initial: 1–2 mg/kg/day (2–3 times a day) Maximum: 4 mg/kg/day–640 mg/day
	Labetalol	Initial:1–3 mg/kg/day (twice daily) Maximum: 10–12 mg/kg/day up to 1,200 mg/day
Diuretics	Hydrochlorothiazide	Initial: 1 mg/kg/day (once daily) Maximum: 3 mg/kg/day up to 50 mg
	Furosemide	Initial: 0.5–2 mg/kg/day (1–2 times a day) Maximum: 6 mg/kg/day
	Amiloride	Initial: 0.4–0.6 mg/kg/day (once daily) Maximum: 20 mg/day
	Spironolactone	Initial: 1 mg/kg/day (1–2 times a day) Maximum: 3.3 mg/kg/day up to 100 mg/day
	Triamterene	Initial: 1–2 mg/kg/day (twice daily) Maximum: 3–4 mg/kg/day–300 mg/day

Table 29-4 (cont)

Class	Agent	Dose
Central alpha blocker	Clonidine	Children >12 y Initial: 0.2 mg/day (twice daily) Maximum: 2.4 mg/day
Vasodilator	Hydralazine	Initial: 0.75 mg/kg/day (4 times a day) Maximum: 7.5 mg/kg/day up to 200 mg/day
	Minoxidil	Children <12 y Initial: 0.2 mg/kg/day (1–3 times a day) Maximum: 50 mg/day Children >12 y Initial: 5 mg/kg/day (1–3 times a day) Maximum: 100 mg/day

From National High Blood Pressure Educational Program Working Group on High Blood Pressure in Children and Adolescents. The Fourth Report on the Diagnosis, Evaluation, and Treatment of High Blood Pressure in Children and Adolescents. *Pediatrics.* 2004;114:555–576.

Most antihypertensive drugs, however, carry a disclaimer relating to their use in children. The trend in the treatment of hypertension in children has been the use of angiotensin-converting enzyme (ACE) inhibitors, long-acting calcium channel blockers, and angiotensin receptor blockers (ARB). The goal of therapy is lowering of blood pressure below the 90th percentile for age, height, and sex with minimal adverse effects (Evidence Level III).

Angiotensin-Converting Enzyme Inhibitors

Angiotensin-converting enzyme inhibitors have been found to demonstrate cardioprotective and renoprotective properties. They have been shown to slow progression of chronic kidney disease in diabetic patients with or without hypertension. They are also considered first-line agents in patients with congestive heart failure and left ventricular dysfunction. One of the more common acute drug effects (ADEs) associated with ACE inhibitors is a dry cough. Hyperkalemia, neutropenia, thrombocytopenia, angioedema, and decreased renal function have been reported in children and adolescents. Renal impairment is typically reversible with ACE inhibitors following discontinuation of the medication and is usually associated with volume depletion. Laboratory studies including a complete blood count, electrolytes level test, serum creatinine concentration test, and blood urea nitrogen concentration test should be monitored shortly (within 2 weeks) after initiation of an ACE

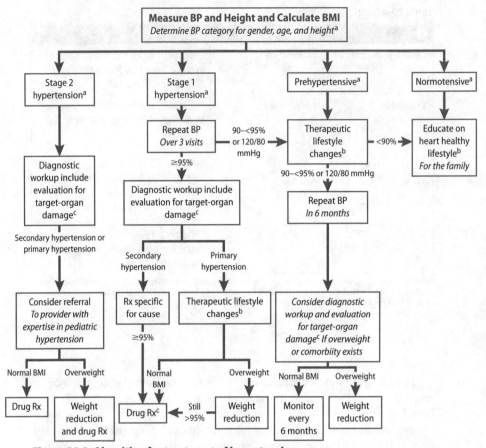

Figure 29-2. Algorithm for treatment of hypertension.

Abbreviations: BMI, body mass index; BP, blood pressure; Rx, prescription.

[a] See appropriate BP tables for gender, age, and height.

[b] Diet modification and physical activity.

[c] Especially if younger, very high BP, little or no family history, or other risk factors.

From National High Blood Pressure Educational Program Working Group on High Blood Pressure in Children and Adolescents. The Fourth Report on the Diagnosis, Evaluation, and Treatment of High Blood Pressure in Children and Adolescents. *Pediatrics.* 2004;114:555–576.

inhibitor or after changes in dosage. In patients on stable therapy, laboratory monitoring every 3 to 6 months is appropriate. The use of ACE inhibitors is contraindicated in patients with bilateral renal artery stenosis, hyperkalemia, and pregnancy. Angiotensin-converting enzyme inhibitors should be avoided in all trimesters of pregnancy because of the risk of cardiac defects as well as renal defects leading to oligohydramnios and pulmonary hypoplasia.

Angiotensin Receptor Blockers

Angiotensin receptor blockers' risk of renal impairment and contraindications in pregnancy discussed previously are similar to ACE inhibitors, so periodic laboratory monitoring is required.

Losartan has been shown to lower blood pressure in children younger than 18 years with minimal adverse events. Irbesartan's safety and efficacy has been studied in children 6 to 16 years of age.

Calcium Channel Blockers

Calcium channel blockers nifedipine, isradipine, and amlodipine are most commonly used in pediatrics. They are particularly useful in patients in which use of an ACE inhibitor or ARB is contraindicated.

Side effects of calcium channel blockers are infrequent and dose related, including peripheral edema, flushing, headache, gingival hyperplasia, and orthostatic hypotension. Short-acting calcium channel blockers including isradipine and nifedipine are often used in the setting of hypertensive urgency for rapid lowering of blood pressure. However, the use of sublingual nifedipine is controversial because it is associated with cerebrovascular and cardiovascular events in adults.

Beta Blockers

Beta blockers should be avoided in specific populations. Because of decreased cardiac output and fatigue, beta blockers should be avoided in athletes. Beta blockers are also contraindicated in patients with asthma because of potential bronchospasm. In diabetic patients, these agents may mask the symptoms of hypoglycemia, including tachycardia and palpitations. Other ADEs include orthostatic hypotension, fatigue, depression, altered lipid profiles, impotence, and hyperkalemia.

Diuretics

In pediatric patients, diuretics are generally no longer considered first-line therapy because of the availability of newer classes of medications such as ACE inhibitors and ARBs but also because of adverse effects. However, diuretics work synergistically with agents such as an ACE inhibitor or ARB and as such are useful in multiple drug regimens. The ADEs associated with these medications include metabolic derangements, such as hyperlipidemia and altered glucose metabolism; electrolyte disturbances (eg, hypokalemia, hypomagnesemia); and dehydration.

Central Alpha Agonists

Clonidine is often limited by its ADEs including dry mouth, sedation, fatigue, and severe rebound hypertension following rapid discontinuation. However, the use of transdermal clonidine may increase adherence in some patients, as patches are changed weekly.

Vasodilators

The common ADEs for hydralazine and minoxidil include headache, tachycardia, flushing, fluid retention, and palpitations.

Long-term Monitoring

Children with prehypertension should be seen in the medical setting every 6 months to monitor and reinforce the importance of nonpharmacologic therapy (Table 29-5). If blood pressures have been controlled for an extended period of time (ie, 12 months), it is not unreasonable to attempt to wean antihypertensive therapy. The use of home and school blood pressure has limited evidence but is particularly helpful when titrating therapy. In addition, ambulatory blood pressure monitoring may assist the clinician in determining if a trial off of antihypertensive therapy is reasonable.

Table 29-5. Suggested Monitoring of Children With Hypertension

Hypertension Category	Monitoring Visits
Prehypertension	Every 6 mo
Stage 1	Every 3–4 mo following appropriate control
Stage 2	Every 2–3 wk, then 3–4 mo following appropriate control

Pediatric patients demonstrate alterations in both cardiac and vascular structure at the time of diagnosis. Moreover, these patients have subtle changes in renal function as well as cerebrovascular reactivity. Hypertension is also associated with poor school performance and learning disabilities. Therefore, prompt recognition and treatment of hypertension in the pediatric population is imperative. Because the prevalence of hypertension is increasing, pediatricians are essential to improving outcomes in this patient population by recognizing, evaluating, and treating patients with this disorder.

Suggested Reading

Demorest RA, Washington RL and the AAP Council on Sports Medicine and Fitness. Athletic participation by children and adolescents who have systemic hypertension. *Pediatrics*. 2010;125(6):1287–1294

Flynn JT. Neonatal hypertension. In: Flynn JT, Inglefinger JR, Portman RJ, eds. *Pediatric Hypertension*. Totowa, NJ: Humana Press; 2011:375–396

Hansen ML, Gunn PW, Kaelber DC. Underdiagnosis of hypertension in children and adolescents. *JAMA*. 2007;298(8):874–879

He FJ, Macgregor GA. Importance of salt in determining blood pressure in children: meta-analysis of controlled trials. *Hypertension*. 2006;48(5):861–869

Kapur G, Mattoo TJ. Primary hypertension. In: Flynn JY, Inglefinger JR, Portman RJ, eds. *Pediatric Hypertension.* Totowa, NJ: Humana Press; 2011:343–356

Messerli FH, Frohlich ED. High blood pressure. A side effect of drugs, poisons, and food. *Arch Intern Med.* 1979;139(6):682–687

National High Blood Pressure Educational Program Working Group on High Blood Pressure in Children and Adolescents. The Fourth Report on the Diagnosis, Evaluation, and Treatment of High Blood Pressure in Children and Adolescents. *Pediatrics.* 2004;114:555–576

CHAPTER 30

Immunization and Vaccines

Karin Hillenbrand, MD, MPH

Key Points

- Most parents who ask questions or express concerns about vaccinating their child can be considered "hesitant" about vaccines rather than resistant. With a patient, collaborative approach that addresses their concerns, parents will usually agree that vaccines are the right choice for their children.

- There are no contraindications to simultaneous administration of any vaccines in the childhood schedule, nor is there a limit to the number of vaccines that can be given at one time. A child should, therefore, simultaneously be given all vaccines for which she is eligible at the time of the visit.

- Physicians should identify valid sources of information and develop a system in the office to remain current with recommendations, address concerns, and manage administrative aspects of the vaccine program.

Overview

Preventing childhood diseases through administration of vaccines is a fundamental component of pediatric practice. Routine childhood vaccination safely and effectively prevents infection with 16 pathogens for most children in the United States (Box 30-1).

Box 30-1. Diseases Against Which All Healthy Children in the United States Should Be Vaccinated

Diphtheria	Mumps
Haemophilus influenzae	Pertussis
Hepatitis A	Pneumococcus
Hepatitis B	Polio
Human papillomavirus	Rotavirus
Influenza	Rubella
Measles	Tetanus
Meningococcus	Varicella

Vaccination refers to the administration of all or part of a microorganism, prepared as a pharmaceutical product ("vaccine"), to induce immunity in the recipient similar to that caused by the natural infection but without the attendant risk of disease. Two major types of vaccines exist: those which are live attenuated (in which the organism is modified to retain the ability to replicate but not to produce illness in the recipient) and those which are inactivated (in which the organism is inactivated by heat or chemicals so that it cannot replicate in the recipient). Live vaccines must replicate in the recipient to be effective. They generally produce long-lasting immunity with a single dose (except the live, oral vaccines); however, in immunocompromised recipients, the vaccine may cause severe or fatal reactions due to uncontrolled replication. Live vaccines may be rendered ineffective by circulating antibodies against the target organism; therefore, systemic live vaccines must be withheld for a period of time following administration of antibody-containing blood products and are typically not administered during the first year after birth, when antibodies received in passive transfer from the mother are present. Inactivated vaccines are not alive and do not replicate. Multiple doses are typically required, as well as periodic boosting to maintain immunity. They are highly purified and have a low incidence of side effects. They are not affected by circulating antibody, and thus can be administered early in infancy. They cannot cause disease by infection, even in immunocompromised individuals.

As drugs, vaccines are subject to regulation and licensure by the US Food and Drug Administration (FDA). Information regarding a vaccine's license, such as approved ages for administration and the manufacturer's recommendations for use, can be found at the FDA Web site, www.fda.gov.

The Centers for Disease Control and Prevention (CDC) determines the US Childhood Immunization Schedule, based on recommendations from the Advisory Committee on Immunization Practices (ACIP), and publishes these recommendations in the *Morbidity and Mortality Weekly Report (MMWR)*. Parallel recommendations for pediatric use are published as policy statements of the American Academy of Pediatrics (AAP) for dissemination to its membership. Updated schedules and recommendations are issued annually in January, with interval recommendations issued as needed.

Laws mandating that children be vaccinated can be instrumental in implementing new vaccine recommendations and in assuring adequate coverage of the population to prevent the spread of disease. All states have immunization laws targeted to school entry, although requirements differ from state to state; states may also require vaccines for children entering day care, middle school, or college. Occurrence of a disease preventable by vaccination should usually be reported through local and state health departments; practitioners should consult state statutes for specific requirements.

Vaccine Administration
· · · · · · · · · · · · · · · · · · · ·

Schedules and Timing

The CDC issues an immunization schedule that provides recommendations for vaccinating children 0 through 18 years of age, as well as a catch-up schedule for children who start late or fall behind. Schedules are typically updated yearly and are available on the CDC's Web site (www.cdc.gov/vaccines). Footnotes accompanying the schedules provide detailed information about timing and administration of each vaccine. Comprehensive immunization recommendations, as well as information about individual vaccines, can be found at the ACIP website (www.cdc.gov/vaccines/acip/recs).

Adherence to a minimum interval between doses of a multi-dose vaccine increases the likelihood of an adequate immune system response; doses given before the minimum interval has elapsed may not be maximally effective and therefore are considered invalid and must be repeated. Conversely, increasing the interval between doses of a multi-dose vaccine does not diminish effectiveness of the vaccine. Therefore, when a child presents later than recommended for vaccines, the next dose in the series should be administered: one need never "start over" in the administration of vaccines, regardless of the time that has elapsed between doses. A catch-up immunization schedule for children who start late, who fall behind, or whose record of immunization is unavailable or inadequate can be found on the CDC Web site.

There are no contraindications to simultaneous administration of any vaccines in the childhood schedule nor a limit to the number of vaccines that can be given at one time. A child should, therefore, simultaneously be given all vaccines for which he is eligible at the time of the visit.

Special Circumstances

Infants born prematurely should be vaccinated according to chronologic age rather than corrected gestational age for most vaccines. An exception to this general approach applies to administration of the initial dose of the hepatitis B series: for preterm newborns weighing less than 2,000 g who are delivered to mothers with a negative test for hepatitis B surface antigen, the initial dose should not be administered until the newborn reaches a chronologic age of 1 month or until hospital discharge.

Immunocompromised children may not be able to receive some vaccines (such as live vaccines) and may benefit from earlier or more frequent administration of others (such as meningococcal or pneumococcal vaccines). Children who travel should receive all usually recommended vaccines. They may also require earlier-than-usual immunization against measles and may benefit from additional immunizations, depending on travel destination.

Infants and children at high risk for serious diseases because of unique exposures or circumstances may benefit from provision of passive immunization using preformed immunoglobulin products. Examples include administration of rabies immunoglobulin (Ig) after exposure to a potentially rabid animal, use of respiratory syncytial virus (RSV) Ig for premature infants during RSV season, and administration of hepatitis B Ig (HBIg) to infants born to mothers infected with the hepatitis B virus.

Comprehensive resources to guide immunization under special circumstances are available from www.cdc.gov/vaccines, www.cdc.gov/travel, and the *Red Book* of the AAP.

Vaccine Selection

A vaccine directed against a specific pathogen may be manufactured by more than one pharmaceutical company. Factors affecting selection of one product over another include price, product availability, age restriction, number of recommended doses, and ease of administration. In most cases, ACIP recommendations do not favor choice of one brand over another. Whenever possible, subsequent doses of a vaccine in a series should be administered using the same brand product that was used at series initiation.

When available, combination vaccines should be used preferentially rather than individual injections of the component vaccines. The use of combination vaccines results in a decreased number of injections a child may require during each visit, which in turn increases acceptability, facilitates timely vaccine administration, decreases the overall number of visits, lowers administrative costs, and allows for consolidation of inventory. When using combination vaccines, the minimum interval as well as the contraindications for each component must be taken into consideration.

Financial Considerations

The funds to purchase vaccines may originate from public or private sources. Public sector funds now purchase more than half of all vaccines administered in the United States, through 3 sources: the Vaccines for Children Program (VFC), Section 317 federal discretionary grants, and state funds. The VFC is a federal entitlement program that allows for the provision of publicly purchased vaccine to eligible children at no cost. All childhood vaccines recommended by the ACIP are included in the program. Vaccines for Children Program–funded vaccines are purchased in bulk by the CDC from manufacturers at reduced cost, and are then distributed through state immunization programs to participating providers. Vaccines for Children Program–purchased vaccine must be provided to eligible children free of charge, although providers may charge an administration fee to offset their costs. Most commercial insurers also provide coverage for recommended childhood vaccines. However, administration fees may not be covered, and families may be required to provide a co-pay for the visit or meet a deductible before the cost of vaccines is covered.

Although payment or reimbursement for nearly all vaccines is available through either public or private sources, the high cost of buying, storing, and administering vaccines threatens the financial stability of many clinics and practices. Maintenance of separate supplies for VFC and privately purchased vaccines can be both costly and confusing, but states often prohibit interchange. The level of administrative cost reimbursement varies tremendously across regions and may not adequately compensate for the time and expense of providing vaccines in the medical home. Providers can consider creating vaccine purchasing pools in their communities to lessen the financial burden on individual practices.

Vaccine Preparation and Administration

Vaccines should be reconstituted according to manufacturer's guidelines. Doses should never be reduced or split, nor should individual vaccines be combined in the same syringe, unless purchased as a combination product. Safety injection devices are recommended for the administration of all injectable vaccines. Hand washing before vaccine preparation and before administration is essential. Gloves do not decrease the risk of needle-stick injury and need not be worn unless the individual administering vaccines is likely to come into contact with infected body fluids or has open sores on the hands. When worn, gloves must be changed between patients.

Recommended routes of administration are stated for each vaccine. Preferred sites for intramuscular (IM) injections are the anterolateral thigh in infants and young children and the deltoid in older children. Subcutaneous injections should be administered in the thigh or upper, outer arm. Injected vaccines should never be administered in the buttocks. Injections should be performed rapidly and smoothly, without aspiration. When multiple vaccines are administered by the IM route, they should be separated by one inch or more. Needles, syringes, and vaccine vials should be disposed of in appropriate medical waste containers.

Young children must be appropriately restrained. Parents should be encouraged to hold the child during vaccine administration, as this is associated with decreased anxiety. Pain and anxiety are less when a child is restrained in a seated position rather than lying down. Other evidence-based strategies to reduce pain and anxiety include breastfeeding prior to vaccination, ingestion of sweet liquids, distraction techniques, provision of topical analgesia using refrigerant spray or lidocaine-containing creams, and tactile stimulation of the skin near the injection site. Antipyretics should not be used before or at the time of vaccine administration, as their use prophylactically has been associated with diminution of the immune response to vaccines in some settings.

Adverse Events

Adverse events following vaccination with an inactivated vaccine occur soon after administration and typically consist of a local injection site reaction, with or without fever. Adverse events following vaccination with a live vaccine are similar to a mild form of the natural illness and typically occur after an incubation period, as the organism in the vaccine must first replicate in the recipient before effect, or adverse effect, occurs. Severe life-threatening reactions, such as anaphylaxis, are very rare. Asking appropriate screening questions prior to vaccination can further decrease the risk.

Parents should be given guidance on the management of adverse events following vaccination. Minor bleeding is addressed by brief pressure and a bandage. Localized soreness, redness, itching, or swelling can typically be managed with a cold compress; oral analgesics or antihistamines may also be useful. Practitioners should be aware of the potential for syncope when older children, adolescents, and young adults receive vaccines. An office protocol should be in place and staff must be prepared to handle anaphylactic reactions if they occur. Minimum preparedness includes the ability to activate the emergency medical services system, administer epinephrine, and perform basic cardiopulmonary resuscitation with airway management.

The National Childhood Vaccine Injury Act requires that any serious adverse event occurring in temporal relationship to administration of a vaccine be reported using the Vaccine Adverse Events Reporting System (www.vaers.hhs.gov).

Contraindications and Precautions

A contraindication to vaccination exists when the recipient is at increased risk for a serious adverse reaction because of an underlying condition. When a contraindication exists, the vaccine should not be given. A precaution to vaccination means that the recipient has a condition which might increase the chances or severity of an adverse reaction or which might make the vaccine less likely to be effective at producing immunity. When a precaution exists, the practitioner should weigh the risk of vaccination against the risk of acquiring the disease. In most cases, when a precaution exists, the vaccine will not be administered. Most contraindications and precautions are temporary, but severe allergy to a vaccine or a component contained within a vaccine is a permanent contraindication to vaccination. Although the list of contraindications and precautions is extensive, they can generally be identified with careful use of just a few screening questions (Box 30-2).

Box 30-2. Screening Questions Useful in Identifying Children With Contraindications or Precautions to Immunization

> **A positive answer to any question warrants further exploration before vaccines are administered.**
>
> - Is the child sick today?
>
> - Does the child have allergies to any medication, food, or vaccine?
>
> - Has the child had a reaction to a vaccine in the past?
>
> - Does the child have a chronic medical problem (including history of seizure or neurologic disorder, asthma or chronic lung disease, heart disease, kidney disease, metabolic disease including diabetes, or a blood disorder)?
>
> - Does the child have cancer, AIDS, or any other immune system problem?
>
> - Has the child taken chemotherapy or corticosteroids recently?
>
> - Has the child received a transfusion of blood or blood products, or immunoglobulins, in the past year?
>
> - Is the child/teen pregnant or does she have a chance to become pregnant during the next month?
>
> - Has the child received any vaccinations in the past 4 weeks?

Modified from Atkinson W, Wolfe S, Hamborsky J, eds. *Epidemiology and Prevention of Vaccine-Preventable Diseases.* 12th ed. Washington, DC: Public Health Foundation; 2012. Available at: www.cdc.gov/vaccines/pubs/pinkbook/index.html. Accessed December 23, 2014

Counseling Parents

Each time vaccines are to be administered, parents should be informed about the benefits and risks and questioned about the existence of contraindications. Since many vaccine-preventable diseases are now very rare, time should be spent educating parents about their seriousness. Following a description of benefits, the most likely adverse events should be reviewed along with guidance for managing them. The counseling process is facilitated by the use of Vaccine Information Statements (VIS). VIS are available in English and Spanish from the CDC's vaccine Web site as well as in many other languages from the Immunization Action Coalition (www.immunize.org). They can be reproduced without permission.

Addressing Parental Concerns

Confusing and often misleading information about vaccines is delivered by television, the Internet, and other media sources. Parents have often heard more about the risk of vaccination than about the risk of disease when they arrive to the office. Many parents will therefore have questions about vaccines. Common parental concerns about vaccines, along with suggested responses, are included in Table 30-1.

Table 30-1. Common Parental Concerns and Suggested Responses

Concern	Response
Too young	Infants can mount an immune response from birth. They are not too young to be affected by the serious diseases prevented by vaccines, so they require protection at an early age.
Too many	Although many more vaccines are available today than in the past, vaccines are highly purified and vaccine antigens represent a very small subset of all the exposures faced by the immune system. Even a very young child's immune system can respond to multiple vaccines at once as well as to the myriad other environmental exposures faced every day.
Natural immunity better	Immunity following recovery from disease typically occurs after a single infection and may persist indefinitely, while immunity from vaccines may require multiple doses and boosters throughout life. However, the cost to the child is experiencing an illness that may cause discomfort, pain, complications, permanent disability, and even death. Vaccines are far safer than the diseases they prevent.
No longer necessary	Vaccines have made many vaccine-preventable diseases very rare. Parents should be counseled about the seriousness of the diseases prevented by vaccines and the risk for resurgence of disease when the vaccination rate in a community drops.
Not safe	Vaccines are medications. No vaccine—and no medication—is completely risk free. Mild side effects, such as fever and injection site pain, occur commonly; more serious side effects, such as anaphylaxis, can also occur, although rarely. Vaccines are closely monitored both before and after licensure for safety concerns. While vaccines are not completely safe, they are as safe as possible. They are safer than most medications and far better than the diseases they prevent.
Contain harmful additives	Additives in vaccines are present in very small amounts. Each is present for a reason: as a preservative, adjuvant, stabilizer, or residual of the manufacturing process. Some additives, such as egg protein and gelatin, have been associated with a risk of allergic reaction, but in general, additives in vaccines have not been associated with safety concerns. Thimerosal is an ethylmercury-based compound used in vaccines as a preservative. Although no side effects have ever been attributed to thimerosal, it has now been eliminated from almost all childhood vaccines.
Can cause chronic diseases	The concern arises because children receive many vaccines during the first 2 years of life, and most children in the United States are vaccinated. Therefore, most children who develop a chronic disease during childhood have been vaccinated. But sequence does not mean consequence, and association does not equal causality. When disease follows vaccination, it occurs at a rate that could be predicted by chance alone. Multiple independent studies show no evidence for a link between vaccines and chronic disease.

Most parents who ask questions or express concerns about vaccines can be considered "vaccine hesitant" rather than "vaccine resistant." When faced with a concerned parent, the physician should listen carefully and respectfully to the specific question and correct any misperceptions and misinformation. Most parents have one or two questions about one or only a few vaccines rather than a global distrust of all vaccines; early identification of specific concerns saves time and allows the physician to provide a targeted, accurate response. Physicians should identify and recommend valid Web sites and books for parents seeking additional information.

It is important to assure that parents understand the risks of choosing *not* to vaccinate: the risk to the child of contracting a vaccine-preventable disease with its attendant morbidity and mortality risks; the risk of spreading a disease to someone who could not be vaccinated because of cancer, immunocompromise, or very young or old age; and the possibility of exclusion from school or other public functions during outbreaks.

Some parents may request that vaccines be administered using an alternative schedule. Parents should be cautioned that the use of alternative or delayed schedules has not been associated with increased safety and has an unknown effect on efficacy. Children for whom vaccination is delayed remain susceptible to disease for a longer period of time. When vaccines are administered over multiple visits, parents incur the cost of additional visits and missed work, and children may suffer from side effects on more days.

Exemptions

Several exemptions from state-mandated vaccination exist. All states allow exemption for a child with a true medical contraindication to vaccination. All states also allow religious exemption, although the definition and procedure varies from state to state. Some but not all states allow parents to express a philosophical objection to vaccination. Providers should be familiar with the types of exemptions allowed in their state and the procedures for each.

Persistent Vaccine Refusal

When parents are persistent in their refusal to accept vaccination for a child, the physician should voice respect for the parent's right to decide on behalf of their child, and assure that they understand the consequences of the decision. Parents should be advised that the importance of vaccines will continue to be addressed at future visits and that they can change their minds at any time. If a parent is opposed to only one or a few vaccines, other vaccines should be given.

Some physicians may consider dismissing parents who refuse to vaccinate from their practices. However, benefits exist for keeping the child in the practice: the opportunity to build a therapeutic alliance over time; a continued ability to provide valid information and perhaps to eventually convince the family to accept vaccination; the ability to provide guidance in the event of an outbreak of a vaccine-preventable disease in the community; and provision of other aspects of care necessary to the maintenance of the child's health and the health of the community. If vaccine refusal is indicative of a larger issue of distrust, difference of philosophy, or persistent poor communication, a practice may suggest that the family find another source of medical care. Unless a child is put at risk of serious harm by parental refusal to vaccinate (such as during an epidemic), reports of child neglect or endangerment should generally not be submitted to state agencies, nor efforts made to involve courts in overturning parental decisions.

Physicians may be concerned about their own potential liability in the case of unimmunized children in their practices. To minimize risk, providers should clearly document their discussion regarding the benefits of vaccination and the risks of remaining unimmunized and may consider having parents sign a "refusal waiver." The AAP has created a "Refusal to Vaccinate" form, which may be useful in providing documentation (www2.aap.org/immunization). Offices may have a policy excluding unvaccinated children from the waiting room when they are ill, especially during an outbreak. It may be desirable to maintain a list of unimmunized children in the community for rapid identification during an outbreak.

Suggested Reading

American Academy of Pediatrics Committee on Bioethics. Responding to parental refusals of immunization of children. *Pediatrics.* 2005;115(5):1428–1431

Centers for Disease Control and Prevention. *Epidemiology and Prevention of Vaccine-Preventable Diseases.* Atkinson W, Wolfe S, Hamborsky J, eds. 12th ed. Washington, DC: Public Health Foundation; 2012

Centers for Disease Control and Prevention. Vaccines and Immunizations Web site. http://www.cdc.gov/vaccines. Accessed November 12, 2014

Centers for Disease Control and Prevention. General recommendations on immunization—recommendations of the Advisory Committee on Immunization Practices (ACIP). *MMWR Recomm Rep.* 2011;60(2):1–64

Section 1. In: Pickering LK, ed. *Red Book: 2012 Report of the Committee on Infectious Diseases.* 29th ed. Elk Grove Village, IL: American Academy of Pediatrics; 2012

CHAPTER 31

Infections in the First Year

Kristina Simeonsson, MD, MSPH

Key Points

- Infections in infancy carry higher morbidity and mortality than in childhood.

- Age of the infant is important in determining likely pathogens as well as appropriate management.

- Many pathogens that used to be leading causes of severe bacterial infections are less common now with widespread use of vaccines; however, these pathogens should still be considered, especially in the unvaccinated infant.

- Congenital infections should be considered in infants with abnormal growth patterns, organomegaly, hearing loss, or developmental delays.

Overview

Worldwide infectious diseases are the leading causes of death in young children. In developed countries, the advent of many vaccines against serious pathogens has reduced the incidence of infectious diseases in younger children; however, considerable morbidity and mortality is still associated with infectious diseases during infancy. In fact, infectious disease hospitalizations account for over 40% of all infant hospitalizations. This chapter will cover some of the more common pathogens responsible for significant morbidity and mortality in the first year of life.

The incidence of serious bacterial infections is more common in the first year of life than during other times in childhood. Routine use of vaccines against *Streptococcus pneumoniae* and *Haemophilus influenzae* type b has significantly reduced the morbidity and mortality of these diseases in infants. Morbidity and mortality from viral infections is higher during infancy than at other times during childhood.

Causes
· · · · · · ·

Viral Infections in Infancy

Infections during the first year of life are caused primarily by viruses, and the most common cause of fever in infants is viral illness. The type of infection, such as bronchiolitis versus gastroenteritis, largely depends on the etiologic agent, but overlap can occur in types of infections caused by the same agent (Table 31-1). Certain viruses, such as influenza and respiratory syncytial virus (RSV), are common pathogens in the wintertime. Enteroviruses predominate in the summer and fall; they can cause a wide variety of illnesses, from aseptic meningitis to nonspecific viral illness, respiratory tract illness, and gastrointestinal tract illness.

Table 31-1. Common Viral Infections in Infancy

Type of Infection	Etiologic Agents
Bronchiolitis	Respiratory syncytial virus Influenza Parainfluenza *Human metapneumovirus* Adenovirus
Pneumonia	Influenza *Human metapnuemovirus* Parainfluenza
Viral syndrome/febrile illness	Herpes simplex virus[a] Influenza[a] Enterovirus *Human herpesvirus 6*
Gastroenteritis	Rotavirus Enterovirus Enteric adenoviruses
Aseptic meningitis/encephalitis	Enterovirus Herpes simplex virus *Human herpesvirus 6*
Upper respiratory tract infection	Adenovirus Respiratory syncytial virus *Human metapneumovirus* Enterovirus
Croup	Parainfluenza Influenza

[a] Agent can cause a sepsis-like syndrome in infants.

Herpes Simplex Virus

In newborns, herpes simplex virus infection can manifest in 1 of 3 ways: disseminated disease, localized central nervous system disease, and disease localized to the skin, eyes, or mouth. Neonatal herpetic infections are often severe, with high morbidity and mortality. Initial signs of herpes simplex virus infection can occur anytime between birth and 6 weeks of life; most cases occur within the first month.

Human Herpesvirus 6

Roseola, caused by *human herpesvirus 6*, is characterized by a high fever that can persist for 3 to 7 days and a characteristic maculopapular rash that occurs after defervescence. Infants can present with febrile seizures, bulging fontanelle, and encephalitis or encephalopathy.

Influenza

While it is well-known that influenza mortality is highest in the very young and very old, infants have the highest rates of hospitalization due to influenza when compared to all other age groups. Complications of influenza in infants can include dehydration, a sepsis-like syndrome, secondary bacterial pneumonia or sepsis, and encephalitis. Influenza vaccine is the single best way to prevent influenza; all infants 6 months and older should receive influenza vaccine annually. Household contacts and caregivers of infants less than 6 months should receive influenza vaccine annually to reduce transmission to these younger infants that cannot be vaccinated.

Parainfluenza

There are 4 types of parainfluenza viruses. While parainfluenza viruses 1 and 2 are most commonly associated with croup, type 3 is more common in infants. Parainfluenza virus 3 usually manifests as a lower respiratory tract infection, such as pneumonia and bronchiolitis.

Respiratory Syncytial Virus

Most infants are infected with respiratory syncytial virus (RSV) during the first year of life. Infants typically will exhibit upper respiratory tract disease symptoms, but 20% to 30% will have lower respiratory tract disease such as bronchiolitis and pneumonia. During the first few weeks of life, signs and symptoms of respiratory tract disease may be minimal or absent. Young infants instead may exhibit poor feeding, irritability, and lethargy as the presenting signs and symptoms. A subset of young infants may present with apnea. Hospitalization for RSV infection may be indicated if the infant is feeding poorly or has an oxygen requirement; infants with RSV are hospitalized at rates higher than other age groups.

Rotavirus

Incidence of clinical illness is highest among infants 3 to 35 months of age. Infants younger than 3 months have relatively low rates of infection because of passive maternal antibody and possibly breastfeeding. Clinical manifestations of rotavirus infection can range from asymptomatic infection to severe dehydrating diarrhea with vomiting and fever. The first infection after 3 months is generally the most severe.

Bacterial Infections in Infancy

Serious bacterial infections such as sepsis, meningitis, pneumonia, septic arthritis, osteomyelitis, and pyelonephritis carry the highest morbidity and mortality. Bacteremia is also of concern because it can often lead to sepsis and meningitis by spread of bacteria from the bloodstream to another site. Risk of infection with *H influenzae* type b and *S pneumoniae* is now less than 1% in unimmunized children. Other pathogens have been identified increasingly in cases of bacteremia including *Escherichia coli*, *Staphylococcus aureus*, and *Neisseria meningitidis*.

When considering bacterial infections in infants, considering the age of the infant is the most important factor to take into account. First, younger infants (<3 months) are more likely to have serious bacterial infections when compared to older infants. Second, the age of the infant can inform the etiology of the infection. For instance, early-onset sepsis (0–7 days) occurs from acquisition of organisms from mother to the infant at the time of delivery. Organisms responsible for early-onset sepsis include group B streptococci, *E coli*, coagulase negative staphylococci, *H influenzae*, and *Listeria monocytogenes*. Although late-onset sepsis (7–90 days) can be caused in part by a later presentation of infection from organisms acquired at delivery, it is more often caused by organisms acquired in the caregiving environment (Table 31-2).

Table 31-2. Serious Bacterial Infections in Infancy

	Common Etiologic Agents by Age		
	Neonates (0–1 mo)	**Young Infants (1–3 mo)**	**Older Infants (3–12 mo)**
Occult bacteremia/septicemia	Enterobacter species Escherichia coli Group B streptococci Klebsiella Listeria monocytogenes Neisseria gonorrhoeae Staphylococcus aureus	Enterococcus Escherichia coli Group B streptococci Staphylococcus aureus Streptococcus pneumoniae	Escherichia coli Haemophilus influenzae Neisseria meningitidis Salmonella Staphylococcus aureus Streptococcus pneumoniae Streptococcus pyogenes
Meningitis	Enterobacter Escherichia coli Group B streptococci Klebsiella Listeria monocytogenes Neisseria gonorrhoeae	Group B streptococci Haemophilus influenzae Listeria monocytogenes Neisseria meningitidis Streptococcus pneumoniae	Haemophilus influenzae Neisseria meningitidis Streptococcus pneumoniae
Urinary tract infection	Enterobacter Escherichia coli Group B streptococci Klebsiella	Enterobacter Escherichia coli	Enterobacter Escherichia coli

Table 31-2 (cont)

Common Etiologic Agents by Age			
	Neonates (0–1 mo)	**Young Infants (1–3 mo)**	**Older Infants (3–12 mo)**
Pneumonia	Escherichia coli Group B streptococci Klebsiella Listeria monocytogenes	Bordetella pertussis Chlamydia trachomatis Group B streptococci Haemophilus influenzae Staphylococcus aureus Streptococcus pneumoniae Streptococcus pyogenes Ureaplasma urealyticum	Bordetella pertussis Haemophilus influenzae Moraxella catarrhalis Staphylococcus aureus Streptococcus pneumoniae Streptococcus pyogenes
Enteritis	Enterobacter Escherichia coli Klebsiella Salmonella Shigella	Campylobacter Escherichia coli Salmonella Shigella Yersinia	Campylobacter Escherichia coli Salmonella Shigella Yersinia
Bone and joint infections	Enterobacter Escherichia coli Group B streptococci Klebsiella Neisseria gonorrhoeae Staphylococcus aureus	Haemophilus influenzae Staphylococcus aureus	Haemophilus influenzae Staphylococcus aureus
Skin and soft tissue infections	Neisseria gonorrhea Staphylococcus aureus	Haemophilus influenzae Staphylococcus aureus Streptococcus pyogenes	Haemophilus influenzae Staphylococcus aureus Streptococcus pyogenes

Group B Streptococci

Group B streptococci are responsible for a significant amount of morbidity and mortality among neonates and young infants. Early-onset group B streptococcal disease (<7 days) most commonly presents as pneumonia or sepsis. Meningitis is the more common presentation of late-onset group B streptococcal disease. Intrapartum prophylaxis has had no demonstrable effect on late-onset group B streptococcal disease (7–90 days).

Gonococcal Infection

Gonococcal infections in infants are limited to the neonatal period. In newborns, gonococcal infections most commonly involve the eye, also known as ophthalmia neonatorum. Treatment of ophthalmia neonatorum requires inpatient admission for parenteral antibiotics and frequent eye irrigation with normal saline until drainage is resolved. Left untreated, *Neisseria gonorrhoeae* in the eye can lead to corneal penetration and permanent blindness. Other sites of infection include scalp abscesses and disseminated infections such as bacteremia, meningitis, and septic arthritis.

Haemophilus Influenzae

H influenzae type b can cause a range of serious infections including pneumonia, bacteremia, meningitis, septic arthritis, and epiglottitis. Other encapsulated strains of *H influenzae* can cause similar infections but are not as common as *H influenzae* type b was in the prevaccine era. Non-typable strains of *H influenzae* typically cause more upper respiratory tract infections, such as otitis media and sinusitis.

Listeria

Early-onset disease can result in preterm birth, pneumonia, and sepsis. A distinct erythematous rash characterized by small pale papules can occur in severe infections; this rash is known as "granulomatosis infantisepticum." Late-onset disease, occurring after the first week of life, usually manifests as meningitis. Hematogenous spread of the organism from the intestine leads to serious infection/disease. Health care–associated outbreaks linked to newborn nurseries have occurred.

Pertussis

Highest annual incidence of pertussis occurs among infants, particularly those younger than 6 months. They are at the highest risk of pertussis-associated complications, such as secondary bacterial pneumonia, apnea, and neurologic complications. Infants younger than 3 months make up most of those who experience pertussis-related deaths as well.

Streptococcus Pneumoniae

Viral upper respiratory tract infections, including influenza, can predispose a person to pneumococcal infection and transmission. Pneumococcal infections are most prevalent during winter months. Pneumococcal meningitis is most common in infants younger than 1 year, with a peak incidence between 3 to 5 months. The case fatality rate for pneumococcal meningitis is higher than meningitis caused by *N meningitidis*, group B streptococci, *L monocytogenes*, and *H influenzae*.

Clinical Features

Infants with infections, even serious infections caused by pathogenic bacteria, can have nonspecific signs and symptoms such as poor feeding, fussiness, irritability, and temperature instability. Taking a thorough history and performing a good physical examination are the cornerstones of determining the cause of infection in the infant. Caregivers should be asked about the infant's temperature, with particular attention paid to the presence of fever or, conversely, an abnormally low temperature, as septic neonates often present with hypothermia. Pertinent features in the past medical history include prematurity, immunization status, and underlying medical conditions. Caregivers should also be asked about the infant's exposure to ill contacts.

Clinical signs of a toxic infant may include lethargy, weak cry, irritability or continuous crying, and poor/absent eye contact. Assess all systems thoroughly, paying particular attention to signs of dehydration such as poor capillary refill and decreased skin turgor. Hypotension is a late finding in septic shock, so tachycardia and poor perfusion should be recognized promptly and treated aggressively. If an infant appears toxic and a source is not found on examination, fever should not be attributed to a nonspecific viral illness such as a viral upper respiratory tract infection. This is particularly true if the infant is not immunized or is underimmunized.

The site of infection may aid in the diagnosis. Meningitis and encephalitis can present with irritability, bulging fontanelle, and poor feeding. Apnea can occur from a respiratory or central nervous system infection. Measuring the respiratory rate is paramount, as pneumonia in infants can present as fever and tachypnea without much in the way of cough. Infants with pneumonia will have tachypnea. Influenza and RSV infections can also present with tachypnea or other symptoms of upper respiratory tract infection, such as cough, nasal congestion, and rhinorrhea. Crackles may be auscultated if the infant has a lower respiratory tract infection. Tachypnea combined with retractions or grunting indicates respiratory distress.

Overlap in the clinical presentation between bacterial and viral processes can occur. Influenza, especially type A; herpes; and enterovirus infections may mimic bacterial sepsis. Examination of the skin can assist with distinguishing a bacterial infection from a viral infection; the presence of an exanthem supports a viral etiology for infection. Viral exanthems may aid the diagnosis. Entero-viruses are responsible for hand-foot-mouth disease as well as herpangina; *human herpesvirus 6* causes the classic rash of roseola, which occurs once the infant has defervesced. The presence of petechiae may signify meningococcemia.

Evaluation

Evaluation of the infant with a suspected infection should focus on identifying the site of infection as well as the etiologic agent. The risk of serious bacterial infections is increased by younger age (ie, infants younger than 3 months and particularly newborns younger than 1 month), height of fever, toxic appear-ance, and presence of underlying chronic conditions such as prematurity, cardiopulmonary conditions, renal conditions, and metabolic syndromes.

Evaluation for serious bacterial infections should occur in these high-risk groups. Infants often present with fever without source. Evaluation and management of these infants will be reviewed here briefly, but more detail can be found in Chapter 24, Fever. A complete blood count and other markers of infection/inflammation such as C-reactive protein concentration, erythrocyte sedimentation rate, or procalcitonin level are often used to evaluate degree of risk of serious bacterial infection. For infants presenting with signs and symptoms of a serious bacterial infection, obtaining cultures of blood, urine, and cerebrospinal fluid may be necessary. Newborns at high risk of serious bacterial infection include those younger than 28 days and those with underly-ing chronic conditions. Chest radiograph should be considered in infants who exhibit respiratory symptoms, such as tachypnea; appear toxic; or have an elevated white blood cell count or C-reactive protein concentration. Cultures of the stool should be considered when diarrhea is bloody or contains pus.

Clinicians should consider herpes simplex virus infection in all neonates with fever and any infant with skin findings or evidence of central nervous system disease. Interestingly, the prevalence of invasive bacterial infections is lower in infants with viral infections, such as enterovirus, RSV, and influenza. Febrile children 3 to 36 months of age with uncomplicated croup, bronchiolitis, varicella, or stomatitis have a very low rate of bacteremia and need not have blood drawn for culture.

Management

Neonates younger than 1 month of age suspected of having a serious bacterial infection require hospitalization. All febrile neonates should receive antibiotics because of the high rates of serious bacterial infections in this population. Ampicillin plus an aminoglycoside is the initial treatment of choice. Febrile infants between 1 to 3 months may require hospitalization. Selection of appropriate antimicrobial therapy will be based on site of infection as well as likely etiology. Infants older than 3 months can likely be managed as outpatients if they are able to take antibiotics by mouth and do not have other complications such as dehydration or respiratory distress.

The management for most viral infections is supportive care. Infants who require intravenous fluids for dehydration or supplemental oxygen for hypoxemia or significant respiratory distress should be hospitalized. Use of acyclovir for herpes infections is recommended for any infant with suspicious skin lesions, an abnormal neurologic examination, pleocytosis on examination of cerebrospinal fluid, or a severe presentation. Recommendations for treating infants with oseltamivir, an antiviral agent to treat influenza, are available.

Long-term Complications

Morbidity from serious bacterial infections can be substantial. Infants with meningitis can have neurologic disabilities, epilepsy, and hearing loss. Infants with urinary tract infections can have renal scarring and an irreversible decrease in renal function. Of the viral etiologies, herpes simplex virus can have the most devastating effects, including permanent neurologic sequelae.

Special Considerations

Congenital infections, commonly referred to as TORCH infections (for toxoplasmosis; other: syphilis, hepatitis B, varicella, human immunodeficiency virus, parvovirus B19; rubella, cytomegalovirus, herpes), should be considered in newborns presenting with microcephaly, hepatosplenomegaly, intrauterine growth retardation, and jaundice. Ordering TORCH titers is no longer recommended. Clinicians should order disease-specific testing based on clinical findings.

These infections carry increased risk to the infant if they are acquired congenitally. For example, developmental delays and hearing loss are common following congenital cytomegalovirus (CMV), rubella, and toxoplasmosis infections. Congenital CMV infection is a frequent cause of sensorineural hearing loss in children; 20% of all hearing loss at birth is attributable to congenital CMV infection, even if the neonate is asymptomatic. In the case of congenitally acquired hepatitis B, as many as 90% of infants who acquire it from their mothers at birth will become chronically infected. Of those with chronic hepatitis B infection, 12% will develop hepatocellular carcinoma. Herpes infections in neonates carry much higher mortality than in older infants and children.

Suggested Reading

Akintemi OB, Roberts KB. Evaluation and management of the febrile child in the conjugated vaccine era. *Adv Pediatr.* 2006;53:255–278

Baraff LJ. Management of infants and young children with fever without source. *Pediatr Annals.* 2008;37(10):673–679

Del Pizzo J. Congenital infections (TORCH). *Pediatr Rev.* 2011;32(12):537–542

Greenhow TL, Hung YY, Herz AM. Changing epidemiology of bacteremia in infants aged 1 week to 3 months. *Pediatrics.* 2012;129(3):e590–e596

Yorita KL, Holman RC, Sejvar JJ, et al. Infectious disease hospitalizations among infants in the United States. *Pediatrics.* 2008;121(2):244-252

CHAPTER 32

Injuries

Kenya McNeal-Trice, MD, and William Mills, MD, MPH

Key Points

- **Frequent injuries include sprains, strains, contusions, open wounds, and other more superficial injuries.**
- **All open wounds and splinters should be assessed for tetanus status and possible antibiotic coverage.**
- **It is important to recognize significant complications from bites and stings such as infection, anaphylaxis, or systemic disease.**
- **Appropriate anticipatory guidance on supervision of the child and environmental hazards to prevent future injury should occur when managing childhood injuries. Follow-up visits provide an excellent opportunity for reinforcing anticipatory guidance.**

Overview

Injury is a common reason for pediatric patients to seek medical attention. The most frequent injuries that present to the primary care office are sprains and strains, contusions, open wounds, and superficial ones such as abrasions, blisters, splinters, and insect bites. For any open wound, the clinician should address the status of tetanus prophylaxis in addition to necessity for antibiotic coverage.

Sprains

Although insufficient data from randomized controlled trials support the effectiveness of applying rest, ice, compression, and elevation, conservative management with rest, the application of ice for 48 hours after injury, and the use of acetaminophen or nonsteroidal anti-inflammatory agents is standard management for sprains. Damage to the physis can cause premature growth arrest and lead to limb length discrepancy. The Salter-Harris classification may be used to help gauge the risk of growth disturbance. Radiographic abnormalities are often absent in patients with type I fractures but should be suspected in patients with tenderness and swelling about the growth plate. Type II fractures are the most common physeal fractures. Both types I and II have low risk of growth disturbance. These patients require immobilization with a splint but may follow up with their pediatrician or an orthopedist on a non-urgent basis within 4 weeks after the injury. Salter Harris type III, IV (both of which are articular fractures), and V (crush injury to the physis) fractures carry a higher risk of growth arrest and require urgent orthopedic follow-up for definitive management.

Nursemaid's Elbow

Nursemaid's elbow, or radial head subluxation, occurs when the annular ligament of the radius becomes trapped between the subluxed head of the radius and the capitellum. Radial head subluxation should be considered in patients who refuse to use their arm and hold it at their side in a partially flexed and pronated position. The arm is typically not swollen or tender to palpation in patients with radial head subluxation; these findings should raise the level of suspicion for fracture.

The subluxated radial head may be reduced by either supination or pronation of forearm. Typically the patient will cry but begin moving the affected arm within several minutes. If the first attempt is unsuccessful, the clinician should reattempt while applying slight axial traction on the forearm. Although both the supination and hyperpronation methods are effective, recent studies suggest the hyperpronation method is more effective and less painful.

Arthropod Bites and Stings

Children are often bitten or stung by arthropods, including spiders, ticks, mites, mosquitoes, fleas, ants, bees, and wasps. Most injuries resulting from bites and stings simply require management of the local site to minimize pruritus and prevent cellulitis. Administration of an oral antihistamine or other antipruritic agent often proves beneficial to patients experiencing pruritus and localized swelling. However, it is important to recognize the more significant complications of arthropod bites, stings, and envenomation, such as infection, anaphylaxis, or systemic disease. As ticks and mosquitoes are recognized arthropod vectors of human disease, it is imperative to follow patients with suspected systemic disease.

Tick Bites

Ticks should be removed from patients as soon as they are discovered to reduce the chance of infection or possible secretion of toxin. Removal by twisting the tick may result in body parts breaking off into the subcutaneous tissue; tick body parts left in the skin can result in chronic site irritation and secondary infection from scratching. It is inappropriate to use substances such as petroleum jelly, lidocaine, or flammable liquid (eg, gasoline) to induce the tick to release. Extreme care should be taken by the individual removing the tick, as the unintentional inoculation of the patient with a disease agent from the tick can result from careless handling. Grasp the tick as close to the skin as possible (with tweezers or forceps) and gently pull. Gloves or a protective covering should be worn over the hands and the tick disposed of properly after removal.

Prophylactic antibiotics are usually not indicated after routine tick removal. However, some clinical studies have demonstrated possible benefit of prophylactic antibiotic treatment after tick bites by *Ixodes scapularis* for prevention of infection with *Borrelia burgdorferi*, the causative agent in Lyme disease.

Spider Bites

Most spider bites result in a local reaction consisting of erythema, pain, and possible papule or blister formation at the site. Maintaining a clean wound site is important to prevent secondary cellulitis.

The 2 species of spiders responsible for nearly all medically significant spider bites in the United States are the *Latrodectus* species (the widow spiders) (Table 32-1) and the *Loxosceles* species (the recluse spiders) (Table 32-2). Envenomation from these species may require advanced medical management because of risk of systemic complications. Patients suspected of envenomation by widow or recluse spiders should be monitored closely for possible progression of symptoms. This is especially important for black widow spider venom, as it lacks cytotoxic agents and envenomation may have minimal cutaneous effects. If progression of clinical symptoms is suspected, patients should be transferred to a facility capable of providing supportive management and acquiring intravenous access.

Table 32-1. Clinical Effects of *Latrodectus* Bites (Widow Spiders)

System Involved	Effect
Cutaneous	Initial (5 minutes–1 hour after bites): local pain 1–2 hours: puncture marks More than 2 hours: regional lymphadenopathy, central blanching at bite site with surrounding erythema
Cardiovascular	Initial tachycardia followed by bradycardia, dysrhythmias, initial hypotension followed by hypertension
Gastrointestinal	Nausea, vomiting
Hematologic	Leukocytosis
Metabolic	Transient hyperglycemia
Musculoskeletal	Hypertonia, abdominal rigidity, "facies latrodectism"
Neurologic	CNS: psychosis, hallucination, visual disturbance, seizure PNS: local pain ANS: increase in all secretions (ie, diaphoresis, salivation, diarrhea, lacrimation, bronchorrhea, mydriasis, miosis, priapism, ejaculation)
Renal	Glomerulonephritis, oliguria, anuria

Abbreviations: ANS, autonomic nervous system; CNS, central nervous system; PNS, peripheral nervous system.
From Hahn IH, Lewin NA. Arthropods. In: *Goldfrank's Toxicologic Emergencies*. 8th ed. New York, NY: McGraw-Hill; 2006:1606, with permission.

Table 32-2. Cutaneous Presentation of *Loxosceles* Bites (Recluse Spiders)

Time From Bite	Symptoms
At time of bite	Painless to mild stinging sensation
1–3 hours post-bite	Vesicles, erythema, pruritis
2–6 hours post-bite	Burning pain at bite site with localized erythema, pruritus, and swelling, possible ulceration
12 hours–1 day post-bite	Bullae, "red, white, and blue sign" (ie, surrounding erythema around area of ischemic blanching with central violaceous necrosis)
1–3 days post-bite	Further necrosis of central ulcer, spreading edema
3–7 days post-bite	Eschar formation, erythema regression
7+ days up to several weeks post-bite	Ulcer possibly continuing to increase in size, gradual healing occurring

Splinter Removal

Splinters most often present as foreign bodies imbedded in superficial or subcutaneous tissue of the extremities. Foreign bodies not completely removed may lead to secondary complications and tissue reactions. In addition, tetanus status of the patient should be appropriately identified to determine the necessity of prophylaxis if risk factors are present. When evaluating the necessity for splinter removal, timing of the injury is a key consideration. Older injuries are more likely to present with tissue reactions and complications and may be more difficult to remove, as an injury track is often no longer patent. Superficial splinters are typically identified by visualization and palpation. Splinters deeper than the superficial and subcutaneous tissue can be more difficult to identify and remove. Indications of the presence of these foreign bodies include early signs of soft tissue reaction or infection (eg, swelling, drainage, erythema). Proper identification for removal of these deeper splinters may require referral for radiologic imaging such as x-ray or ultrasound.

Objects with highest probability of causing infection or inflammation should be removed as soon as possible. These often include organic objects such as wood, thorns, soil, stones, and vegetative objects. The overlying skin should be cleaned with a povidone-iodine solution and, when necessary, a local anesthetic of 1% or 2% lidocaine should be used. For larger or less superficial splinters, regional anesthesia, such as a digital block, should be considered.

After splinter removal, the area should be flushed with normal saline or cleaned with povidone-iodine solution. Following subungual splinter removal, a topical antibiotic and occlusive dressing should be used. Sutures are often unnecessary, especially if there is concern the wound may have been contaminated. Patients should follow up with an office visit or phone call within 48 hours to evaluate for post-procedure infection or retained foreign body.

Subungual Hematoma
· · · · · · · · · · · · · · · · · · · ·

Management of subungual hematoma of the finger or toe can be divided into 3 basic strategies: watchful waiting, nail trephination, and nail removal with nail bed repair. Watchful waiting may not be an option for patients with significant pain, and nail removal is a potentially painful and time-consuming process. In patients without other significant injury to the phalanx, nail trephination will provide good functional and cosmetic results.

Although often not necessary, consideration should be given to the administration of local anesthesia by means of digital block. The nail should be cleaned with povidone-iodine or chlorhexidine (one must ensure proper drying, as chlorhexidine, like isopropyl alcohol, is flammable). Avoiding the lunula, trephine (ie, puncture) the nail with a hot wire, such as an electrocautery device, or a size-21 gauge or larger needle. After the hematoma has been evacuated, dress the nail with antibiotic ointment and sterile gauze.

Although fractures are seen in up to one-half of fingernail injuries, infection is uncommon, and prophylactic antibiotics are not recommended. Patients should, however, be advised to monitor for signs of infection. Furthermore, they should be counseled that the nail will likely fall off, may take months to regrow, and may be permanently deformed or never regrow. Referral to a hand specialist should be considered if fracture is suspected.

Abrasions
· · · · · · · · · ·

Abrasions are the result of tangential force or trauma to the epidermis and dermis resulting in varying thickness of skin loss. Based on the resistant surface that caused the injury, abrasions can be contaminated with foreign bodies including soil or debris. Management should focus on the prevention of infection and promotion of healing. The wound should be thoroughly cleaned to promote healing and prevent infection. A phenomenon known as "traumatic tattooing" can result if retained foreign material is not removed from the wound. This occurs when the healing process encloses debris or foreign material in the epidermis or dermis. Depending upon the degree of epidermis and dermis involvement, abrasions may resemble burns and can be exquisitely painful and sensitive to manipulation. Gentle cleansing with water, saline, or non-detergent containing products (ie, povodone-iodine) are most effective when used within 6 hours of injury. Some authors suggest the use of local anesthetic applied circumferentially around small abrasions (ie, a field block) to assist with pain management and allow for adequate scrubbing of wounds with significant amounts of debris. If managed appropriately, most abrasions heal without significant cosmetic sequelae. It is important that abrasions be kept clean during healing. Smaller wounds can be covered with a nonadherent dressing and topical antibiotic cream or ointment.

Lacerations

. . . .

Laceration management depends on multiple factors such as size, depth, location, and timing of the injury. Ideally, most wounds should be closed within 6 to 12 hours. Because of the excellent blood supply, wounds on the scalp and face are less likely to become infected and may be closed up to 24 hours after the injury. Older wounds should be allowed to heal by secondary intention to reduce the risk of infection. Closure of punctures and bite wounds should be addressed on a case-by-case basis, weighing the risk of infection against cosmetic implications. All lacerations should be irrigated extensively; a good rule of thumb is 100 mL of fluid for each 1 cm of laceration delivered via a 60 mL syringe to provide adequate pressure. Most providers irrigate with normal saline; however, tap water may be as effective. The edges of the wound should be cleansed with either povodone-iodine or chlorhexidine gluconate.

Prior to closure, local anesthesia with either a topical anesthetic such as LET (lidocaine, tetracaine, epinephrine) or locally injected lidocaine should be considered. The maximum dose of lidocaine is 5 mg/kg when used alone or 7 mg/kg when administered with epinephrine.

For smaller lesions under minimal to no tension, multiple closure methods are possible. Tissue adhesive is a relatively simple means of wound closure. The face is the most common area onto which tissue adhesive is applied. Adhesive is not recommended for high moisture surfaces (ie, hands, feet, or joints) since moisture and repetitive motion may cause the bond to break. Deeper wounds in which adequate elimination of subcutaneous dead space cannot be assured should not be closed with tissue adhesive, as healing and scar contracture can lead to wound inversion into the dead space. Care should be taken to keep tissue adhesive out of the patient's eyes. Lacerations near the eye may be safely closed after the eyelashes are protected with topical antibiotic ointment. Another helpful trick is to draw the tissue adhesive into a small pipette, such as those used to test a finger stick blood glucose, which will allow for more controlled and pinpoint application. After closure, avoid application of antibiotic ointment or petroleum jelly, as these can degrade tissue adhesive. Advise patients to keep the wound areas dry; it is likely not a problem for these areas to get splashed, but they should not become saturated (ie, swimming pool wet).

Suture size and timing until removal vary based on wound location. Obviating the need for a return visit for suture removal has multiple benefits for pediatric patients. Staples are a means of rapid wound closure. In the pediatric population, they are primarily used to close scalp lacerations because of ease of application and appropriate wound edge eversion.

Except for wounds closed with tissue adhesive, apply a thin coating of antibiotic ointment and a dressing after wound closure. Advise patients to leave the dressing in place approximately 24 hours and clean with soapy water followed by application of antibiotic ointment 1 to 2 times a day (keep dry if tissue adhesive is used). Healing wounds should be kept out of the sun, as they are at increased risk of sunburn to the area. Most wounds, if cleaned and prepared properly, do not require systemic antibiotics (Table 32-3); prophylaxis should be addressed on an individualized basis (Figure 32-1).

Table 32-3. Common Wound Infections and Suggested Systemic Treatment

Wound Type	Common Pathogens	Systemic Antibiotic	Recommended Dosing
Lacerations, abrasions	Staphylococci, streptococci	Cephalexin **or**	25–50 mg/kg/day, every 6 hours
		Dicloxacillin **or**	50 mg/kg/day, every 6 hours
		Erythromycin (if patient is sensitive to penicillin)	30–50 mg/kg/day, every 6–8 hours
Puncture wounds	Staphylococci, streptococci, *Pseudomonas* species (osteochondritis)	Cephalexin **or**	25–50 mg/kg/day, every 6 hours
		Dicloxacillin **or**	50 mg/kg/day, every 6 hours
		Erythromycin (if patient is sensitive to penicillin)	30–50 mg/kg/day, every 6–8 hours
		Antipseudomonal agent (eg, ceftazidime) given intravenously	100–150 mg/kg/day, every 8 hours
Human bites	Staphylococci, streptococci, anaerobes	Amoxicillin-clavulanic acid **or** Clindamycin **and**	30–50 mg/kg/day, twice a day 10–30 mg/kg/day, every 8 hours
		Trimethoprim sulfamethoxazole (if patient is sensitive to penicillin)	8–10 mg/kg/day, twice a day
Animal bites	Staphylococci, streptococci, *Pasteurella* species, *Eikenella* species	Amoxicillin-clavulanic acid **or** Clindamycin **and**	30–50 mg/kg/day, twice a day 10–30 mg/kg/day, every 8 hours
		Trimethoprim sulfamethoxazole (if patient is sensitive to penicillin)	8–10 mg/kg/day, twice a day

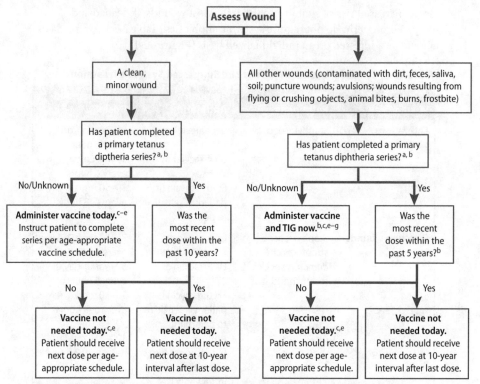

Figure 32-1. Tetanus prophylaxis algorithm for routine wound management.

Abbreviations: DT, diphtheria and tetanus toxoids; DTaP, diphtheria and tetanus toxoids and acellular pertussis; DTP, diphtheria and tetanus toxoids and pertussis; IM, intramuscularly; Td, tetanus and diphtheria toxoids; Tdap, tetanus toxoid, reduced diphtheria toxoid, and acellular pertussis; TIG, tetanus immune globulin; TT, tetanus toxoid.

[a] Primary series consists of a minimum of 3 doses of tetanus- and diphtheria-containing vaccine (DTaP/DTP/Tdap/DT/Td).

[b] Persons who are HIV positive should receive TIG regardless of tetanus immunization history.

[c] Age-appropriate vaccine:
  • DTaP for infants and children 6 weeks up to 7 years of age (or DT pediatric if pertussis vaccine is contraindicated).
  • Td for persons 7 through 9 years of age and ≥65 years of age.
  • Tdap for persons 10 through 64 years, unless the person has received a prior dose of Tdap.*

[d] No vaccine or TIG is recommended for infants <6 weeks of age with clean, minor wounds. (And no vaccine is licensed for infants <6 weeks of age.)

[e] **Tdap*** is preferred for persons age 10 through 64 who have never received Tdap. Td is preferred to TT for persons 7 through 9 years, those ≥65 years, or those who have received a Tdap previously. If TT is administered, an absorbed TT product is preferred to fluid TT. (All DTaP/DTP/Tdap/DT/Td products contain absorbed tetanus toxoid.)

[f] Give TIG 250 U IM for all ages. It can and should be given simultaneously with the tetanus-containing vaccine.

[g] For infants <6 weeks of age, TIG (without vaccine) is recommended for "dirty" wounds (wounds other than clean, minor).

Suggested Reading

Chan C, Salam GA. Splinter removal. *Am Fam Physician.* 2003;67(12):2557–2562

Sagerman PJ, McBride AS, Halvorson EH. Management of wounds in the pediatric emergency department. *Pediatr Emerg Med Pract.* 2010;7(9):1–24

Trott AT. *Wounds and Lacerations: Emergency Care and Closure.* 4th ed. Philadelphia, PA: Elsevier Saunders; 2012:161–191

CHAPTER 33

Joint and Extremity Pain

Scott Vergano, MD

Key Points

- Arthritis in a child is never normal and always deserves further testing.

- A septic joint is an orthopedic emergency. Decreased range of motion is the hallmark of the disease. Refusal to bear weight, fever, and elevated erythrocyte sedimentation rate (ESR), C-reactive protein (CRP) concentration, and white blood cell count are all suggestive of septic arthritis of the hip.

- The pain of osteomyelitis may develop over several days to 1 to 2 weeks. Point tenderness and an elevated ESR and CRP concentration accompany most cases of osteomyelitis, but fever and leukocytosis are often absent.

- Although growing pains are ubiquitous, bone pain is a common presentation of acute leukemia. Presence of fever, bruising, systemic signs, or decreased activity suggest the need for further evaluation.

Overview

Painful joints and extremities are a common occurrence in children. Often pain cannot reliably be localized. Because the differential diagnosis is extensive and the diagnosis may be urgent or serious, these children present a dilemma to the clinician. A logical approach is required for appropriate evaluation.

When facing a child with pain in the joints or extremities, the clinician can use an algorithm (Figure 33-1 and Box 33-1) to help guide differential diagnosis and evaluation. The starting point is a thorough and careful evaluation of the joints for presence of joint effusion/synovial swelling or tenderness with decreased range of motion as signs of arthritis. Pain without swelling, known as arthralgia, is often less ominous than arthritis, in which inflammation is present.

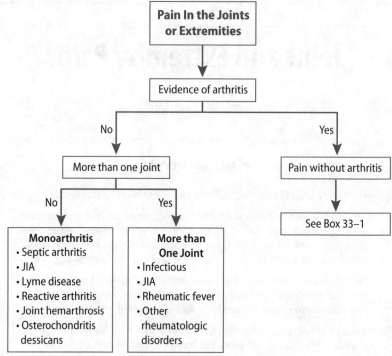

Figure 33-1. Evaluation of joint and extremity pain algorithm.

Abbreviation: JIA, juvenile idiopathic arthritis.

Box 33-1. Differential Diagnosis of Extremity Pain Without Arthritis

Hip pain
- Septic hip
- Transient synovitis
- Legg-Calvé-Perthes disease
- Slipped capital femoral epiphysis

Knee pain
- Patellofemoral syndrome
- Osgood-Schlatter disease
- Ligamentous injury
- Meniscal injury
- Osteochondritis dissecans
- Referred pain from hip

Foot pain
- Sprains
- Strains
- Fractures
- Overuse injuries (eg, Achilles tendonitis, Sever disease)
- Tarsal coalition
- Kohler disease
- Accessory navicular
- Stress fracture

Box 33-1(cont)

Bone pain
- Osteomyelitis
- Bone tumor
- Sprains
- Strains
- Fractures
- Intentional trauma
- Complex regional pain syndrome
- Growing pains

Upper extremity pain
- Sprains
- Strains
- Fractures
- Dislocations
- Intentional trauma
- Overuse injuries (of the shoulder, elbow, or wrist)
- Osteomyelitis
- Bone tumor
- Complex regional pain syndrome

Generalized pains
- Growing pains
- Juvenile fibromyalgia syndrome
- Amplified musculoskeletal pain
- Leukemia
- Viral infection
- Lyme
- Hypermobility syndromes (Ehlers-Danlos syndrome, generalized joint hypermobility)

Arthritis
· · · · · · · ·

Monoarthritis

Septic arthritis is an orthopedic emergency and requires urgent evaluation of synovial fluid and parenteral antibiotic therapy to minimize long-term joint dysfunction. Fever, erythema, and elevated acute-phase reactants are common, but the hallmark of the disease is significantly decreased range of motion. The arthritis of Lyme disease involves the knee in 90% of cases, and although range of motion may not be significantly limited, the degree of joint inflammation is generally prominent. Both reactive arthritis and juvenile idiopathic arthritis (JIA) may present with monoarthritis of a large joint. Reactive arthritis generally follows gastrointestinal, respiratory, or genitourinary tract infections and resolves quickly, whereas JIA persists for 6 weeks or longer. A careful and thorough physical examination looking for at least one other joint with arthritis can be very helpful in making a diagnosis, as oligoarthritis affecting 2 to 4 joints has a more limited differential diagnosis than monoarthritis. Joint hemarthrosis, as present for example in an anterior cruciate ligament injury to the knee or a clotting disorder, and osteochondritis dissecans of the knee or elbow may also present with swelling to a single joint. Magnetic resonance imaging with contrast can often be useful in distinguishing the etiology of monoarthritis.

Polyarthritis

Viral infections commonly cause polyarthritis of the large joints, with *human parvovirus B19* particularly responsible among teenagers and young adults. Gonorrhea, rubella, Epstein-Barr virus, cytomegalovirus, and herpes simplex viruses may produce a similar clinical picture. Subsets of juvenile idiopathic arthritis typically presenting as polyarthritis include rheumatoid factor (RF) positive and RF negative polyarthritis, psoriatic arthritis, and enthesitis-related arthritis. Other rheumatologic conditions to consider include lupus, inflammatory bowel disease, Henoch-Schönlein purpura, and other connective tissue disorders. Migratory polyarthritis is a major criterion for acute rheumatic fever. Diagnosis requires at least one other of the major Jones criteria (ie, carditis, chorea, erythema marginatum, subcutaneous nodules) or 2 minor criteria (ie, fever, previous rheumatic fever or rheumatic heart disease, acute phase reactions: ESR/CRP concentration/leukocytosis, prolonged PR interval), not including arthralgia, plus evidence of an antecedent group A streptococcal infection.

Pain Without Arthritis

When approaching a child with extremity pain, the clinician should consider whether the pain is localized to a particular area or generalized (see Box 33-1). Hip arthritis is discussed within this section because inflammation within the hip joint, while suggested by decreased range of motion, can never be visualized on physical examination. Each region will be discussed separately, starting with the lower extremities and ending with generalized extremity pain.

Lower Extremities

The Hip

The most critical distinction in the child with acute hip pain is between septic arthritis and transient synovitis. Transient synovitis is suggested by a history of recent upper respiratory infection, age between 2 and 6 years, lack of fever, and spontaneous resolution in 1 to 2 days. Recent prediction rules have identified the following factors as suggestive of septic arthritis:

- Refusal to bear weight
- Fever >38.5
- ESR >40 or CRP >20
- White blood cell count >12,000

The presence of no risk factors indicates a likelihood of septic arthritis of 2% to 13%; 3 risk factors, a likelihood of 73% to 83%; and 4 risk factors, a likelihood of 93% to 97% (Evidence Level II-2). Two additional conditions that require urgent orthopedic evaluation are Legg-Calvé-Perthes disease (LCP) and slipped capital femoral epiphysis (SCFE). A boy between the ages of 4 and 10 years, particularly in the setting of prothrombic conditions (ie, protein C and S deficiencies, factor V defects) or with a history of transient synovitis, use of systemic corticosteroids, indolent onset of unilateral hip pain, is likely to have LCP, an avascular necrosis of the femoral head. An overweight early adolescent or a child with hypothyroidism or growth hormone deficiency who experiences acute or subacute onset of hip pain and antalgic gait may have SCFE, a growth-plate fracture of the hip that may require urgent surgical stabilization.

The Knee

When evaluating the child with isolated knee pain, it is critical to exclude both conditions that present with arthritis as well as the hip pathologies mentioned previously, each of which may present with referred pain to the knee. Anterior knee pain is common in the older child and adolescent and in the absence of point tenderness, laxity of knee stabilizers, and arthritis may be diagnosed as patellofemoral syndrome. The treatment of patellofemoral syndrome is conservative, with a period of rest, anti-inflammatory medications, and physical therapy. Osgood-Schlatter disease causes swelling and point tenderness at the proximal tibial tubercle unilaterally or bilaterally and may be diagnosed clinically based on examination. Acute ligamentous injuries are suggested by increased motion upon stress applied to knee stability, often accompanied by hemarthrosis. Meniscal injuries often cause pain, grinding, locking, or increased motion with internal and external rotation of the knee. Osteochondritis dissecans, an avascular necrosis of the knee, usually presents with pain worsened with activity or frequently associated with joint swelling, catching, or locking.

The Ankle and Foot

Acute foot pain in children is commonly caused by sprains and strains that resolve with rest and anti-inflammatory therapy, though significant swelling or point tenderness indicate evaluation for a fracture. Importantly, growth-plate fractures of the ankle will not be evident on plain radiographs and must be considered with point tenderness over the malleolus or if conservative management fails to produce improvement in 2 to 4 days. Chronic foot pain in children commonly results from overuse injuries. Achilles tendonitis causes tenderness over the Achilles tendon, and Sever disease causes tenderness over the calcaneus bone medially or laterally in late childhood or early adolescence. Both may be suspected based on history and physical examination findings and treated with reassurance, decreased activity, and appropriate footwear. Tarsal coalition may cause a flat foot and decreased range of motion, and accessory navicular or Kohler disease, an avascular necrosis of the navicular bone, may cause medial foot pain. All 3 conditions are diagnosed with radiographs. In a child with chronic foot pain not resolving with conservative management, stress fracture must be considered, often requiring a magnetic resonance imaging, bone scan, or orthopedic or sports medicine consultation.

The Legs

The etiology of pain localized to the bones of the legs varies, from referred hip pathology previously discussed to serious conditions such as osteomyelitis, myeloid cancers, and bone tumors to benign conditions such as growing pains. Osteomyelitis typically presents with pain worsening over several days to 1 to 2 weeks. In younger children, it may manifest as limp, refusal to bear weight, and refusal to move the affected area. With fever being variable and leukocytosis present in only 35% of cases, the strongest indicators of osteomyelitis are point tenderness at the site and an elevated ESR or CRP in 90% of cases (Evidence Level II-3). Bone tumors or malignancy should be suspected in the presence of visible swelling or point tenderness of the extremity, pain worse at night, systemic symptoms, or pathologic fracture. Sprains and strains are common, but fractures, intentional trauma, and complex regional pain syndrome (formerly termed *reflex sympathetic dystrophy*) must be considered in select cases. Perhaps the most common etiology, growing pains, may be empirically diagnosed in the school-aged child whose pain is bilateral, worse at night, not associated with swelling or systemic symptoms, and not interfering with daytime activity.

Upper Extremities

Pain in the upper extremities often parallels the etiologies already mentioned in the legs. Trauma is a common cause, including sprains, strains, fractures, and dislocations. In the younger child, intentional trauma must also be considered. Most common overuse injuries include shoulder pain from baseball, softball, tennis, and volleyball and elbow pain from baseball and tennis. Osteomyelitis and bone tumors, as discussed, remain important considerations, as does complex regional pain syndrome and carpal tunnel syndrome in the wrist. Several features of upper extremity injuries are unique to childhood.

Shoulder

Rotator cuff tears are rare in the pediatric population. Instead, shoulder injuries in infants and young children are more likely to be fractures through the proximal growth plates of the humerus, while shoulder dislocations occur commonly in older children and adolescents. Neurovascular integrity must be carefully assessed, and shoulder dislocations must be referred promptly for correction.

Elbow

School-aged children who fall onto an outstretched arm are at risk for a supracondylar fracture, which may appear on a radiograph only as a widened anterior fat pad ("sail sign") or as a visible posterior fat pad. Because of the potential for neurovascular compromise or compartment syndrome, the child's arm must be stabilized and referred urgently for orthopedic evaluation.

Wrist

In adolescents, tenderness and swelling over the anatomical snuff-box of the hand may be indicative of a scaphoid fracture, which requires immobilization in a cast even if the bony abnormality is not evident on a radiograph.

Generalized

Children and adolescents may present with generalized achiness and extremity pains not localized to a specific region. When accompanied by fever, bruising, or other systemic symptoms, bone pain is a common presentation of acute leukemia. Every such child warrants a complete blood count with differential, and many require further testing (eg, comprehensive metabolic panel, lactate dehydrogenase level, uric acid level, bone marrow examination) for evaluation of malignancy. Influenza, adenovirus, and other viral infections are well recognized causes of diffuse musculoskeletal pain, as is early disseminated Lyme disease or other tick-borne illnesses. Hypermobility syndromes such as Ehlers-Danlos syndrome and generalized joint hypermobility commonly cause nonspecific pain in the extremities, particularly when accompanied by hyperelastic skin, easy bruising, and atrophic scarring. The diagnosis of Ehlers-Danlos syndrome is established by a score of 5 out of 9 or higher on the Beighton scale and may be confirmed with genetic testing. Joint pain may be managed by a strengthening and joint protection exercise program offered by physical therapy.

Additional considerations for children with global pain include juvenile fibromyalgia syndrome, characterized by tender trigger points; sleep disturbance and physical inactivity; and also amplified musculoskeletal pain, characterized by a normal physical examination and lack of response to pain medications. These conditions may be managed by increased aerobic conditioning (including cognitive behavioral therapy), improved sleep hygiene, psychological counseling, and treatment of psychiatric comorbidities such as depression.

Conclusion

In summary, the causes of pain in the joints and extremities are diverse, and a thoughtful and organized approach to evaluation is necessary. Knowledge of common etiologies, ages of presentation, and location can be helpful. The presence or absence of arthritis should be the starting point for consideration, and further evaluation will depend upon the location of disease, age of the patient, history of presentation, and presence or absence of systemic symptoms. Suggested diagnostic evaluation and treatment for the conditions discussed in this chapter are listed in Table 33-1.

Table 33-1. Diagnostic Evaluation and Recommended Therapy for Selected Joint and Extremity Conditions

Condition	Diagnostic Evaluation	Treatment
Monoarthritis		
Septic arthritis	CBC, ESR, CRP concentration Joint aspiration for cell count and culture	Emergent joint aspiration Hospitalization and IV antibiotics
Lyme disease	Lyme ELISA with confirmatory Western blot	Oral antibiotics
Reactive arthritis	CBC, ESR, CRP concentration	Supportive care
JIA	CBC, ESR, CRP concentration +/− ANA +/− rheumatoid factor	Rheumatologic evaluation NSAIDs Disease-modifying anti-rheumatic drugs Steroid injections OT/PT
Polyarthritis		
Viral infections	CBC, ESR, CRP concentration Parvovirus titers EBV, CMV, rubella titers	Supportive care
JIA	CBC, ESR, CRP concentration +/− ANA +/− rheumatoid factor	Rheumatologic evaluation NSAIDs Disease-modifying anti-rheumatic drugs Steroid injections OT/PT
Rheumatic fever	CBC, ESR, CRP ECG, echocardiogram Anti-streptococcal antibodies	Antibiotics ASA, NSAIDs, +/− steroids Long-term antibiotic prophylaxis

Table 33-1 *(cont)*

Condition	Diagnostic Evaluation	Treatment
Extremity Pain		

Septic arthritis hip	CBC, ESR, CRP concentration
	Hip ultrasound
	Joint aspiration for cell
	  count and culture
		Emergent joint aspiration
		Hospitalization and IV
		  antibiotics

Transient synovitis	CBC, ESR, CRP concentration	NSAIDs Supportive care
Legg-Calvé-Perthes	X-ray MRI, bone scan	Orthopedic referral Brace, traction, PT +/− surgery
SCFE	X-ray	Emergent surgery
Patellofemoral syndrome	None	NSAIDs Rest, exercises, PT
Osgood-Schlatter disease	None	NSAIDs, cold compresses
Ligament injury knee	MRI	Rest Orthopedic evaluation +/− surgery
Meniscal injury knee	MRI	Rest Orthopedic evaluation +/− surgery
Osteochondritis dissecans	X-ray MRI	Rest Orthopedic evaluation +/− surgery

Overuse injury
  (of the ankle, elbow, or
  shoulder)
	None	Decrease activity
		Supportive care

Tarsal coalition	X-ray	Orthopedic or podiatry evaluation +/− surgery
Accessory navicular	X-ray	Orthopedic or podiatry evaluation +/− surgery
Kohler disease	X-ray	Rest Orthopedic or podiatry evaluation
Stress fracture	MRI Bone scan	Rest Cast, brace Gradual return to activity

Table 33-1 *(cont)*

Condition	Diagnostic Evaluation	Treatment
Extremity Pain		
Osteomyelitis	CBC, ESR, CRP concentration MRI Bone aspirate for culture	Orthopedic referral Hospitalization and IV antibiotics
Bone tumor	X-ray	Oncology or orthopedic referral
Shoulder dislocation	+/− x-ray	Urgent reduction
Supracondylar fracture	X-ray	Immobilization Urgent orthopedic evaluation
Hypermobility syndromes	Physical examination +/− genetic testing	Physical therapy Consider orthopedic or genetics referrals
Complex regional pain syndrome Juvenile fibromyalgia Amplified musculoskeletal pain	None	Referral for multidisciplinary intervention

Abbreviations: ANA, antinuclear antibody; ASA, acetylsalicylic acid (aspirin); CBC, complete blood count; CMV, cytomegalovirus; CRP, C-reactive protein; EBV, Epstein-Barr virus; ELISA, enzyme-linked immunosorbent assay; ESR, erythrocyte sedimentation rate; IV, intravenous; JIA, juvenile idiopathic arthritis; MRI, magnetic resonance imaging; NSAIDs, nonsteroidal anti-inflammatory drugs; OT, occupational therapy; PT, physical therapy; SCFE, slipped capital femoral epiphysis.

Suggested Reading

Berard R. Approach to the child with joint inflammation. *Pediatr Clin North Am.* 2012;59(2):245–262

Carson S, Woolridge DP, Colletti J, Kilgore K. Pediatric upper extremity injuries. *Pediatr Clin North Am.* 2006;53(1):41–67

Duey-Holtz AD, Collins SL, Hunt LB, Husske AM, Lange AM. Acute and non-acute lower extremity pain in the pediatric population: part I. *J Pediatr Health Care.* 2012;26(1):62–68

Duey-Holtz AD, Collins SL, Hunt LB, Cromwell PF. Acute and non-acute lower extremity pain in the pediatric population: part II. *J Pediatr Health Care.* 2012;26(3):216–230

Duey-Holtz AD, Collins SL, Hunt LB, Cromwell PF. Acute and non-acute lower extremity pain in the pediatric population: part III. *J Pediatr Health Care.* 2012;26(5):380–392

Frank G, Mahoney HM, Eppes SC. Musculoskeletal infections in children. *Pediatr Clin N Am.* 2005;52(4):1083–1106

Frick SL. Evaluation of the child who has hip pain. *Orthop Clin N Am.* 2006;37(2): 133–140

Gutierrez K. Bone and joint infections in children. *Pediatr Clin North Am.* 2005;52(3):779–794

John J, Chandran L. Arthritis in children and adolescents. *Pediatr Rev.* 2011;32(11): 470–480

Taekema HC, Landham PR, Maconochie I. Towards evidence based medicine for paediatricians. distinguishing between transient synovitis and septic arthritis in the limping child: how useful are clinical prediction tools? *Arch Dis Child.* 2009;94(2): 167–168

Tse SML, Laxer RM. Approach to acute limb pain in childhood. *Pediatr Rev.* 2006;27(5):170–180

CHAPTER 34

Lymphadenopathy

Chad Thomas Jacobsen, MD, MS

Key Points

- Lymphadenopathy is a common finding in children; it can be localized or generalized.

- Evaluation should be driven by the patient's history and physical examination, and children presenting with prolonged generalized lymphadenopathy or worrisome clinical features (eg, weight loss, protracted fevers, organomegaly, petechiae/bruising) will need a more extensive evaluation directed by findings.

- Benign, localized lymphadenopathy typically will regress by 4 to 6 weeks without intervention.

- Subacute/chronic bilateral cervical lymphadenitis is usually caused by Epstein-Barr virus or cytomegalovirus and should be managed symptomatically.

- Acute localized lymphadenitis with moderate to severe symptoms (eg, fever, overlying warmth, tenderness, or erythema or fluctuant lymph nodes) should be treated with empiric antibiotics directed against *Staphylococcus aureus* or group A streptococci. Patients with periodontal disease should have their coverage broadened to include anaerobes.

- Management of generalized lymphadenopathy should have therapy directed to the underlying etiology.

Overview

Lymphadenopathy, the presence of abnormally enlarged lymph nodes, is a very common finding in the pediatric practice. In most cases, these enlarged lymph nodes are benign; however, lymphadenopathy may be the first clue to a serious underlying illness.

The lymphatic system is comprised of lymph, lymphatic vessels, lymph nodes, the spleen, tonsils, adenoids, Peyer patches, and the thymus.

Lymph node enlargement can be caused by a number of factors. It can be caused by an appropriate response to antigenic stimulation within the node (reactive lymphadenopathy), infection of the node itself (lymphadenitis), swelling of the node caused by local cytokine release, deposit of foreign material within the histiocytic cells of the node (eg, in lipid storage disease), or malignant infiltration of the node itself.

In general, most "normal" lymph nodes are usually less than 1 cm in their longest diameter; the normal size limits of lymph nodes, however, can differ very much by their regional location. Lymph nodes in the axillary and cervical regions typically are up to 1 cm in size, whereas normal lymph nodes in the inguinal regions may be up to 1.5 cm and in the epitrochlear region, only up to 0.5 cm in size.

Approach to Adenopathy

The history obtained for patients with enlarged lymph nodes should focus on the patient's age, the time course of the adenopathy, associated symptoms, a thorough social history (including travel history, dietary history, and pets/animal contacts), a complete family history, concurrent medications, and a complete past medical history.

One clinic-based review noted that 44% of children younger than 5 years who were seen for well-child visits had lymphadenopathy, as did 64% of those seen for sick visits. Most of the children who were found to have adenopathy during sick visits were between the ages of 3 and 5 years.

The potential causes of lymphadenopathy can change significantly with age. For example, inguinal adenopathy in an adolescent may be caused by a sexually transmitted infection, whereas in younger children it is most likely caused by locoregional infection due to trauma. A pathologically enlarged cervical lymph node in an otherwise well-appearing patient is more likely to be Hodgkin lymphoma in an adolescent than in a child 3 to 5 years of age, as Hodgkin lymphoma is rarely seen before 10 years of age.

Benign enlarged lymph nodes typically show signs of regression within 4 to 6 weeks; therefore, nodes that have not decreased in size after 4 to 6 weeks warrant further investigation.

Associated findings/symptoms of weight loss (ie, greater than 10% of body weight), fevers, night sweats, and pruritus raise the concern of malignancy (in particular, lymphoma) and warrant a more immediate referral/evaluation by a subspecialist.

The history should also explore the patient's social history and should include any travel history (eg, to areas of endemic tuberculosis), a thorough dietary history (ie, consumption of uncooked meats, unprocessed cheese, and unpasteurized milk, as these foods can be associated with bacterial illnesses), and animal exposure (especially exposure to cats/kittens and the subsequent risk for cat-scratch disease). In addition, one should ask if any ill family members are in the household. A medication review should be performed, as lymphadenopathy has been noted to develop following the use of a number of medications; the lymphadenopathy is thought to be due to a hypersensitivity-like reaction to the offending medication (Box 34-1). Finally, adolescents should be questioned about sexual activity and other risk factors for human immuno-deficiency virus (HIV).

Box 34-1. Medications Associated With Lymphadenopathy

- Allopurinol
- Atenolol
- Captopril
- Carbamazepine
- Cephalosporins
- Gold
- Hydralazine
- Penicillins
- Phenytoin
- Primidone
- Pyrimethamine
- Quinidine
- Sulfonamides
- Sulindac

A complete physical examination is essential to developing the differential diagnosis for lymphadenopathy in a child and should include palpation of all areas that commonly present with lymphadenopathy, the location(s) of the enlarged node(s), the size and character of the enlarged node(s), the general appearance of the child, and a full general examination, including the abdominal examination.

A well-appearing child with an upper respiratory tract infection associated with a solitary enlarged lymph node is most likely to have reactive lymphadenopathy. An ill-appearing child with generalized adenopathy and associated systemic symptoms (eg, weight loss, fevers) is most likely to have a systemic illness (eg, infection, malignancy, inflammatory disorder).

Enlarged cervical lymph nodes are often associated with infections of the head and neck. Enlarged supraclavicular lymph nodes are usually pathologic and require immediate evaluation. Supraclavicular lymph nodes that are palpated on the right are typically associated with tumors or infections involving the mediastinum; those palpable on the left are typically associated with intra-abdominal malignancy (usually lymphoma). Unilaterally enlarged epitrochlear lymph nodes are usually the result of infection involving that hand or arm. Bilaterally enlarged epitrochlear lymph nodes are more likely due to systemic illness and require further evaluation. Enlarged inguinal lymph nodes are common in children and are most often caused by frequent occurrence of minor trauma and infections in the lower extremities. Significant inguinal adenopathy (eg, greater than 2.5 cm in diameter), however, may indicate the presence of a sexually transmitted infection, a urinary tract infection, lymphoma, or an abdominal tumor.

Generalized lymphadenopathy is defined as lymphadenopathy that is present in 2 or more noncontiguous regions. It is often one of many clinical features in a number of systemic diseases (Table 34-1).

Table 34-1. Causes of Generalized Lymphadenopathy in Children

Infectious	
Bacterial	Brucellosis, group A streptococcal infection, leptospirosis, tularemia
Fungal	Blastomycosis, coccidioidomycosis
Parasitic	Leishmaniasis, malaria, toxoplasmosis
Spirochetal	Lyme disease, syphilis
Viral	Adenovirus, Epstein-Barr virus, cytomegalovirus, hepatitis B virus, herpes simplex virus, human immunodeficiency virus, rubella, rubeola, varicella-zoster virus
Noninfectious	
Drugs	Allopurinol, atenolol, captopril, carbamazepine, cephalosporins, gold, hydralazine, penicillins, phenytoin, primidone, pyrimethamine, quinidine, sulfonamides, sulindac
Immunologic	Chronic granulomatous disease, Kawasaki disease, serum sickness, vasculitis syndromes (eg, systemic lupus erythematosus, rheumatoid arthritis)
Malignant	Acute lymphocytic leukemia or acute myelogenous leukemia, Hodgkin lymphoma, non-Hodgkin lymphoma, neuroblastoma, rhabdomyosarcoma
Metabolic	Gaucher disease, Niemann-Pick disease
Other	Kikuchi disease, Langerhans cell histiocytosis, Rosai-Dorfman disease, sarcoidosis

It has been shown that the risk of malignancy increases with increasing size of the lymph node, with cervical lymph nodes that are greater than 2 cm in maximal diameter being at greater risk for the presence of malignant disease.

Benign lymph nodes are typically soft, compressible, and freely mobile. Tender lymphadenopathy is most frequently caused by infection, particularly if there is overlying erythema, warmth, induration, or fluctuation. Hard, matted, immobile and nontender nodes are often found in malignancy or with prior inflammatory disease that resulted in fibrosis of the nodes. Firm, rubbery, nontender nodes are often associated with lymphoma.

Differential Diagnosis

Localized Lymphadenopathy

Cervical lymphadenopathy is particularly common in the school-aged child, and the differential diagnosis is expansive (Table 34-2). One recommended approach to considering patients who present with swollen lymph nodes of the neck is to distinguish between acute (several days) and subacute/chronic (over weeks to months) lymphadenopathy and whether the adenopathy is unilateral or bilateral.

Table 34-2. Causes of Cervical Lymphadenitis in Children

Infectious	
Bacterial	Anaerobic bacteria, *Bartonella henselae*, group A streptococci, group B streptococci, mycobacterium, nontuberculous mycobacteria, *Pasteurella multocida*, *Staphylococcus aureus*, tularemia, *Yersinia pestis*
Fungal	Aspergillosis, histoplasmosis
Parasitic	Toxoplasmosis
Viral	Adenovirus, cytomegalovirus, enterovirus, Epstein-Barr virus, herpes simplex virus, hepatitis B virus, human immunodeficiency virus, parvovirus, rubella, rubeola, roseola, varicella-zoster virus
Noninfectious	
Immunologic	Juvenile idiopathic arthritis, systemic lupus erythematosus
Malignancy	Leukemia, lymphoma, neuroblastoma, rhabdomyosarcoma, thyroid cancer
Miscellaneous	Kawasaki disease, Kikuchi disease, histiocytosis, sarcoidosis

Acute bilateral cervical lymphadenopathy is most commonly caused by a self-limited viral process (eg, influenza, adenovirus, parainfluenza, rhinovirus, enterovirus). Most patients will present with current or recent concerns of nasal congestion, rhinorrhea, or a sore throat. The lymph nodes associated with this illness typically are small, rubbery, and mobile and minimally tender. The clinical course is self-limited, but the adenopathy may persist for several weeks.

Bacterial infections of the oropharynx can also lead to acute bilateral cervical lymphadenitis. The pathogen most commonly responsible for acute bilateral cervical lymphadenitis is group A streptococci (GAS). These patients typically present with bilaterally enlarged, tender, and non-erythematous cervical lymph nodes, a sore throat, and occasionally a sandpaper-like skin rash or erythematous tonsils with palatal petechiae. These patients should be further evaluated for GAS by throat culture or rapid antigen detection.

Other causes of acute bilateral cervical lymphadenitis may include herpes simplex virus (presenting as primary gingivostomatitis with lymphadenitis), Epstein-Barr virus (EBV), or cytomegalovirus (CMV). Epstein-Barr virus and cytomegalovirus usually cause generalized lymphadenopathy but may occasionally present with acute bilateral cervical lymphadenitis.

Acute unilateral cervical lymphadenitis occurs much less frequently than acute bilateral cervical lymphadenitis and is usually caused by bacterial infections. Up to 80% of cases of acute unilateral cervical lymphadenitis are caused by either *Staphylococcus aureus* or group A streptococcal infections. Most of these cases occur in younger children (ie, younger than 5 years) who appear nontoxic. The involved lymph nodes typically are tender, warm, erythematous, and poorly mobile. Up to one-third of infected nodes may suppurate and become fluctuant. The management of these nodes will be described later in the chapter.

Cervical lymphadenitis in the newborn and young infant is most frequently caused by late-onset infection with group B streptococci. These infants are typically between 3 and 7 weeks of age, male, febrile, and irritable. The involved lymph nodes are typically tender and erythematous and have ill-defined margins.

Acute unilateral cervical lymphadenitis in patients with evidence of periodontal disease is usually caused by an infection with anaerobic bacteria. The involved lymph nodes are indistinguishable from those infected with GAS or *S aureus*.

Tularemia is a febrile zoonotic disease caused by the organism *Francisella tularensis* that can also present with acute unilateral cervical lymphadenitis.

Subacute/chronic bilateral lymphadenitis is most frequently caused by EBV or CMV. Epstein-Barr virus typically presents as infectious mononucleosis, which is characterized by fever, exudative pharyngitis, lymphadenopathy, and hepatosplenomegaly.

Subacute/chronic unilateral lymphadenitis in children is usually caused by infections with nontuberculous mycobacteria (NTM) or *Bartonella henselae,* the causative agent of cat-scratch disease. It is less commonly due to tuberculosis or toxoplasmosis.

Cat-scratch disease is caused by infection with *B henselae* following a cat bite or scratch. Enlargement of the lymph node draining the site of inoculation occurs anywhere from 1 to 9 weeks following the scratch. The affected nodes are typically warm and tender and slightly erythematous.

Pediatric infection with *Mycobacterium tuberculosis* is rare in the United States, with involvement of the cervical nodes usually caused by extension from the paratracheal lymph nodes. Toxoplasmosis is typically transmitted by ingestion of poorly cooked meat (particularly lamb or pork) that contains cysts from *Toxoplasma gondii* or by contact with mature oocysts from soil, litter boxes, or contaminated food. The nodes most typically affected are the anterior and posterior cervical and axillary ones. They are sometimes tender, are typically non-fluctant, and may persist for months.

Other important noninfectious causes of cervical lymphadenitis may include malignancy (eg, acute leukemia, lymphoma) or connective tissue disease (eg, juvenile idiopathic arthritis, systemic lupus erythematosus). Other potential causes can include Kawasaki disease, Langerhans cell histiocytosis, Kikuchi disease (tender cervical lymphadenopathy and fever of unknown etiology), Rosai-Dorfman disease, autoimmune lymphoproliferative disorder, and sarcoidosis.

As noted earlier, supraclavicular lymphadenopathy is strongly suspicious for malignancy when noted in children. Right-sided supraclavicular adenopathy is usually associated with cancer involving the mediastinum, while left-sided supraclavicular adenopathy is often associated with intra-abdominal malignancy (eg, lymphoma). Patients with identified supraclavicular adenopathy warrant immediate referral to a pediatric oncologist for further evaluation.

Axillary lymphadenopathy is most often due to infections involving the arm, thoracic wall, or breast. Cat-scratch disease is one of the more common causes of axillary lymphadenopathy in children.

Unilateral epitrochlear lymphadenopathy (ie, epitrochlear nodes greater than 0.5 cm in diameter) is most frequently associated with infections of the hand or forearm. Bilateral epitrochlear lymphadenopathy, however, is very unusual and is concerning for an underlying malignancy.

Finally, inguinal lymphadenopathy in children is not usually associated with a specific etiology unless the lymph nodes are quite large (ie, >3 cm). Possible etiologies include sexually transmitted infections, acute leukemia, and lymphoma.

Generalized Lymphadenopathy

Generalized lymphadenopathy is defined as enlargement of lymph nodes in 2 or more noncontiguous regions. It is not seen as often as localized lymphadenopathy in the pediatric practice and can be the first sign of a serious underlying systemic illness. The possible etiologies of generalized lymphadenopathy in children are listed in Table 34-1, and several of these will be discussed next.

Systemic infection with bacterial or viral pathogens is the most common cause of generalized lymphadenopathy in children. Common causes include EBV and CMV. Measles and rubella are also potential causes and should be considered in unimmunized children or those who have come from areas of the world where these illnesses are endemic.

Primary infection with HIV can be associated with generalized lymphadenopathy during the acute symptomatic phase of HIV infection. It usually involves the cervical, occipital, and axillary regions in the setting of fever and malaise. The involved lymph nodes are typically nontender. These enlarged lymph nodes may persist for some time beyond the acute phase while other symptoms of chronic infection develop.

Serum sickness presents with generalized lymphadenopathy along with fever, arthralgias, malaise, pruritus, and rash. The enlarged lymph nodes are typically tender in character. Several medications have been associated with serum sickness and include carbamazepine, cephalosporins, penicillins, phenytoin, and sulfonamides. A more comprehensive list of medications associated with adenopathy can be found in Box 23-1.

Autoimmune diseases such as systemic lupus erythematosus, juvenile idiopathic arthritis, and dermatomyositis can cause generalized lymphadenopathy. The nodes are typically nontender and discrete and vary in size from 0.5 cm to several centimeters in diameter.

Malignancy is another rare, but important, consideration when evaluating someone with generalized lymphadenopathy. Malignancy should be high on the differential diagnosis in patients who also present with weight loss (>10% of body weight), generalized adenopathy without a clear cause, fevers, lack of upper respiratory tract infection symptoms, and an abnormal complete blood count (CBC) or chest radiograph. Acute leukemia is the most common pediatric malignancy and may present with generalized lymphadenopathy that is usually nontender and has developed rapidly. Other associated features may include fever, pallor, petechiae/bruising, or hepatosplenomegaly. Lymphomas may also present with regional or generalized lymphadenopathy. Other malignancies that may have associated regional lymph node enlargement include rhabdomyosarcoma and neuroblastoma.

Diagnostic Evaluation

In most cases of acute localized lymphadenopathy, no laboratory or imaging studies will be needed and these patients can be observed over 4 to 6 weeks if no features of malignancy are on either the history or physical examination. In cases when worrisome features on history or physical examination are present, extensive testing may be indicated.

Acute cervical lymphadenopathy accompanied by pharyngitis in children older than 2 years may require a throat culture or rapid antigen screen. Patients who also present with hepatomegaly or splenomegaly should be further evaluated for EBV. These patients should also be tested for a CBC with differential and EBV titers (or monospot test in patients older than 8 years).

Patients with acute cervical adenopathy with respiratory symptoms, prolonged cervical lymphadenopathy, or supraclavicular adenopathy warrant further laboratory and radiographic evaluation. These patients should undergo a CBC with differential diagnosis along with a chest radiograph (to evaluate for mediastinal or hilar adenopathy) as part of their initial evaluation. In addition, placement of a tuberculin skin test (TST) should be considered.

Children suspected of having bacterial lymphadenitis should first undergo an empiric course of antibiotics (first- or second-generation cephalosporin) and be reevaluated in 2 weeks. If there is no response to therapy, those patients should have further testing with a CBC/differential, have a TST placed, and have their antibiotic coverage broadened. Other serologic testing (eg, *B henselae,* tularemia, toxoplasmosis) may need to be obtained at that time as indicated by a repeat history and examination. If still no response (or if enlarging despite therapy) over the next 2 weeks, they should be referred for biopsy.

Children presenting with prolonged generalized lymphadenopathy or worrisome clinical features (ie, weight loss, protracted fevers, organomegaly, petechiae/bruising) will need a more extensive evaluation directed to findings on the clinician's history and physical examination. Basic evaluation should include a chest radiograph, a test for CBC with a differential, liver function tests, a test for erythrocyte sedimentation rate (ESR), a test for lactate dehydrogenase concentration (can be a marker of malignancy), and placement of a TST. Human immunodeficiency virus, EBV, CMV assays may need to be obtained in some children. Patients with suspected malignancy should be referred to a pediatric oncologist for further evaluation, which may include biopsy of a suspicious lymph node or bone marrow aspiration and biopsy. Patients with suspected autoimmune disorders, such as systemic lupus erythematosus, should have serologic screening that includes an antinuclear antibody panel and anti-double-stranded DNA antibody.

Biopsy should be considered for patients whose lymph nodes show continued progression or lack of any regression after 4 to 6 weeks of observation or empiric therapy. In addition, it should be considered immediately in patients with an enlarged supraclavicular lymph node and for patients with findings concerning for malignancy. For patients with multiple enlarged lymph nodes, most experts have recommended excisional biopsy of the largest and most abnormal lymph node, preferably in the supraclavicular or lower cervical chain (if abnormal) as those are often associated with the highest yield for diagnostic information (Evidence Level III).

Management

Acute Cervical Lymphadenopathy

Children with isolated acute cervical lymphadenopathy less than 1 cm in diameter without associated concerning clinical symptoms or findings can be observed clinically over a 4- to 6-week period (Evidence Level III). Children with nodes between 1 and 3 cm in diameter that are concerning for bacterial lymphadenitis (eg, associated tenderness, warmth, erythema) should receive an empiric 10- to 14-day course of oral antibiotics that cover streptococcal and staphylococcal infections (Evidence Level III). Children with concomitant periodontal disease should have their antibiotic coverage broadened to include anaerobic organisms (Evidence Level III). Most patients should have a clinical response within 2 to 3 days from the initiation of antimicrobial therapy.

Children with fevers and nodes that are fluctuant should be referred for ultrasonography to identify a possible abscess which may require incision and drainage. Those with acute unilateral cervical lymphadenitis who appear toxic should be referred for bacterial cultures, consideration of incision and drainage of the inflamed node, and empiric coverage with parenteral antibiotics (Evidence Level III).

Children with lymph node enlargement greater than 3 cm in diameter, those who have had no decrease in size of their lymph nodes after 4 to 6 weeks, those who fail to respond to antibiotic therapy, and those with systemic symptoms (eg, fever, weight loss, hepatosplenomegaly) should be referred for excisional biopsy to further evaluate the adenopathy.

Subacute/Chronic Unilateral Cervical Lymphadenopathy

Subacute/chronic unilateral cervical lymphadenitis is usually caused by NTM infections or those of *B henselae*, the causative agent of cat-scratch disease.

Some experts have recommended only symptomatic treatment in immuno-competent patients with cat-scratch disease; those with painful, suppurative lymph nodes may need fine needle aspiration for symptomatic relief.

Immunocompetent children with NTM or suspected NTM lymphadenitis who have no evidence of pulmonary or disseminated disease may be treated with surgical excision without antimicrobial therapy as the first-line therapy, as surgical excision is both diagnostic and curative (Evidence Level I). Incision and drainage should be avoided because of the high risk of developing a chronic draining sinus tract and increased risk of recurrence.

Children with NTM or suspected NTM lymphadenitis who are not candidates for surgical excision (eg, those with an established draining sinus tract or who are at risk for a poor neurologic outcome such as facial nerve damage) may be offered empirical antimicrobial therapy with a macrolide in combination with either a rifamycin (rifampin or rifabutin) or ethambutol (Evidence Level I). This approach has been shown to be moderately successful but may be associated with risk for the development of a fistulous sinus tract. The optimal duration of antimicrobial therapy is unknown, but many experts recommend that patients receive therapy until their symptoms resolve, usually within 3 to 6 months (Evidence Level III).

Subacute/Chronic Bilateral Cervical Lymphadenitis

Most cases of subacute/chronic bilateral cervical lymphadenitis are caused by viral infections (eg, EBV, CMV) and should be managed symptomatically.

Axillary Lymphadenopathy

Axillary adenopathy in children is most commonly due to regional infections, including cat-scratch disease. Patients with adenopathy thought to be second-ary to cat-scratch disease may be observed and treated symptomatically. Those with adenopathy secondary to a regional infection should receive a 10- to 14-day course of empiric antibiotics covering staphylococcal and streptococcal infections. Children with concerning systemic symptoms (eg, weight loss, protracted fevers, organomegaly, petechiae/bruising) should receive a chest radiograph and referral for further evaluation/excisional biopsy.

Inguinal Lymphadenopathy

Inguinal lymphadenopathy in children is usually not associated with a specific etiology unless the nodes are very large (>3 cm). Those with large, tender lymph nodes and no history of sexual activity should receive a 10- to-14 day course of empiric antibiotics covering staphylococcal and streptococcal infections. Those with large lymph nodes and a history of sexual activity should be further evaluated for sexually transmitted infections and have their therapy directed by their work-up.

Generalized Lymphadenopathy

Patients with generalized lymphadenopathy should have a detailed evaluation as detailed. Therapy should be directed to the underlying etiology of their disease.

Suggested Reading

Friedmann AM. Evaluation and management of lymphadenopathy in children. *Pediatr Rev.* 2008;29(2):53–60

Henry M, Kamat D. Integrating basic science into clinical teaching initiative series: approach to lymphadenopathy. *Clin Pediatr (Phila).* 2011;50(8):683–687

Loeffler AM. Treatment options for nontuberculous mycobacterial adenitis in children. *Pediatr Infect Dis J.* 2004;23(10):957–958

Nield LS, Kamat D. Lymphadenopathy in children: when and how to evaluate. *Clin Pediatr.* 2004;43(1):25–33

Rajasekaran K, Krakovitz P. Enlarged lymph nodes in children. *Pediatr Clin N Am.* 2013;60(4):923–936

Stutchfield CJ, Tyrrell J. Evaluation of lymphadenopathy in children. *Paediatr Child Health.* 2012;22(3):98–102

Timmerman MK, Morley AD, Buwalda J. Treatment of non-tuberculous mycobacterial cervicofacial Lymphadenitis in children: critical appraisal of the literature. *Clin Otolaryngol.* 2008;33(6):546–552

CHAPTER 35

Neonatal Hyperbilirubinemia

Keri A. Marques, MD

Key Points

- Neonatal hyperbilirubinemia is a common disorder that affects approximately 60% of all full-term infants.

- Physiologic jaundice of the newborn differs from pathologic causes of neonatal hyperbilirubinemia, which includes an extensive differential and may require further diagnostic evaluation.

- All infants should be routinely monitored for jaundice. Laboratory evaluation is indicated if jaundice is present within the first 24 hours of life.

- Acute bilirubin encephalopathy can occur with severe hyperbilirubinemia, leading to chronic and permanent sequelae for the infant. Therefore, pathologic bilirubin levels should be monitored until stable or trending downward.

- Assessment of each infant's risk for developing hyperbilirubinemia should be completed by obtaining transcutaneous bilirubin or serum total bilirubin measurements or by assessing the infant's clinical risk factors prior to discharge from the nursery.

Overview

Neonatal hyperbilirubinemia is a common disorder affecting approximately 60% of all full-term infants. While most cases of neonatal hyperbilirubinemia are benign, severe hyperbilirubinemia can occur and result in permanent central nervous system damage.

Causes and Differential Diagnosis

Neonates produce 2 to 3 times the amount of bilirubin than that of an adult because of an increased production and decreased uptake of bilirubin, which is compounded by decreased conjugation and excretion of bilirubin in the immature systems of a neonate. Production of bilirubin is increased due to the presence of an increased number and turnover of red blood cells. These normal alterations in the neonate's physiology lead to a transient increase in unconjugated bilirubin level, which is termed *physiologic jaundice*. Physiologic jaundice peaks between 48 and 96 hours for a full-term infant with total serum bilirubin levels most commonly remaining under 15 mg/dL. The peak can be delayed in a near-term infant. Physiologic jaundice usually resolves by the end of the first week of life; however, this can be slightly prolonged in infants of Asian decent.

There are several pathologic causes for both unconjugated and conjugated neonatal hyperbilirubinemia (Boxes 35-1 and 35-2). Any jaundice in the first 24 hours of life is considered pathologic and requires further investigation for a pathologic cause. In addition, evaluation for pathologic hyperbilirubinemia should be done if the total serum bilirubin is crossing percentiles or exceeds 0.2 mg/dL per hour.

Box 35-1. Indirect Hyperbilirubinemia

Increased Production of Bilirubin or Increased Load on the Liver	Decreased Clearance of Bilirubin
Hemolytic immune mediated: Coombs positive ■ Rh disease ■ ABO incompatibility ■ Minor blood group incompatibilities **Heritable disorders** **Red blood cell membrane defects** ■ Hereditary spherocytosis, elliptocytosis, pyropoikilocytosis, stomatocytosis **Red blood cell enzyme deficiencies** ■ Glucose-6 phosphate dehydrogenase deficiency[b] ■ Pyruvate deficiency ■ Other erythrocyte enzyme deficiencies **Hemoglobinopathies** ■ Alpha-thalassemia ■ Beta-thalassemia **Unstable hemoglobins** ■ Congenital Heinz body hemolytic anemia **Increased enterohepatic circulation** ■ Breast milk jaundice ■ Pyloric stenosis[b] ■ Small or large bowel obstruction or ileus **Other** ■ Sepsis[a] ■ Disseminated intravascular coagulation ■ Extravasation of blood: hematomas, pulmonary, abdominal, cerebral, or other occult hemorrhage ■ Polycythemia ■ Macrosomic infant of diabetic mothers	**Inborn errors of metabolism** ■ Crigler-Najjar syndrome, types I and II ■ Gilbert syndrome ■ Galactosemia[a] ■ Tyrosinemia[a] ■ Hypermethioninemia[a] **Metabolic** ■ Hypothyroidism ■ Hypopituitarism[a] **Other** ■ Prematurity ■ Glucose-6 phosphate dehydrogenase deficiency[b] ■ Pyloric stenosis

[a] Can cause both direct and indirect hyperbilirubinemia.

[b] Decreased clearance and increased production/load on liver are part of pathogenesis.

From Maisels MJ. Jaundice. In: MacDonald MG, Seshia MMK, Mullet MD, eds. *Neonatology: Pathophysiology and Management of the Newborn*. 6th ed. Philadelphia, PA: Lippincott Williams & Wilkins; 2005:798, with permission.

Box 35-2. Direct Hyperbilirubinemia

Sepsis[a]
TORCH (toxoplasmosis, other pathogens, rubella, cytomegalovirus, and herpes simplex)
Shock/hypovolemia
Enterovirus, varicella, echovirus, adenovirus, and *parvovirus B19*
Prolonged total parental nutrition
Hypothyroidism
Hypopituitarism[a]
Galactosemia[a]
Fructosemia
Tyrosinemia[a]
Hypermethioninemia[a]
Cystic fibrosis
Alpha$_1$-antitrypsin deficiency
Choledochal cyst
Extrahepatic biliary atresia
Nonsyndromic paucity of interlobar bile ducts
Congenital hepatic fibrosis
Progressive familial intrahepatic cholestasis types 1–3
Inspissated bile/mucus plug
Cholelithiasis
Tumor/mass
Neonatal sclerosing cholangitis
Spontaneous perforation of the bile ducts
Intestinal obstruction
Alagille syndrome
Disorders of lipid metabolism or bile metabolism
Mitochondrial disorders
Citrin deficiency
Gestational alloimmune liver disease
Idiopathic neonatal hepatitis

[a] Can cause both direct and indirect hyperbilirubinemia.

One of the most common causes of early pathologic hyperbilirubinemia is immune mediated hemolytic disease from ABO incompatibility. If an incompatibility is present, the infant's blood type will be either A or B and must also have a positive Coombs test.

Major blood group Rh and minor blood groups (Kell, Duffy, MNS system, and P system) can also cause alloimmune hemolytic disease of the newborn in utero, which can result in hydrops fetalis. Rh disease is associated with the most severe form of immune mediated hemolytic disease. If the mother does not have a transfusion history, Rh disease will not occur for the first pregnancy, but the mother will remain at risk for subsequent pregnancies and should receive prophylaxis.

Sepsis should always be considered as a cause for early hyperbilirubinemia in an infant and can result in indirect or direct hyperbilirubinemia. Urinary tract infection can be associated with unexplained hyperbilirubinemia in the first week of life and may result in an elevation of direct bilirubin. The infant may not present with typical symptoms of urinary tract infection; therefore, a urinalysis and urine culture should be included if there is an elevation of direct bilirubin (Table 35-1).

Table 35-1. Laboratory Evaluation for Jaundiced Infant of 35 or More Weeks' Gestation

Indications	Assessments
Jaundice in first 24 hours of life	Measure TcB and/or TSB
Jaundice appears excessive for infant's age	Measure TcB and/or TSB
Infant receiving phototherapy or TSB rising rapidly (ie, crossing percentiles and unexplained by history and physical examination)	Blood type and Coombs test Complete blood count and smear Option to perform reticulocyte count, G6PD, and ETCO, if available Repeat TSB in 4–24 hours depending on infant's age and TSB level
TSB concentration approaching exchange levels or not responding to phototherapy	Perform reticulocyte count, G6PD, albumin, ETCO, if available
Elevated direct bilirubin level	Do urinalysis and urine culture. Evaluate for sepsis if indicated by history and physical examination.
Jaundice present at or beyond 3 weeks of age or sick infant	Total and direct bilirubin level If direct bilirubin level is elevated, evaluate for cholestasis Check results of newborn galactosemia and thyroid screen, evaluate for signs and symptoms of hypothyroidism

Abbreviations: ETCO, end-tidal carbon dioxide; G6PD, glucose-6 phosphate dehydrogenase; TcB, transcutaneous bilirubin; TSB, total serum bilirubin.

From Maisels MJ, Baltz RD, Bhutani V, et al. Management of hyperbilirubinemia in the newborn infant 35 or More Weeks of Gestation. *Pediatrics.* 2004;114:297.

Glucose-6 phosphate dehydrogenase (G6PD) deficiency is an X-linked disorder and a common cause of pathologic neonatal hyperbilirubinemia. It usually presents with high total serum bilirubin level requiring treatment, often with an exchange transfusion. Approximately 30% of cases of kernicterus in the United States are associated with G6PD deficiency. Vitamin K, which is routinely given after delivery, may trigger hemolysis for an infant with class I G6PD deficiency. Testing for G6PD deficiency should be performed for a jaundiced infant receiving phototherapy with a suspicious family history or ethnic background for G6PD and also for any jaundiced infant having a poor response to phototherapy. G6PD testing may have a false-negative result if there is significant hemolysis at the time of testing and therefore should be repeated at 3 months after the hemolytic episode if strongly suspected. Not all infants with

G6PD and jaundice will have overt hemolysis, as there is also decreased ability to conjugate bilirubin resulting in high indirect bilirubin levels.

Breastfeeding jaundice occurs in the first week of life and results from decreased caloric and volume intake due to inadequate maternal milk supply. These infants can present with weight loss and hypovolemia and may require inpatient treatment with phototherapy and hydration. Infants receiving phototherapy should continue to breastfeed, if at all possible, but may require supplementation with expressed human milk or formula until breastfeeding is well established. Breastfeeding jaundice differs from breast milk jaundice, which is a common cause of prolonged jaundice in the newborn, presenting in the second to third weeks of life. Halting breastfeeding for 24 hours will improve the hyperbilirubinemia in the case of breast milk jaundice; however, interruption of breastfeeding is not routinely recommended. With breastfeeding jaundice, the total serum bilirubin level is often not high enough to require phototherapy.

Some inborn errors of metabolism can cause decreased clearance of bilirubin and therefore present with jaundice in the newborn period. Examples of disorders that are included in newborn screening programs that can cause jaundice include congenital hypothyroidism, galactosemia, and tyrosinemia.

Congenital hypothyroidism (CH) is a cause of prolonged jaundice in a newborn. Initial signs and symptoms of congenital hypothyroidism at birth can be subtle or even absent. This is because of residual circulating transplacental maternal T4 and often combined with inadequate functioning thyroid tissue. Common clinical signs of CH include feeding difficulties, prolonged jaundice, hoarse cry, constipation, dry skin, hypothermia, lethargy, large fontanels, macroglossia, abdominal distension with an umbilical hernia, and hypotonia. Some infants with thyroid dyshormonogenesis may have a goiter present at birth. Congenital hypothyroidism is associated with increased risk of congenital anomalies of the heart, kidneys, urinary tract, and gastrointestinal and skeletal systems.

Galactosemia is an autosomal recessive disorder involving decreased activity of galactose-1-phosphate uridyl transferase (GALT). The most common signs and symptoms for an infant with classic galactosemia include jaundice, hepatomegaly, feeding difficulties, poor weight gain, vomiting, diarrhea, lethargy, hypoglycemia, hypotonia, cataracts, encephalopathy, full fontanelle, and bleeding or excessive bruising. Infants with galactosemia may have liver dysfunction, renal dysfunction, hemolytic anemia, and septicemia. Septicemia is commonly secondary to *Escherichia coli*. If a diagnosis of galactosemia is suspected, any human milk, human-derived formula, or bovine-derived formula should immediately be discontinued and replaced with a soy-based formula. Lactose-free formulas should not be used, as they have not been proven to be safe in this population. Continue a galactose-free diet until the diagnosis is confirmed, and then refer the patient to a center with pediatric and dietary specialties.

Any jaundice that persists for more than 3 weeks in duration is considered prolonged jaundice. Any infant with prolonged jaundice should be evaluated for neonatal cholestasis by obtaining a direct and total serum bilirubin level (see Table 24-1). The most common cause for unconjugated prolonged jaundice at 2 weeks of age is benign breast milk jaundice. If the unconjugated bilirubin is markedly elevated, other causes of indirect bilirubin should be considered (see Box 24-1). An elevated direct bilirubin level indicates neonatal cholestasis and is defined as a direct bilirubin level greater than 1.0 mg/dL when the total serum bilirubin level is less than 5.0 mg/dL or a direct bilirubin greater than 20% of the total serum bilirubin when the total is greater than 5.0 mg/dL.

Biliary atresia is a cause of neonatal cholestasis that requires prompt diagnosis and surgical treatment. Patients with biliary atresia usually present with prolonged jaundice, dark urine, pale-colored stools, and hepatospleno-megaly. They may also have coagulopathy due to malabsorption of vitamin K, which can lead to an intracranial bleeding.

Clinical Features

Jaundice is defined as yellow tinting of the skin due to deposition of bilirubin in the skin and subcutaneous tissue. Neonatal jaundice usually presents in a cephalocaudal pattern and can include yellow tinting of the sclera and mucus membranes. Applying light pressure to the skin with a finger can help reveal jaundice on physical examination. Physical examination should also include evaluation for an extravascular collection of blood, such as a cephalohematoma, pallor, bruising, and hepatosplenomegaly, as the presence of these findings can increase the risk of developing hyperbilirubinemia.

Acute bilirubin encephalopathy (ABE) describes the acute manifestations that occur because of severe hyperbilirubinemia and then progresses into kernicterus, a chronic and permanent stage of sequelae. Acute bilirubin encephalopathy presents in 3 stages: initial, intermediate, and advanced. Initial symptoms of ABE include slight stupor, hypotonia, poor suck, and high-pitched cry. Clinical features of the intermediate phase include moderate stupor with irritability, tone variability that is usually increased with retrocollis-opisthoto-nos, minimal feeding, and high-pitched cry. The advanced stage of ABE includes deep stupor or coma, hypertonia with retrocollis-opisthotonos, no feeding, and a shrill cry.

Transition from the acute phase to kernicterus, the chronic phase, occurs during the first year of life. These infants will have residual difficulties with feeding, motor delay, and increased reflexes with hypotonia and will continue to have a high-pitched cry. The infants go on to develop choreoathetoid cerebral palsy, sensorineural hearing loss, dental enamel dysplasia, and gaze abnormali-ties. Hypotonia is present until school age and then progresses into hypertonia in the teenage years. Cognitive function is usually spared.

Evaluation and Management

Management of jaundice in the newborn nursery requires the physician to use a systemic assessment of the risk for severe hyperbilirubinemia, close follow-up, and prompt intervention when needed. The American Academy of Pediatrics (AAP) has published recommendations that help guide physicians through management of neonatal hyperbilirubinemia for neonates 35 or more weeks in gestation.

All neonates should be routinely monitored for jaundice and assessed along with the infant's vital signs at least every 8 to 12 hours. If jaundice is present on examination and the neonate is younger than 24 hours of age, a measurement of total serum bilirubin (TSB) or a transcutaneous bilirubin (TcB) is needed. The results of the TSB or TcB should be interpreted using the hourly nomogram for designation of risk. If the bilirubin is above the 95th percentile, further evaluation for a cause of the hyperbilirubinemia is required. Laboratory evaluation for the jaundiced neonate in the nursery is summarized in Table 24-1.

TcB is a quick and useful tool in the newborn nursery and should correlate well with an institution's total serum bilirubin levels. In some situations, a TcB should be confirmed with a TSB, and an hourly TcB nomogram for healthy infants can be useful (Figure 35-1)

If the total serum bilirubin is elevated, treatment may be indicated. There are 2011 AAP guidelines of when to initiate treatment of phototherapy and exchange transfusion for neonates who are 35 or more weeks' gestation. These guidelines require the assessment of risk factors, which include gestational age, presence of isoimmune hemolytic disease, G6PD deficiency, asphyxia, significant lethargy, temperature instability, sepsis, acidosis, or albumin less than 3.0 mg/dL.

When a TSB level is at exchange level, the infant needs to be immediately admitted directly to a pediatric hospital service and should not go through the emergency department; this only delays the initiation of intensive phototherapy and exchange transfusion. Exchange transfusion should be done for any patient who presents with jaundice and signs consistent with intermediate or advanced stages of ABE. If an exchange transfusion is being considered, a bilirubin-albumin ratio can be measured and used along with the TSB level to help determine the need for an exchange transfusion.

Intravenous immunoglobulin has been shown to decrease the need for exchange transfusion with ABO or Rh isoimmune hemolytic disease. Administration of intravenous immunoglobulin is recommended if the TBS is rising despite phototherapy or if the TSB is within 2 mg/dL of exchange transfusion level.

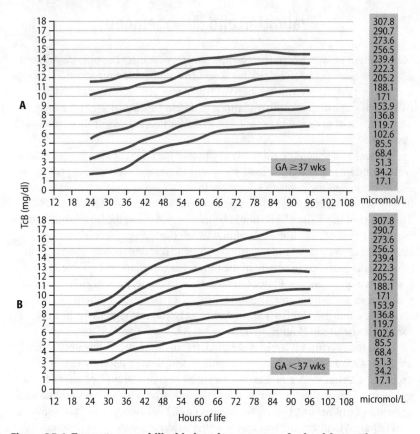

Figure 35-1. Trancutaneous bilirubin hourly nomogram for healthy newborns.

Nomograms showing curves of the 10th, 25th, 50th, 75th, 90th, and 95th percentiles for TcB (BiliChek) in 2,198 healthy normal European neonates ≥35 weeks of gestation. (A) and (B) show nomograms for term (≥37 weeks) and near-term (≥35 but <37 weeks) babies, respectively. Bilirubin values on the left are expressed in mg/dL and on the right (grey boxes) in μmol/L.

From De Luca D, Romagnoli C, Tiberi E, Zuppa AA, Zecca E. Skin bilirubin nomogram for the first 96 h of life in a European normal healthy newborn population, obtained with multiwavelength transcutaneous bilirubinometry. *Acta Paediatr.* 2008;97(2):46–150, with permission.

Discharge and Follow-up

Prior to discharge home from the newborn nursery, the AAP recommends assessing each infant for risk of developing hyperbilirubinemia using either a TSB or TcB measurement or assessing clinical risk factors. If an infant has no clinical risk factors, the risk of that infant developing severe hyperbilirubinemia is very low. The risk factors that are most frequently associated with severe hyperbilirubinemia include breastfeeding, gestation at less than 38 weeks, significant jaundice in a sibling, and jaundice noted prior to discharge home from the nursery.

If an infant is discharged home prior to 24 hours of life, outpatient follow-up should be completed by 72 hours of life. Infants discharged between 24 and 47 hours of life need a follow-up visit scheduled by 96 hours of life. An infant discharged between 48 and 72 hours of life should have a follow-up appointment scheduled by 120 hours of life. Earlier and additional appointments for follow-up may be needed for infants with clinical risk factors or for infants that are discharged prior to 48 hours of life. The period of greatest risk for developing severe hyperbilirubinemia is between 72 and 96 hours of life. Therefore, if there is doubt about the parent's ability to bring the infant for follow-up, then delaying discharge from the nursery beyond 72 hours may be needed to ensure there is no development of hyperbilirubinemia prior to discharge.

Upon discharge, parents should be educated about jaundice with verbal and written information (www.healthychildren.org).

The outpatient follow-up assessment should include the infant's weight with percentage of change since birth weight, adequacy of intake, pattern of voiding and stooling, and presence or absence of jaundice. Clinical judgment should be used to determine whether a TSB or TcB measurement should be done at the follow-up visit, keeping in mind that visual estimation of bilirubin levels can lead to errors, particularly in darkly pigmented infants. If there is any doubt about the bilirubin level, a TSB or TcB should be measured.

Suggested Reading

American Academy of Pediatrics Subcommittee on Hyperbilirubinemia. Management of hyperbilirubinemia in the newborn infant 35 or more weeks of gestation. *Pediatrics.* 2004;114(4);297–316

De Luca D, Romagnoli C, Tiberi E, Zuppa AA, Zecca E. Skin bilirubin nomogram for the first 96 h of life in a European normal healthy newborn population, obtained with multiwavelength transcutaneous bilirubinometry. *Acta Paediatr.* 2008;97(2):46–150

Kobayashi H, Stringer MD. Biliary atresia. *Semin Neonatol.* 2003;8(5):383–391

Maisels MJ, Bhutani VK, Bogen D, Newman TB, Stark AR, Watchko JF. Hyperbilirubinemia in the newborn infant > or =35 weeks' gestation: an update with clarifications. *Pediatrics.* 2009;124(4):1193–1198

Maruo Y, Nishizawa K, Sato H, Sawa H, Shimada M. Prolonged unconjugated hyperbilirubinemia associated with breast milk and mutations of the bilirubin uridine diphosphate-glucuronosyltransferase gene. *Pediatrics.* 2000;106(5):E59

Polin RA, Yoder MC, eds. *Workbook in Practical Neonatology.* 4th ed. Philadelphia, PA: Saunders Elselvier; 2007

CHAPTER 36

Newborn Care After Delivery

Keri A. Marques, MD

Key Points

- Most term infants at birth will not require immediate neonatal resuscitation efforts and will qualify for routine care.

- Routine care can be provided for term infants that have good tone and that are spontaneously breathing or crying.

- It is standard for all infants in the newborn nursery to receive prophylaxis for neonatal ophthalmia, vitamin K prophylaxis, hepatitis B vaccination, metabolic screening, audiology screening, and screening for critical congenital heart disease.

- Breastfeeding provides optimal nutrition for newborns and should be advocated and supported by the medical team.

- Prior to discharging a newborn from the nursery, the physician should ensure all recommended discharge criteria have been met and the appropriate anticipatory guidance has been reviewed with parents.

Delivery Room Care

The delivery of a newborn is a miraculous event that initiates her transition from intrauterine to extrauterine life. When resuscitation is required, one should follow the 3 basic steps in any resuscitation (ABC): airway (ensure airway is open and clear), breathing (ensure breathing is occurring with or without assistance), and circulation (assess heart rate and oxygenation). It is also vitally important to keep the newborn warm to prevent radiant heat loss. It is recommended that the providers caring for her after delivery be trained in neonatal resuscitation.

The presence of antepartum and intrapartum risk factors can help predict which newborns may need resuscitation; however, at times, even those without risk factors may need resuscitative measures (Box 36-1).

Box 36-1. Antepartum and Intrapartum Risk Factors That May Be Associated With Need for Neonatal Resuscitation

Antepartum Factors	Intrapartum Factors
Maternal diabetes	Emergency c-section
Gestational hypertension or preeclampsia	Forceps or vacuum-assisted delivery
Chronic hypertension	Breech or other abnormal presentations
Fetal anemia or isoimmunization	Premature labor
Previous fetal or neonatal death	Precipitous labor
Bleeding in second or third trimester	Chorioamnionitis
Maternal infection	Prolonged rupture of membranes
Maternal cardiac, renal, pulmonary,	(>18 hours before delivery)
thyroid, or neurologic disease	Prolonged labor (>24 hours)
Polyhydramnios	Macrosomia
Oligohydramnios	Category 2 or 3 fetal heart rate patterns
Premature rupture of membranes	Use of general anesthesia
Fetal hydrops	Uterine tachysystole with fetal heart rate
Post-term gestation	changes
Multiple gestation	Narcotics administered to mother within
Size-dates discrepancy	4 hours of delivery
Drug therapy, such as magnesium	Meconium-stained amniotic fluid
Adrenergic agonists	Prolapsed cord
Maternal substance abuse	Abruptio placentae
Fetal malformation or anomalies	Placenta previa
Diminished fetal activity	Significant intrapartum bleeding
No prenatal care	
Mother older than 35 years	

From Kattwinkel J, ed. *Textbook of Neonatal Resuscitation.* 6th ed. Elk Grove Village, IL: American Academy of Pediatrics; 2011. © 2011 American Heart Association, Inc, and American Academy of Pediatrics.

Routine care is a modified version of resuscitation that allows for the newborn to stay with the mother. If there are secretions, the physician can clear the airway by wiping the newborn's mouth and nose. Suctioning is not routinely recommended for newborns receiving routine care and should be provided only for those that are experiencing airway obstruction and are in need of resuscitation efforts.

Apgar scores should be assigned to newborns following delivery at 1 and 5 minutes of life. This gives a standardized approach to recording the transition to extrauterine life for a newborn. If his 5-minute score is less than 7, additional scores should be done at 5-minute intervals until a score greater than 7 is achieved or until 20 minutes of life.

Transitional Period

The transitional period continues after delivery until 6 hours of age. During this critical time, is it important to provide continued evaluation of the newborn, focusing on respirations, temperature, heart rate, color, and tone. Abnormalities in these key areas can indicate underlying illness, which may require further evaluation and intervention.

Oxygen saturation values slowly rise over the first 10 minutes of life to reach values greater than 90%. Most infants immediately after delivery have saturations of 60% to 70% and exhibit central cyanosis, which is blue color to the lips, tongue, and torso for the first few minutes of life. Central cyanosis is caused by low oxygen levels, as opposed to acrocyanosis, a blue color to the hands and feet that indicates decreased circulation and does not correlate with oxygen levels. Targeted pre-ductal pulse oximetry values for the first 10 minutes of life are presented in Table 36-1. Of note, preterm infants have a slower rise in oxygen saturation to achieve saturation values greater than 90% when compared to term infants.

Table 36-1.Targeted Pre-ductal Oximetry Values After Birth

Minutes of Life	Pre-ductal Pulse Oximetry, %
1 min	60–65
2 min	65–70
3 min	70–75
4 min	75–80
5 min	80–85
10 min	85–95

From Dawson JA, Kamlin CO, Vento M, et al. Defining the reference range for oxygen saturation for infants after birth. *Pediatrics*. 2010;125(6):e1340–e1347.

Physical Examination of the Newborn

Estimation of gestational age is possible by performing a physical maturity and neuromuscular maturity examination, called the New Ballard score. The New Ballard score should be performed with precision and as soon as possible following delivery, preferably within 12 hours for a preterm infant.

Observation of the newborn is one of the most important entities to his examination. When starting the inspection, it is helpful to start with the general assessment and work from head to toe to ensure all systems are assessed properly.

Routine Care of the Newborn

Prophylaxis for Neonatal Ophthalmia

Newborns with conjunctivitis in the first 4 weeks of life are considered to have neonatal ophthalmia. A newborn with conjunctivitis should be evaluated and treated promptly. Prevention of neonatal ophthalmia is a standard part of routine care of the newborn after delivery. A prophylaxic agent should be placed in the eyes of every newborn following delivery. Three available agents can be used: 1% silver nitrate solution, 0.5 % erythromycin ointment, and 1%

tetracycline ophthalmic ointment. These solutions will cover infection from *Neiserria gonorrhoeae* but will not be effective against *Chlamydia trachomatis.*

Vitamin K

Intramuscular vitamin K is recommended to be given to all newborns following delivery to prevent early and late vitamin K deficiency bleeding (VKDB). The optimal dose for preterm infants has yet to be established requiring further research. Late VKDB (ie, 2–12 weeks of age) can be prevented with parental vitamin K prophylaxis; however, late VKDB can still occur in newborns who have a severe malabsorption syndrome.

Umbilical Cord Care

Omphalitis can be a serious condition and cause severe morbidity and mortality in a newborn. When aseptic techniques are used during the delivery, only dry cord care is needed for the newborn following delivery. In settings where aseptic technique does not occur, the use of antiseptic agents on the cord should be used.

Newborn Feeding

Breastfeeding is the recommended choice for optimal infant nutrition because of the known short-term and long-term benefits to both mother and baby (see Chapter 9).

Hepatitis B

Universal hepatitis B vaccination at birth and prenatal maternal hepatitis B screening are the standard of care to prevent perinatal hepatitis B transmission. All infants with a birth weight greater than 2,000 g should begin the hepatitis B vaccination series with an initial vaccine at birth. Infants weighing less than 2,000 g should have the initial hepatitis B vaccine at 1 month of age or at hospital discharge, whichever comes first. The hepatitis B vaccination series should be completed by 6 to 18 months of age.

If the mother is hepatitis B surface antigen (HBsAg) positive, the infant will require both hepatitis B vaccine and hepatitis B immunoglobulin prior to 12 hours of life regardless of his birth weight. If the mother is HBsAg positive and the infant is less than 2,000 g, the initial hepatitis B vaccine given will not count in the 3-dose series; the infant will need to continue with a full 3-dose series starting at 1 to 2 months of age.

If the mother is HBsAg unknown, the hepatitis B vaccine should be given as routine after birth (ie, less than 12 hours of life), and maternal serology for hepatitis B should be sent. Hepatitis immunoglobulin can be given up to 7 days following delivery if the mother's serology results are positive. It is recommended that the infant not be discharged until the mother's hepatitis B serology is known and appropriate actions have been taken. Follow-up testing for the infant is recommended once the vaccination series is complete with anti-HBs and HBsAg.

Screening in the Nursery

Newborn Metabolic Screening

The newborn metabolic screening is a blood test performed on all newborns in the United States, providing screening results for several disorders that may become symptomatic later in life, leading to significant morbidity or mortality. If the screen is collected prior to 24 hours of life, a repeat screen needs to be obtained at 1 to 2 weeks of life. For preterm or sick newborns, the screen should be collected near the seventh day of age and the screening repeated at 28 days or prior to discharge, whichever time comes first.

Audiology

Universal screening for hearing in newborns is recommended by the US Preventive Task Force. It has been shown that early detection and early intervention in patients with congenital hearing loss improves linguistic outcomes. The Joint Committee on Infant Hearing recommends that all newborns receive a hearing screening prior to 1 month of age. Two methods currently meet the standards for infant hearing screening: the auditory brainstem responses and the otoacoustic emissions. Both of these screens evaluate the peripheral auditory system and the cochlea but do not evaluate the central auditory system. Any newborn who fails the hearing screening will need further audiology assessment to evaluate and determine if there is hearing impairment. It is recommended by the Joint Committee on Infant Hearing that infants who fail the hearing screening have an audiology assessment performed prior to 3 months.

Screening for Critical Congenital Heart Disease

Screening for critical congenital heart disease (CCHD) is recommended by the Secretary of Health and Human Services and supported by the American Academy of Pediatrics (AAP). Pulse oximetry is readily available, painless, and a useful tool in detecting patients with CCHD. Relying on prenatal ultrasound and postnatal physical examination will prevent diagnosis of a number of patients with CCHD, leading to significant morbidity and mortality. The targeted population for this screening is all newborns in the newborn nursery. The pulse oximetry screening should be done when the patient is older than 24 hours or as close to discharge as possible if he is going home prior to 24 hours, to reduce false-positive results. The saturations should be taken in the right hand as well as in one foot.

A positive screen is defined as a saturation in either the right hand or foot of less than 90%, which requires immediate evaluation with echocardiogram and evaluation for hypoxemia. If saturation is greater than or equal to 95% in either extremity with a difference less than or equal to 3% between upper and lower extremities, this is defined as a negative screen. If the results are 90% to 95% in either extremity or greater than 3% in difference between upper and lower extremities, the screening should be repeated. If this pattern continues after 3 checks, evaluation with echocardiogram and hypoxemia work-up should be provided (Figure 36-1). The AAP emphasizes that the saturation thresholds may vary at high altitude, and these values are yet to be determined.

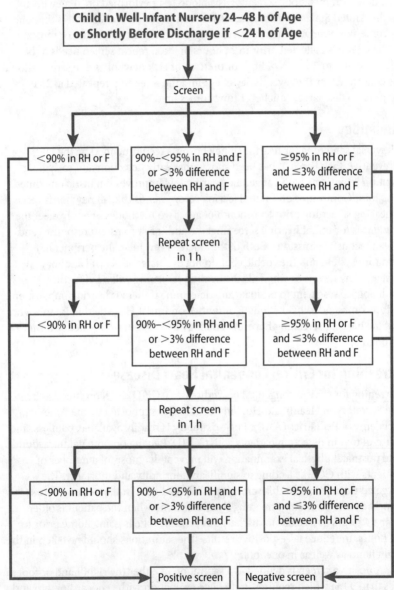

Figure 36-1. Algorithm for pulse oximetry screening for critical congenital heart disease.

Abbreviations: F, foot; RH, right hand.

From Kemper AR, Mahle WT, Martin GR, et al. Strategies for implementing screening for critical congenital heart disease. *Pediatrics*. 2011;128(5):e1259–e1267.

Screening for Neonatal Hypoglycemia

Term infants in the newborn nursery are not routinely screened for hypoglycemia unless risk factors or symptoms are present. Infants who are at risk for neonatal hypoglycemia include those who are small and large for their gestational age, preterm infants, and infants of diabetic mothers. The most common symptom of hypoglycemia for an infant is jitteriness. Other symptoms include lethargy, hypotonia, irritability, high-pitched cry, exaggerated Moro reflex, tremor, apnea, cyanosis, poor feeding, stupor, coma, and seizures.

Hyperbilirubinemia

All newborns should be routinely monitored for development of jaundice (see Chapter 35). Any newborn with jaundice in the first 24 hours of life requires further evaluation for etiology of the jaundice.

Risk Factors for Developmental Dysplasia of the Hip

Developmental dysplasia of the hip (DDH) should be screened for by assessing the newborn's risk factors and performing serial physical examinations. Risk factors for DDH include breech intrauterine position, family history of DDH, female sex, and limited fetal mobility. All newborns should be evaluated for hip instability by physical examination, and referral to an orthopedic surgeon should be made if instability is noted. Hip ultrasound is the preferred method of imaging in the newborn period to evaluate for DDH and should be scheduled for approximately 4 to 6 weeks of age for newborns who are at high risk for DDH.

Circumcision

Male circumcision in the newborn nursery is an elective procedure that is chosen by the parents for a variety of reasons including cosmetic, religious, and medical reasons. Parents should be given information regarding the risks and benefits of circumcision so they can make an informed decision about this elective procedure, even prenatally.

The 2012 statement from the AAP task force on male circumcision concluded that the health benefits of male circumcision outweigh the risks, justifying parents having access to the procedure if they so choose.

Discharge and Anticipatory Guidance

The decision to discharge an infant is a team approach and should include the pediatrician, nursing staff, any support staff involved, the obstetrician, and, most importantly, the family caring for the infant. The AAP describes the readiness for discharge being unique for each infant and should focus on the infant's health, as well as the mother's health, stability, competence, and ability to care for the infant, in addition to the availability of a social support system and access to health care for follow-up. Box 36-2 gives the AAP Committee on Fetus and Newborn minimum criteria for discharge for a term infant defined as 37 to 41 weeks' completed gestation. This table also gives information about when to schedule follow-up with the medical home and the purpose of the follow-up visit.

Box 36-2. Minimum Discharge Criteria for Term Newborn (37 to 41 Weeks' Completed Gestation)

1. Clinical course and physical examination at discharge have not revealed abnormalities that require continued hospitalization.

2. The infant's vital signs are documented as being within reference ranges, with appropriate variations based on physiologic state, and stable for the 12 hours preceding discharge. These ranges include a respiratory rate below 60 per minute and no other signs of respiratory distress, a heart rate of 100 to 160 beats per minute, and axillary temperature of 36.5°C to 37.4°C (97.7–99.3°F) measured properly in an open crib with appropriate clothing.

3. The infant has urinated regularly and passed at least 1 stool spontaneously.

4. The infant has completed at least 2 successful consecutive feedings, with assessment to verify that the infant is able to coordinate sucking, swallowing, and breathing while feeding.

5. There is no significant bleeding at the circumcision site.

6. The clinical risk of development of subsequent hyperbilirubinemia has been assessed, and appropriate management or follow-up plans have been instituted as recommended in American Academy of Pediatrics clinical practice guidelines for management of hyperbilirubinemia. (See Chapter 35 on neonatal hyperbilirubinemia.)

7. The infant has been adequately evaluated and monitored for sepsis on the basis of maternal risk factors and in accordance with current guidelines for prevention of perinatal group B streptococcal disease.

8. Maternal blood test and screening results are available and have been reviewed, including
   • Maternal syphilis and hepatitis B surface antigen status
   • Screening tests, including a test for HIV, performed in accordance with state regulations

9. Infant blood tests are available and have been reviewed such as cord or infant blood type and direct Coombs test results, as clinically indicated.

10. Initial hepatitis B vaccine has been administered according to the current immunization schedule.

11. Newborn metabolic and hearing screenings have been completed per hospital protocol and state regulations.

Box 36-2 *(cont)*

12. The mother's knowledge, ability, and confidence to provide adequate care for her infant have been assessed for competency regarding
    - Breastfeeding or bottle-feeding (the breastfeeding mother and infant should be assessed by trained staff regarding breastfeeding position, latch-on, and adequacy of swallowing)
    - The importance and benefits of breastfeeding for both mother and infant
    - Appropriate urination and defecation frequency for the infant
    - Cord, skin, and genital care, including circumcision care, for the infant
    - The ability to recognize signs of illness and common infant problems, particularly jaundice
    - Infant safety (such as use of an appropriate car safety seat, supine positioning for sleeping, maintaining a smoke-free environment, and room sharing)
13. Family, environmental, and social risk factors have been assessed, and the mother and her other family members have been educated about safe home environment. If risk factors are identified, discharge should be delayed until they are resolved or a plan to safeguard the infant is in place. This plan may involve discussions with social services or state agencies such as child protective services. These risk factors include but are not limited to
    - Untreated parental substance abuse or positive urine toxicology results in the mother or newborn
    - History of child abuse or neglect
    - Mental illness in a parent who is in the home
    - Lack of social support, particularly for single, first-time mothers
    - Mothers who live in a shelter, a rehabilitation home, or on the street
    - History of domestic violence, particularly during this pregnancy
    - Communicable illness in a parent or other members of the household
    - Adolescent mother, particularly if other above-listed conditions apply
14. A medical home for continuing medical care for the infant has been identified and a plan for timely communication of pertinent clinical information to the medical home is in place. For newborns discharged less than 48 hours after delivery, an appointment should be made for the infant to be examined by a licensed health care professional, preferably within 48 hours of discharge based on risk factors but no later than 72 hours in most cases. If this cannot be ensured, discharge should be deferred until a mechanism for follow-up evaluation is identified. The follow-up visit can take place in a home or clinic setting as long as the health care professional who examines the infant is competent in newborn assessment and the results of the follow-up visit are reported to the infant's physician or his or her designee on the day of the visit.

Box 36-2 *(cont)*

15. Barriers to adequate follow-up care for the newborn, such as lack of transportation to medical care services, lack of easy access to telephone communication, and non–English-speaking parents, have been assessed and, whenever possible, assistance has been given to the family to make suitable arrangements to address them. The purpose of the follow-up visit is to

- Weigh the infant; assess the infant's general health, hydration, and extent of jaundice; identify any new problems; review feeding pattern and technique; and obtain historical evidence of adequate urination and defecation patterns for the infant.
- Assess quality of mother-infant attachment and details of infant behavior.
- Reinforce maternal or family education in infant care, particularly regarding infant feeding and safety such as breastfeeding, back to sleep, and child safety seats.
- Review the results of outstanding laboratory tests, such as newborn metabolic screens, performed before discharge.
- Perform screening tests in accordance with state regulations and other tests that are clinically indicated, such as bilirubin measurement.
- Verify the plan for health care maintenance, including a method for obtaining emergency services, preventive care and immunizations, periodic evaluations and physical examinations, and necessary screenings.
- Assess for parental well-being including postpartum depression in the mother.

16. Obstetrical care, newborn nursery care, and follow-up care should be considered independent services to be reimbursed as separate packages and not as part of a global fee for maternity-newborn labor and delivery services.

From American Academy of Pediatrics Committee on Fetus and Newborn. Hospital stay for healthy term newborns. *Pediatrics.* 2010;125(2):405–409.

Parental education on caring for the infant as well as safety is a key step in the discharge on an infant. The family should have baseline knowledge of when to be concerned and seek medical care for their newborn. Signs and symptoms of illness should be reviewed with the families and they should know to seek medical care when any of the following are present: vomiting, diarrhea, fever or temperature instability, irritability, lethargy, poor feeding, jaundice, decreased urine output, and bleeding/discharge from umbilical stump or circumcision site. Box 36-3 outlines parental anticipatory guidance that can be included in your education session with the family prior to discharging a newborn from the newborn nursery.

Box 36-3. Newborn Discharge—Anticipatory Guidance

Safety
Car Safety
- Infants should always ride in car seat.
- Car seat should be rear-facing in the middle seat of the back seat in all vehicles.
- Never smoke with infant in the car.
- Read instructions on installation of car seat and have car seat inspected to ensure optimum safety.

Safe Sleeping
- Provide safe sleep environment.
  - Place infant on his or her back to sleep.
  - Infant should sleep alone in crib or bassinet.
  - Crib should not include any loose/soft bedding or toys.
  - Crib slats should be equal or less than $2^{3}/_{8}$ inches apart.

Water Temperature
- Water heater should be set at or lower than 120°F.
- Water should be lukewarm and tested prior to placing infant in water.

Parent Well-being
- Parents should seek medical assistance if they are feeling overwhelmed, sad, or blue for more than a few days.
- Take time to sleep when possible, and accept help from social support system.

Smoking
- Keep your home and car smoke free.

Caring for Your Baby
Infection
- Keep your infant away from anyone who is sick.
- Always have visitors wash their hands prior to holding the newborn.
- Use an rectal thermometer to take temperature.
- If your baby has a temperature greater than 100.4°F/38.0°C, seek medical care immediately.
- If your infant is lethargic, irritable, not consolable, refusing to feed, or having decreased number of wet diapers, seek medical care.

Umbilical Cord Care
- Umbilical cord remnant generally will fall off within the first week.
- Keep this area dry and clean.
- If you see any redness, discharge, or bleeding from the umbilical remnant, seek medical care.

Circumcision Care
- If you see any swelling, bleeding, or unusual discharge or odor seek medical care.

Jaundice
- *Jaundice* is a medical term for yellowing of the skin.
- If you notice yellowing of the eyes or skin, notify your medical home.

Box 36-3 *(cont)*

Caring for Your Baby *continued*

Crying
- Crying is a way for your infant to communicate.
- A crying infant may be bored, tired, hot or cold, wet, uncomfortable, overexcited, distressed, or in pain.
- If you are feeling impatient with your crying infant, hand over the baby to another caregiver or ensure your infant is in a safe environment and step away from the situation.
- *Never* shake a baby.

Feeding
- Breastfeeding
  - Feed your infant 8–12 times a day.
  - Seek lactation support through your medical home if problems arise.
- Formula Feeding
  - Offer approximately 2 oz of iron-fortified formula every 2–3 hours or more often if the baby is still hungry.
  - Follow instructions on label to prepare formula.
  - Never use a microwave oven to warm formula.
  - Throw out any remaining formula left in bottle after feeding.

Bowel Movements/Voiding
- Bowel movements vary in size, color, consistency, and frequency.
- Infants may have a bowel movement following each feed.
- At first the stools will be black and thick, then transition to yellow and seedy.
- Contact your medical home if your baby is having excessive watery or hard stools.
- Your baby should have 6–8 wet diapers per day.

Spitting Up/Vomiting
- All infants will spit up to some degree.
- Try to burp your baby during and after feeding.
- Spit-ups are generally milk-like in nature.
- Seek medical care if your baby is having excessive vomiting, forceful vomiting, bloody vomit, green color to vomit.

From *Bright Futures: Guidelines for Health Supervision of Infants, Children, and Adolescents.* 3rd ed. Elk Grove Village, IL: American Academy of Pediatrics; 2008.

Suggested Reading

American Academy of Pediatrics Joint Committee on Infant Hearing. Year 2007 position statement: principles and guidelines for early hearing detection and intervention programs. *Pediatrics.* 2007;120(4):898–921

American Academy of Pediatrics Task Force on Circumcision. Circumcision policy statement. *Pediatrics.* 2012;130(3):585–586

Dawson JA. Kamlin CO, Vento M, et al. Defining the reference range for oxygen saturation for infants after birth. *Pediatrics.* 2010;125(6):e1340–e1347

Finster M, Wood M. The Apgar score has survived the test of time. *Anesthesiology.* 2005;102(4):855–857

Kattwinkel J, ed. *Textbook of Neonatal Resuscitation.* 6th ed. Elk Grove Village, Il: American Academy of Pediatrics; 2011

Mahle WT, Martin GR, Beekman RH 3rd, et al. Endorsement of Health and Human Services recommendation for pulse oximetry screening for critical congenital heart disease. *Pediatrics.* 2012;129(1):190–192

Narvey M, Fletcher MA. Physical assessment and classification. In: Macdonald MG, Mullen MD, Seshia MMK, eds. *Avery's Neonatology: Pathophysiology and Management of the Newborn.* 6th ed. Philadelphia, PA: Lippincott Williams & Wilkins; 2005: 327–350

CHAPTER 37

Nutrition

Kathleen V. Previll, MD

Key Points

- Every well-child visit is an opportunity to review the dietary habits of a family. Parents and caregivers should be encouraged to choose which foods they offer their infants and children; the infant and child should choose how much to eat.

- The social and health benefits of good nutrition are vital for optimal growth and development.

- Breastfeeding remains the optimal feeding for newborns and infants.

- Offer children 5 servings a day of fruits and vegetables.

- Sugar-sweetened beverages are not indicated.

- Half of grains offered should be whole grains.

- Frequent meals in restaurants may exceed the energy, sodium, sugar, and saturated fat requirements of children.

Overview

Medical professionals must arm themselves with nutrition knowledge that respects the cultural beliefs of their patients and achieves professional recommendations from nutrition research. Because good nutrition helps every child attain optimal growth and cognitive development, pediatricians should be especially competent in identifying nutritional issues and managing them. Through healthy eating, the infant and child lower their risk for chronic disease, especially cardiovascular complications, and on a social level, mealtimes can enhance the emotional bond between child and caregiver.

Feeding practices are influenced by cultural habits, socioeconomic status, experience in cooking, demands placed on caregivers from work, and the growing convenience of commercially prepared foods. Understanding these influences and integrating them with current nutrition guidelines remains a challenging aspect of medical practice (Tables 37-1 and 37-2).

Table 37-1. Feeding Guide for Birth to 2 Years[a]

Age in Months	Average kcal/day	Dairy	Protein Foods	Vegetables	Fruits	Grains
0–4	400–550 90–120 per kilogram	Breast milk: 8–12 times/day Iron-fortified formula	Supplied from milk	None	None	None
4–6	550–650	Breast milk: 5–7 times/day Iron-fortified formula	None	None	None	None
6–12	680–830	Breast milk: 4–6 times/day Iron-fortified formula	Pureed meats Yogurt after 9 months Soft foods	Pureed or mashed: ½ to 1 jar/day	Pureed or mashed: ½ to 1 jar/day 100% juice in cup: 2–3 oz/day	Mixed cereals fortified with iron Baby biscuits
12–24	830–1,000	Whole or 2% milk: 16–32 oz/day (Use cup.)	Soft, small pieces meat; yogurt, cheese, or beans; or fish: 1 serving/day Finger foods Utensils 15–18 months	Soft cooked: 2 servings/day	Fresh or canned: 2 servings/day	Mixed cereals Bread, pasta, or rice (Whole grains = half of grains given.)

Adapted from Kleinman RE, Greer FR, eds. *Pediatric Nutrition.* 7th ed. Elk Grove Village, IL: American Academy of Pediatrics; 2013:125,153 and Holt K, Wooldridge NH, Story M, Sofka D, eds. *Bright Futures: Nutrition.* 3rd ed. Elk Grove Village, IL: American Academy of Pediatrics; 2011.
[a] Timing of introduction of complementary foods based on development of child and is not evidence based.

Table 37-2. Feeding Guide for Children 2 to 12 Years

Age in Years	Average kcal/day[a]	Dairy	Protein Foods	Vegetables	Fruits	Grains
2–3	1,000	Low-fat milk: 4 oz/serving (2½ cups/day total)	Meats, beans, or fish: 1–2 oz/serving (2–4 oz/day)	2–3 tbsp/serving (1–1½ cup/day) Raw only if able to chew	½–1 small piece 100% juice: 4–6 oz/day Fresh, canned, or juice: 1–1½ cup/day	½ to 1 slice bread or ¼–½ cup cooked or dry cereal: 3–5 oz/day
4–8	1,200–1,400	Low-fat milk: 4–6 oz/serving (2½–3 cups/day)	1–2 oz or 4–6 tbsp/serving (3–5 oz/day)	4–6 tbsp/serving (1½–2½ cups/day)	4–6 tbsp/serving (1–1½ cups/day)	1 slice or ½–1cup/serving (4–6 oz/day)
9–12	1,600–1,800	Low-fat milk: 4–8 oz/serving (2½–3 cups/day)	2 oz/serving (4–5½ oz/day)	¼–½ cup/serving (1½–2½ cups/day)	¼–½ cups/serving (1½–2 cups/day)	1 slice or ½–1 cup/serving (5–6 oz/day)
Comments		Fat-free or 1% is low fat. Milk, yogurt, cheese or nonfat dry milk.	Lean or low-fat meats 1 oz = 1 egg, 2 tbsp peanut butter, or 4 tbsp cooked beans.	Choose dark green and orange: carrots, spinach, broccoli, squash greens. Limit starchy vegetables like potatoes, peas.	Less than half of total should be juice.	1 oz = 1 slice bread; ½ cup pasta or rice; 5 saltine crackers; ½ English muffin; or ½ bagel. Half of grains = whole grains.

[a] Based on meeting nutritional needs of sedentary children at younger age of each group.

Adapted from Kleinman RE, Greer FR, eds. *Pediatric Nutrition.* 7th ed. Elk Grove Village, IL: American Academy of Pediatrics; 2013.

Nutrition Guidelines

Several government, nonprofit, and industry agencies contribute to national dietary guidelines in the United States. The original dietary guidelines were instituted in 1980 by federal Public Law 100-445. This federal mandate requires the secretary of the US Department of Agriculture (USDA) and the Department of Health and Human Services to review all federal publications and create a report every 5 years. The most recent *Dietary Guidelines for Americans* were published in 2010 and represent the first evidence-based, public health approach to nutrition guidelines. The level of evidence for each recommendation may be found in the nutrition evidence library www.nel.gov. New *Dietary Guidelines for Americans* will be published in the fall of 2015.

The Institute of Medicine, an independent nonprofit, generates a major influence on nutrition guidelines in the United States through their diverse professional committee analysis and publications (www.iom.edu/global/topics /food-nutrition.aspx).

Surveillance of Nutrition Outcomes

By measuring what children and adolescents eat, we learn better ways to implement good nutrition. The Centers for Disease Control and Prevention Pediatric Nutrition Surveillance System (www.cdc.gov/pednss) includes data on more than 8 million children served by the federal programs for low-income children.

All surveillance systems indicate we continue to inappropriately feed our young children sugar-sweetened beverages and too much salt. Infant and toddler diets are low in iron and zinc, and breastfeeding rates fall below the national recommendation by Healthy People 2010 of 75%. The American lifestyle promotes working parents to provide meals away from home, especially in fast-food restaurants. In general, these meals exceed the energy, sugar, saturated fat, and sodium needs of the child.

Newborn and Early Infancy

Breastfeeding remains the optimal feeding for all newborns. Human milk is sufficient in protein, carbohydrate, and fat and meets the micronutrient needs of infants except for vitamin D. Iron stores are sufficient in full-term breastfed infants until 4 months when iron supplementation should be added at 1 mg/kg/ day for term infants. After 6 months the diet should be enriched to include iron-rich foods.

Breastfeeding decreases the risk of illness in newborns and infants and enhances the health outcomes of the mother. Some immune protections benefits from breastfeeding cannot be replicated by any other feeding practice (see Chapter 9).

The best alternative to breastfeeding in the first 12 months is iron-fortified formula. Formula content has been regulated since 1986 by the Infant Formula Act (Public Law 99-570), and all contain a standard concentration of 20 kcal/oz with supplemental micronutrients. Formulas are manufactured in powder, concentrate, and ready-to-feed preparations. Most formulas consumed by infants are modified cow's milk. Formulas based on soy protein and also protein-hydrolyzed cow's milk are also available for infants with special digestive needs. Soy formulas may be preferred by vegetarian caregivers. They are appropriate for infants with galactosemia because the carbohydrate is not lactose but rather corn syrup solids and sucrose. Soy formula may be fed to infants with IgE-associated reactions to cow's milk, such as a rash, but not to infants with cow's milk protein allergy, which more commonly presents as blood in the stools. Soy formula is not felt to prevent atopy; however, atopic infants may benefit from a protein-hydrolyzed formula.

Preterm Infants

Preterm infants on enteral feeds require close monitoring for growth and development. Human milk remains the ideal milk for feeding because of the immunologic and antimicrobial components. It is generally not adequate in protein requirements and micronutrients, however, and human milk fortifier is highly recommended if the preterm infant is less than 1,500 g and until they reach a weight of 2,000 g. If formula is given, it should be premature formula designed to meet their unique protein, carbohydrate, fat, and micronutrient needs. Soy protein is not recommended because of lack of evidence that it meets the optimal absorption and utilization of preterm infants. Premature formula contains higher calcium and phosphorus content than traditional formulas to meet the stores the preterm infant has not acquired in the last trimester. These premature formulas should be fed for the first year of life. The powdered preparations of formula are also discouraged because of their nonpathogenic microorganism content, which the preterm immune system is not prepared to resist.

Cow's Milk

The American Academy of Pediatrics (AAP) and the American Heart Association recommend low-fat cow's milk for toddlers older than 2 years. Low-fat cow's milk is fat-free or contains only 1% of fat. From 12 to 24 months, 2% cow's milk may be offered in a cup. Before 12 months, cow's milk is inappropriate because of its increased solute load, inadequate fatty-acid profile, and insufficient amounts of iron, zinc, and vitamin E.

Starting Complementary Foods

Complementary foods may be introduced when an infant achieves developmental milestones which make the foods easy to feed and digest and is recommended to start at approximately 6 months of age.

Full-term infants have good head control at 4 months and trunk control at 5 months. The tongue thrust which interferes with spoon feeding is extinguished at about 4 months. By 6 months, infants have developed a more sophisticated suck-swallow reflex, and the gag reflex is diminished. At 12 months, the suck-swallow reflex is gone and the infant swallows from a cup well. The gastrointestinal digestive enzymes are available at about 3 months, and the salivary gland produces digestive enzymes by 4 months.

Just as with breast or formula feeding, it is important for parents to learn satiety cues from their infants. Pursing the lips, turning the head away, and showing interest in other activities means it is time to stop the feeding.

Developmentally, infants and toddlers may touch, taste, and spit out foods as they explore new textures. Food acceptance is improved by offering the food as many as 10 to 15 times to adjust to taste and texture. New foods are generally offered every 3 to 5 days. No special sequence of food groups is necessary and there is no need to delay any food group in children older than 6 months due to allergy concerns. By 7 to 8 months all food groups should be represented in the diet.

Choosing First Complementary Foods

Both the AAP *Pediatric Nutrition* (2013) and *Bright Futures: Nutrition* (2011) advise a single-grain cereal fortified with iron or meat as a first food. There are recommendations to offer meat as a first food because of its iron and zinc content. If the mother exclusively breastfeeds, the introduction of these iron-rich complementary foods at 6 months fulfills the infant's need to build her own iron stores.

Increased consumption of fruits and vegetables is recommended by nutritionists. Five servings per day are optimal, and serving size is age dependent (¼–½ cup/serving). These foods contain the micronutrients which fulfill dietary intake recommendations (adequate intake [AI] and recommended daily allowance [RDA]) for infants and toddlers. Juice should be pasteurized 100% juice, and 4 to 6 oz/day may represent one serving of fruit. Juice should be served in a cup and not just before bedtime to prevent cavities.

Calcium and Vitamin D

The recommendations for RDA (>2 years) and AI (<2 years) for calcium and vitamin D were updated in the 2010 report by the Food and Nutrition Board of the Institute of Medicine. Its report was accepted by the AAP Committee on Nutrition in 2012. Deficiencies of vitamin D are linked to hypertension, immune dysfunction, cancer, diabetes, cardiovascular disease, and poor bone mineralization. The definition of vitamin D deficiency is currently a 24(OH) VitD blood level below 20 ng/mL.

Iron

Full-term infants achieve their iron stores in the last trimester. Preterm infants less than 1,800 g need attention to restoring the iron stores, and, if breastfed, require 2 mg/kg/day from 1 to 12 months. Breastfed infants may benefit from starting iron-rich complementary foods, such as single-grain cereal or meats, after 6 months. Iron supplementation for full-term breast feed infants is recommended at 4 months at 1 mg/kg/day.

Supplemental Vitamins

The AAP and the American Dietetic Association do not routinely recommend daily multivitamins for infants and children older than 12 months. Infants and children who might benefit from multivitamins are listed in Box 37-1.

Box 37-1. Characteristics of Children for Whom Multivitamins Are Beneficial

Has eating disorder

Is obese on restricted diet

Is on fad diet

Has failure to thrive

Has parental neglect

Has chronic illness such as cystic fibrosis, renal disease, or inflammatory bowel disease

Is vegetarian with no dairy

Is extremely picky with low vegetable and fruit intake

National School Lunch Program

The National School Lunch Program (www.nap.edu) was initiated in 1946 by Congress under Public Law 79-396. The Breakfast Program was added in 1975. Analysis by the Institute of Medicine in 2009 helped make this program a national model for balanced nutrition, meeting the USDA *Dietary Guidelines for Americans of 2005* (Evidence Level III). As a result, school meals now contain more fruits and vegetables, are lower in sodium content, and emphasize whole grains.

Suggested Reading
· · · · · · · · · · · · · · · · · ·

Expert Panel on Integrated Guidelines for Cardiovascular Health and Risk Reduction in Children and Adolescents; National Heart, Lung, and Blood Institute. Expert panel on integrated guidelines for cardiovascular health and risk reduction in children and adolescents: summary report. *Pediatrics.* 2011;128(Suppl 5):S213–S256

Gidding SS, Dennison BA, Birch LL, et al. Dietary recommendations for children and adolescents: a guide for practitioners. *Pediatrics.* 2006;117(2):544–559

Holt K, ed. *Bright Futures: Nutrition.* 3rd ed. Elk Grove Village, IL: American Academy of Pediatrics; 2011

Institute of Medicine. *Dietary Reference Intakes for Vitamin D and Calcium.* Washington, DC: National Academies Press; 2012

Kleinman RE, Greer FR, eds. *Pediatric Nutrition.* 7th ed. Elk Grove Village, IL: American Academy of Pediatrics; 2013

US Department of Agriculture. Choose My Plate Web site. http://www.choosemyplate. gov. Accessed November 24, 2014

US Department of Agriculture. Nutrition evidence library. http://www.nel.gov. Accessed February 18, 2015

US Department of Agriculture, US Department of Health and Human Services. *Dietary Guidelines for Americans, 2010.* 7th ed. Washington, DC: US Government Printing Office. http://www.health.gov/dietaryguidelines. Accessed November 24, 2014

US Department of Agriculture Food and Nutrition Service. National school lunch program. US Department of Agriculture Web site. http://www.fns.usda.gov/nslp /national-school-lunch-program-nslp. Accessed November 24, 2014

CHAPTER 38

Obesity

Indrajit Majumdar, MD, MBBS, and Teresa Quattrin, MD

Key Points

- Body mass index percentiles are used for appropriate categorization and management of youth with abnormal weight gain.
- Exogenous obesity is the most prevalent etiology for abnormal weight gain in youth.
- Growth rate is a sensitive indicator to rule out other causes of abnormal weight gain.
- Family-based nutritional counseling and behavioral modification is the backbone of management.
- Drug therapy is limited to the management of comorbidities associated with obesity.
- Weight loss surgery should only be considered for selected youth whose medical management has failed.

Overview

The prevalence of obesity in the 2 to 19 years of age population is 16.9%, with 31.7% being overweight. The diagnosis of overweight and obesity requires accurate measurement of weight and height and calculation of body mass index (BMI). BMI is calculated as follows:

- Weight (in kilograms) divided by height (in centimeters) squared or
- Weight (in pounds) divided by height (in inches) squared $\times$ 703

Adults with a BMI between 25 and 29.9 kg/m² are categorized as overweight and those with BMI equal to or greater than 30 kg/m², as obese. For children and adolescents, age- and sex-specific BMI percentile curves are similar to those in use for height and weight. Between ages 2 and 20 years, children and young adults are considered overweight or obese if their BMI is equal to or greater than the 85th percentile or 95th percentile, respectively. In children younger than 2 years, BMI is not an accurate tool to assess adiposity but may be useful to monitor the child's growth and the potential onset of early increase in BMI, which puts youth at higher risk for being persistently overweight in later years.

Causes

Exogenous obesity, the most common cause of abnormal weight gain, is often the result of an imbalance between energy intake and expenditure. Endogenous obesity, which accounts for only a minority of overweight children, adolescents, and young adults, is defined as obesity associated with medical conditions such as Cushing syndrome, or hypothyroidism or genetic conditions, such as Prader-Willi syndrome (Table 38-1). When medical conditions are responsible for endogenous obesity, they are associated with defined physical findings.

Table 38-1. Endocrine Disorders and Syndromes Associated With Obesity and Growth Failure

Endocrine Disorders	Syndromes
• Cushing syndrome • Hypothyroidism • Growth hormone deficiency • Pseudohypoparathyroidism type 1a • Melanocortin-4 receptor mutation	• Prader-Willi syndrome • Bardet-Biedl syndrome • Alström syndrome • Cohen syndrome • Carpenter syndrome

In children and adolescents, plotting height-growth velocity in relation to weight gain is useful to differentiate between exogenous and endogenous obesity. The former is almost always associated with normal or increased height-growth velocity. On the other hand, most endogenous conditions associated with obesity, such as Cushing syndrome and hypothyroidism, are usually characterized by growth deceleration (Evidence Level I). The increased growth velocity in exogenous obesity may be secondary to hyperinsulinemia, with insulin being a well-known growth factor. Because of the increased growth velocity, the obese phenotype may not be evident initially, as excessive weight gain is masked by the increased growth in height. This is particularly true in the preschool years when height-growth velocity is still fast. With excessive weight gain, the child's height percentile often switches to a higher channel than that predicted by the mid-parental height.

Clinical Features

The clinical evaluation of youth with abnormal weight gain should focus on differentiating exogenous obesity from endogenous conditions associated with obesity. Health care professionals should be familiar with the child's dietary history, physical and sedentary activities, and family history of obesity, diet, exercise habits, and home environment, which may increase the likelihood of the child being inactive. A careful evaluation of the growth pattern is important in reaching the correct etiologic diagnosis.

Common comorbidities include impaired glucose metabolism and undiagnosed type 2 diabetes (T2DM), other endocrinologic abnormalities (listed on the next page), and orthopedic, pulmonary, gastrointestinal, neurologic, cardiovascular, and psychological complications of obesity (Table 38-2).

Table 38-2. Signs and Symptoms of Obesity-Associated Comorbidities

Comorbidities	Symptoms	Signs
Insulin resistance and diabetes mellitus	Polyuria, nocturia, polydipsia, weight loss	Acanthosis nigricans
Hypertension	Often asymptomatic	BP elevation >95th percentile for age, sex, and height
Hyperlipidemia	Asymptomatic	None unless hyperlipidemia is secondary to familial hyperlipidemia syndromes
Obstructive sleep apnea	Tiredness, sleepiness, enuresis, poor school performance, snoring	Enlargement of tonsils and adenoids, narrow upper airway
Nonalcoholic fatty liver disease	Asymptomatic	Hepatomegaly and signs of portal hypertension
Gastroesophageal reflux, gall bladder abnormalities, constipation	Abdominal pain	Abdominal tenderness
Polycystic ovarian syndrome	Oligomenorrhea, amenorrhea, acne, excess body hair, alopecia	Signs of androgen excess including acne, frontal hair loss, hirsutism
Premature adrenarche	Premature onset of sweat, body odor, axillary and pubic hair	Presence of body odor, sweat, pubic/axillary hair in boys <9 y and girls <8 y, growth acceleration
Orthopedic complication	Back pain, hip pain, abnormal gait	Joint tenderness (ie, hips and knees), limited range of motion of hips or groin tenderness suggestive of slipped capital femoral epiphysis
Dermatologic abnormalities	Coarse and dark skin, "stretch marks"	Acanthosis nigricans (insulin resistance) Light (exogenous obesity)/ violaceous striae (Cushing syndrome)
Neurologic abnormalities	Headache	Papilledema (pseudotumor cerebri)
Psychosocial	Reports of teasing, bullying	Signs suggestive of depression, low self-esteem

Abbreviation: BP, blood pressure.

The most significant obesity-related comorbidity is the spectrum of insulin resistance with or without acanthosis nigricans. Glucose abnormalities range from impaired fasting glucose to undiagnosed T2DM, dyslipidemia, and hypertension (Evidence Level I). Metabolic syndrome, a compilation of these metabolic disturbances, is a significant risk factor for the development of T2DM and atherosclerotic cardiovascular disease. For the pediatric population, several defining criteria for the metabolic syndrome are available. Metabolic syndrome is defined by the presence of 3 or more of 5 criteria, which include waist circumference equal to or greater than the 90th percentile for age and sex; blood pressure equal to or greater than the 90th percentile for age, sex, and height; fasting serum triglyceride level equal to or greater than 150 mg/dL; fasting high-density lipoprotein cholesterol level equal to or less than 40 mg/dL; and fasting glucose equal to or greater than 100 mg/dL. The prevalence of metabolic syndrome in obese adolescents is between 12% to 44% (Evidence Level I).

Other endocrinologic comorbidities include premature onset of adrenarche in boys and girls (often associated with advanced bone age) and irregular menstrual cycles with or without polycystic ovarian syndrome in adolescent girls.

The gastrointestinal system complications include nonalcoholic fatty liver disease, gastroesophageal reflux, gall bladder disease, and constipation.

Orthopedic complications include slipped capital femoral epiphysis, back pain, gait abnormalities, and acute fractures. Pulmonary complications may include sleep apnea and hypoventilation syndrome.

Obesity has significant psychological effect. Overweight youth often face bullying and teasing, which adversely affects their self-esteem. They are at increased risk for depression, which may set up a vicious cycle of binge eating, comfort eating, and obesity (Evidence Level II).

Evaluation

After rule-out of endogenous obesity (see Table 38-1), the assessment of a child with obesity should focus on behaviors related to dietary intake and activity (particularly sedentary behavior).

Dietary History

A dietary history should focus on the following topics (Evidence Level I):
- Consumption of sugar-sweetened beverages and juices
- Consumption of fruits and vegetables
- Food group portion sizes
- Eating habits including fast-food intake, family meals (and breakfast habits (Eating in front of the TV is related to higher energy consumption, and skipping breakfast is associated with weight gain.)
- Eating disorders including binge eating and comfort eating
- Sleeping habits (Overweight youth often have a TV in the bedroom, and many calories are ingested at night in front of the TV.)

A 3-day food record that includes weekdays and weekends, with a parent as a proxy reporter, may be an accurate method to assess overall energy intake in youth (Evidence Level I). History of energy-dense snack intake may be useful but may not correlate with weight change in youth (Evidence Level I). The use of cellular phone camera to document a meal is another reported strategy.

Activity Behavior Assessment

Activity behavior assessment should focus on the following topics:

- Amount of moderate-to-vigorous physical activity per day and involvement in greater than 60 minutes of moderate-to-vigorous physical activity (see Box 38-1) per day (Evidence Level I)
- Extent of sedentary activity: recreational screen time exposure greater than 2 hours per day (including TV viewing, computer use, video game use) (Evidence Level I)

Assessment of the Whole Family Unit

Assessment of the child's and family's attitude toward obesity, including readiness to change, affects success of any obesity management program. An effort should be made to assess parental attitude toward obesity, including their understanding of healthy eating habits and recognition of obesity as a health risk. Family-based interventions have been shown to be more effective than obesity management programs focusing only on the obese child. The family history should focus on any history of obesity in parents and siblings, including a maternal history of obesity, T2DM, or gestational diabetes; a family history of hyperlipidemia; and any instance of early myocardial infarction and stroke.

Physical Examination

The physical examination begins with an accurate measurement of height and weight followed by calculation of BMI and BMI percentile. A significant shift in height or weight percentiles should prompt the health care professional to verify measurements, especially in view of the height acceleration often observed following weight gain, as described above. An accurate record of vital signs is essential to diagnose hypertension, and blood pressure should be measured with an appropriately sized cuff. A thorough and systematic evaluation should be done to assess for stigmata of conditions associated with endogenous obesity (see Table 38-1) and other signs of obesity-related comorbidities (see Table 38-2).

Laboratory Evaluation

Laboratory evaluation of youth with abnormal weight gain is focused on the assessment of potential comorbidities associated with obesity (Table 38-3).

Table 38-3. Recommended Initial Laboratory Evaluation in Children 10 Years or Older

	FLP	ALT/AST	FBG
BMI >85th–94th percentiles			
Negative risk factor(s)[a]	Yes	No	No
Positive risk factor(s)[a]	Yes	Yes	Yes[b,c]
BMI ≥95th percentile	Yes	Yes	Yes[b,c]

Abbreviations: ALT, alanine aminotransferase; AST, aspartate aminotransferase; BMI, body mass index; FBG, fasting blood glucose; FLP, fasting lipid panel.

[a] Parent, grandparent, aunt/uncle, or sibling with myocardial infarction, angina, stroke, coronary artery bypass graft/stent/angioplasty at younger than 55 years in males, younger than 65 years in females.

[b] American Diabetes Association recommended indications for screening (Evidence Level III):
- Family history of type 2 diabetes in first- or second-degree relative
- Race/ethnicity (ie, Native American, African American, Latino, Asian American, Pacific Islander)
- Signs of insulin resistance or conditions associated with it (eg, acanthosis nigricans, hypertension, dyslipidemia, polycystic ovary syndrome, or small-for-gestational-age birth weight)
- Maternal history of diabetes or gestational diabetes during the child's gestation

[c] Hemoglobin A1c and 2-hour post-prandial glucose test may be used alternatively, but higher cost associated with these tests should be kept under consideration.

Modified from National Institute for Children's Health Quality. *Expert Committee Recommendations on the Assessment, Prevention and Treatment of Child and Adolescent Overweight and Obesity - 2007: An Implementation Guide from the Childhood Obesity Action Network.* Published 2007. Available at: obesity.nichq.org/resources/expert%20committee%20recommendation%20implementation%20 guide. Accessed February 9, 2015.

In addition to the studies outlined in Table 38-3, the following tests should be ordered based on history and physical examination findings:
- Orthopedic: radiographs of joints as needed for evaluation of joint pain
- Respiratory: polysomnography for obstructive sleep apnea
- Pulmonary function tests: for breathing difficulty from obesity hypoventilation syndrome
- Endocrine:
  - Routine endocrine testing in not necessary unless other endocrinopathy is clinically evident, such as premature adrenarche or growth failure. Bone age, assessed with a radiograph of the left hand and wrist, is often advanced in obese children.
  - Striae are frequently seen in obese youth and do not warrant an investigation for Cushing syndrome unless associated with growth failure and hypertension (Evidence Level I).
  - To assess for polycystic ovarian syndrome evaluation, measure serum androgen (testosterone total and free), gonadotropin (luteinizing hormone and follicle-stimulating hormone), and sex hormone–binding globulin concentrations. Pelvic ultrasound may be indicated if clinical and laboratory study findings are inconclusive.

Management
· · · · · · · · · · · ·

The management of obesity is challenging. The main treatment modality is lifestyle modification with nutritional counseling and encouragement of regular exercise (Box 38-1).

Box 38-1. Suggested Family-Based Lifestyle Modification for Youth With Obesity

Nutritional
- Decreasing/eliminating sugar-sweetened beverages
- Ensuring 3 meals daily, including breakfast
- Encouraging consumption of 5 servings of fruits (2) and vegetables (3) per day
- Controlling portion size
- Limiting consumption of fast-food intake and "eating out"
- Having a set routine for family mealtime, avoiding distractions such as TV viewing
- Removing junk food from the household, having healthy food readily available

Physical-Sedentary Activity
- Encouraging ≥60 min of moderate[a] to vigorous[b] physical activity/day to be incorporated in the daily routine (eg, parking far away from the store, taking stairs, walking to friend's house)
- Limiting screen viewing, including computer use and video games, to <2 h per day
- Removal of TV from the bedrooms

[a] Examples of moderate physical activity include playing baseball or jogging.
[b] Examples of vigorous physical activity include running or playing soccer.

Various methods can be used to explain portion size. Picturing the serving sizes is effective and may help contain the portion size, even when an unhealthy choice, such as french fries, is made. It is important that health care professionals point out that one container may hold more than one serving. Additionally, children, adolescents, and their parents may benefit from an explanation about the energy content of a specific food portion in relation to total daily energy requirements as determined by age, sex, and physical activity level (Table 38-4).

In 2007, the expert committee published recommendations for the assessment, prevention, and treatment of overweight and obesity in children and adolescents. They define "a staged approach to obesity treatment," which includes weight loss targets (Table 38-5). The treatment algorithm starts at "Stage 1 Prevention Plus" and escalates to the next stage if weight/BMI or velocity has not improved after 3 to 6 months.

Table 38-4. Energy Daily Requirement Based on Age, Sex, and Physical Activity Level[a]

Age (y)	Daily Kilocalories per Activity Level					
	Sedentary[b]		Moderate[b]		Active[b]	
	Female	Male	Female	Male	Female	Male
2–3	1,000–1,200	1,000–1,200	1,000–1,400	1,000–1,400	1,000–1,400	1,000–1,400
4–8	1,200–1,400	1,200–1,400	1,400–1,600	1,400–1,600	1,400–1,800	1,400–1,800
9–13	1,400–1,600	1,600–2,000	1,600–2,000	1,800–2,200	1,800–2,200	2,000–2,600
14–18	1,800	2,000–2,400	2,000	2,400–2,800	2,400	2,800–3,200
19–21	1,800–2,000	2,400–2,600	2,000–2,200	2,600–2,800	2,400	3,000

[a] Based on estimated energy requirements (EER) equations, using reference heights (average) and reference weights (health) for each age/sex group EER equations.

[b] *Sedentary* is a lifestyle that includes only the light physical activity (PA) associated with typical day-to-day life. *Moderate* is a lifestyle that includes PA equivalent to walking about 1.5 to 3 miles/day at 3–4 miles/hour, in addition to the light PA associated with typical day-to-day life. *Active* is a lifestyle that includes PA equivalent to walking >3 miles/day at 3–4 miles/hour, in addition to the light PA activity associated with typical day-to-day life.

[c] Estimates for females do not include women who are pregnant or breastfeeding.

Modified from the National Heart, Lung, and Blood Institute. *Integrated Guidelines for Cardiovascular Health and Risk Reduction in Children and Adolescents*. Bethesda, MD: US Department of Health and Human Services; 2012. NIH publication 12-7486A. October 2012. Available at: www.nhlbi.nih.gov/guidelines/cvd_ped/index.htm. Accessed February 9, 2015.

Table 38-5. Weight Loss Goals per the Expert Committee Recommendations, 2007

BMI	Age (y)		
	2–5	6–11	12–19
85th–94th percentile	Decrease weight velocity or weight maintenance.	Decrease weight velocity or weight maintenance.	Decrease weight velocity or weight maintenance.
94th–99th percentile	Weight maintenance	Weight loss: 1 lb/mo	Weight loss: 1 lb/wk
≥99th percentile	Gradual weight: ½ lb/wk	Weight loss: 2 lb/wk	Weight loss: 2 lb/wk

Abbreviation: BMI, body mass index.

Modified from National Institute for Children's Health Quality. *Expert Committee Recommendations on the Assessment, Prevention, and Treatment of Child and Adolescent Overweight and Obesity - 2007: An Implementation Guide from the Childhood Obesity Action Network*. Published 2007. Available at: obesity.nichq.org/resources /expert%20committee%20recommendation%20implementation%20guide. Accessed February 9, 2015.

The various stages of the treatment algorithm are as follows:

- *Stage 1 Prevention Plus.* Involves family visits with a health care professional with some training in pediatric weight management/behavioral counseling. The whole family should be involved in the lifestyle modification process.
  - *Family-based life style modifications:* Selected goals are defined in Table 38-5.
  - *Weight goal:* The main goal is weight maintenance or a decrease in BMI velocity. The long-term BMI target is equal to or less than the 85th percentile, although some children can be healthy with a BMI of between the 85the and 94th percentile.
- *Stage 2 Structured Weight Management.* At this stage, the family visits (monthly) a health care professional specifically trained in weight management.
- *Stage 3 Comprehensive, Multidisciplinary Intervention.* The family is referred to a multidisciplinary team with experience in childhood obesity. Follow-up is often weekly for 8 to 12 weeks with follow-up.
- *Stage 4 Tertiary Care Intervention.* This stage involves the use of medications (Orlistat), very-low-calorie diets, and weight control surgery (gastric bypass or banding). It is recommended for selected patients only if provided by experienced programs with established clinical or research protocols.

In November 2011, the National Heart, Lung, and Blood Institute published the *Integrated Guidelines for Cardiovascular Health and Risk Reduction in Children and Adolescents* (Evidence Level I–III), which provide further details about the dietary treatment of children and adolescents with abnormal weight gain. While the focus of this committee was on children and adolescents at elevated cardiovascular risk, the recommended Cardiovascular Health Integrated Lifestyle Diet (CHILD 1) can be used as a first-step diet for all children and youth with abnormal weight gain (Box 38-2).

The Center for Nutrition Policy and Promotion, an organization of the US Department of Agriculture, recently developed a simplified food guidance system called MyPlate (http://choosemyplate.gov). The main messages of this program are

- *Balancing calories.* Eat less and avoid oversized portions.
- *Foods to be increased.* Make half the plate fruits and vegetables, make at least half the grains whole grains, switch to fat-free or low-fat (1%) milk, and vary the protein food choices.
- *Foods to be reduced.* Reduce high-sodium foods such as soup, bread, and frozen items, and drink water instead of sugary drinks.

Box 38-2. Cardiovascular Health–Integrated Lifestyle Diet (CHILD 1)

Birth–6 mo
- Exclusively breastfeed (no supplemental formula or other foods) until age 6 mo.[a]

6–12 mo
- Continue breastfeeding[a] until at least age 12 mo. Gradually add solid foods; transition to iron-fortified formula if reducing breastfeeding.
- Fat intake should not be restricted without medical indication.
- *Encourage water.* Limit 100% fruit juice to <4 oz/day, with no sweetened beverages.

After 12 mo
- Transition to reduced-fat[b] (2% to fat-free) unflavored cow's milk.[c]
- *Encourage water.* Avoid sugar-sweetened beverage intake.
- Transition to table food
  - *With* total fat 30% of daily kcal/EER,[d] saturated fat 8%–10% of daily kcal/EER, monounsaturated and polyunsaturated fat up to 20% of daily kcal/EER
  - With *limited* cholesterol <300 mg/day
  - *Without* trans fat as much as possible

Supportive actions
- The fat content of cow's milk to be introduced at age 12–24 mo should be decided together by parents and health care professionals based on the child's growth/obesity risk, intake of other nutrient-dense foods, and other sources of fat.
- Continue limiting 100% fruit juice (from a cup) to <4 oz/day.
- Limit sodium intake.
- Consider DASH-type diet (**D**ietary **A**pproaches to **S**top **H**ypertension) rich in fruits, vegetables, whole grains, low-fat/fat-free milk and milk products; lower in sugar. Be mindful that excessive fruit intake leads to excessive carbohydrate/calories.
- Teach portions based on EER for age/sex; use tools such as age-appropriate smaller plates, cups, and bowls.
- Encourage regular moderate-to-vigorous physical activity, with parents modeling it.
- Encourage dietary fiber from foods: age plus 5 g/day.[e]

[a] Infants that cannot be fed directly at the breast should be fed expressed milk pumped and stored properly. Infants for whom expressed milk is not available should be fed iron-fortified formula.

[b] For toddlers 12–24 months of age with a family history of obesity, heart disease, or high cholesterol, parents should discuss possibility of transition to reduced-fat milk with the pediatric care professional after 12 months of age.

[c] Continued breastfeeding is still appropriate and nutritionally superior to cow's milk. Milk reduced in fat should be used only in the context of an overall diet that supplies 30% of calories from fat.

[d] EER is estimated energy requirements per day for age/sex (see Table 38-4).

[e] Naturally fiber-rich foods are recommended (fruits, vegetables, whole grains); fiber supplements are not advised. Limit refined carbohydrates (sugars, white rice, and white bread).

Modified from the National Heart, Lung, and Blood Institute. *Integrated Guidelines for Cardiovascular Health and Risk Reduction in Children and Adolescents.* Bethesda, MD: US Department of Health and Human Services; 2012. NIH publication 12-7486A. October 2012. Available at: www.nhlbi.nih.gov/guidelines/cvd_ped/index.htm. Accessed February 9, 2015.

Medical Management of Obesity and Related Complications

Pharmacotherapy may be considered for youth with a BMI equal to or greater than the 95th percentile (or an absolute BMI greater than 35 kg/m^2) whose comprehensive lifestyle modification weight loss program has failed and who have significant insulin resistance. The following medications can be considered:

- *Metformin (Evidence Level II).* Metformin is currently US Food and Drug Administration approved for use in youth 10 years or older for T2DM only.
- *Orlistat (Evidence Level I).* Orlistat is US Food and Drug Administration approved for weight loss in youth older than 12 years. Note: Orlistat safety information now includes a warning about the risk of severe liver injury.

Box 38-3. Medical Therapy of Obesity-Related Comorbidities

Diabetes mellitus (Evidence Level I)
- Medical management is guided by the level of diabetes control and the HbA1c.
- Metformin standard release or extended release: 500–2000 mg per day
- Other oral hypoglycemic agents that are US FDA approved for use in patients >18 y (eg, biguanides, DPP-4 inhibitors, thiazolidinediones, GLP-1 agonists such as exenatide, liraglutide)
- Insulin analogs using basal- and bolus-insulin regimen (preferable) vs fixed-dose mixed insulin regimens

Hyperlipidemia (Evidence Level I-II)
- CHILD 2 diet and lifestyle changes for 6 months.
- Pharmacotherapy with statins/HMG CoA inhibitors to be considered ≥10 years based on the LDL concentration, number and level of risk factors.
- Triglyceride concentration more than 1,000 mg/dL are treated with omega-3 fatty acid/fibrates/niacin in patients >18 y.

Hypertension (Evidence Level III)
- CHILD 1 diet along with low-sodium diets
- In children 6–17 y: may use losartan, amlodipine, felodipine, fosinopril, lisinopril, metoprolol, and valsartan
- In African American youth: may need fosinopril for effective blood pressure control

PCOS (Evidence Level II)
- Metformin at maximum tolerated dose +/−
- Oral contraceptive pills +/−
- Medications with antiandrogenic effects (eg, spironolactone)

OSA (Evidence Level II)
- Tonsillectomy and adenoidectomy
- CPAP device use overnight

NAFLD (Evidence Level II)
- Nutritional management (See above.)
- Behavioral modification (See above.)
- Metformin
- Thiazolidinediones

Abbreviations: CHILD, cardiovascular health-integrated lifestyle diet; CPAP, continuous positive airway pressure; DPP, dipeptidyl peptidase; FDA, Food and Drug Administration; GLP, glucagon-like peptide; HbA1c, hemoglobin A1c; HMG CoA, 3-hydroxy-3-methyl-glutaryl-CoA; NAFLD, nonalcoholic fatty liver disease; LDL, Low density lipoprotein cholesterol; OSA, obstructive sleep apnea; PCOS, polycystic ovary syndrome.

Weight Loss Surgery/Bariatric Surgery in Adolescents

Youth with extreme obesity often do not respond to lifestyle changes or medical management. Weight loss surgery (WLS) has become an alternative management for patients with extreme obesity and significant obesity-related comorbidities. Remarkable improvement in, or even resolution of obesity-related comorbidities (ie, diabetes, hyperlipidemia, hypertension, and sleep apnea), is seen after bariatric surgery. For example, obese adults with uncontrolled type 2 diabetes show significant reduction of their insulin requirements and may discontinue insulin therapy following gastric bypass surgery. However, all bariatric surgical procedures are associated with long-term complications and require prolonged periods of monitoring. Therefore, youth should be carefully selected for bariatric surgery only when benefits clearly outweigh the unknown potential complications and need for long-term follow-up (Table 38-6).

Recently, modified selection criteria for WLS were published (Evidence Level II-III). Health care professionals should also keep in mind that the long-term outcomes and effects of WLS are unknown.

Table 38-6. Selection Criteria for Weight Loss Surgery in Adolescents

Comorbidities	BMI (kg/m^2) >35	BMI (kg/m^2) >40
Type 2 diabetes mellitus	✓	✓
Moderate or severe obstructive sleep apnea (AHI >15 events/h)	✓	✓
Pseudotumor cerebri	✓	✓
Severe steatohepatitis	✓	✓
Mild obstructive sleep apnea (AHI ≥5 events/h)		✓
Hypertension		✓
Insulin resistance, glucose intolerance, dyslipidemia		✓
Impaired quality of life or activities of daily living, among others		✓

Table 38-6 (cont)

Eligibility Criteria[a]	
Tanner Stage	IV or V (unless severe comorbidities indicate WLS earlier)
Skeletal maturity	Completed at least 95% of estimated growth (only if planning a diversional or malabsorptive operation, including RYGB)
Lifestyle changes	Demonstrates ability to understand what dietary and physical activity changes will be required for optimal postoperative outcomes
Psychosocial	Evidence of • Mature decision-making, with appropriate understanding of potential risks and benefits of surgery. • Appropriate social support without evidence of abuse or neglect. • If psychiatric condition (eg, depression, anxiety, or binge-eating disorder) is present, it is under treatment. • Family and patient have the ability and motivation to comply with recommended treatments preoperatively and postoperatively, including consistent use of micronutrient supplements.

Abbreviations: AHI, apnea-hypopnea index; BMI, body mass index; RYGB, Roux-en-Y gastric bypass; WLS, weight loss surgery.

[a] All of the eligibility criteria must be fulfilled irrespective of BMI.

Modified from Pratt JS, Lenders CM, Dionne EA, et al. Best practice updates for pediatric/adolescent weight loss surgery. *Obesity (Silver Spring)*. 2009;17(5):901–910, with permission.

Various WLS surgical procedures include
- Roux-en-Y gastric bypass, which is considered a safe and effective option for extremely obese adolescents. However, appropriate long-term follow-up should be provided (Evidence Level II).
- Sleeve gastrectomy, which should be considered investigational.
- Adjustable gastric band, which is not approved by the US Food and Drug Administration for use in adolescents.
- Biliopancreatic diversion and duodenal switch procedures, which are not recommended in adolescents.

Suggested Reading

Cook S, Auinger P, Li C, Ford ES. Metabolic syndrome rates in united states adolescents, from the National Health and Nutrition Examination Survey, 1999-2002. *J Pediatr*. 2008;152(2):165–170

Davis MM, Gance-Cleveland B, Hassink S, Johnson R, Paradis G, Resnicow K. Recommendations for prevention of childhood obesity. *Pediatrics*. 2007;120(Suppl 4):S229–S253

Epstein LH. Family-based behavioural intervention for obese children. *Int J Obes Relat Metab Dis*. 1996;20(Suppl 1):S14–S21

National Heart, Lung, and Blood Institute. *Integrated Guidelines for Cardiovascular Health and Risk Reduction in Children and Adolescents.* Bethesda, MD: US Department of Health and Human Services; 2012. NIH publication 12-7486A. http://www.nhlbi.nih.gov/guidelines/cvd_ped/index.htm. Published October 2012. Accessed February 9, 2015

Nicklas TA, Yang SJ, Baranowski T, Zakeri I, Berenson G. Eating patterns and obesity in children. The Bogalusa Heart Study. *Am J Prev Med.* 2003;25(1):9–16

Pratt JS, Lenders CM, Dionne EA,et al. Best practice updates for pediatric/adolescent weight loss surgery. *Obesity (Silver Spring).* 2009;17(5):901–910

Quattrin T, Liu E, Shaw N, Shine B, Chiang E. Obese children referred to the pediatric endocrinologist: characteristics and outcome. *Pediatrics.* 2005;115(2):348–351

Quattrin T, Roemmich JN, Paluch R, Yu J, Epstein L, Ecker M. Efficacy of family-based weight control program for preschool children in primary care. *Pediatrics.* 2012;130(4):660–666

Rafalson L, Eysaman J, Quattrin T. Screening obese students for acanthosis nigricans and other diabetes risk factors in the urban school-based health center. *Clin Pediatr.* 2011;50(8):747–752

Strong WB, Malina RM, Blimkie CJ, et al. Evidence based physical activity for school-age youth. *J Pediatr.* 2005;146(6):732–737

CHAPTER 39

Orthopedics: The Limp

Steven L. Frick, MD

Key Points

- The most common cause of limp in a child is trauma; the most concerning is musculoskeletal infection or neoplasm.

- Some diagnoses are time-sensitive and failure to make a timely diagnosis can lead to further harm (eg, septic arthritis [permanent joint damage], leukemia/malignant tumor [spread of malignancy], slipped capital femoral epiphysis [further slip progression and risk of osteonecrosis], muscular dystrophy [failure to offer genetic counseling prior to another pregnancy].

- A good history and physical examination, radiographs, and laboratory studies (complete blood count with differential, erythrocyte sedimentation rate, or C-reactive protein) can result in correct diagnosis in the vast majority of cases.

Overview

The limping child presents a diagnostic challenge. The most important task for the clinician is to make a presumptive diagnosis explaining the etiology of the limp. Limping children should be followed until the limp resolves and should be referred for evaluation by a specialist if limping persists. Common causes of limp can be grouped by ages to assist clinicians in formulating the differential diagnosis: younger children (ages 1 to 3 years), children (ages 4 to 10), and adolescents (ages 11 to 17) (Table 39-1).

Table 39-1. Common Causes of Limping in Skeletally Immature Patients, Grouped by Typical Age of Presentation

Toddlers	Children	Adolescents
Septic arthritis	Septic arthritis	Septic arthritis
Transient synovitis	Transient synovitis	—
Osteomyelitis	Osteomyelitis	Osteomyelitis
Fracture	Fracture	Fracture
DDH	Perthes	SCFE
JIA	JIA	—
Muscular dystrophy	Muscular dystrophy	—
Cerebral palsy	Cerebral palsy	—
ALL	ALL	—
—	Overuse syndromes	Overuse syndromes
—	Tarsal coalition	Tarsal coalition
—	Growing pains	—
—	Discoid meniscus	Osteochondritis dessicans

Abbreviations: ALL, acute lymphoblastic leukemia; DDH, developmental dislocation of the hip; JIA, juvenile idiopathic arthritis; SCFE, slipped capital femoral epiphysis.

Definition

Physical examination of the musculoskeletal system should always include an observation of the gait pattern in children of walking age.

A limp can be simply defined as an abnormal gait. The most common limp is an antalgic gait, defined as a shortened stance phase. This typically indicates a painful condition in which the child is spending less time weight bearing on the injured side and thus will lift the foot on the injured side early. Another commonly seen form of limp is the abductor lurch, or Trendelenburg gait, caused by weakness of the hip and pelvic musculature, resulting in the pelvis tilting downward. A short-limbed gait can be noted by compensation for the limb length discrepancy with toe walking on the short side, or flexion of the hip and knee on the longer side, to maintain a level pelvis during gait. An uncompensated short-limb gait will show pelvic tilt from step to step, as if the patient were stepping into a hole on the short side. Children with spastic muscles can have very complicated gait patterns, as they compensate for abnormal muscle and neurologic function. Common presentations are toe walking, crouched gait (ie, increased knee flexion throughout the stance phase), and stiff knee gait. A stiff knee gait is indicated by toe walking on the opposite side, with outward rotation of the involved limb, circumduction of the involved limb (ie, swinging outward), or elevation of pelvis on the involved side. Common causes of a stiff knee gait include spasticity as well as knee injuries. Children with a stiff knee gait will have difficulty clearing the foot on the involved side, as knee flexion is the most critical motion to allow foot clearance during swing. An important gait pattern to recognize is proximal muscle weakness gait. This is commonly seen in children with muscular dystrophy, and, thus, most are young boys who present with increased lordosis (ie, hyperextension) of the lumbar spine during gait to compensate for weak hip extensors and will maintain knee extension during gait to prevent loading of the quadriceps muscles. Children suspected of having this gait pattern should undergo a test for Gowers sign, in which the child is asked to sit on the floor and stand up without assistance. A positive Gowers sign is noted if the child climbs up himself by placing his hands on his knees and thighs and uses his upper extremities to push his trunk up into an extended position, as the hip extensor muscles are too weak to easily get the trunk into an erect position without help.

Causes and Differential Diagnosis

A key fact to remember when evaluating children with a limp is that trauma is the most common cause. This is usually a minor fracture or a simple contusion; significant fractures typically present with a refusal to bear weight on the involved limb rather than a limp. The most concerning causes of limp are musculoskeletal infection or neoplasm. Making a timely diagnosis is most critical for septic arthritis, as delay in diagnosis may allow the infection to permanently damage the articular cartilage of the joint, resulting in loss of function and potential growth disturbance. Because of the potential for spread and systemic infection, the diagnosis of acute osteomyelitis in a timely fashion is also important to limit morbidity and speed resolution with appropriate therapy. Malignant bone tumors are rare, but making the correct diagnosis as soon as possible is obviously desired. The most common malignancy involving bone is acute leukemia. In one study, almost 20% of children with acute lymphoblastic leukemia (ALL) presented with the chief concern of limp or extremity pain. In children evaluated for limp due to proximal muscle weakness, a timely diagnosis of a genetic disorder may affect family planning.

Younger Children (Ages 1 to 3 Years)

The history is often provided by the parents but is often inaccurate as well. Minor traumas may not be witnessed, as well as other events that may precipitate a limp. The list of the differential diagnosis includes fracture of the foot or lower extremity, foreign body in the foot, lower extremity or foot contusion, transient synovitis, septic arthritis, osteomyelitis, discitis, neurologic disorders, cerebral palsy, muscular dystrophy, developmental dysplasia of the hip, coxa vara, juvenile idiopathic arthritis, neoplasms, and leukemia.

Children (Ages 4 to 10)

In this age group, it is usually easier to get a more complete history from the patient. As secondary gain issues are less common in children than adults, concerns of lower extremity pain or limping should be investigated thoroughly.

A common concern in this age group is bilateral lower extremity "growing pains" that may present with concerns of a limp or abnormal gait, even when the main issue is recurring episodes of self-limited pain (actual limping during examination is uncommon). This is most frequently present after vigorous daytime activities, occurs just before bedtime, and is relieved by parental massage or mild over-the-counter analgesics. The next morning, the child is typically normal and has another active day, but the pattern is frequently recurring and is typical for the diagnosis of growing pains. Reassurance is all that is needed for this diagnosis. Instructions to the parents should emphasize that if the concerns worsen, the limp persists throughout the daytime (particularly if it results in the child refusing to participate in activities that are enjoyable), or the pain begins to awaken the child from a sound sleep, further evaluation may be needed and a return visit is recommended. In children, the differential diagnosis list for limping still includes possible infection of joints or bones, traumatic conditions including minor fractures, and transient synovitis. Other diagnoses are a limb length discrepancy that is progressive or a discoid meniscus. Mild cerebral palsy is often not appreciated until children reach an age where youth sports begin, and it becomes noticeable that during running the children have an abnormal pattern or are unable to keep up with their peers. This age is also the time when Legg-Calve-Perthés disease is typically first symptomatic.

Adolescents (Ages 11 to 17)

Typically 2 different groups of patients are in this age group: those who minimize their injury and want a rapid return to sports or other physical activities and those who emphasize their symptoms and are seeking a medical excuse to avoid physical activity. In addition to the differential diagnoses considered in the first 2 age groups, adolescents often present with overuse symptoms, including stress fractures and apophysitis, as well as other musculoskeletal conditions related to maturation and the stresses placed by active young people on growth plates and developing bones. These include slipped capital femoral epiphysis and osteochondroses such as Osgood-Schlatter disease, tendinitis, and stress fractures. Some other diagnoses commonly presenting with symptoms in this age group are symptomatic hip dysplasia, tarsal coalition, and osteochondritis dissecans.

Clinical Features

Septic Arthritis

Children with septic arthritis typically present with sudden onset of symptoms, frequently localized to the joint involved. Many children presenting with septic arthritis will provide a history of a recent mild trauma. The clinician should remember to consider septic arthritis in the differential diagnosis of the limping child, even when a clear history of trauma preceding the onset of symptoms has been given. Early in the onset of the infection, limping will occur and may progress to complete refusal to bear weight on the involved limb as the child seeks to keep the involved joint immobile. Motion of the involved joint typically causes severe pain. Swelling and erythema may be notable if the joint is superficial, but for deep joints, such as the hip, the physical appearance can be very benign. Younger patients tend to have more severe presentation with rapid onset of joint immobility, whereas older patients and in particular adolescents may continue to ambulate and limp on infected joints. While a fever and progression to a febrile systemic illness commonly occur in septic arthritis, some children present without fever and may appear well with the exception of a limp or extremity pain. Septic arthritis can occur in any age group, with a slight predilection for toddlers and children younger than 2 years.

In certain endemic areas of the United States, children presenting with joint swelling and pain should be evaluated for infection with *Borrelia burgdorferi*.

Transient Synovitis

Transient or toxic synovitis also presents with acute onset of joint pain and limp and may also progress to a failure to bear weight on the involved limb. Patients will restrict the range of motion of the involved joint to limit pain. It is most commonly seen between the ages of 3 and 8 and thus less common in toddlers and adolescents. Typically, patients do not have a fever or systemic illness, and the severity of symptoms is usually less severe than patients with septic arthritis. Frequently, there is a history of a recent viral upper respiratory tract illness. Transient synovitis is believed to be an immunologic response to a viral illness or a trauma and usually has a gradual course with complete resolution following symptomatic treatment with anti-inflammatory medications.

Osteomyelitis

Acute hematologic osteomyelitis can occur in any age group but is most frequently seen in patients with open growth plates. The location of osteomyelitis is most frequent in the metaphyseal region of long bones and is related to the vascular anatomy at the junction between the metaphysis and the growth plate. Patients usually present with acute onset of pain and often fever. They present with limp, refusal to move the involved bone, and diminished range of motion in the adjacent joints. Swelling and erythema, as well as warmth, may be present over the involved area, and tenderness to palpation on the involved area of bone is almost always present.

Subacute hematogenous osteomyelitis has a very different presentation and accounts for almost one-third of primary bone infections. The onset is insidious, with very few symptoms, and it is typically present for a longer duration. Patients often present with minimal physical examination findings but complain of mild persistent pain and limp.

Chronic multifocal osteomyelitis is a rare condition of unknown etiology. These patients often have vague constitutional symptoms along with localized bone pain. They also may have skin lesions, such as psoriasis or pustulosis. Many believe that this is a inflammatory disorder and not infectious etiology. Multiple regions are involved with characteristic bone lesions, often in the diaphyseal region of long bones, especially the clavicle.

Discitis

Discitis may present in toddlers who have difficulty walking or even refuse to walk, but it can be seen in other age groups as well. *Infectious spondylodiscitis* is now the preferred terminology. Patients frequently present with a limp or refusal to bear weight, and this may progress to pseudoparalysis. Frequently, these patients do not appear ill and often are not febrile. They typically have elevated inflammatory blood markers and when diagnosed early have a rapid response to antibiotic therapy.

Fractures

The most common fracture that will present in the limping toddler is a non-displaced fracture of the tibia from a torsional injury, without an associated fibula fracture. This is termed a "toddler's fracture." There may be no witnessed trauma, and the presentation is sudden unexplained onset of a limp or refusal to bear weight. Symptoms should be localized to the tibia, and frequently the physical examination findings are positive only for tenderness to palpation, without any swelling or deformity. Other fractures that are common in young children are fractures that occur near or through the growth plates (eg, in the foot at the base of the first metatarsal, in the ankle at the lateral malleolus). Typically, motion of the involved bone causes increased pain, as does palpation over the fracture.

Pyomyositis

Pyomyositis is an infection of muscle and frequently can mimic septic arthritis, particularly in the hip. Patients present similarly, with acute onset of the pain and discomfort with motion. Stretching the most involved muscle will cause pain and thus the patient will try to limit this motion. The symptoms are usually not as severe as septic arthritis but can be difficult to differentiate. Commonly involved muscles include the psoas muscle and other muscles around the pelvis and thigh. Many of these muscles are deep and are not able to be easily palpated; thus, tenderness and swelling are difficult to appreciate. It is important to consider this diagnosis when findings from studies performed to diagnose septic arthritis are negative, but the patient's presentation and examination suggest an infectious etiology.

Myositis

Patients with myositis often present with limited, focal tenderness and limited motion. In addition to infection, inflammatory problems can affect the muscles and create a situation in which the patient presents with a limp.

Cerebral Palsy

Patients with cerebral palsy usually present with a history of delayed motor milestones and concerns of an abnormal gait. Mild gait abnormalities may be present in these patients, such as toe walking, lack of coordination, or frequent tripping and falling. Careful physical examination may reveal signs of spasticity, such as increased muscle tone, resistance during rapid flexion and extension of joints, hyperreflexia, and clonus. In addition to examining the child during walking, asking her to run can magnify subtle abnormalities of gait and make the diagnosis easier. This will commonly be seen in the child with mild hemiplegic cerebral palsy, in which asking her to run will exaggerate posturing of the involved upper extremity, with diminished arm swing during the gait cycle.

Muscular Dystrophy

Muscular dystrophy often presents in the toddler age group with delayed ambulation, stumbling, falling, and, in particular, difficulty climbing or ascending stairs. Frequently, these children are having difficulty keeping up with their peers during play. Examination may reveal toe walking and proximal muscle weakness. Tightness of the calf muscles may have an effect on the foot architecture, and often the chief concern in these young boys is of flat feet, along with abnormal gait. Thus, every toddler boy presenting with a concern of flat feet should be examined with a Gowers sign. In classic cases, pseudohypertrophy of the calf muscles will also be present.

Developmental Hip Dislocation

Children with dislocated hips from birth will typically not have any pain. They often have an abnormal gait related to the altered biomechanics, with the dislocated hip causing the abductor muscles to have an ineffective lever arm. These children may present with seemingly benign chief concerns of intoeing and an abnormal gait. The Galeazzi sign is helpful in diagnosing unilateral or asymmetric bilateral cases; a positive Galeazzi sign is demonstrated with the patient lying supine and the hips flexed to 90 degrees, when lengths of the femoral segments are not equal.

Juvenile Idiopathic Arthritis

Juvenile idiopathic arthritis is classified based on the number of joints involved. The most common presentation for limping children will occur in patients with pauciarticular juvenile arthritis. It most commonly presents around the age of 2 years, and the knee, ankle, or subtalar joint is the most frequent cause of symptoms and limping.

Bone Tumors

Malignant bone tumors are very rare in children presenting with a limp. The most common malignant bone tumors in the pediatric age group will be small round blue cell tumors, such as Ewing sarcoma or peripheral neuroectodermal tumors; in adolescents, osteogenic sarcoma will be more common. Benign tumors, such as nonossifying fibromas; simple bone cysts; and aneurysmal bone cysts may also cause pain, particularly if they are large enough to structurally weaken the bone. Another rare benign bone tumor that often causes pain is an osteoid osteoma; classically, this presents with pain present at night that is dramatically relieved with aspirin or other nonsteroidal medications.

Leukemia

Acute leukemia is the most frequent neoplasm in children younger than 16 years, with musculoskeletal concerns as the presenting feature in approximately 20% of these patients. Bone pain in the lower extremities and a limp are common chief concerns. Frequently, night pain is present, as well as pain at rest. Occasionally, a leukemic infiltration will cause a joint effusion.

Legg-Calvé-Perthes Disease

Legg-Calvé-Perthes disease is most common in children between ages 4 to 8 years, although it can occur in older children. It results from a disruption of the blood supply to the growing femoral head (known as proximal femoral epiphysis), leading to eventual collapse of the femoral head to varying degrees depending on the severity. The cause of the disorder is unknown, but boys are more commonly affected than girls and are typically small for their age and often very active. They frequently present with a limp and concerns of groin pain, although often the pain may be referred to the knee region. An antalgic gait is often present, and physical examination findings typically show increased pain at the extremes of motion, particularly internal rotation or abduction of the hip. These physical findings will localize the symptoms to the hip joint and allow for targeted radiographic imaging to make the diagnosis. The symptoms frequently wax and wane but are persistent and will last for months to years, depending on the severity of involvement.

Limb Length Discrepancy

There are multiple possible causes of limb length discrepancy: congenital growth disturbances, acquired growth disturbances following trauma or infection, vascular malformations and overgrowth, overgrowth following fractures, and neurologic disorders resulting in diminished growth on one side. Physical findings are an uneven pelvis when standing with the feet together, unequal limb lengths as measured from the anterior superior iliac spine to the medial malleolus, or different femoral and tibial lengths when measured supine with the hips and knees flexed.

Slipped Capital Femoral Epiphysis

Slipped capital femoral epiphysis is the most common disorder of the hip in adolescents and is typically seen in overweight children. The cause is thought to be a combination of obesity, skeletal alignment, and hormonal effects of puberty leading to a gradual mechanical failure of the proximal femoral growth plate, resulting in the femoral head slipping off the femoral neck. Boys typically present around the age of 14; and girls, around the age of 12. Physical findings in addition to an increased body mass index are limited internal rotation of the hip, pain with attempted active straight leg raising, and a hip limp (known as an abductor lurch). Frequently, the pain is referred to the knee, supporting the axiom that knee pain equals hip pain in the skeletally immature patient until proven otherwise.

Overuse Syndromes

Overuse syndromes are commonly seen in older children and adolescents, especially as participation in youth sports has increased. These most commonly involve areas of tenderness over growth plates at the site of tendon insertions. The medical terminology for this is *apophysitis,* commonly seen at the heel (ie, Severs syndrome) and the knee (ie, Osgood-Schlatter syndrome). Stress fractures are now also more commonly seen and result when the growing bone is subjected to repetitive stresses that exceed the bone's ability to mechanically support the stress. These occur most commonly in the foot, ankle, and leg. Rest, activity modification, and anti-inflammatory medications result in resolution. In young patients with true stress fractures, an assessment of bone health with a nutritional history, menstrual history in girls, and possible work-up of bone mineral chemistry may be indicated.

Discoid Meniscus

The abnormal shape and thickness of the lateral meniscus can limit knee motion (usually the knee cannot be fully extended) and predispose the meniscus to trauma and tearing. Children often present between ages 4 and 7 years, commonly when the meniscus has torn, with limp, pain, and swelling.

Osteochondritis Dissecans

Osteochondritis dissecans most commonly occurs in adolescents and presents typically with knee pain, although it may involve the ankle. Repetitive stress is believed to be the cause. Patients typically present with joint pain and occasionally swelling/effusions.

Tarsal Coalitions

Tarsal coalitions are a failure of segmentation of the tarsal bones of the foot. Depending on the bones involved, presentation with a limp and foot pain typically occurs between the ages of 8 and 12 years. These patients typically present with a mild limp and are found to have significantly limited inversion and eversion movements of the foot.

Evaluation

· · · · · · · · · · ·

History

The goal of history taking is to clarify the onset of symptoms, the duration of symptoms, and the severity of symptoms and to ask specific questions to determine the acuity of the problem. Most important is to rule out septic arthritis, as failure to quickly treat an infectious process may result in permanent destruction of articular cartilage and, in severe cases, epiphyseal cartilage, with resultant growth disturbances. Second, questions directed at the presence of possible neoplasm are important in making the diagnosis when a malignant process is present so that appropriate therapy can begin rapidly. Inquiries should be made into the presence of a fever; a history of any recent illnesses, weight loss or constitutional symptoms, increases in activity, or falls or trauma; a history of night or rest pain; and whether the child can climb stairs easily or keep up with peers.

Physical Examination

Physical examination begins with observational gait analysis, observing the child walking toward and away from the physician and also from the side as the child walks by the physician. Attention should be paid to how the foot strikes the floor; the amount of time spent in stance phase; motion at the ankle, knee, and hip; whether the pelvis remains level; the ability to clear the foot in swing phase; and if reciprocal arm swing is present. The ability to balance the trunk and head centered over the pelvis during the gait cycle is also noted. When the child is on the examination table, attention should be paid to the resting position of the joints. In the presence of large joint effusions, typically the hip and knee are held in a position of flexion; and the ankle, in plantar flexion. The presence or absence of active movement, or resistance to passive movement at each joint, should be noted.

When supine, the ability of the patient to actively lift the heel off of the examination table within the leg extended (an active straight leg raise test) will load the hip joint and is a good quick test for irritability of the hip joint. For hip pathology, internal rotation is frequently the first passive motion that will become restricted, so testing internal rotation of the hip to see if it causes pain is excellent for hip pathology. Careful palpation of the skeleton should be performed in the limping child, beginning in the lumbar spine, along the pelvis, down the femur, over the knees, down the legs over both the tibia and fibula, and then to the ankle and the feet. The knee, ankle, and subtalar joints should be assessed for the presence or absence of effusion. Palpation of the soft tissues of the lower extremities should be completed to assess for the presence or absence of swelling or masses. Skin should be assessed for erythema or other rashes. Frequently, areas of tenderness, swelling, or limited motion will be noted in the examination of the joints, and this will allow for targeting of radiographic imaging studies.

Imaging and Laboratory Studies

Importantly, if the physical examination findings are unremarkable, and, based on the history, the level of clinical suspicion for a specific diagnosis is low, plain radiographs of the lower extremities in limping children have been shown to have a low yield. In these situations, radiographic studies may be deferred, with timely follow-up arranged to make sure the limp resolves. In cases with focal physical examination findings, or if the limp does not resolve, imaging is indicated. Indications for radiography are tenderness on bone, focal swelling or effusion, or limited range of motion of a joint. Radiographic imaging should begin with orthogonal views (anteroposterior and lateral) of the bone or joint suspected as the source of the limp. Radiographs should be carefully scrutinized for fracture, areas of abnormally increased or decreased density (indicating possible infection or neoplasm), or periosteal reaction. Certain conditions have characteristic radiographic findings, including Legg-Calvé-Perthes disease, slipped capital femoral epiphysis, osteochondritis dissecans, developmental hip dysplasia, and Osgood-Schlatter syndrome.

When plain radiography findings are non-diagnostic or normal, and the clinical presentation suggests either a neoplastic, inflammatory, or infectious etiology, laboratory studies can be very helpful.

One of the most challenging diagnostic dilemmas when evaluating limping children is to differentiate between transient synovitis of the hip or septic arthritis of the hip. Kocher et al developed a predictive algorithm based on 4 criteria: inability to weight bear, presence of fever, elevated erythrocyte sedimentation rate, and elevated white blood cell count. When all 4 were present, greater than 90% of patients had septic arthritis. When zero or one criteria were met, a very small percentage of patients had septic arthritis. The need to combine multiple variables when assessing patients for possible infectious etiology points to the challenges of clinical decision-making in these patients.

At this stage, if the combination of history, physical examination, plain radiography, and standard blood work have not made a diagnosis, and the child is worsening or has a persistent limp, advanced imaging may be helpful. If the symptoms can be localized to a specific joint or anatomic area, ultrasound evaluation is painless, simple, and safe to obtain. For evaluation of the limping child in which localization of the source of the symptoms is difficult, magnetic resonance imaging has largely replaced the use of bone scans. Magnetic resonance imaging screening views in the coronal plane can be obtained from the lumbar spine to the ankles in younger children, with further imaging performed in areas where abnormalities are noted. As patients are often under anesthesia during the examination, it is possible to proceed with aspiration or needle biopsy of any suspicious areas to make the diagnosis of either infection or neoplasm—usually the 2 diagnoses the clinician is most concerned about.

Management

Most limps are self-limited and are the result of minor trauma. Even some minor fractures may resolve without the need for immobilization or specific treatment. Most fractures that present with a limp will be minor and will heal uneventfully with simple immobilization using a cast or splint. Activity modification, and restriction from sporting activities for a few weeks, will result in resolution. It is important to notify parents that it may frequently take a fracture-related limp several weeks, and sometimes a few months, to completely resolve. It is very unusual for a child to have a permanent limp as a result of the fracture. Limps caused by repetitive stress and overuse are typically treated with rest and activity modification.

Limps that are caused by infection will be treated differently if the infection involves the joint, compared to infections involving muscle or bone. Because of the risk of permanent damage to articular cartilage in the joint, it is more important to make the diagnosis rapidly and begin treatment early in septic arthritis. The principle of treatment is to relieve the pressure within the joint and remove infected joint fluid so that potentially damaging inflammatory products of the infection are removed. Decompression of the joint will also allow the antibiotics to reach the source of the infection. Most commonly, infected joints are treated with surgical decompression and debridement, but certain joints may be amenable to aspiration, sometimes repeatedly. For all bone and joint infections, it is important to try to obtain diagnostic material for cultures and sensitivities prior to the start of antibiotics, except in cases of florid sepsis in which antibiotics should be started immediately on presentation. This is atypical for the limping child. The clinician should attempt to get cultures by aspiration of focal areas of tenderness, or aspiration of fluid collections identified by imaging, whenever possible. In addition, for musculoskeletal infections, it is important to obtain a blood culture prior to the initiation of antibiotic therapy, as frequently the blood culture is the only culture that will be positive. Often the blood culture can be positive even in the absence of fever at the time the blood culture is drawn.

When no diagnosis has been found despite the initial work-up as described above, if the limp persists or worsens, specialist referral is indicated to make a diagnosis. Children with persistent limping who are difficult to diagnose sometimes end up having subtle neurologic abnormalities or rare muscle diseases.

Suggested Reading

Flynn JM, Widmann RF. The limping child: evaluation and diagnosis. *J Am Acad Orthop Surg.* 2001;9(2):89–98

Glotzbecker MP, Kocher MS, Sundel RP, Shore BJ, Spencer SA, Kasser JR. Primary lyme arthritis of the pediatric hip. *J Pediatr Orthop.* 2011;31(7):787–790

Howard PK, Broering B. Use of the Ottawa ankle scale in pediatric patients. *Adv Emerg Nurs J.* 2009;31(4):264–268

Kim HK. Legg-Calvé-Perthes disease. *J Am Acad Orthop Surg.* 2010;18(11):676–686

Kocher MS, Zurakowski D, Kasser JR. Differentiating between septic arthritis and transient synovitis of the hip in children: an evidence-based clinical prediction algorithm. *Journal Bone Joint Surg Am.* 1999;81(12):1662–1670

Pavone V, Lionetti E, Gargano V, Evola FR, Costarella L, Sessa G. Growing pains: a study of 30 cases and a review of the literature. *J Pediatr Orthop.* 2011;31(5):606–609

Luhmann SJ, Jones A, Schootman M, Gordon JE, Schoenecker PL, Luhmann JD. Differentiation between septic arthritis and transient synovitis of the hip in children with clinical prediction algorithms. *J Bone Joint Surg Am.* 2004;86-A(5):956–962

Sawyer JR, Kapoor M. The limping child: a systematic approach to diagnosis. *Am Fam Physician.* 2009;79(3):215–224

CHAPTER 40

Pain, Chronic

Laurie Hicks, MD

Key Points

- Chronic, persistent pain is underestimated, underdiagnosed, and undertreated.
- There are emotional, cognitive, behavioral, psychological, and social influences on pain that must be addressed during evaluation and management.
- WHO guidelines for treatment of pain (by the lader, by the clock, by the child, and by the appropriate route) should be followed.
- Complementary and alternative medical therapies should be used in addition to pharmacologic treatment of pain.

Overview

While many issues confront a pediatrician's knowledge base and cause anguish, few cause as much frustration as chronic pain. Not only is there disagreement among pediatricians about the best approach to the work-up for a child who presents with unexplained chronic pain, but there is also uncertainty about treatment approach and the ability to positively affect outcomes. This is particularly the case when no tissue injury, pathology, or other physiologic explanation for the pain is apparent. As a result, physicians are often at a loss for how best to proceed, and, unfortunately, in these situations, children and families often get the distinct impression that the physician does not believe the pain is real but rather that the child is exaggerating or has a psychologic problem.

The reasons a child can present to the primary pediatric office with chronic pain are numerous and multifactorial. Pain may be the main reason for seeking help, or it may be secondary to another problem. It may be acute, or it may be chronic but presenting for evaluation for the first time. Or it may be chronic but acutely worse. Evaluation and management of persistent pain in children starts with acknowledging its existence. Part of the healing process starts when the primary care physician believes the problem and offers hope that that the pain can be successfully managed and the child can find relief.

This chapter will present an approach to thinking about and helping manage chronic pain but will not be an exhaustive treatise on pharmacologic management of pain. The term *chronic pain* will be used interchangeably with the term *persisting pain* as used by the 2012 World Health Organization (WHO) guidelines.

Definition

Chronic pain is often defined as pain that has persisted for longer than 3 months. In children, this often has very little meaning because one should not wait some arbitrary length of time before dealing with the issue. The WHO defines chronic pain as "continuous or recurrent pain that persists beyond the normal expected time of healing." It may start as acute tissue injury but persist even after the injury has healed. Ongoing pain can lead to rerouting and reshaping of pain fibers so that pain can occur after the initial injury has healed. New research on pain has led to the knowledge that pain can persist after the stimulus is gone. So it is possible that children may have no physical or laboratory manifestations to account for their pain; however, that does not make the pain any less real to the child. On the other hand, physical changes, along with pain, may exceed what one would expect from the known insult such as complex regional pain syndrome and gut dysmotility. Pain can be nociceptive or neuropathic. Nociceptive pain comes from tissue injury and is either somatic (ie, skin, mucosa, or the musculoskeletal system) or visceral (ie, internal organs). Neuropathic pain is injury to or nerve cell dysfunction of the peripheral and central nervous system. Both types of pain can be present in the same child.

Persistent pain in children has been underestimated and therefore underdiagnosed and treated. Presenting symptoms may be vague and nonspecific. Many of the patients we encounter are unable to talk with us, either because of age or disability. Children with pain do not often conform to our adult expectations of how someone in pain should behave or act. Fragmentation of care within a large group pediatric practice as well as having multiple subspecialists involved in the care of a child with a chronic complex problem is a barrier to good pain management: Who assumes primary responsibility for helping the child and family with the issue of pain?

Pain is an inherently subjective experience. What one child experiences as pain may be inconsequential to another. Pain is complex and multifactorial with sensory, emotional, cognitive, behavioral, psychological, and social overlays to the experience of pain. The child's developmental stage, environment, social and cultural background, and previous experience of pain and the context of the situation in which the pain occurs all have bearings on how the child experiences pain. How the brain interprets the neural input from an injury will be influenced from neural input from all these other sources. For the purposes of dealing with children, pain is something that makes a child hurt and it is what the child says it is, regardless of whether one thinks pain should or shouldn't be present.

The Meaning of Pain

In addition to assessing the pain itself, one must also assess the meaning of the pain to the child and family. A simple stomachache that does not really bother the child may become much worse if the parent expresses great concern. The reason for such concern may be that the parent is worried the pain represents the presenting symptom. Is this a neuroblastoma with which another child in the neighborhood was recently diagnosed? Is this the first indication that the child will have ulcers just like her grandfather? Without knowing this information, reassurance alone may not be enough to alleviate the parent's concern, whereas reassurance with specific information about why the pain is not an ominous diagnosis may provide adequate relief. Many people may not readily admit what really worries them (ie, it is too frightening or embarrassing), and the longer the pain has been present, the more their fears grow. Asking is simple; not asking does the patient and family a disservice and dismisses their concerns.

Types of Persistent Pain

Persistent pain can be divided into 3 groups. Although the common factor of pain is present in all categories, the approach to evaluation and management may be vastly different.

One group includes otherwise healthy children with common persistent pain syndromes, including abdominal pain, headaches, and chest pain. Complex regional pain syndrome would also fit into this category. The second group includes children with chronic illnesses known to be associated with persistent pain, such as cancer, sickle cell disease, cystic fibrosis, and juvenile idiopathic arthritis. The third group encompasses children with complex chronic medical problems not necessarily characterized by pain, but the underlying condition predisposes the child to problems associated with pain (ie, gastroesophageal reflux disease, constipation, muscle spasms, hip dislocation). This group also includes children with hypoxic-ischemic encephalopathy, cerebral palsy, mitochondrial disorders, degenerative neurologic disorders, and developmental disabilities, such as autism spectrum disorder.

Common Persistent Pain Syndromes

Most pediatricians are familiar with common persistent pain syndromes such as chronic recurrent abdominal pain, chronic headaches, and chronic chest pain. However, evaluation and diagnosis are not straightforward, treatment is not always easy or effective, and both are time-consuming. Effective management requires a multidisciplinary approach.

It is essential to take a thorough history, including a detailed psychosocial history, to pinpoint any stressors that may be the source of pain or contributing to the child's experience of pain. A complete physical examination should be performed so the parents and child can see that nothing is being overlooked or missed. This "performance" of the physical examination can be part of the healing process. Remember to start away from the body part causing the most pain. Appropriate studies are ordered only as suggested by history and physical examination findings.

Discussing pain theory can help the child and family make sense of any persistence of pain. Pain can be present even after the initial insult has resolved. The goal of treatment should be recovery of function with limited diagnostic testing. This must be dealt with and explained at the initial meeting with child and parents. One might say something to the following effect:

> *We know that chronic pain can cause anxiety because there is fear that the pain represents a symptom of a life-altering diagnosis. Fortunately, this is rare in children. I know the pain is real because pain can persist even after the original cause has resolved. Think of it like a software glitch: hardware is OK, but the software has an error (Coakley R, Schecter N. Pediatr Pain Letter. 2013;15[1]:1–8). Therefore, my approach will be to do a thorough physical examination but the least invasive work-up that will give me all the information I need to find out if anything is wrong and to rule out the worst possible diagnoses. Then we will work out a plan to help with the pain. I can't promise to make the pain go away completely, but I will work with you to get the pain to a level that is tolerable so you can get back to doing all the things you like to do and to stop worrying so much about what is wrong, which is known to make pain worse.*

Chronic Illnesses With Pain as a Primary Problem

One or more subspecialists usually manage children with chronic diseases that have pain as a primary problem. Sickle cell disease and juvenile idiopathic arthritis are beyond the scope of this chapter. Pain in children with cystic fibrosis is not the first thing that comes to mind with this disease, but chest pain, headaches, limb pain, abdominal pain, and back pain are not uncommon, particularly as the disease progresses. Pain in cancer patients can be disease related or treatment related. Pain is often the presenting symptom that resolves with treatment. However, often ongoing pain issues require pain management for extended periods of time, and pain is often a major symptom at the end of life. The current knowledge of principles of pain management for all types of pain in children and adults stems from efforts put forth to find better ways to treat cancer pain. With this in mind, the later sections dealing with specifics of evaluation and treatment can be directly applied to children with cancer.

It is important for the primary care pediatrician to understand the basics of pain management in this population because these kids come to the office for their well-child checks and for acute illnesses, giving the pediatrician as the medical home a perfect opportunity to address this important issue and assess whether pain control is adequate. Being available to address the issue of pain in these kids will help ensure they have a better quality of life.

Children With Complex Chronic Medical Problems

The primary care pediatrician is increasingly encountering more children with complex chronic medical conditions with ongoing pain issues. Pain issues may have been addressed and managed as inpatients but now require follow-up, or new pain issues are developing as their chronic condition progresses.

A challenging population of children who may have chronic pain is that with those who have neurodevelopmental disabilities. Some of these children will be graduates from the neonatal intensive care unit and have problems stemming from extreme prematurity or extremely low birth weight. Others will have genetic syndromes, metabolic disorders, neurodegenerative disorders, or mitochondrial disorders. Some children may be survivors from traumatic brain injury or have autism spectrum disorder. Although these children will have many subspecialists involved in their care, it will often fall to the primary care pediatrician to initially diagnose and manage pain in these patients.

First of all, it is important to realize that this group of children has pain that too frequently goes unrecognized. This subset of children experience more pain than children who are physically and developmentally healthy. Some behavioral signs that might indicate pain include increased seizure activity, increased agitation, change in sleep patterns, behavioral problems that are out of the norm, increased crying, and decreased appetite. If confronted with any of these signs/symptoms, one should ask specifically about pain. Are you in pain? Do you think your child is in pain?

However, children with neurodevelopmental disorders often have chronic pain from problems that are not easy to figure out. Musculoskeletal problems such as hip dislocation, muscle spasms, and dystonia may not be readily apparent. Many of these children have decreased mobility leading to osteoporosis, making them susceptible to fractures, which may occur during physical therapy. Fractures in this population may go unrecognized for days or even weeks. In addition to causing pain, fractures often bring up the specter of abuse when this is not the case.

Children with neurodevelopmental disabilities have many problems arising from the gastrointestinal tract and have an "increased frequency of sensitizing gastrointestinal tract experiences" that can cause chronic pain. They frequently have had gastrostomy tube or gastrojejunal tube placement and fundoplication. Gastroesophageal reflux, feeding problems related to gastric dysmotility and distention, and chronic constipation may contribute to persistent pain. Sometimes, even after proper management of these problems, pain, irritability, and feeding problems persist. This can be explained by the concept of visceral hypersensitivity or visceral hyperalgesia resulting in increased sensitivity to visceral stimulation. Although the initial pain response is nociceptive, the persistent painful stimulation leads to an alteration in pain pathways creating a neuropathic-type pain. Gabapentin, which is used for neuropathic pain syndromes in adults, such as diabetic neuropathy and trigeminal neuralgia, has been used empirically with success in children to treat visceral hyperalgesia. It has provided relief for some children with neurologic impairment unrelated to the gastrointestinal tract problem.

Behavioral scales developed for use in children with verbal or communication disorders that rely on the caregiver for input can be helpful. If old enough and cognitively intact, some children will be able to use the Wong-Baker Faces Pain Rating Scale or the numerical analog scale to rate their pain.

Evaluation

Pain assessment includes a thorough history and careful physical examination. Was there any preceding injury or illness? What is the current level of functionality of the child? It is important to ask about response to current and previous treatments including medications, surgeries, and any complementary or alternative therapies. What worked and what didn't work? Were there any side effects and what were they?

Self-report of pain is the gold standard, and it is critical to believe what the child says. Try to find out what words the child uses to talk about pain and use those words. A 3-year old will not often answer the question. For children who are verbal, it is best to ask them these questions with supplemental input from parents or caregivers.

Location, timing, duration, quality, and severity of pain are assessed. How and when the pain started, how long it has been going on, where on the body it is located, what makes it worse or better, and how long it lasts must all be detailed. Always ask about how pain affects daily activities such as school, play, after-school activities, and sleep.

A pitfall in evaluation of pain is what the child or their caregivers may say about their pain compared to how they appear to the physician. It is easy and tempting to dismiss concerns when our eyes tell us one thing but our patients, another. That is one reason why, historically, pain in children has been underestimated. It is important to remember that behind the smile there can be pain. Children with persistent pain learn to live and deal with their disease and may play or sleep through the pain as a coping mechanism. The converse is true too. It may be obvious to the casual observer that a child is in pain but not telling the truth to avoid painful treatment.

Measurement of severity using age-appropriate pain scales can help with evaulation. The Faces Pain Scale-Revised, Poker Chip Tool, Visual Analogue Scale (VAS), Oucher Photographic, and Numerical Rating Scale (NRS) are some scales that have been validated for acute and persistent pain. The VAS and NRS can be used for children older than 8 years. The others have been validated down to 3 to 4 years of age depending on maturity of the child. For infants, the FLACC scale is helpful. It looks at face, legs, activity, cry, and consolability. For children who are preverbal or cognitively impaired, there are tools that quantify and rate behavior such as the r-FLACC. All pain scales are an attempt to quantify pain in little ones who cannot communicate and to give older children and adolescents a voice. It is important when using a scale to use the same one consistently over time in the same patient to measure effectiveness of interventions.

Management

In 2012, the WHO published guidelines on pain management that are simple and elegant and have become the standard of care. The guidelines call for pain in children to be treated by the ladder, by the clock, by the child, and by the appropriate route.

According to the WHO guidelines, "by the ladder" refers to a stepwise approach to the use of medications, starting with mild analgesic and stepping up to stronger analgesics as the pain gets worse. The WHO now uses a 2-step approach. For mild pain, start with acetaminophen or ibuprofen. When this no longer adequately controls the pain, switch to opioids in low doses for moderate pain and higher does for severe pain.

"By the clock" refers to using scheduled dosing of pain medications instead of "PRN" dosing. PRN (from the latin *pro re nata* or "as needed") dosing is not recommended unless pain is truly episodic. If an ongoing reason for pain is expected to be persistent for any length of time, better control will be achieved and less medication used overall if the medication is given around the clock. If the pain is allowed to escalate, it will take more medication to reduce it to an acceptable level than if the medication is given on a schedule. Also, when a lag time occurs between the time of asking for a drug and the time of administration, unnecessary pain and anxiety occur. When pain is inadequately treated, a pattern of behaviors, including moaning, clock watching, and repeated requests for medication, can occur, called "pseudo-addiction." These behaviors usually go away when the pain medication is dosed and scheduled appropriately.

"By the child" means tailoring treatment to the individual child and titrating doses based on the child's response. It means listening to and believing what the child or parent says about the pain and the effectiveness of treatment.

"By the appropriate route" means choosing "the simplest, most effective and least painful route" of drug administration that is suitable for the child and the situation. Medications can be given orally, enterally by feeding tubes, intravenously, subcutaneously, by rectum, transdermally, by mucosa, intranasally, and intramuscularly. Intramuscular injections are discouraged, and the rectal route has unreliable bioavailability and should be used as a last resort.

Step 1 medications include acetaminophen and ibuprofen (Table 40-1). Both are used frequently in children and are well tolerated but have limitations. Acetaminophen can cause liver damage if the dose is too high. Ibuprofen can cause bleeding problems and gastrointestinal tract irritation.

Table 40-1. Suggested Medications

Gabapentin[a]
Day 1–3: 5.0 mg/kg/dose qhs po or via tube
Day 4–6: 2.5 mg/kg qam, 2.5 mg/kg midday, and 5 mg/kg qhs
Day 7–9: 2.5 mg/kg qam, 2.5 mg/kg midday, and 10 mg/kg qhs
Day 10–12: 5 mg/kg qam, 5 mg/kg midday, and 10 mg/kg qhs
May continue to increase by 5 mg/kg/day until effective analgesia is achieved up to 75 mg/kg/day (maximum total dose of 3,600 mg) or limiting adverse effects occur. May titrate more rapidly for severe pain. Give half of total daily dose at night to take advantage of gabapentin's sedating properties. It is well tolerated with a very low frequency of severe adverse effects. Occasional patients will report mood or behavioral changes. If there is a need to stop, taper off over 1–2 weeks.

Nortriptyline[a]
Day 1–4: 0.2 mg/kg qhs po or by tube
Day 4–8: 0.4 mg/kg qhs po or by tube
Increase as tolerated every fifth day by 0.2 mg/kg to a maximum of 1 mg/kg/day or 50 mg/day. If using past 1 mg/kg/day, check plasma concentration and ECG. Consider twice daily dosing with 25% in morning and 75% in evening. May titrate more rapidly for severe pain. If there is a need to stop, wean off over 1–2 weeks to avoid irritability and bothersome vivid dreaming from REM rebound. Adverse effects to watch for include sedation, dry mouth, orthostatic hypotension, constipation, and urinary retention.

Acetaminophen
Neonates: 10–15 mg/kg po or by tube q 6–8 h, maximum dose of 60 mg/kg/day from all sources
Infants: 10–15 mg/kg/days po q 4–6 h, maximum dose of 75/mg/kg/day up to 1 g/4 h and 4 g every day from all sources
>12 y: 325–650 mg po or via tube, maximum dose of 1 g/4 h and 4 g/day from all sources

Ibuprofen
6 mo–12 y: 5–10 mg/kg po or via tube q 6–8 h, maximum dose of 40 mg/kg/day
>12 y: Use adult dosings.

Hydrocodone/acetaminophen
Elixir, 7%, alcohol. Many dosages with various amounts of acetaminophen.
2 mg/kg/day acetaminophen from all sources
>2 y, .50 kg: 2.5–10 mg hydrocodone po q 4–6 h/not to exceed 1 g/4 h and 4 g/day acetaminophen from all sources

Table 40-1 *(cont)*

Oxycodone
0.05–0.15 mg/kg po or via tube q 4–6 h

Morphine
<6 mo: po or tube 0.1 mg/kg q 4–6 h
IV: 0.05–0.2 mg/kg q 4 h
>6 mo–12 y: po or via tube 0.2–0.5 mg/kg q 4–6 h
IV: 0.1–0.2 mg/kg q 4 h

Abbreviations: ECG, electrocardiogram; IV, intravenously; po, orally; REM, rapid eye movement; q, every; qam, every day before noon; qhs, every night at bedtime.

ᵃ Data from Hauer JM, Wical BS, Charnas L. Gabapentin successfully manages chronic unexplained irritability in children with severe neurological impairment. *Pediatrics*. 2007;119(2):519–522.

Step 2 medications include opioids. Morphine is the most common opioid. Oxycodone and hydrocodone are other opioids that can be used effectively in children. Hydrocodone is only found in combination with acetaminophen in the United States. Though used commonly, its use is limited by the amount of acetaminophen, which can easily reach a ceiling dose. Hydromorphone, fentanyl, methadone, and meperidine are other opioids that require someone experienced in advanced pain management to use. Meperidine is not used in children because of propensity to cause seizure. Methadone is often a good choice, but it has a variable half-life and is metabolized differently from person to person, requiring monitoring by an experienced provider. Fentanyl patches can be used when chronic pain is stable and under good control; oral route is no longer available.

Codeine is no longer recommended for children. The WHO calls it "an excluded medicine for pain relief."

Using opioids in children can be safe and effective if misconceptions and fears are overcome. Tolerance, dependence, and addiction need to be understood. Tolerance means the body can become adapted to doses such that higher does will be needed to achieve the same amount of pain control. Dependence is a physical response to use of opioids and is characterized by physical withdrawal symptoms if the drug is stopped abruptly. Dependence can develop after 5 to 7 days of use. Weaning the dose slowly and watching for adverse effects can prevent withdrawal symptoms such as fever, sweating, yawning, and vomiting. Addiction is a psychological and pathologic response to drug use and involves criminal behavior to obtain the drug.

Adjuvant medications for persistent pain can be used in addition to any of the step 1 or step 2 medications. If neuropathic pain or visceral hyperalgesia are the predominate causes of pain, these medications may be used alone. A few of the most common drugs for neuropathic pain include gabapentin, amitriptyline, and clonidine. Other adjuvants include steroids for bone pain and inflammation, benzodiazepines for anxiety that may accompany or exacerbate pain, and dantrolene and baclofen for spasticity and dystonia.

When management of chronic pain with systemic medications is limited by adverse effects or is ineffective, regional anesthesia approaches to pain can be explored in patients with advanced cancer, complex regional pain syndrome, or spasticity and dystonia.

Complementary and Alternative Medicine

While the pharmacologic treatment of pain is the mainstay of treatment, other aspects of chronic pain need to be addressed. Complementary and alternative medicine (CAM) therapies should be used in addition to pharmacologic treatments to maximize the child's quality of life. Living in chronic pain can have emotional, behavioral, and psychological consequences that may need to be addressed. In addition, some children and adolescents with chronic pain have significant problems with fatigue that contribute to poor quality of life. Complementary and alternative therapies, such as cognitive-behavioral therapy, hypnosis, guided imagery, and others, can be used for these issues, which, in turn, can help reduce pain burden and give children some control over their level of pain. In some cases, CAM therapies may be the best way to treat pain, such as physical therapy for complex regional pain syndrome or muscle spasms. Advocating for an increased availability of CAM therapies would benefit many pediatric patients and perhaps decrease reliance on medications.

Conclusion

Chronic or persistent pain in children is real. For the primary care physician who encounters a child with chronic pain, evaluation and treatment can be challenging but rewarding. Even if a subspecialist manages the child's pain, knowledge of the principles of pain management can make the primary care physician a better and more caring advocate for the child and family. Just knowing relief is available can help a patient cope with the pain. The goal should be to reduce the pain to an acceptable level at which the child can participate in activities that are age appropriate and important for the continued growth and development of the child.

Suggested Reading

Avery ME, First LR. *Pediatric Medicine*. 2nd ed. Philadelphia, PA: Lippincott Williams & Wilkins; 1993

Coakley R, Schecter N. Chronic pain is like…the clinical use of analogy and metaphor in the treatment of chronic pain in children. *Pediatr Pain Letter*. 2013;15(1):1–8

Gold JI, Mahrer NE, Yee J, Palermo TM. Pain, fatigue, and health-related quality of life in children and adolescents with chronic pain. *Clin J Pain*. 2009;25(5):407–412

Hauer J. Identifying and managing sources of pain and distress in children with neurological impairment. *Pediatr Ann*. 2010;39(4):198–205

Hauer JM, Wical BS, Charnas L. Gabapentin successfully manages chronic unexplained irritability in children with severe neurological impairment. *Pediatrics.* 2007;119(2):519–522

Kelly LE, Rieder M, van den Anker J, et al. More codeine fatalities after tonsillectomy in North American children. *Pediatrics.* 2012;129(5):e1343–e1347

Knoll AKI, McMurtry CM, Chambers CT. Pain in children with autism spectrum disorder: experience, expression, and assessment. *Pediatr Pain Letter.* 2013;15(2):1–6

Konijnenberg AY, De Gradff-Meeder ER, Kimpen JL, et al. Children with unexplained chronic pain: do pediatricians agree regarding the diagnostic approach and presumed primary cause? *Pediatrics.* 2004;114(5):1220–1226

Penner M, Xie WY, Binepal N, Switzer L, Fehlings D. Characteristics of pain in children and youth with cerebral palsy. *Pediatrics.* 2013;132(2):e407–e413

Ravilly S, Robinson W, Suresh S, et al. Chronic pain in cystic fibrosis. *Pediatric.* 1996;98(4):741-747

Rork JF, Berde CB, Goldstein RD. Regional anesthesia approaches to pain management in pediatric palliative care: a review of current knowledge. *J Pain Symptom Manage.* 2013;46(6):859–873

Schechter NL, Berde CB, Yaster M. *Pain in Infants, Children, and Adolescents.* 2nd ed. Philadelphia, PA: Lippincott Williams & Wilkins; 2003

World Health Organization. *WHO Guidelines on the Pharmacological Treatment of Persisting Pain in Children With Medical Illnesses.* Geneva, Switzerland: World Health Organization; 2012

CHAPTER 41

Pallor

Beng Fuh, MD

Key Points

- Pallor generally becomes evident at hemoglobin levels less than 8 to 9 g/dL and is influenced by skin complexion.

- The presence of a heart murmur may suggest anemia or heart disease, while lymphadenopathy, palpable masses, or hepatosplenomegaly may suggest a malignancy.

Overview

Pallor is a common physical finding in children. Pallor results from anemia or a decrease in blood flow to the body surface. Pallor can be chronic (and subtle) or acute. Chronic pallor may be asymptomatic, may not be readily apparent to the child's caregiver, and may be first noticed by someone who does not see the child regularly. Acute pallor is more likely to be symptomatic and may present as an emergency. Pallor may arise from hematologic causes, such as anemia, bone marrow failure, or malignancy, or it may be secondary to non-hematologic causes, such as respiratory failure, asphyxia, hypothermia, anaphylactic reaction, or circulatory collapse as seen in shock. Most causes of pallor are easily treatable, but in a few cases pallor may be caused by serious medical conditions necessitating rapid diagnosis and intervention. The ease with which pallor is recognizable is often dependent on the skin complexion. Individuals with very light skin complexion may be erroneously diagnosed as having pallor, and mild pallor may be missed in children with dark complexion if close attention is not paid to the conjunctivae, lips, palms, and nail beds.

Causes

The causes of pallor in children can be divided into hematologic and non-hematologic.

Hematologic Causes

Pallor generally becomes evident at hemoglobin levels less than 8 to 9 g/dL and is influenced by skin complexion, but it should be noted that the sensitivity of pallor in detecting anemia is low (Evidence Level II-1). Table 41-1 shows common hematologic causes of pallor.

Table 41-1. Common Hematologic Causes of Pallor

Blood Loss	Hemolysis	Sickle Cell Disease
■ Acute blood loss ■ Hemangioma ■ Chronic blood loss	■ Immune hemolysis ■ Red blood cell enzyme defects ■ Red blood cell membrane defects	■ Hemolytic anemia ■ Splenic sequestration ■ Aplastic anemia
Hypoproliferative Anemia	**Nutritional Anemia**	**Others**
■ Aplastic anemia ■ Diamond-Blackfan anemia ■ Transient erythroblastopenia of childhood ■ Fanconi anemia	■ Iron deficiency anemia ■ Vitamin B12 deficiency ■ Folate deficiency	■ Malignancy (leukemia or metastatic to bone marrow) ■ Anemia of chronic illness ■ Lead poisoning

Other hematologic causes include diseases that can infiltrate the bone marrow, such as histiocytosis, osteopetrosis, storage diseases, and myelofibrosis. Other forms of bone failure, including medications that result in anemia, infection, pregnancy, transient depression secondary to acute infections, and radiation, can also cause pallor.

Non-hematologic Causes

These conditions generally cause pallor by decreasing the amount of blood floor to the surface. Box 41-1 shows common non-hematologic causes of pallor.

Box 41-1. Common Non-hematologic Causes of Pallor

Asphyxia	Anaphylactic shock
Septic shock	Hypoglycemic shock and other metabolic disorders
Hypovolemic shock	CNS injury
Cardiogenic shock	Skin edema
Respiratory failure	Skin infiltration
Cystic fibrosis	Renal disease
Pheochromocytoma	Lack of sun exposure
Hypothermia	Lead poisoning

Abbreviation: CNS, central nervous system.

Pseudo-pallor can occur when individuals with very light skin are inaccurately diagnosed as having pallor.

Diagnosis and Evaluation

Pallor is a physical diagnosis. When pallor is detected in a child, a rapid assessment should be done to determine if the child's health is clinically unstable. If the health is unstable, immediate measures should be taken to stabilize the child. After stabilizing the child and in children who are clinically stable on presentation, a thorough evaluation should be done to establish the cause of pallor. The following approach is suggested.

History and Physical Examination

A thorough history is needed to establish the onset, course, and associated symptoms of the pale child. Acute pallor associated with dark-colored urine, jaundice, or splenomegaly is more likely to be secondary to hemolytic anemia. Acute pallor with no symptoms of hemolysis is more likely to be secondary to acute blood loss or non-hematologic causes of anemia. A more chronic course of pallor is most commonly identified by the primary care physician or a family member who has not recently seen the child. If chronic, the pallor is more likely to be secondary chronic blood loss, hypoproliferative anemia, or nutritional anemia.

A good family history helps in the diagnosis of familial pallor commonly secondary to inherited anemia. Family history of cholecystectomy or splenectomy may suggest an inherited hemolytic anemia, such as red blood cell enzyme disorders and red blood cell membrane defects.

Pallor should be obvious on physical examination. In children with dark skin, attention should be paid to the conjunctivae, lips, palms, and nail beds. Vital signs should be carefully reviewed for presence of tachycardia, hypotension, fever or hypothermia, tachypnea, or respiratory depression.

   The presence of a heart murmur may suggest anemia or heart disease, while lymphadenopathy, palpable masses, or hepatosplenomegaly, may suggest a malignancy. Jaundice and scleral icterus suggest hemolytic anemia. Surface hemangiomas may hint at internal hemangiomas causing occult blood loss. Skin edema may suggest perfusion related causes of pallor.

Laboratory Studies

A complete blood count and a reticulocyte count should be obtained in every child with pallor. All other studies should be tailored based on the history, physical examination, and findings on the complete blood count. Because reticulocyte count is frequently expressed as a percentage of red blood cells, an absolute reticulocyte count or a corrected reticulocyte count should be obtained. The following step-by-step approach is suggested in analyzing the complete blood count (Table 41-2).

Table 41-2. Complete Blood Count Analysis

Laboratory Finding	Implication
Expected blood counts	Is pseudo-pallor or non-hematologic pallor.
Low hemoglobin level and other abnormal blood cell lines	Consider bone marrow pathology. Bone marrow biopsy or chromosome breakage studies may be warranted.
Low hemoglobin level and expected WBC and platelet counts	Check reticulocyte count and proceed as below.
Elevated reticulocyte count	Evaluate for hemolysis or blood loss.
Low reticulocyte count	Consider red blood cell aplasia (DBA, TEC, viral suppression). May get parvovirus B19 and EBV titers and consider bone marrow biopsy.
Elevated MCV (macrocytic anemia)	Check vitamin B12 and folate levels.
Low MCV (microcytic anemia)	Order iron studies and evaluation for thalassemia

Abbreviations: MCV, mean corpuscular volume; WBC, white blood cell.

Management

Given that pallor is a physical finding and not a specific diagnosis, treatment should be directed at the cause of pallor (Figure 41-1).

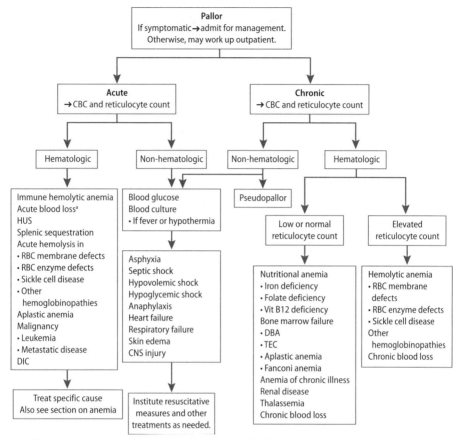

Figure 41-1. Evaluation and management of pallor.

Abbreviations: CBC, complete blood count; DIC, diffuse intravascular coagulation; HUS, hemolytic-uremic syndrome; RBC, red blood cell; vit, vitamin.

[a] CBC and reticulocyte count may initially be normal in individuals with acute blood loss.

Life-threatening conditions such as shock must be recognized promptly and treated with fluid resuscitation, blood transfusions, antibiotics, dextrose, supplemental oxygen, intubation, vasopressors, and other specific interventions as needed. Fluid overload may worsen the clinical symptoms and outcomes in children with cardiopulmonary disorders. The hypovolemic/hypothermic child must be warmed as the fluid resuscitation precedes. All symptomatic patients with pallor need frequent reassessment with treatment adjustments as needed.

Non–life-threatening anemia can be treated according to etiology specific guidelines.

Suggested Reading

Berard R, Matsui D, Lynch T. Screening for iron deficiency anemia in at risk children in the pediatric emergency department: a survey of Canadian pediatric emergency department physicians. *Pediatr Emerg Care.* 2007;23(5):281–284

Chalco JP, Huicho L, Alamo C, et al. Accuracy of clinical pallor in the diagnosis of anaemia in children: a meta-analysis. *BMC Pediatr.* 2005;5:46

Ezer A, Torer N, Nursal TZ, et al. Incidence of congenital hemolytic anemias in young cholelithiasis patients. *World J Gastroenterol.* 2010;16(43):5457–5461

Kalter HD, Burnham G, Kolstad PR, et al. Evaluation of clinical signs to diagnose anaemia in Uganda and Bangladesh in areas with and without malaria. *Bull World Health Organ.* 1997;75(Suppl 1):103–111

CHAPTER 42

Proteinuria

Amanda W. Dale-Shall, MD, MS, and Leonard G. Feld, MD, PhD, MMM

Key Points

- Orthostatic proteinuria is the most common form of proteinuria in children and adolescents and has an excellent prognosis.

- Transient proteinuria resolves within 48 hours or when the acute illness resolves.

- First-morning urine evaluation is the most accurate approach in the evaluation of orthostatic proteinuria.

- Urine protein-to-creatinine ratio less than 0.2 is normal for children older than 2 years.

- Pathologic proteinuria requires prompt evaluation and treatment by a pediatric nephrologist.

Overview

Proteinuria is a common urinary dipstick finding in children. Low-grade and transient proteinuria is usually of little clinical significance. Higher-grade or persistent proteinuria should be monitored more closely. In most cases, further evaluations demonstrate benign transient or orthostatic proteinuria rather than a pathologic kidney disease such as nephrotic syndrome. When proteinuria is associated with microscopic or macroscopic hematuria, hypertension, hypoalbuminemia, edema, oliguria, decreased renal function, or systemic findings, a detailed investigation should be performed. Accurately quantifying the degree of proteinuria is a critical step in the evaluation process (Table 42-1). The evaluation may prompt a renal biopsy to be performed for further diagnostic and prognostic information, which will aid in the determination of initiation of possible medications, such as immunosuppressive agents.

Table 42-1. Measurement of Urinary Protein

Method	Technique	Range	Comments
Dipstick testing	Random *or* first-morning specimen	**Negative or trace** (<20 mg/dL) **Abnormal** ≥1+ (30 mg/dL)	**False-positive results** Reagent strip immersed too long in urine specimen, alkaline or highly concentrated urine, pyuria, gross hematuria, and certain detergents **False-negative results** Very dilute urine specimens or urinary protein that is not albumin
U$_{Pr}$:U$_{Cr}$	Random *or* first-morning specimen	**Reference** <0.8: <6 mo <0.5–6: 24 mo <0.2: >2 y **Abnormal** (>2 y) >0.2–0.49: mild >0.5–0.99: moderate >1–2: pathologic	Falsely elevated with malnutrition or low muscle mass due to low GFR
24-h urine collection	Total *or* recumbent versus upright collection	**Reference** <150 mg/m^2/24 h (= **U$_{Pr}$:U$_{Cr}$** <0.2) <4 mg/m^2/h **Abnormal** >4–10 mg/m^2/h: mild >11–39: moderate >40: pathologic	Inadequate collection that leads to inaccuracy and is difficult to perform if patient is incontinent and in young children

Abbreviations: GMR, glomerular filtration rate; U$_{Pr}$:U$_{Cr}$, urine protein-to-creatinine ratio.

Various types of protein are detected on the urinary dipstick and include albumin, beta$_2$-microglobulin, immunoglobulins, and Tamm-Horsfall mucoproteins, although the urinary dipstick test is most sensitive to albumin detection. Abnormalities occurring at various locations of the nephron will lead to various types and degrees of proteinuria.

The urine protein-to-creatinine ratio (U$_{Pr}$:U$_{Cr}$) is very useful to estimate the magnitude of proteinuria in the pediatric population. Timed urinary collections (12 or 24 hour) can be inaccurate because of inadequate or incomplete collections and are not feasible in infants and toddlers who have not achieved continence. Studies have demonstrated the direct correlation of the urine protein-to-creatinine ratio and 24-hour urine protein collection results in various renal diseases (Evidence Level II-1). The main advantage of the $U_{Pr}:U_{Cr}$ is the ability to use a random, or untimed, urine specimen or a first-morning urine specimen that is collected via bag, clean catch, or catheterization instead of relying on a 24-hour collection. First-morning urine analysis is the preferred method to reduce the effect of postural proteinuria or exercise on the urinary protein measurement.

In children with severe malnutrition or low muscle mass, creatinine excretion is expected to be low, resulting in a falsely elevated $U_{Pr}:U_{Cr}$. In cases with variable $U_{Pr}:U_{Cr}$ results, a timed 24-hour urine collection should be used to assess the degree of urinary protein excretion.

Alternative urinary protein measurements are necessary in 2 situations. First, in cases of low-molecular-weight proteinuria (tubular or interstitial renal diseases), urinary protein electrophoresis is used to determine the percentage of albumin, beta$_2$-microglobulin, and other protein components. Second, to assess renal injury staging in patients with diabetes mellitus, urinary albumin excretion or urinary albumin-to-creatinine ratio ($U_{Alb}:U_{Cr}$) is calculated. Normal urinary albumin excretion is less than 20 mcg per min or less than 30 mg per day. Microalbuminuria is defined as greater than 20 mcg per min but less than 200 mcg per min. In comparison, significant albumin or overt nephropathy (proteinuria with positive dipstick results) is a value greater than 200 mcg per min or 300 mg per day. The current recommendation is to follow the $U_{Alb}:U_{Cr}$ on a periodic basis in patients with diabetes mellitus rather than a timed urine collection or a urinary dipstick test (Evidence Level II-1).

Evaluation and Management

Proteinuria may be a normal finding in children; however, pathologic proteinuria has various causes in children. It is important to differentiate among transient, orthostatic, isolated, and persistent proteinuria (Box 42-1 and Figure 42-1).

Transient Proteinuria

Transient proteinuria is a benign form of proteinuria that generally resolves within hours or days of the onset and is not associated with recurrence. Examples include proteinuria that occurs during or soon after strenuous activities or during episodes of an acute illness such as dehydration in which the proteinuria resolves with the resolution of the acute problem. Results of a repeat urine dipstick test performed within a few weeks after initial testing will be normal; therefore, no further work-up is necessary. If the proteinuria persists, additional testing should be performed and is outlined below.

Box 42-1. Causes of Proteinuria (Asymptomatic or Symptomatic)

Transient Proteinuria	Pathologic or Persistent Proteinuria

■ Abdominal surgery
■ Congestive heart failure
■ Dehydration
■ Emotional stress
■ Epinephrine infusion
■ Exercise
■ Extreme cold
■ Fever
■ Seizures
	■ Benign (sporadic or familial)
	■ Acute glomerulonephritis
	■ Chronic
	  – Primary glomerular diseases with or without nephrotic syndrome
	    • Minimal-change nephrotic syndrome
	    • Focal segmental glomerulosclerosis
	    • Hereditary nephritis (Alport syndrome)
	    • IgA nephropathy
	    • Membranous nephropathy
	    • Membranoproliferative glomerulonephritis

Orthostatic or Postural Proteinuria
■ Transient or fixed
	– Secondary glomerular or systemic disease
	    • Acute poststreptococcal or infectious glomerulonephritis
	    • Antiphospholipid syndrome
	    • Diabetes mellitus
	    • Henoch-Schönlein purpura
	    • Hepatitis
	    • Systemic lupus erythematosus
	■ Interstitial nephritis or tubular proteinuria
	■ Cystinosis
	■ Dent disease
	■ Lowe syndrome
	■ Heavy metal intoxication
	■ Congenital or acquired abnormalities of the urinary tract
	  – Autosomal dominant polycystic kidney disease
	  – Congenital nephrotic syndrome
	  – Hydronephrosis
	  – Reflux nephropathy
	  – Renal hypoplasia/dysplasia

Modified with permission from Feld LF, Schoeneman MJ, Kaskel FJ. Evaluation of a child with asymptomatic proteinuria. *Pediatr Rev*. 1984;5:248–254.

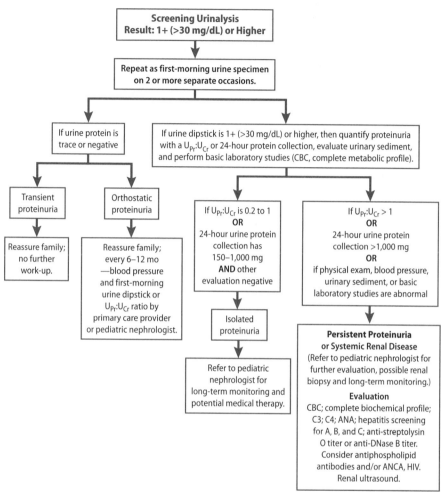

Figure 42-1. Algorithm of the stepwise diagnostic approach for the evaluation of proteinuria.

Abbreviations: ANA, antinuclear antibodies; ANCA, antineutrophil cytoplasmic antibodies; CBC, complete blood count; $U_{Pr}:U_{Cr}$, urine protein-to-creatinine ratio.

Modified from Dale-Shall AW, Feld LG. Approach to a child with proteinuria. In: Elzouki AY, Harfi HA, Stapleton FB, Oh W, Whitney RJ, eds. *Textbook of Clinical Pediatrics*. London, England: Springer; 2012:2711–2722 (Evidence Level II-3–Level III), with permission.

Orthostatic or Postural Proteinuria

Orthostatic or postural proteinuria is the most common form of proteinuria in children and adolescents. Orthostatic proteinuria is defined as elevated protein excretion in an ambulatory or erect position that is within range values during recumbency. The total urinary protein excretion in orthostatic proteinuria rarely exceeds 1 g in a 24-hour urine collection. The most accurate way to evaluate for orthostatic proteinuria is via either a split-timed urine collection (separate recumbent and ambulatory specimens) or with $U_{Pr}:U_{Cr}$ testing on a first-morning urine specimen (Box 42-2). It is essential to properly perform this testing to distinguish between orthostatic and pathologic proteinuria. Long-term follow-up studies have observed that orthostatic proteinuria is a benign process with no apparent long-term renal sequelae. However, yearly urine dipstick testing and blood pressure measurements are suggested.

Box 42-2. Urine Collection Instructions and Interpretation for Orthostatic Proteinuria Evaluation

Instructions
1. Child has limited activity on the day of the test (no exercise, food, or fluids after 8:00 pm).
2. Child voids at bedtime (consider voiding twice before bed, 30 min apart). Discard urine.
3. When child awakes in the morning, urine specimen is collected in the cup prior to getting out of bed or with limited ambulation. Label specimen no. 1 (or FMU) and place in refrigerator.
4. Child should then ambulate. Collect another urine specimen 2–4 h later. Label specimen no. 2 (random specimen) and place in refrigerator.
Interpretation (Evidence Level I)
1. *Diagnosis is orthostatic proteinuria* if urine specimen no. 1 is negative or trace on the dipstick or the $U_{Pr}:U_{Cr}$ is <0.2, and urine specimen no. 2 has ≥1+ on the dipstick or the $U_{Pr}:U_{Cr}$ is ≥0.2. (Perform orthostatic testing at least twice to confirm diagnosis.)
2. *Diagnosis is not orthostatic proteinuria* if urine specimen no. 1 is has ≥1+ on the dipstick or the $U_{Pr}:U_{Cr}$ is ≥0.2, and urine specimen no. 2 has ≥1+ on the dipstick or the $U_{Pr}:U_{Cr}$ is ≥0.2

Abbreviation: FMU, first-morning urine.

Pathologic Proteinuria

Pathologic proteinuria is defined as persistent, abnormal urinary dipstick results or a $U_{Pr}:U_{Cr}$ result above range values as outlined previously (see Table 42-1). This type of proteinuria suggests acute or chronic renal disease and warrants a further evaluation and a referral to a pediatric nephrologist. If an increased urinary protein is present on dipstick testing, a $U_{Pr}:U_{Cr}$ on a first-morning urine specimen should be performed. If the patient is continent, a 24-hour urine collection should be considered as well. Many renal and systemic diseases have pathologic proteinuria, making the differential diagnosis broad (Table 42-2; see Box 42-1 and Figure 42-1). The evaluation for pathologic proteinuria includes a detailed patient and family history and physical examination, followed by more extensive and focused laboratory and renal imaging studies with consideration for a renal biopsy. The approach is similar whether the proteinuria is asymptomatic or symptomatic and with or without associated systemic manifestations. The investigation requires a prompt evaluation with a possible hospitalization and renal biopsy.

Table 42-2. Clinical Manifestations of Systemic Renal Diseases Associated With Persistent Proteinuria

Systemic Disease	Renal Findings	Physical Findings	Laboratory Tests
Postinfectious GN	Macroscopic or microscopic hematuria, pyuria, urine cellular casts, elevated serum creatinine level	Streptococcal pharyngitis or skin lesions or other infectious symptoms 2–4 wk prior to renal findings	Positive anti-streptolysin O or anti-DNase B titer, decreased complement C3 level
IgA nephropathy	Macroscopic or microscopic hematuria, rarely elevated creatinine level	Abdominal or flank pain, fever, URTI symptoms 2–3 d prior to renal findings	Normal complement—C3 and C4 levels
Henoch-Schönlein purpura	Macroscopic or microscopic hematuria	Abdominal pain, lower extremity and buttock purpura, arthralgia, arthritis, peripheral edema	Normal complement—C3 and C4 levels
Hemolytic uremic syndrome	Macroscopic hematuria, oliguria, elevated BUN and creatinine levels	Bloody diarrhea, abdominal pain, emesis, pallor, anorexia	Anemia, thrombocytopenia, elevated LDH level, normal complement—C3 and C4 levels
Systemic lupus erythematosus	Microscopic hematuria, urine cellular casts, elevated creatinine	Fever, weight loss, alopecia, facial rash, chest pain, shortness of breath, arthralgia, arthritis	Positive ANA and anti-DS DNA titer, decreased complement C3 and C4 levels, elevated ESR
Interstitial nephritis	Elevated urine eosinophil level, sterile pyuria, dysuria, microscopic hematuria, elevated creatinine level	Fever, rash, nausea, emesis, infectious symptoms, recent exposure to antibiotics or other medications, back pain	Elevated ESR level, eosinophilia, anemia

Abbreviations: ANA, antinuclear antibodies; ANCA, antineutrophil cytoplasmic antibodies; CBC, complete blood count; U_{Pr}:U_{Cr}, urine protein-to-creatinine ratio.
Modified from Dale-Shall AW, Feld LG. Approach to a child with proteinuria. In: Elzouki AY, Harfi HA, Stapleton FB, Oh W, Whitney RJ, eds. *Textbook of Clinical Pediatrics.* London, England: Springer; 2012:2711–2722 (Evidence Level II-3–Level III), with permission.

The treatment of each pathologic entity is outside the scope of this chapter. Table 42-3 outlines some treatments options which may be selected by a pediatric nephrologist.

Table 42-3. Possible Treatments for Primary and Secondary Renal Disease With Proteinuria (Evidence Level I–II-2)

Supportive therapy	Antihypertensive agents, diuretics, albumin infusions for serum albumin concentrations <1.5 g/dL, hyperlipidemia therapy, infection/immunization and thromboembolic risk assessment; PPD prior to immunosuppressive therapy
Non-immunosuppressive approaches to reduce proteinuria and preserve renal function	Angiotensin-converting enzyme inhibitors, angiotensin receptor–blocking agents, or both (to assess renal function and serum potassium prior to initiating, at 10–14 d after initiation and then every 3–6 mon; patients must be informed of teratogenic risks)
Immunosuppressive agents	Glucocorticoids Oral: prednisone/prednisolone, 60 mg/m² per day for 4–6 wk followed by 40 mg/m² on alternate days for 4–6 wk Parenteral: methylprednisolone pulses, 10–30 mg/kg up to 1 g per dose, maximum of 3 doses) Cyclophosphamide (alkylating agent; need to consider maximal dose) Chlorambucil (alkylating agent; need to consider maximal doses—8.2–16.8 mg/kg) Calcineurin inhibitors (cyclosporine or tacrolimus; need to monitor trough blood levels) Mycophenolate mofetil (reversible inhibitor of inosine monophosphate dehydrogenase in purine biosynthesis) Levamisole (immunomodulator belonging to a class of synthetic imidazothiazole derivative; not approved for use in the United States)

Abbreviation: PPD, purified protein derivative.

Suggested Reading

Ettenger RB. The evaluation of the child with proteinuria. *Pediatr Ann.* 1994;23(9): 486–494

Feld LG, Schoeneman MJ, Kaskel FJ. Evaluation of the child with asymptomatic proteinuria. *Pediatr Rev.* 1984;5(8):248–254

Gipson DS, Massengill SF, Yao L, et al. Management of childhood onset nephrotic syndrome. *Pediatrics.* 2009;124(2):747–757

Guder WG, Hofmann W. Clinical role of urinary low molecular weight proteins: their diagnostic and prognostic implications. *Scand J Lab Invest Suppl.* 2008;241:95–98

Hogg RJ, Portman RJ, Milliner D, Lemley KV, Eddy A, Ingelfinger J. Evaluation and management of proteinuria and nephrotic syndrome in children: recommendations from a pediatric nephrology panel established at the National Kidney Foundation conference on proteinuria, albuminuria, risk, assessment, detection, and elimination (PARADE). *Pediatrics*. 2000;105(6):1242–1249

Lin CY, Sheng CC, Chen CH, Lin CC, Chou P. The prevalence of heavy proteinuria and progression risk factors children undergoing urinary screening. *Pediatr Nephrol*. 2000;14(10-11):953–959

Price CP, Newall RG, Boyd JC. Use of protein:creatinine ratio measurements on random urine samples for prediction of significant proteinuria: a systematic review. *Clin Chem*. 2005;51(9):1577–1586

Wilmer WA, Rovin BH, Hebert CJ, Rao SV, Kumor K, Hebert LA. Management of glomerular proteinuria: a commentary. *J Am Soc Nephrol*. 2003;14(12):3217–3232

CHAPTER 43

Pruritus

Jeana Bush, MD

Key Points

- Pruritus is the most common of all dermatologic complaints and encountered frequently in pediatric practice.

- Pruritus can be classified as dermatologic, systemic, neurologic, or psychogenic.

- Most causes can be identified with a thorough history and physical examination.

- The possibility of a systemic disorder should be considered in patients presenting with generalized pruritus without an obvious source.

- Therapy should be directed toward the underlying cause along with extensive education on appropriate skin care.

Overview

Pruritus can be defined as a sensation that elicits the desire to scratch and is most commonly referred to as *itching*. It is a common symptom but in itself is not a disease. It occurs in the setting of many disease processes and can originate from numerous organ systems. As the most common of all dermatologic concerns, it can interfere with sleep, concentration, and daily function; severity can range from being an annoyance to physically debilitating.

Pruritus is classified as acute (ie, lasting less than 6 weeks) or chronic (ie, lasting longer than 6 weeks). The International Forum for the Study of Itch divides pruritus into 2 primary tiers, the first tier used when the origin of the itch is unknown and the second tier for known etiologies of pruritus (Box 43-1).

Box 43-1. Pruritus Tiers

Tier 1
- Group I: pruritus on diseased skin (ie, inflamed)
- Group II: pruritus on non-diseased skin
- Group III: pruritus presenting with severe chronic secondary scratch lesions

Tier 2
- Dermatologic: pruritus from a primary skin disorder
- Systemic: pruritus with origin from disorders affecting other organ systems
- Neurologic: pruritus related to disorders of the peripheral or central nervous system
- Psychogenic: psychiatric disorders in which people complain of pruritus
- Mixed: pruritus attributed to one or more causes

Dermatologic Disorders

Atopic Dermatitis

Atopic dermatitis is a chronic inflammatory disorder of the skin. The pruritus of atopic dermatitis can have a significant effect on quality of life if left untreated. The hallmark of this disease is allokinesis, in which a normally innocuous stimulus induces intense pruritus. Examples of such stimuli can include sweating, temperature change, and skin contact with certain types of clothing or fibers. Another hallmark of this condition is a vicious "itch-scratch" cycle where excoriations from scratching induce intense pruritus.

Atopic dermatitis is a clinical diagnosis with a broad differential diagnosis. Patients report chronic and relapsing pruritus and dermatitis. Physical findings include sparing of the central face (headlight sign), xerosis (dryness), creases under the lower eyelids (Dennie-Morgan lines), periorbital darkening, and accentuation of the palmar skin lines. The dermatitis may vary in presentation depending on the age of the patient. In infants, it often presents on the cheeks and extensor surfaces of the arms and legs. Older children have the more typical flexural surface involvement of the antecubital and popliteal fossae, back of the neck and hands, wrists, and ankles.

Treatment is directed at decreasing skin dryness using moisturizers, avoiding excessive bathing and education on appropriate skin products. Avoiding fragrant or dye-containing soaps, detergents, and fabric softeners can be helpful. The inflammation can be treated with topical corticosteroids, preferably ointments over lotions because of the high water concentration and emollience. Starting with low potency topical steroids and moving up in strength is the standard treatment, being sure to avoid oral or systemic steroids due to rebound flares and long-term adverse effects. Symptomatic treatment with antihistamines (Table 43-1) is important for breaking the itch-scratch cycle of this disease. Children with atopic dermatitis are at high risk for multiple widespread skin infections including molluscum contagiosum, herpes simplex (specifically, eczema herpeticum), and *Staphylococcus aureus*.

Table 43-1. H1-Antihistamines With Pediatric Oral Dosing

Trade Name	Generic Name	Typical Usage	Recommended Dosing
First Generation			
Benadryl	Diphenhydramine	Symptomatic relief of allergic symptoms caused by histamine release; anti-motion sickness; antitussive; mild nighttime sedative; adjunct to epinephrine in the treatment of anaphylaxis	2 to <6 years: 6.25 mg every 4–6 hours, max 37.5 mg/day 6 to <12 years: 12.5–25 mg every 4–6 hours, max 150 mg/day >12 years and adults: 25–50 mg every 4–6 hours, max 300 mg/day
Dramamine	Dimenhydrinate	Treatment and prevention of nausea, vertigo, and vomiting associated with motion sickness	2 to 5 years: 12.5–25 mg every 6–8 hours, max 75 mg/day 6 to 12 years: 25–50 mg every 6–8 hours, max 150 mg/day >12 years and adults: 50–100 mg every 4–6 hours, max 400 mg/day
Tavist	Clemastine	Allergic rhinitis and other allergic symptoms including urticaria	Infants and children <6 years: 0.05 mg/kg/day as clemastine base or 0.335 to 0.67 mg/day of clemastine fumarate divided into 2–3 doses 6 to 12 years: 0.67–1.34 mg clemastine fumarate twice daily, max 4 mg/day >12 years and adults: 1.34 mg clemastine fumarate twice daily, max 8 mg/day
Chlor-Trimeton, Teldrin	Chlorpheniramine maleate	Allergic rhinitis and other allergic symptoms including urticaria	2 to 5 years: 1 mg every 4–6 hours 6 to 11 years: 2 mg every 4–6 hours, not to exceed 12 mg/day or timed-release 8 mg every 12 hrs >12 years and adults: 4 mg every 4–6 hours, not to exceed 24 mg/day or timed-release 8–12 mg every 12 hours

Table 43-1 (cont)

Trade Name	Generic Name	Typical Usage	Recommended Dosing
First Generation			
Polaramine	Dexchlorpheniramine	Allergic rhinitis and other allergic symptoms including urticaria	2 to 5 years: 0.5 mg every 4–6 hours, not to exceed 3 mg/day 6 to 11 years: 1 mg every 4–6 hours, not to exceed 6 mg/day >12 years and adults: 2 mg every 4–6 hours, not to exceed 12 mg/day
Rynatan	Chlorpheniramine tannate; pyrilamine tannate	Allergic rhinitis and other allergic symptoms including urticaria	2 to 6 years: 2 mg twice daily, not to exceed 8 mg in a 24-hour period 6 to 12 years: 4–8 mg twice daily, not to exceed 16 mg in a 24-hour period >12 years and adults: 8–16 mg twice daily, not to exceed 32 mg in a 24-hour period
Atarax; Vistaril	Hydroxyzine	Antipruritic; antiemetic; anxiolytic; preoperative sedation	<6 years: 50 mg/day in divided doses or 2 mg/kg/day divided every 6–8 hours >6 years: 50–100 mg/day in divided doses
Phenergan	Promethazine	Symptomatic treatment of various allergic conditions; motion sickness; sedative; antiemetic	(as an antihistamine) Children >2 years: 0.1 mg/kg/dose (not to exceed 12.5 mg) every 6 hours during the day and 0.5 mg/kg/dose (not to exceed 25 mg) at bedtime as needed Adults: 6.25–12.5 mg 3 times/day and 25 mg at bedtime

Periactin	Cyproheptadine	Allergic rhinitis and other allergic symptoms including urticaria; appetite stimulant; prophylaxis for cluster and migraine headaches; spinal cord damage associated with spasticity	2 to 6 years: 2 mg every 8–12 hours, not to exceed 12 mg/day 7 to 14 years: 4 mg every 8–12 hours, not to exceed 16 mg/day Adults: 4–20 mg/day divided every 8 hours, not to exceed 0.5 mg/kg/day
Second Generation			
Zyrtec, All Day Allergy	Cetirizine	Perennial and seasonal allergic rhinitis; uncomplicated skin manifestations of chronic idiopathic urticaria	6 to 12 months: 2.5 mg once daily 12 to 23 months: initially 2.5 mg once daily; may be increased to 2.5 mg twice daily 2 to 5 years: 2.5 mg/day may be increased to max 5 mg/day as single dose or divided doses >6 years to adult: 5–10 mg/day as single dose or divided into 2 doses
Allegra	Fexofenadine	Seasonal allergic rhinitis and chronic idiopathic urticaria	6 months to <2 years: 15 mg twice daily 2 to 11 years: 30 mg twice daily >12 years to adult: 60 mg twice daily or 180 mg once daily
Alavert, Claritin, Loradamed, Tavist ND Allergy	Loratadine	Nasal and non-nasal symptoms of allergic rhinitis; chronic idiopathic urticaria	2 to 5 years: 5 mg daily >6 years to adult: 10 mg daily

Abbreviations: max, maximum.

Data from Taketomo C, ed. *Pediatric and Neonatal Dosage Handbook*. 21st ed. Hudson, OH: Lexi Comp; 2014.

Xerosis

Xerosis is most commonly referred to as "dry skin." It is a common cause of pruritus in the pediatric population, especially during the winter months. Xerosis is characterized by dry, scaly skin and most commonly occurs on the lower extremities. Risk factors for development of xerosis include genetic predisposition, frequent bathing, and ambient high temperatures with low humidity (which is common inside heated homes during cold winter months). The primary treatment of xerosis is limitation of factors that dry the skin and increasing moisture.

Contact Dermatitis

Contact dermatitis arises from direct skin contact with any foreign substance. It may be primary irritant dermatitis or allergic contact dermatitis. Primary irritant contact dermatitis is a nonallergic reaction to prolonged or repetitive contact with a variety of irritants, which can include detergents, soaps, saliva, acidic products, or excrement. Common examples of allergic triggers include metals (eg, nickel, chromium), oleoresin from plants (eg, poison ivy, oak, or sumac), and topical medications (eg, neomycin, bacitracin). Treatment depends on the source of dermatitis. Irritant dermatitis treatment involves restoring the water and lipid to the skin surface using moisturizers at least twice daily (Table 43-2). Allergic contact dermatitis must be treated for at least 14 to 21 days, and the offending allergen must be identified and avoided to prevent recurrence. Dermatitis of less than 10% of skin surface can be treated with topical corticosteroids of moderate potency in ointment preparations for 2 to 3 weeks. If the dermatitis involves greater than 10% of the skin surface, systemic steroids are necessary.

Urticaria

Urticaria is a rash most commonly referred to as *hives*. The typical lesion is well circumscribed, blanchable, raised, and erythematous with central pallor. It is characterized by marked pruritus. The lesions may enlarge and coalesce, transiently appearing and disappearing and resolving most often over a few hours. Acute urticaria is defined as lasting less than 6 weeks, while chronic urticaria refers to persistent or recurring lesions lasting 6 weeks or more.

Acute urticaria is usually an allergic reaction, while chronic urticaria has various causes including systemic disorders. Common causes of acute urticaria include allergens (eg, foods, medications, pollens, stinging insects), physical factors (eg, cold, heat, pressure as in dermatographism, exercise-induced), and infections. Papular urticaria is a common cause in children caused primarily by stinging insects (eg, fleas, mosquitoes, bedbugs) and characterized by papular or vesicular linear clusters. Chronic urticaria occurs more often in adults than children. Unlike adults, the association of chronic urticaria with malignancy is not well established, so evaluation for malignancy is usually not necessary. However, if malignancy is suspected, the patient should be referred to an oncologist.

Table 43-2. Types of Moisturizers

Type	Mechanism	Indication	Examples	Comments
Occlusive	Blocks trans-epidermal water loss	Xerosis AD Prevention of irritant CD	Petrolatum Zinc oxide Lanolin Mineral oil Silicones	Messy Comedogenic May cause folliculitis (mineral oil) or dermatitis (lanolin)
Humectant	Attracts water to the stratum corneum	Xerosis Icthyosis	Urea Alpha-hydroxy acids Glycerin Sorbital Lactic Acid	May cause irritation (urea, lactic acid)
Emollient	Smoothes skin	Decrease skin roughness	Cholesterol Squalene Fatty acids	Not always effective
Replacement of deficiencies in "raw materials" of the intact stratum corneum	Claims to replenish essential skin components	Possible skin rejuvenation	Ceramides Natural moisturizing factor	Unproven benefits; may improve skin moisturization and barrier function

Abbreviations: AD, atopic dermatitis; CD, contact dermatitis.

Treatment of urticaria focuses on avoiding underlying triggers and histamine blockers (see Table 43-1). If maximal doses of H_1-receptor antagonists do not relieve symptoms, an H_2-receptor antagonist, such as ranitidine or cimetidine, may be added. For severe or refractory cases, oral glucocorticosteroids may be used in short bursts (0.5–1 mg/kg/day for 5 days). If there are any signs or symptoms of anaphylaxis (eg, angioedema, respiratory distress, or gastrointestinal distress), a self-injectable epinephrine pen should be prescribed. Chronic urticaria or refractory cases should be referred to an allergist for further evaluation and management.

Miliaria Rubra

More commonly referred to as *prickly heat* or *heat rash,* miliaria rubra is caused by blocked eccrine sweat glands at the granular layer of the skin. This leads to leakage of sweat into the surrounding dermis. The rash is characterized by intense erythema with maculopapular vesicles and pruritus. It occurs in hot, humid environments often on intertriginous areas or surfaces of the body covered by clothing.

Infections

Superficial fungal infections due to dermatophytes (tinea) are common causes of localized pruritus. Tinea cruris (or jock itch) typically presents with bilateral, crescent-shaped lesions extending from the inguinal folds to the upper thighs. Tinea pedis (or athlete's foot) typically presents with white macerations; dry, scaly skin; or localized blisters between the toes. Tinea capitis occurs commonly in children and presents with an itchy scalp. Most fungal skin infections are treated with topical antifungal creams (eg, miconazole, clotrimazole, terbinafine). However, tinea capitis requires oral therapy (eg, griseofulvin, fluconazole, terbinafine, or itraconazole).

Viral infections (ie, varicella, molluscum) and bacterial infections (ie, folliculitis) are also recognized causes of pruritus.

Insect Bites and Infestations

Insect bites (especially mosquitos, fleas, and scabies) can be markedly pruritic. Some children develop papular urticaria, a delayed hypersensitivity reaction to insect bites that is more common in warmer months. The rash of papular urticaria is characterized by erythematous, or umbilicated papules most commonly found in groups on the trunk and extensor surfaces of the extremity.

Scabies is a common infestation in the pediatric population caused by the mite *Sarcoptes scabiei*. The pathognomonic finding is the threadlike burrow (ie, thin gray, red, or brown line 2–15 mm long) produced from the mite traveling through the epidermis. Most often lesions are located on the intertriginous areas of the neck, axillae, groin, and webs of fingers and toes. Patients report intense pruritus worse at night, which is a result of delayed hypersensitivity to the mite protein and may persist for weeks after eradication.

Another common infestation in pediatric patients is pediculoses, more commonly known as lice. Pediculosis capitis (or "head lice"), corporis (or "body lice"), and pubis (or "pubic lice") cause significant pruritus from a delayed hypersensitivity reaction to the saliva of the louse. The infecting organism is named based on the body part it infests (*Pediculus humanus capitis, Pediculus humanus corporis,* and *Pediculus humanus pubis).* Diagnosis is clinical. In the case of head or pubic lice, nits are usually visible along the hair shaft. Body lice may present with a pruritic papular rash with excoriations. It is important to search the inner seams of clothing for lice and eggs. Body lice occur most commonly in the setting of poor hygiene, while pubic lice are typically transmitted via sexual contact and occur mainly in adolescents. Pubic lice may be associated with small bluish-grey macules around the groin, lower abdomen, and thighs. Treatment options include topical pediculicides such as permethrin, pyrethrin, malathion, lindane, benzyl alcohol, spinosad, and ivermectin. It is important to know the resistance patterns of louse in the geographical area of practice.

Lastly, enterobiasis (or *pinworms*) is a helminthic infection caused by *Enterobius vermicularis* that causes intense perianal pruritus. It is spread by ingestion of eggs, which can be aerosolized or located on surfaces such as contaminated hands and toys. Diagnosis is by visualization of worms in the perianal region or positive "scotch tape test" with recovery of worms. Treat the entire family with mebendazole (100 mg) or albendazole (400 mg) in a single dose, and repeat treatment in 2 weeks. All linens and clothes should be laundered in hot water.

Psoriasis

Approximately one-third of initial presentations of psoriasis occur in children younger than 20 years. Eighty percent of patients with psoriasis report pruritus, most commonly with a cyclic nature worse at night. Interestingly, it tends to be generalized pruritus rather than localized to the psoriatic plaques and poorly responsive to antipruritic medications. The most common form of this condition involves silvery scales over characteristic, erythematous skin lesions. The Koebner phenomenon is common (ie, psoriasis outbreak in the area of an abrasion) and often presents in a linear fashion.

Several forms of psoriasis are seen in the pediatric population. Guttate psoriasis presents with small, scaly papules and plaques on the face, trunk, and proximal extremities. It has been associated with streptococcal infections as a trigger. Erythrodermic psoriasis is an exfoliative-type of skin reaction with warmth, erythema, and widespread scaling. It can be associated with difficulty maintaining body temperature (eg, hypothermia/hyperthermia), dehydration, hypoalbuminemia, and anemia of chronic disease. Pustular psoriasis is characterized by numerous small coalescing pustules most often localized to the palms and soles.

The mainstay of treatment for psoriasis is immune-modulators. Plaques are treated with topical glucocorticoids, calcipotriene (vitamin D analog), tazarotene gel (retinoid), tar, or anthralin in combination with UVB therapy. PUVA (oral psoralen and UVA light) is effective but associated with increased risk of skin cancer so generally not recommended in children. Dermatology consultation is recommended for children with a diagnosis of psoriasis.

Systemic Disorders

Renal Disease (Uremic Pruritus)

Pruritus resulting from uremia is more common in the adult population but is a markedly disabling symptom in patients with end-stage renal disease. Symptoms tend to be most intense during or at the end of dialysis or in the evening and night.

Gastrointestinal Disease (Cholestatic Pruritus)

The combination of jaundice and generalized pruritus is nearly pathognomonic for biliary obstruction. It can be associated with intrahepatic or extrahepatic biliary obstruction, drug-induced cholestasis (eg, oral contraceptives, anabolic steroids, erythromycin), viral hepatitis or primary biliary cirrhosis. Choleretic agents (eg, ursodeoxycholic acid), opiate antagonists, antihistamines, and antibiotics (eg, rifampin) have also been found to be effective. The generalized pruritus of liver disease tends to start with an acral distribution over the palms and soles, which is an unusual site in most other forms of pruritus. It is also interesting to that the pruritus is unrelated to the degree of hyperbilirubinemia, as patients with intense jaundice are often unaffected.

Endocrine Diseases

Patients with thyrotoxicosis can present with pruritus. Patients with hypothyroidism may also experience pruritus secondary to xerosis. In diabetic patients, infections with *Candida albicans* can predispose to localized pruritus, especially in the genital and perineal areas.

Hematologic and Oncologic Disorders

Iron deficiency, even without anemia, can cause pruritus that improves with iron supplementation. Myeloproliferative disorders such as polycythemia vera may produce pruritus, particularly after a hot bath (known as aquagenic pruritus). Patients may describe a "skin prickling" sensation more so than an itch. The pruritus can last from minutes to hours and tends to be generalized. Aquagenic pruritus has also been associated with myelodysplastic disorders and T-cell lymphomas.

Leukemia and Hodgkin disease can cause pruritus. Itching may be a primary symptom in Hodgkin lymphoma (up to 30% of patients) and may precede presentation of lymphoma by up to 5 years, although this is more common in the adult population.

Rheumatologic Disorders

Patients with dermatomyositis will frequently experience intense pruritus that interferes with sleep and daily activity. Pruritus is also a common concern in systemic sclerosis (ie, scleroderma). Itching is not typically a cutaneous characteristic of lupus erythematosis, so if a patient reports itching with presumed lupus, the diagnosis should be reconsidered.

Neurologic Disorders

The neurologic disorders associated with pruritus are not typically seen in the pediatric population. Brachioradialis pruritus presents with pruritus in the proximal dorsolateral forearm and is typically seen in fair-skinned, middle-aged adults who spend significant amounts of time outdoors. Notalgia paresthetica is characterized by unilateral, localized pruritus. Postherpetic neuralgia is a common phenomenon following infection with herpes zoster and may lead to chronic localized pruritus. Multiple sclerosis can infrequently cause recurrent, severe episodes of generalized pruritus.

Psychiatric Disorders

Psychogenic Pruritus

Pruritus can be a manifestation of stress, anxiety, obsessive-compulsive disorder, personality disorder, depression, or psychosis. Psychogenic/neurotic excoriation is characterized by excessive picking or scratching of normal skin. Patients report significant pruritus, but the source of itch is not apparent. Examination will reveal scattered, linear excoriations anywhere on the body but most often on the extremities. Delusional parasitosis is a manifestation of hypochondriacal psychosis (often presenting with pruritus) that the patient attributes to a nonexistent parasitic infection.

Evaluation and Treatment

The presence of skin lesions usually points towards a dermatologic cause. Itching localized to one anatomic region usually suggests a specific local cause or exogenous exposure. Generalized pruritus often, but not always, points to a systemic etiology. Timing of occurrence and chronicity can be very revealing. Pruritus in general tends to worsen at night, but this is especially true with scabies and pinworms. If pruritus awakens a child from sleep, the cause is most likely organic. Recent, acute onset suggests infection, insect bite, urticaria, contact dermatitis, or sunburn. Chronic dermatitis occurs in the setting of atopic dermatitis and other systemic disorders. Certain associated symptoms such as weight loss, fever, weakness, or polyuria should raise flags for systemic illnesses such as renal failure or malignancy. Social history is important to elicit recent sick contacts in the case of infestations or foreign travel in the case of certain infections. Family history can be revealing in the case of atopic disease, psoriasis, thyroid, or renal disorders.

The physical examination should be comprehensive, not just focusing on the skin. Weight and height should be plotted on standard growth charts, looking for signs of systemic disease such as growth failure in chronic renal disease. Clues to other disorders include pallor in the case of anemia, hepatomegaly in obstructive biliary disease, nail changes in psoriasis, or goiter in hyperthyroidism. The skin examination should pay close attention to the details of rashes or accompanying findings (eg, excoriations, scars, hypo- or hyperpigmentation). Table 43-3 can be helpful in characterizing skin findings. Lastly, lack of skin findings can also be very revealing, suggesting other diagnoses such as psychogenic pruritus.

Table 43-3. Pruritic Dermatologic Conditions That Are Usually Apparent on Physical Examination

Physical Findings	Possible Etiology
Erythematous lesion with vesiculation, papulation, oozing, crusting, scaling, and sometimes lichenification	Atopic dermatitis
Erythematous lesion limited to the area of contact with an offending substance	Contact dermatitis
Circumscribed, raised wheals	Urticaria
Minute papulovesicles with intense erythema, usually localized to areas covered by occlusive clothing	Miliaria rubra
Macules, papules, vesicles, pustules appearing in crops with a centrifugal distribution	Chickenpox
Dome-shaped pustules with an erythematous base, lesions centered on hair follicles	Folliculitis
Erythematous, elevated, scaly, annular lesion with central clearing	Tinea corporis (ringworm)
Urticaria wheal with central punctum	Insect bite
Wheals, papules, vesicles, and threadlike burrows	Scabies
Nits on hair shafts	Pediculosis
Dry and cracked skin with fine scales	Xerosis

From Leung, AKC. Pruritus in children. *JR Soc Promot Health*.1998;118(5):280-286, with permission.

Treatment of pruritus should be tailored to the suspected etiology or diagnosis. Known precipitating or contributing factors should be avoided. In general, H_1-receptor antagonists are the mainstay of treatment (see Table 43-1). Histamine is one of the primary mediators of the itch sensation in the skin. In addition to blocking H_1 receptors in the dermis, many antihistamine medications such as hydroxyzine or diphenhydramine have the added benefit of sedation. This is particularly helpful in most conditions where pruritus is worse at night. H_2 receptors are not involved with pruritus, so H_2-receptor antagonists are generally not helpful. Behavioral modifications such as avoiding long, hot baths are helpful to prevent over-drying of the skin. Soothing lotions or emollients (see Table 43-2) are helpful in most conditions. Fingernails should be kept short to avoid excessive trauma to the skin. Topical steroids such as hydrocortisone can be used in steroid-responsive dermatoses. Consultation with appropriate subspecialists is recommended when the underlying diagnosis warrants expert opinion.

Suggested Reading

Greco PJ, Ende J. Pruritus: a practical approach. *J Gen Intern Med.* 1992;7(3):340–349

Langley EW, Gigante J. Anaphylaxis, urticaria, and angioedema. *Pediatr Rev.* 2013;34(6):247–257

Leung AK, Wong BE, Chan PY, Cho HY. Pruritus in children. *J R Soc Promot Health.* 1998;118(5):280–286

Stander S, Weisshaar E, Mettang T, et al. Clinical classification of itch: a position paper of the International Forum for the Study of Itch. *Acta Derm Venereol.* 2007;87(4): 291–294

CHAPTER 44

Rashes

Charles F. Willson, MD

Key Points

- Examine the entire body, unclothed, to determine distribution.
- Describe the rash to yourself in dermatologic terms (eg, macular, papular, pustular, vesicular).
- Exclude or manage life-threatening conditions. Generalized rashes are likely caused by a systemic infection or reaction.
- Use only mild steroids on areas where the skin is thin (eg, face, eyelids, ears, scrotum).
- Complications due to prolonged steroid applications may be lessened by applying them only on weekdays and resting the skin on weekends (avoid high potency steroid preparations).

Overview

Rashes account for about 30% of visits to pediatric offices but also are encountered in nurseries, intensive care units, and pediatric inpatient settings. Developing a systematic approach to a rash will make identification much easier and more accurate. Rashes are often very helpful as a sign at the onset of illness and help direct work-up for a sick child.

Causes

The skin is the boundary to our environment, and many rashes are related to external factors such as environmental substances, trauma, heat exposure, infectious agents, and infestations. The skin may also react to internal stimuli brought to it via the blood or lymph. Consider the depth of the skin involvement and what manifestations are the primary rash and what may be secondary to scratching or topical therapy. The condition causing the rash may be localized to the skin, or the rash may be a manifestation of a systemic disease or process. Hair and nails are specialized components of the skin and should be

carefully examined. Age and sex of the child may be important in the differential diagnosis of a rash, especially within the neonatal period.

When considering a child with a rash, a careful history will often focus the
differential diagnosis to only a few conditions. Always ask

▶ When and where did the rash start?

▶ Has the rash spread?

▶ Are there any associated symptoms (eg, fever, cough, conjunctivitis,
  pruritus, pain locally or elsewhere)?

▶ Is the rash getting better or worse?

▶ Has the parent given any treatment, topical or systemic?

▶ Has the rash occurred before in this child or another family member?

▶ Has the child been exposed to anyone with an illness or rash (always positive for a child in a day care setting)?

▶ Any recent trauma?

▶ Has there been environmental exposures?

▶ Any new foods?

▶ Any new topical contactants such as soaps, shampoos, bubble baths, lotion,
  or new clothing?

▶ Has the child had all recommended vaccines for her age?

▶ What does the parent or caregiver think is causing the rash?

When examining a child with a rash, it is crucial to examine the entire
child, looking for patterns, distribution, and signs of systemic illness or a
genetic condition. Also, determine which lesions are the primary lesions and
what lesions may be secondary to scratching, medication, or even an infectious
disease reaction. A generalized rash is more often caused by internal factors,
while a localized rash may reflect a specific trauma or exposure. Figure 44-1
shows typical distribution patterns for common rashes seen in childhood. Once
you have come to a preliminary diagnosis, construct a differential diagnosis list
and consider why you do not think it is the rash on the differential.

Because many rashes start centrally and spread peripherally, presence of
the rash on palms and soles may be helpful in accurately diagnosing the rash.
Table 44-1 lists common rashes that are often found in an acral distribution.

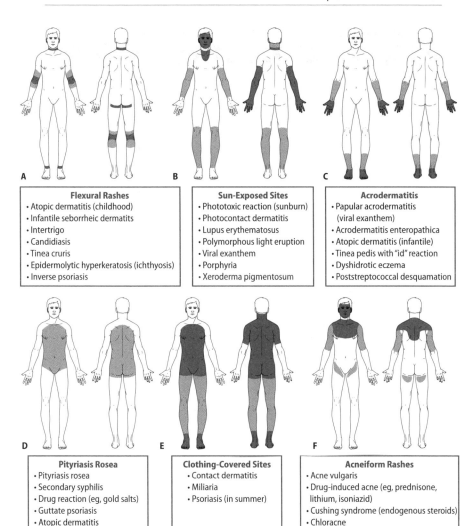

Figure 44-1. Pattern diagnosis.
A, Flexural rashes. B, Sun-exposed sites. C, Acrodermatitis. D, Pityriasis rosea. E, Clothing-covered sites. F, Acneiform rashes.

Table 44-1. Generalized Rash With Involvement of Palms and Soles

Common	Variable	Rare
Rocky Mountain spotted fever	Lichen planus	Guttate psoriasis
Rubella	Meningococcemia	Insect bites
Scabies	Psoriasis (plaques)	Keratosis pilaris
Secondary syphilis	Urticaria (hives)	Lyme disease
Staph scalded skin		Miliaria rubra
Tinea corporis		Nummular eczema
Toxic epidermal necrolysis		Pityriasis rosea
Toxic shock syndrome		Scarlet fever
		Seborrheic dermatitis
		Varicella
		Viral exanthems

From Ely JW, Seabury Stone M. The generalized rash: part II Diagnostic approach. *Am Fam Physician.*
2010;81(6):735–736, with permission.

Figures 44-2 and 44-3 outline an approach to the rash of a sick neonate and
a sick child older than 2 months in the outpatient setting.

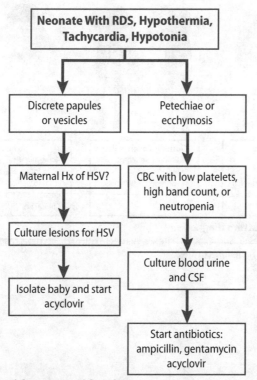

Figure 44-2. The sick neonate with rash.

Abbreviations: CBC, complete blood count; CSF, cerebrospinal fluid; HSV, herpes simplex virus; Hx, history;
RDS, respiratory distress syndrome.

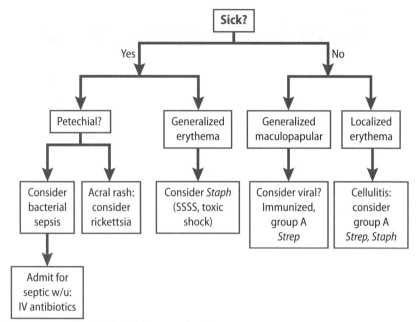

Figure 44-3. The child with fever and rash.

Abbreviations: IV, intravenous; SSSS, staphylococcal scalded skin syndrome; *Staph, Staphylococcus; Strep, Streptococcus*; w/u, work-up.

When cause of the rash is unclear but the patient is stable, we should fall back on the medical model of a thorough history, a comprehensive review of systems, and a complete physical examination to further focus the potential diagnoses. Always consider diseases that may cause significant morbidity and even mortality first.

Despite study and experience, some rashes are often confused or misdiagnosed (Table 44-2).

Clinical Features and Management

Neonatal Rashes

In the neonatal nursery, the first consideration of any rash should be for any acute infectious process such as neonatal herpes, group B streptococcal infection, or a TORCH disease (toxoplasmosis, other [syphilis, varicella-zoster, parvovirus B19], rubella, cytomegalovirus, herpes). Any vesicle should be cultured for herpes simplex virus. Petechiae on the back after rubbing in the delivery room may signal a group B streptococcal infection or autoimmune thrombocytopenia.

Table 44-2. Often Confused Rashes

Condition	Similar Rashes (Distinguishing Features)
Atopic dermatitis	Contact dermatitis (not associated with dry skin)
	Keratosis pilaris (nonpruritic, involves posterolateral upper arms)
	Psoriasis (well-defined plaques, silvery white scale, flexural areas)
	Scabies (involves genitalia, axillae, finger webs; look for burrows)
	Seborrheic dermatitis (greasy scale, nonpruritic, distribution)
Contact dermatitis	Atopic dermatitis (symmetric distribution, family history, allergic triad)
	Dermatitis herpetiformis (vesicles on extensor areas, painful)
	Psoriasis (patches on knees, elbows, scalp, gluteal cleft; silver scale)
	Seborrheic dermatitis (greasy scale on eyebrows, nasolabial folds)
Drug eruption (morbilliform)	Erythema multiforme (target lesions)
	Viral exanthem (more common in children, less intense erythema, less likely to be dusky red, more focal systemic symptoms)
Pityriasis rosea	Drug eruption (no scale, lesions coalesce)
	Erythema multiforme (target lesions)
	Guttate psoriasis (thicker scale, history of group A Streptococcus)
	Lichen planus (violaceous, involves wrists and ankles)
	Nummular eczema (larger round lesions, not oval)
	Psoriasis (thick white scale, involves extensor surfaces)
	Secondary syphilis (positive serology, involves palms and soles)
	Tinea corporis (+KOH, scale at periphery rather than within border)
	Viral exanthema (no scale, lesions coalesce)
Psoriasis	Atopic dermatitis (atopic features, flexural areas, lichenification)
	Lichen planus (violaceous, minimal scale, involves wrists and ankles)

Abbreviation: KOH, potassium hydroxide.

Adapted from Ely JW, Seabury Stone M. The generalized rash: part I. Diagnostic approach. *Am Fam Physician.* 2010;81(6):726–734, with permission.

A common rash with no significant sequelae, despite its ominous-sounding name, is erythema toxicum neonatorum. These raised, erythematous lesions are often widely distributed and regress after a few hours only to reappear elsewhere. Pustular melanosis may be identified by a superficial bleb that is easily wiped off, leaving a pigmented macule in its place. Maternal systemic lupus erythematosus may cause a rash and arrhythmias in the neonate.

Vascular anomalies are fairly frequent, such as flame nevi, salmon patches, and port wine stains. Pigmented nevi and mongolian spots are common. Cutaneous angiomas (or strawberry marks) are often not present at birth, but their development may be predicted by a superficial blood vessel in the neonatal period. Over the ensuing weeks, a classic strawberry angioma may develop at that site, enlarging throughout the first year and then regressing. For angiomas that may impair vision or threaten the airway, a course of propranolol may cause early resolution. These lesions may also be ablated by laser treatment. Pigmented nevi and mongolian spots are common. Large "bathing suit" pigmented nevi may be distressing to parents and present a heightened risk of malignancy in adulthood.

Certain inherited or genetic syndromes cause typical rashes that may be the first manifestation of the process of each respective syndrome such as café au lait spots (as seen in neurofibromatosis), ash leaf, shagreen patches, or a port wine stain in the ophthalmic distribution of cranial nerve V.

Papulosquamous Lesions

Psoriasis is relatively uncommon in childhood but must be considered with a persistent rash that has an acral and extensor surface distribution, often involving the scalp, elbows, knees and genitalia. It has a pearly scale that bleeds when lifted. Guttate psoriasis is a form of psoriasis often with an onset following a streptococcal infection. Pityriasis rosea is often announced by a herald patch, followed by oval lesions with scales attached at the periphery of the lesions that follow the lines of tension of the skin. Giannotti-Crosti syndrome involves polygonal lesions with an acral distribution.

The Dermatitis Group

Atopic Dermatitis

Atopic dermatitis is the most common chronic rash in childhood, found in 10% to 15% of children. There is often an associated familial inheritance pattern of sensitization called atopy: dry skin, asthma, and allergic rhinitis. Presence of atopic dermatitis does not imply that the child will have the other hypersensitivity conditions or that the rash is IgE mediated. There is an infantile presentation and a more typical childhood presentation. Dry skin is the underlying hallmark of atopic dermatitis. Because of the dryness, the skin is pruritic (ie, "the itch that rashes"). As the skin is scratched, the typical pattern of redness, edema, erosions, inflammatory papules, serous drainage, and crusts develops.

Infantile atopic dermatitis often involves the face and exposed areas. The diaper area is typically spared because of the more humid environment and the inability of the infant to scratch the area under the diaper.

Childhood atopic dermatitis has the characteristic distribution in the flexural creases and behind the neck.

Management of atopic dermatitis. For both the infantile and childhood varieties of atopic dermatitis, the critical features of management include

1. A parental understanding that the goal of management is to control symptoms. There is no cure; daily treatment will bring best results.
2. Moisturize the entire skin. Choose an inexpensive product such as Vaseline intensive care.
3. Control the itch. Choose a cost-effective antihistamine such as hydroxyzine or cetirizine.
4. Apply an anti-inflammatory medication to the most involved areas. Use low potency on thin skin, such as that of the face, ears, and genitals, and moderate potency on the arms, legs, trunk, and back.
5. Use a mild soap, and make baths a quick dip; many dermatologists advise for unscented soap.
6. Consider if excoriated areas are infected. If so, consider a topical antibiotic such as mupirocin or a systemic antibiotic such as erythromycin.

Close follow-up after initiating treatment is essential because many parents become frustrated with a lack of immediate results. To lessen adverse effects of long-term application of topical steroids, parents can apply the steroid on weekdays (after work) and none on the weekends (to allow for rest). Antihistamines and moisturizers are used daily.

Seborrhea

While the cause of seborrhea is still debated and probably multifactorial, it clearly is related to an excess production of oil in the sebaceous glands with a possible fungal component (ie, *Malassezia furfur*). There are infantile and adult presentations. Distribution of the rash overlaps with atopic dermatitis and psoriasis. Unlike as with atopic dermatitis, bathing with soap and water and mild rubbing to remove scales is the mainstay of treating seborrhea. Also unlike atopic dermatitis, seborrhea is often found in the diaper area. As the stimulation of the sebaceous glands by transplacental passage of maternal hormone subsides, infantile seborrhea resolves usually by 3 months of age only to recur during the hormone-rich period of adolescence with dandruff and acne.

Management of seborrhea. Reassurance that excessive oil production will subside over time is a mainstay. Daily care includes gentle brushing during bathing to remove scales. An antiseborrheic shampoo such as Selsun Blue or Head and Shoulders may be used on the scalp. For inflamed areas, a mild potency steroid may be used on weekdays.

Contact Dermatitis

Contact dermatitis may be divided into irritant dermal effects and allergic dermal reactions. Except for irritant rash due to diapering and new underclothing, both occur primarily on exposed skin. A detailed history of all possible exposures to agents that may irritate skin (eg, alcohols, hydrocarbons, exposures such as excessive sun or wind that traumatize or dry the skin) should be considered. New clothing is often implicated because of fabric brighteners that will be removed with the first washing. When cloth diapers were used routinely, laundry detergent was a common cause of contact dermatitis and should be considered in some cases. A new disposable diaper brand may contain an irritant that the previous brand did not. Common contacts of an allergic nature in children include: plants (which can cause rhus dermatitis), nickel (in items such as jewelry, belts, and metal fasteners on jeans), soaps, shoes, and medications.

Management of contact/irritant dermatitis. Once an offending agent is suspected, the management is fairly simple. Remove the offending agent and soothe the irritated skin with emollients and, in more severe cases, topical steroids. For a favorite pair of jeans, a piece of cloth tape may be placed over the metal snap each time the jeans are worn to prevent nickel allergy. For diaper dermatitis, exposure to the air and rapid changing of the wet/soiled diaper is crucial. Because yeast prefer warm, dark, moist areas, an anti-candidal agent is often used and then covered with an ointment to prevent exposure to moisture.

Systemic Allergic Syndromes

Urticaria

Urticaria (or hives) is an IgE-mediated rash that occurs acutely after exposure to an allergen. Intense pruritus and a plaque-like erythematous rash that appears, then disappears within hours, only to reappear in another location, is the hallmark of urticaria. Antihistamines are the treatment of choice acutely. Urticaria should be differentiated from angioedema, which also arises acutely but is not pruritic. Angioedema near the mouth and nose is of immediate concern because of the potential for swelling occluding the airway.

Erythema Multiforme

Like urticaria, erythema multiforme arises acutely with erythema and swelling often in a target pattern. Pruritus is minimal, but vesicles, bullae, and microhemorrhage (ie, ecchymosis) may be present. Unlike urticaria, the erythema multiforme rash stays in one spot and simply enlarges over time. Facial swelling and joint swelling may also occur. A search for the allergen and prompt removal from the environment is critical. Antihistamines and steroids are often used.

Stevens-Johnson Syndrome

Sometimes referred to as erythema multiforme major, Stevens-Johnson syndrome involves not just the skin lesions of erythema multiforme (minor) but also systemic involvement with conjunctiva, oral, and recto-genital mucous membranes. Referral to an ophthalmologist is indicated for conjunctival involvement because panophthalmia may lead to blindness. Reactions to medications and viral infections are the most common triggers for erythema multiforme major. Treatment is supportive with nonsteroidal anti-inflammatory agents and antihistamines. Steroids may be helpful if started early in the course of the hypersensitivity reaction.

Toxic Epidermal Necrolysis

With toxic epidermal necrolysis, the initial rash rapidly progresses to generalized sloughing of the skin. Removal of the offending agent is critical to survival. Prompt admission to an intensive care or burn unit is indicated.

Infectious Rashes and Infestations

Viral

A viral infection is probably the most often implicated diagnosis for a generalized erythematous maculopapular rash accompanied by fever. The astute clinician will always attempt to specify which virus would cause the rash. By specifying which virus, we can advise the parent how long the rash will last and other manifestations that may develop. In the case of roseola caused by *herpesvirus 6*, the rash develops at the end of the illness after 4 or 5 days of fever, so only clinical suspicion will aid in the initial diagnosis. On the other extreme, Kawasaki disease, although suspected, should not be diagnosed before the fifth day of fever. If a specific virus cannot be implicated, another causative agent should be suggested (eg, erythroderma due to staphylococcal infection–scalded skin or toxic shock syndrome). A common mimicker of varicella is the vesicles due to mosquito bites. Other vesicular rashes may be caused by reactivation of varicella in a dermatomal distribution (eg, herpes zoster) or in clusters (eg, herpes simplex).

Wart viruses are problematic because of their propensity to spread before finally yielding to host defenses. Local irritants such as liquid nitrogen and the daily application of tape are effective therapies. The vaccine for human papillomavirus should decrease the risk of cervical cancer in sexually active girls and may decrease the incidence of common warts in teens.

Bacterial

Group A staphylococci and streptococci are common pathogens present on our skin that can invade the dermis because of moisture (around the mouth and nose), friction (caused by excoriation from atopic dermatitis), or burns (thermal or chemical). Once a lesion develops on the skin, the pathogen can quickly spread to surrounding areas and then remotely through scratching. Methicillin-resistant *Staphylococcus aureus* is responsible for an epidemic of deeper cutaneous abscesses that are best treated by incision and drainage.

During warm months in certain locations, ticks may transmit Rocky Mountain spotted fever. A petechial rash that begins on the distal extremities, accompanied muscle aches and increasingly elevated fever, are hallmarks for Rocky Mountain spotted fever. The rash usually appears on the fourth day of fever, with increasing morbidity, and even mortality, if not treated accurately and promptly.

Fungal

Candida albicans is a common colonizer of the mouth (and can lead to thrush) and diaper areas until cellular immunity develops in the second year of life. In older children, the dermatophytes cause tinea in many locations. Most areas can be treated topically, but tinea capitis usually requires oral anti-fungal medications such as griseofulvin. Tinea capitis may lead to a localized hypersensitivity reaction called a kerion. Hair loss and pustules along a tight braid line (known as braid dermatitis) may mimic tinea capitis. Tinea pedis, tinea cruris, and tinea versicolor are most commonly found in adolescents.

Infestations

Pediculosis (or lice) and scabies are frequent causes of highly pruritic rashes. Lice prefer the hair-bearing areas, while scabies like the thin skin between the fingers, toes, and axilla. Scabies are suspected with a generalized pruritus, and a careful search for the characteristic burrows may confirm the diagnosis. Treatment with an insecticide will eliminate the organism, but the rash is caused by a hypersensitivity reaction to the scabies excreta and will persist for a week or more after the treatment. Likewise, with pediculosis the nits will persist on the hair shaft long after the organism has been eliminated. Over-treatment with the insecticide is frequent and can cause toxicity.

Cutaneous larva migrans is another infestation but due to the cat tapeworm. The characteristic linear burrow on the lower extremities is highly pruritic.

Other

In any child with a prolonged fever and rash, Kawasaki disease must be considered. Thought to be a hypersensitivity response to an infectious agent, Kawasaki disease may cause dilatation and thrombosis of the coronary arteries, a rare cause of myocardial infarction in a child. The rash is a generalized exanthem that may often be confused with scarlet fever or a common viral exanthema. Fever must be present for 5 days. Inflammatory markers are extremely elevated, with platelet counts approaching 1 million per microliter and sedimentation rates greater than 100 mm/hour. Intravenous immunoglobulin will block the inflammatory response. A pediatric cardiologist should perform an echo of the coronary arteries and follow up if they are inflamed. This is one of the rare indications for prolonged aspirin therapy in children.

Atypical presentations of Kawasaki disease may occur when nonsteroidal anti-inflammatory drugs have been used to treat the fever.

Vascular Lesions

Superficial hemangiomas often arise within weeks of birth, expanding throughout the first year, then regressing slowly over the next few years. When a hemangioma affects the vision, more aggressive therapy for ablation with lasers may be attempted. Recently, reports indicate that beta-blockers, such as propranolol, may cause early and complete resolution of large and bothersome angiomas. Deep hemangiomas may persist, and, if closely associated with growth plates of the bone, may cause overgrowth of the bone. Salmon patches on the face in an ophthalmic nerve distribution may indicate intracranial hamartomas (eg, Sturge-Weber syndrome).

Hypo-pigmented Lesions

Melanocytes are sensitive to disturbances of the skin such as dryness in atopic dermatitis leading to pityriasis alba, blanching from topical steroids applied over a period of time, and immune response to dysplastic nevi with halo nevi. True vitiligo is difficult to miss because of the complete lack of pigment causing a pure white hue. Albinism is rare but must be considered when the hair and eyes also lack pigment.

Disorders of the Hair and Nails

Loss of hair is always troubling to the patient and the parent. While alopecia areata is rare in children, other causes such as tinea infections of the scalp, traction, and systemic illness (eg, telogen effluvium) will be routinely encountered. Children may inherit dystrophic nails or hair. Similar to tinea pedis, fungal infection of the nails is rare until adolescence. Psoriasis and albinism have typical patterns of nail involvement.

The Pros and Cons of Topical Steroids

Inflammation of the skin is uncomfortable, and topical steroids help relieve that discomfort. However, proper treatment depends on an accurate diagnosis. Putting a steroid on an undiagnosed rash should be avoided because of the risk of it masking the true diagnosis. It may also cause the rash to acutely worsen if an infection is present. The highest potency steroids should be avoided in most cases and reserved for the dermatologist. Ointments tend to penetrate the skin better and provide a more potent effect. Complications of steroid overuse include thinning of the skin, increased superficial vascularization, acne, and striae formation. Injections of steroids into the superficial dermis can lead to atrophy and subcutaneous tissue loss. One way to avoid complication when a prolonged course of topical steroid is contemplated is to apply the steroid for only 5 days and rest on the weekend to allow for skin recovery. A good strategy may be to choose a product from each potency category and become familiar with it in your practice (Box 44-1).

Box 44-1. Examples of Topical Steroid Potency From Highest to Lowest.

   I. Diprolene gel/ointment, Psorcon ointment, Temovate cream/ointment

  II. Cyclocort ointment, Diprosone ointment, Elocon ointment

 III. Aristocort ointment, Cultivate ointment, Diprolene cream

  IV. Cordran ointment, Cyclocort cream, Elocon cream/lotion

   V. Aristocort cream, Cloderm cream, Cordran cream

  VI. Aclovate ointment, DesOwen cream, Locorten cream

 VII. Topical hydrocortisone, dexamethasone, flumethasone, prednisolone

Conclusion

Rashes and skin disorders are visible markers of many disorders, some life threatening that demand immediate and aggressive treatment; some persistent, uncomfortable, or even disfiguring; and some merely inconvenient. The clinician will become familiar with the more common rashes and become friendly with an astute dermatologist with a good manner with children and their parents when a new rash is encountered or a familiar rash does not respond as expected.

Suggested Reading

Chan M, Goldman RD. Erythema multiforme in children: the steroid debate. *Can Fam Physician*. 2013;59(6):635–636

Ely JW, Seabury Stone M. The generalized rash: part II. Diagnostic approach. *Am Fam Physician*. 2010;81(6):735–739

Hurwitz S, ed. *Clinical Pediatric Dermatology*. 2nd ed. WB Saunders: Philadelphia, PA; 1993

Krowchuk DP, Mancini AJ, eds. *Pediatric Dermatology: A Quick Reference Guide*. 2nd ed. American Academy of Pediatrics: Elk Grove Village; 2012

Miller M, Miller AH. Incomplete Kawasaki disease. *Am J Emerg Med*. 2013;31(5):894. e5–894.e7

Zitelli BJ, Davis HW, eds. *Atlas of Pediatric Physical Diagnosis*. 3rd ed. Mosby-Wolfe: Philadelphia, PA; 1997

Zuniga R, Ngyen T. Skin conditions: common skin rashes in infants. *FP Essent*. 2013;407:31–41

CHAPTER 45

Syncope

Randi Teplow-Phipps, MD; Alan J. Meltzer, MD; and Betsy Pfeffer, MD

Key Points

- Syncope is defined as a sudden loss of consciousness and postural tone, typified by an abrupt onset and spontaneous recovery.

- The majority of syncopal episodes can be determined by the history and physical examination findings alone.

- All patients should have an evaluation for orthostatic hypotension and should be measured while lying down and then monitored in a standing position for 2 to 3 minutes.

- Those with neurocardiogenic syncope should be encouraged to drink plenty of fluids, preferably water, and to avoid beverages with caffeine, as they may cause dehydration.

Overview

Syncope is defined as a sudden loss of consciousness and postural tone, typified by an abrupt onset and spontaneous recovery. This is caused by transient cerebral hypoperfusion and may be associated with a prodrome. It is often accompanied by dizziness, pallor, tachycardia, changes in vision (eg, blurry, graying, or blacking out), sweating, or nausea. The event may be precipitated by pain, defecation, exercise, micturition, or stress. Syncope can be thought of in 3 main categories: neurocardiogenic, cardiac, and "other," which includes neurologic and psychogenic. Neurocardiogenic syncope, the most common form of syncope in children and adolescents, is associated with autonomic dysfunction and orthostatic intolerance. Cardiac syncope, while rare, should be taken seriously, as the consequences may be life threatening. As many as 15% to 20% of children and adolescents may experience at least one syncopal episode in their lifetime. While syncope is traditionally considered a benign condition, it can result in significant morbidity and mortality if it occurs during activities such as driving, swimming, or diving.

Causes and Differential Diagnosis

Pre-syncope is the sensation of dizziness with possible change in sensory function but without a total loss of consciousness or loss of postural tone. Pseudo-syncope, often occurring in patients with a history of true syncope, is the apparent sudden loss of consciousness and postural tone but with intact brain activity. Vertigo is a sense of whirling or spinning motion of external objects and is not associated with loss of consciousness. Other conditions often mistaken for syncope include seizures, breath-holding spells, drop attacks, cardiac-associated conditions, and psychiatric disorders. See Table 45-1 for differential diagnosis and associated history and physical examination findings.

Table 45-1. Differential Diagnosis, Etiology, Associated History, and Physical Examination Findings of Syncope

Differential Diagnosis	Specific Etiology	Associated on History	Physical Examination
Neurocardiogenic/vasovagal	• Autonomic dysfunction • Orthostatic hypotension • Inappropriate vasodilation with low cerebral blood flow	• Precipitated by emotion, prolonged standing, dehydration • Prodrome associated (eg, nausea, vomiting, pain, fear, dizziness, lightheaded, sweating, short of breath)	• Orthostatic hypotension • Abnormal if change in BP of >20 mm Hg from laying to standing or >20 BPM increase in pulse • Recurrence of symptoms
Cardiogenic	• Long QT syndrome • WPW • HCM • Dilated cardiomyopathy • Myocarditis • Brugada syndrome and other channelopathies • Heart block: second degree • Congenital heart disease sequelae • Aortic stenosis • Coronary artery anomaly • Primary pulmonary hypertension	• Occurs with exercise • Known family history of sudden cardiac death • Known or suspected heart disease • Palpitations, SOB, chest pain	• Murmur • Abnormal ECG

Table 45-1 (cont)

Differential Diagnosis	Specific Etiology	Associated on History	Physical Examination
Neurologic	• Epilepsy/seizures • Atypical migraine • Sleep disorder: narcolepsy, cataplexy	• Postictal state, disoriented • Prolonged tonic/clonic or rhythmic movements • Aura • Unconscious >5 minutes	• Focal neurologic deficits
Psychological	• Factitious disorder • Conversion disorder • Generalized anxiety disorder • Panic attack/hyperventilation • Depression • Alcohol/substance abuse	• Not usually associated with physical symptoms of sweating or pallor • Not associated with LOC	• No injury with collapse
Breath-holding spells	• Precipitated by pain/anger	• Children 6–60 months of age • Typical pattern of pain/anger followed by brief cry, then breath-holding, resulting in pallor/cyanosis/LOC or seizure	• Normal ECG
Other	• Eating disorder • Pregnancy • Drugs/medication effects • Hypoglycemia		• Abnormal electrolyte levels or other laboratory values • Resting bradycardia associated with anorexia and drug ingestion

Abbreviations: BP, blood pressure; BPM, beats per minute; ECG, electrocardiogram; HCM, hypertrophic cardiomyopathy; LOC, loss of consciousness; SOB, shortness of breath; WPW, Wolff-Parkinson-White disease.

Most syncopal episodes can be determined by the history and physical examination findings alone. Key components of the history should include precipitating factors, position and activities at time of event (eg, cough, urination, defecation, exercise), cardiac- or neurologic-associated symptoms, evidence of a postictal state, and history of an abnormal respiratory pattern. Specific "red flag" questions (Box 45-1) should be addressed to help rule out life-threatening causes of syncope associated with cardiac disease. Identifying these causes on history can help identify those who require further evaluation and management. In addition, questions about behaviors such as strangulation and the "choking game" may be important. In the choking game, individuals purposely attempt self-strangulation or allow strangulation by others to produce a euphoric state just before loss of consciousness. Failure to release the pressure may result in death secondary to cerebral hypoxia.

Box 45-1. Red Flag Questions When Evaluating Syncope

Concerns for Cardiac Disease

- Was there a prodrome?
- Did the episode occur while supine or sleeping?
- Was the event preceded by chest pain or exercise?
- Is there a family history of sudden cardiac death (<30 y) or familial heart disease?
- Was the syncope in response to loud noise, fright, or stress?

Concerns for Seizures

- Was it associated with tonic/clonic movements?
- Did the patient have a postictal state?
- Are there residual neurologic abnormalities?

Past medical history should inquire about cardiac, psychiatric, and chronic diseases such as diabetes mellitus, iron deficiency anemia, and epilepsy. Menstrual history for post-menarchal girls is important to determine likelihood of pregnancy, which may be associated with hypotension and a tendency toward syncope. Family history for specific cardiac-related disease, syncope, epilepsy, deafness associated with prolonged QT syndrome, and sudden/early death is indicated. Certain medications and other licit and illicit drugs may be associated with resting bradycardia or hypotension and therefore may help determine the cause of syncope.

Evaluation

Physical examination findings are almost always normal when a patient presents with syncope. During and immediately after a syncopal event, vital signs should be monitored. Patients with neurocardiogenic syncope are usually bradycardic and hypotensive at the time of the event as opposed to patients with cardiac syncope who are usually tachycardic and hypotensive. All patients should have an evaluation for orthostatic hypotension and should be measured while lying down and then monitored in a standing position for 2 to 3 minutes. Abnormal results are defined as a decrease in blood pressure of greater than 20 mm Hg, an increase of heart rate greater than 20 beats per minute, or a recurrence of symptoms, such as lightheadedness or syncope upon standing. A cardiac examination should carefully evaluate for a new murmur. In aortic stenosis, a systolic ejection murmur and ejection click would be heard. In hypertrophic cardiomyopathy, a systolic ejection murmur will be heard with decrease from a standing to a sitting/lying position. A four-limb blood pressure is indicated to evaluate for coarctation of the aorta and is considered positive if there is greater than 20 mm Hg difference between the arms and legs. A thorough neurologic examination should be conducted to evaluate for any focal deficits or persistent changes in neurologic status.

Diagnostic studies should be guided by the results of the history and physical examination. Routine use of electrocardiograms (ECGs) in all cases of syncope has been promoted (Evidence Level III). An ECG is helpful to identify a non-sinus rhythm such as bradycardia, atrioventricular block, and other arrhythmias. In addition, the following may be identified on an ECG: Wolff-Parkinson-White syndrome (delta wave), prolonged QT interval, bundle branch block, and ventricular hypertrophy in hypertropic cardiomyopathy. A referral to a cardiologist would be indicated for an abnormal ECG if the event occurred with exercise, if there is a strong family history of cardiac disease, or with recurrent syncopal events. Additional Holter monitoring may be indicated when suspicion level is higher for a cardiac arrhythmia as the etiology. Routine use of echocardiography in the absence of clinical suspicion for cardiac syncope is not recommended, as it has shown little benefit (Evidence Level II-2). Head-up tilt table test should only be done in consultation with a cardiologist; its utility has been suggested in cases of non-cardiac syncope where the etiology is still in question (sensitivity 75%, specificity 90%, Evidence Level II-1). It has shown some value in predicting response to medication therapy.

Other laboratory tests and imaging are not routinely recommended because of low yield. If a specific finding is on history or physical examination, the following tests may be helpful: (a) complete blood count to evaluate for anemia; (b) electrolyte levels for hyponatremia and other renal dysfunction; (c) glucose levels to determine hypoglycemia related to diabetes; (d) an electroencephalogram (EEG) if prolonged loss of consciousness, seizure activity, or postictal phase (Evidence Level III); and (e) neuroimaging for head trauma and injury, persistent altered mental status, or focal neurologic deficits.

Management

Management of syncope should be based on the underlying etiology (Table 45-2). Those with neurocardiogenic syncope should be encouraged to drink plenty of fluids, preferably water, and to avoid beverages with caffeine, as they may cause dehydration. A good indication of adequate hydration is dilute or clear urine in a patient with normal renal function. In addition, salt is recommended to achieve a "regular" dietary level in patients who may have salt-restricted diets. Reassurance should be given to patients who do not have any positive "red flag" questions and otherwise benign history and physical examination. Recurrent syncope, despite hydration and adequate salt intake, may be an indication for medication initiation with mineralocorticoids or beta-blockers if a thorough evaluation has ruled out underlying life-threatening diseases. Management for cardiac and other causes of syncope are specific to the identified etiology.

Table 45-2. Management of Syncope Based on Etiology

Etiology of Syncope	Recommended Therapy
Vasovagal/neurocardiogenic	First line: Lie down, elevate legs. Increase salt and water intake to maintain hydration, avoid precipitating stimuli. Reassurance. Second line: mineralocorticoids, beta-blockers
Cardiogenic	Directed by etiology (eg, antiarrhythmics, radio frequency ablation, surgery, pacing)
Neurologic	Anticonvulsants if indicated
Psychological	Therapy directed by psychiatric evaluation
Breath-holding spells	Reassurance
Other	Indicated by etiology

Suggested Reading

Alehan D, Celiker A, Osme S. Head-up tilt test: a highly sensitive, specific test for children with unexplained syncope. *Pediatr Cardiol.* 1996;17(2):86–90

Driscoll D, Jacobsen S, Porter CJ, Wollan PC. Syncope in children and adolescents. *J Am Coll Cardiol.* 1997;29(5):1039–1045

Lewis DA, Dhala A. Syncope in the pediatric patient. The cardiologist's perspective. *Pediatr Clin North Am.* 1999;46(2):205–219

McLeod K. Dizziness and syncope in adolescence. *Heart.* 2001;86(3):350–354

Salim MA, Ware LE, Barnard M, Alpert BS, DiSessa TG. Syncope recurrence in children: relation to tilt-test results. *Pediatrics.* 1998;102(4 Pt 1):924–926

Strickberger SA, Benson DW, Biaggioni I, et al. AHA/ACCF Scientific Statement on the evaluation of syncope. *Circulation.* 2006;113(2):316–217

Zhang Q, Zhu L, Wang C, et al. Value of history taking in children and adolescents with cardiac syncope. *Cardiol Young.* 2013;23(1):54–60

CHAPTER 46

Torticollis

Kevin S. Carter, MD

Key Points

- Congenital muscular torticollis (CMT) is the most common etiology for torticollis, occurring in up to 2% of infants.
- Ultrasound is the preferred initial imaging modality for CMT.
- Physical therapy with passive stretching is sufficient to treat most cases of CMT.
- Acquired torticollis in children is most commonly the result of trauma or infection but may also arise from a number of other conditions.

Overview

The term *torticollis* is derived from Latin, meaning "twisted neck," and refers to a deformity related to an effective unilateral shortening of the sternocleidomastoid muscle (SCM). The condition results in inclination of the head toward the ipsilateral shoulder and rotation of the neck to the contralateral side. In children, this asymmetry most commonly arises from a problem intrinsic to the muscle itself, but several nonmuscular conditions can mimic the characteristic head tilt. The presence of torticollis should therefore alert the clinician to search for an underlying etiology for the "wry neck."

Differential Diagnosis

The primary differentiation of the etiology of torticollis relates to whether the condition is deemed congenital or acquired. Congenital torticollis is defined by its presence at or shortly after birth, though no specific time frame is designated for its diagnosis. Some studies undertaken to characterize congenital torticollis include cases with presentations up to 1 year of age, potentially including confounding factors in their analyses.

Box 46-1 lists several of the causes of congenital torticollis, which occurs in up to 2% of infants. Most of these cases are the result of a grouping of conditions referred to collectively as congenital muscular torticollis (CMT).

Congenital muscular torticollis includes fibromatosis coli, also referred to as pseudotumor of infancy, in which a fibrous mass is palpable within the affected muscle. Also included in the spectrum of CMT is SCM tightness without pseudotumor, as well as postural torticollis, wherein neither palpable mass nor tightness is present.

Box 46-1. Etiologies of Congenital Torticollis

Congenital Muscular Torticollis
Sternomastoid tumor (pseudotumor of infancy) Muscular torticollis Postural torticollis
Skeletal/Ligamentous
Klippel-Feil syndrome and other cervical vertebral abnormalities Craniosynostosis Occipitoatlantal fusion Ligamentous laxity (Down syndrome, osteogenesis imperfecta)
CNS/Ocular
Strabismus Congenital nystagmus Cranial nerve palsies Syringomyelia Benign paroxysmal torticollis
Skin
Pterygium colli

Abbreviation: CNS, central nervous system.

Congenital torticollis may arise from nonmuscular conditions as well. Infants with ocular abnormalities, such as strabismus or nystagmus, can develop torticollis as a means of compensation for visual loss. Cervical vertebral anomalies, such as in the case of Klippel-Feil syndrome, will also result in head tilt. Infants with Sandifer posturing as a result of gastroesophageal reflux may also exhibit torticollis.

In older children and some infants, torticollis is acquired as a result of either trauma or through disease processes affecting the SCM and the accessory nerve that provides its innervation. Infection local to the SCM, such as lymphadenitis or retropharyngeal abscess, can cause muscle spasm. Such inflammation can also result in laxity of ligaments connecting C1 and C2, leading to subluxation, and is referred to as atlantoaxial rotatory fixation (AARF). When this occurs in the absence of trauma, the condition is referred to as Grisel syndrome. Central nervous system diseases, such as stroke or tumor, can also manifest with torticollis.

Evaluation
· · · · · · · · · · ·

As the conditions responsible for torticollis in children range from benign and self-limited to potentially life threatening, the clinician must take care in evaluating the patient presenting with new head tilt. This is particularly true in the older infant, as CMT becomes less likely. Acquired torticollis is generally acute or subacute in onset, and a careful history and examination should point the investigator to the correct underlying diagnosis (Box 46-2). In cases where AARF is suspected, plain radiographs are warranted, but dynamic computed tomography of the neck (in cases with no history of trauma) may be necessary to confirm the diagnosis. Magnetic resonance imaging of the brain and neck is useful if osteomyelitis or central nervous system pathology is suspected.

Box 46-2. Etiologies of Acquired Torticollis

Trauma
Fracture/dislocation Muscular spasm CNS (spinal hematoma)
AARF
Ligamentous laxity
Infectious
Retropharyngeal abscess Cervical lymphadenitis Mastoiditis Meningitis/encephalitis
Neoplastic
CNS tumor Bone tumor (including metastatic disease)
Miscellaneous
Dystonia (drug reactions, idiopathic spasmodic torticollis) Sandifer posturing Chiari malformation

Abbreviations: CNS, central nervous system; AARF, atlantoaxial rotatory fixation.

In infants, CMT is largely diagnosed by physical examination. Patients may have notable SCM tightness or a palpable fibrous sternomastoid tumor, though in cases of postural torticollis, these findings may be absent. It remains unclear what actually causes pseudotumor of infancy; suggested theories include birth trauma as well as intrauterine malpositioning leading to ischemia and subsequent fibrosis of the muscle. Pseudotumor is not always palpable at birth, but the characteristic mass and associated tightness may emerge as fibrosis occurs within the affected tissue.

The preferred modality for imaging in CMT has shifted from plain cervical radiographs to ultrasound of the affected SCM. In a retrospective study of plain radiographs for initial evaluation of torticollis in infants, the rate of false-positive findings leading to further unnecessary studies was 50% higher than the rate of actual cervical abnormalities. Additionally, patients with osseous abnormalities had other findings on examination and history to suggest a diagnosis other than CMT, indicating that pretest probability should play a large role in considering conventional radiography as an initial modality for evaluation (Evidence Level III).

Management

Acquired torticollis is typically relieved by treatment of the underlying condition, once discovered. Most acute cases are painful in nature, and rest and analgesics are generally sufficient adjuncts to therapy for the etiology of the torticollis. Muscle relaxants or benzodiazepines can also be used in older children for persistent muscular spasm. Atlantoaxial rotatory fixation is generally managed with analgesics and rest, often with a soft collar for support. However, in severe cases or if neurologic findings are present, orthopedic and neurosurgical consultation should be obtained.

While some cases of CMT resolve spontaneously, untreated cases may cause patients to develop craniofacial asymmetry. Any infant with tightness in the SCM or limitation of movement should be referred to physical therapy. Most cases are treated with passive stretching of the affected muscle, which can be performed by the parents at home once they have been instructed in technique by a physical therapist. Parents should be warned that infants with sternomastoid tumor frequently experience some tearing of the SCM during therapy, but this is typically painless and carries no increased risk of long-term complications. Most cases will resolve fully within 4 months; if head tilt is persistent after 6 months of therapy, surgical consultation is recommended for SCM lengthening (Evidence Level II-2).

Suggested Reading

Cheng JC, Tang SP, Chen TM, Wong MW, Wong EM. The clinical presentation and outcome of treatment of congenital muscular torticollis in infants: a study of 1,086 cases. *J Pediatr Surg.* 2000;35(7):1091–1096

Do TT. Congenital muscular torticollis: current concepts and review of treatment. *Curr Opin Pediatr.* 2006;18(1):26–29

Haque S, Bilal Shafi BB, Kaleem M. Imaging of torticollis in children. *RadioGraphics.* 2012;32(2):557–571

Ohman A, Nilsson S, Beckung E. Stretching treatment for infants with congenital muscular torticollis: physiotherapist or parents? A randomized pilot study. *PM R.* 2010;2(12):1073–1079

Ohman A, Nilsson S, Lagerkvist AL, Beckung E. Are infants with torticollis at a risk of delay in early motor milestones compared with a control group of healthy infants? *Dev Med Child Neurol.* 2009;51(7):545–550

Vomiting

John M. Olsson, MD

Overview

Vomiting is a physical act that results in the forceful expulsion of stomach contents through the mouth. This should be distinguished from regurgitation, which results from more passive passage of stomach contents into the esophagus without use of gastrointestinal motor activity.

Causes and Differential Diagnosis

A variety of conditions, both physical and psychological/behavioral, can cause vomiting in children. In addition to systemic and metabolic conditions, physical causes include conditions affecting the gastrointestinal, nervous, urinary, and endocrine systems (Box 47-1). Psychological/behavioral causes include rumination, bulimia, psychogenic vomiting, and cyclic vomiting syndrome.

Box 47-1. Differential Diagnosis of Vomiting by Systems

Gastrointestinal	Neurologic	Endocrine
■ **Esophagus** (stricture, web, ring, atresia, tracheo-esophageal fistula, achalasia, foreign body)	■ Tumor	■ Diabetic ketoacidosis
	■ Cyst	■ Adrenal insufficiency
	■ Hematoma	**Respiratory**
	■ Cerebral edema	
■ **Stomach** (pyloric stenosis, web, duplication, peptic ulcer, gastroesophageal reflux)	■ Hydrocephalus	■ Pneumonia
	■ Pseudotumor cerebri	■ Sinusitis
	■ Migraine headache	■ Pharyngitis
	■ Abdominal migraine	**Miscellaneous**
■ **Intestine** (duodenal atresia, malrotation, duplication, intussusceptions, volvulus, foreign body, bezoar, NEC	■ Seizure	
	■ Meningitis	■ Sepsis syndromes
	Renal	■ Pregnancy
		■ Rumination
	■ Obstructive uropathy (ureteropelvic junction obstruction, hydronephrosis, nephrolithiasis)	■ Bulimia
■ **Colon** (Hirschsprung disease, imperforate anus, foreign body, bezoar)		■ Psychogenic
		■ Cyclic vomiting syndrome
■ **Acute gastroenteritis**	■ Renal failure	■ Overfeeding
■ *Helicobacter pylori* infection	■ Glomerulonephritis	■ Medications/vitamin/drug toxicity
	■ Urinary tract infection	
■ **Parasitic infection** (ascariasis, giardiasis)	■ Renal tubular acidosis	■ Superior mesenteric artery syndrome
■ **Appendicitis**	**Metabolic**	■ Child abuse
■ **Milk/soy protein allergy**		
■ **Inflammatory bowel disease**	■ Galactosemia	
	■ Hereditary fructosemia	
■ **Pancreatitis**	■ Amino acidopathy	
■ **Cholecystitis, cholelithiasis**	■ Organic acidopathy	
	■ Urea cycle defect	
■ **Hepatitis**	■ Fatty acid oxidation disorder	
■ **Peritonitis**	■ Lactic acidosis	
■ **Trauma** (duodenal hematoma)	■ Lysosomal storage disorder	
	■ Peroxisomal disorder	

Abbreviation: NEC, necrotizing enterocolitis.
From Chandran L and Chitkara M. Vomiting in children: reassurance, red flag, or referral? *Pediatr Rev.* 2008;29(6):183–192.

It is useful to separate causes of vomiting by age and by the presence/absence of bilious vomiting. Congenital and acquired obstructive lesions are more common causes of vomiting during infancy (Table 47-1), while vomiting from acute gastroenteritis is more common in older children and adolescents. Bilious vomiting suggests an intestinal obstruction distal to the ligament of Treitz and warrants emergency evaluation and consultation with a pediatric surgeon (Box 47-2). Bloody emesis can be caused by esophagitis/gastritis, peptic ulcer disease, Mallory-Weiss tears, bleeding varices, or Dieulafoy lesions.

Table 47-1. Age-Related Differential Diagnosis of Vomiting in Children Younger Than 12 Months

Age	Common Causes	Type of Vomiting	Comment/Associated Features
Newborn	Intestinal atresia/webs	Bilious, depending on level of lesion	May occur at level of esophagus, duodenum, jejunum
	Meconium ileus	Bilious	Consider cystic fibrosis, genetic testing suggested
	Hirschsprung disease	Bilious or nonbilious	History non-passage of stools in nursery, suction rectal biopsy may show lack of intestinal ganglion cells
	Necrotizing enterocolitis	Bilious or nonbilious	Plain films of abdomen may show intestinal pneumatosis
	Inborn errors of metabolism	Bilious or nonbilious	May have acidosis or hypoglycemia
0–3 months	Pyloric stenosis	Nonbilious	Hypochloremic metabolic alkalosis
	Malrotation with midgut volvulus	Bilious	Abdominal distension may be present, plain radiographs of abdomen may show air-fluid levels and paucity of distal bowel gas, emergent surgical consultation indicated
	Inborn errors of metabolism	Bilious or nonbilious	Newborn metabolic screening may be abnormal, may have acidosis or hypoglycemia
	Milk/soy protein allergy	Bilious or nonbilious, may have gross or occult blood	History of extreme fussiness may be present, fecal occult blood may be positive
	Gastroesophageal reflux	Nonbilious, may have gross or occult blood	Emesis usually within 30 minutes of feeding, symptoms worse in supine position
	Child abuse	Nonbilious	Anterior fontanelles fullness may be present, abdominal distension/tenderness may be present, imaging of central nervous system or abdomen may be necessary

Table 47-1 *(cont)*

Age	Common Causes	Type of Vomiting	Comment/Associated Features
3–12 months	Gastroenteritis	Nonbilious initially, may progress to bilious	Stool studies may help establish offending pathogen
	Intussusception	Bilious	Abdomen distension may be present, plain radiographs of the abdomen may show air-fluid levels and paucity of distal bowel gas, stools may be grossly bloody with "currant jelly" appearance, emergent surgical consultation indicated, may be reduced by contrast enema
	Child abuse	Nonbilious	Anterior fontanelles fullness may be present, abdominal distension/tenderness may be present, imaging of central nervous system or abdomen may be necessary
	Intracranial mass lesion	Nonbilious	Anterior fontanelles fullness may be present, CNS imaging studies diagnostic

Abbreviation: CNS, central nervous system.

From Chandran L, Chitkara M. Vomiting in children: reassurance, red flag, or referral? *Pediatr Rev.* 2008;29(6): 183-192.

Box 47-2. Conditions That Can Cause Bilious Vomiting in Infancy

- Intestinal atresia and stenosis
- Malrotation with or without volvulus
- Meconium ileus
- Necrotizing enterocolitis
- Hirschsprung disease
- Inborn errors of metabolism
- Intussusception

Evaluation
· · · · · · · · · · ·

Two key clinical considerations in the evaluation and management of vomiting are determining hydration status and identifying the cause of the vomiting.

The immediate concern is the patient's hydration status and overall hemodynamic stability. Oral rehydration may be attempted for patients with mildly or moderately dehydration secondary to acute gastroenteritis. For those patients with severe dehydration, whose diagnosis is uncertain, or who have acute gastroenteritis and have failed oral rehydration, parenteral rehydration is required. In addition to restoring normal hydration, other supportive measures should be considered prior to beginning a diagnostic evaluation (ie, placement of a nasogastric tube).

Evaluation of the patient with vomiting begins with a thorough history and physical examination. A detailed history of the vomiting includes its onset, frequency, duration, relationship to feeding, presence of bile, character of the vomiting, and whether there is blood in the emesis. Additional details about feeding include changes in appetite, type of proteins being ingested, introduction of new foods, overall intake, formula preparation, and frequency of feedings. Signs such as fever, nausea, abdominal pain, diarrhea, rhinorrhea, otalgia, rash, cough, chest pain, or difficulty breathing may help identify causes. Past medical history may suggest conditions that may predispose a child to future obstructive disease (eg, necrotizing enterocolitis with consequent intestinal stricture).

Family history compatible with metabolic disease or conditions that have an increased familial prevalence (eg, Hirschsprung disease or pyloric stenosis) are important considerations. In addition to assessing hemodynamic status, the examination should focus on the abdomen to note its appearance, such as distension. Bruising of the abdomen might suggest the possibility of trauma, either as a result of an accident or child abuse. Auscultation of the abdomen before palpation may determine whether an ileus or other obstruction is present. In addition to noting the presence and location of any abdominal tenderness, palpation for masses is very important. Olive-shaped masses in the epigastric area are suggestive of pyloric stenosis, and sausage-shaped masses in the right lower quadrant suggest intussusception.

When evaluating an infant for vomiting (Figure 47-1), it is important to determine whether the vomiting has an acute onset or an abrupt change in character, as opposed to vomiting that is chronic in nature. In cases of acute vomiting, delineation of whether the emesis is bilious or non-bilious is key, with the presence of bilious emesis being more often associated with an obstructive lesion warranting immediate evaluation. Work-up for bilious emesis includes plain radiographs of the abdomen and a work-up for possible sepsis, another life-threatening cause of bilious emesis in infancy. Further work-up will be dictated by results of these studies. Pediatric surgery consultation is suggested in cases where prompt operative intervention may be required.

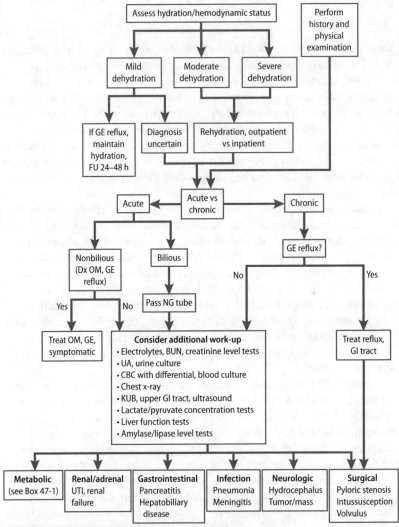

Figure 47-1. Vomiting in the first 12 months of life.

Abbreviations: BUN, blood urea nitrogen; CBC, complete blood count; Dx, diagnosis; FU, follow up; GE, gastro-esophageal; GI, gastrointestinal; KUB, kidney, ureter, and bladder; NG, nasogastric; OM, otitis media; UA, urinalysis; UTI, urinary tract infection; vs, versus.

Infants with non-bilious vomiting may have an identified associated condition, such as otitis media or gastroenteritis, not requiring further evaluation. However, in infants with an uncertain diagnosis, additional work-up should include assessment of electrolyte levels, renal and hepatic function, pancreatic enzymes, and metabolic studies (ie, ammonia, lactate, pyruvate), as well as a screen for sepsis. Radiographic studies may also be warranted if the history or physical examination findings suggest possible surgical diagnoses (eg, pyloric stenosis, intussusception). Continuing management of these infants will be based on the results of these tests and ongoing clinical assessments.

For infants with chronic or persistent vomiting, differentiation of the more common gastroesophageal reflux from other causes of vomiting is important. The vomiting observed in gastroesophageal reflux is usually not forceful, does not interfere with weight gain, and is a nuisance rather than a significant concern. However, more severe cases of gastroesophageal reflux and chronic vomiting that fail to meet the criteria for gastroesophageal reflux merit the same work-up for potential systemic causes recommended for infants with acute non-bilious vomiting.

Evaluation of the child/adolescent beyond infancy (Figure 47-2) also requires a thorough history and physical examination with attention to age-specific concerns. For example, an adolescent girl who presents with vomiting may be pregnant, thereby prompting appropriate history and obtaining of urine for a pregnancy test. The presentation should provide details about the nature of the vomiting, frequency, associated symptoms, color, and presence/absence of blood in the emesis or stool. The past medical history including past surgeries, current medical conditions, and current medications is important, as is family history that includes inflammatory bowel disease and peptic ulcer disease, as these become more relevant in older children and adolescents.

The approach to the child/adolescent with vomiting should distinguish acute from chronic presentations. The most common presentation of acute vomiting in the child or adolescent is acute gastroenteritis. Diarrhea is almost always associated with the vomiting in cases of gastroenteritis. When vomiting is the only presenting symptom, one must carefully consider alternative diagnoses. Constipation, toxic ingestions, food poisoning, strep throat, and otitis media are also common causes of vomiting identifiable by history and physical examination findings. If, however, the patient does not meet the clinical criteria for these diagnoses or presents with disease that is chronic or lasts longer than is consistent with acute gastroenteritis, the differential diagnosis should be expanded. In such cases, electrolyte concentration tests, renal and liver function tests, urinalysis and urine culture, metabolic studies (eg, venous pH, glucose, ketones), and pancreatic enzyme concentration tests would be performed. Imaging studies of the head, chest, and abdomen may be required based on the patient's examination and status.

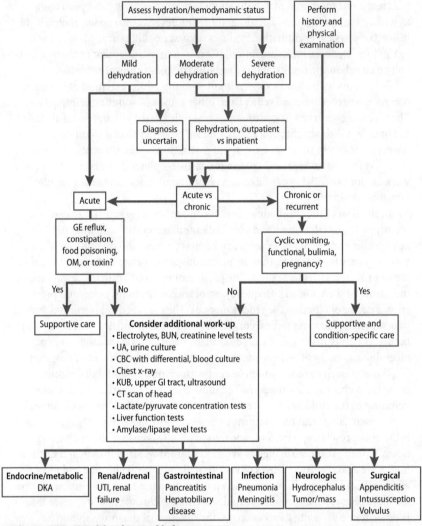

Figure 47-2. Vomiting beyond infancy.

Abbreviations: BUN, blood urea nitrogen; CBC, complete blood count; CT, computed tomography; DKA, diabetic ketoacidosis; GE, gastroesophageal; KUB, kidney, ureter, and bladder; OM, otitis media; UA, urinalysis; UTI, urinary tract infection.

Management

Treatment is directed at correcting the underlying etiology of the vomiting and restoring normal hydration status. If the disease is mild and no specific etiology has been identified, the patient should be treated symptomatically with fluid therapy to maintain hydration. In general, antiemetic medications should be avoided because of the serious potential adverse effects of phenothiazines and metoclopramide, often used in adults. A recent Cochrane Review provided Level I evidence for the use of ondansetron in the treatment of children and adolescents with vomiting associated with acute gastroenteritis in the emergency department, showing that those who were treated with ondansetron were less likely to be admitted to the hospital, were less likely to require intravenous rehydration, and were more likely to achieve cessation of vomiting. Antiemetic treatment with ondansetron should be limited to management of vomiting caused by acute gastroenteritis in the emergency department. Evidence supporting its benefit on a continuing outpatient basis is lacking. Ondansetron has been shown to reduce vomiting in children receiving chemotherapy and radiation therapy and who have postoperative nausea and vomiting.

Suggested Reading

Allen K. The vomiting child: what to do and when to consult. *Aust Fam Physician.* 2007;36(9):684–687

Chandran L, Chitkara M. Vomiting in children: reassurance, red flag, or referral? *Pediatr Rev.* 2008;29(6):183–192

Culy CR, Bhana N, Plosker GL. Ondansetron: a review of its use as an antiemetic in children. *Paediatr Drugs.* 2001;3(6):441–479

DeCamp LR, Byerley JS, Doshi N, Steiner MJ. Use of antiemetic agents in acute gastroenteritis: a systematic review and meta-analysis. *Arch Pediatr Adolesc Med.* 2008;162(9):858–865

Fedorowicz Z, Jagannath VA, Carter B. Antiemetics for reducing vomiting related to acute gastroenteritis in children and adolescents (Review). *Cochrane Database Syst Rev.* 2011;9:CD005506

Murray KF, Christie DL. Vomiting. *Pediatr Rev.* 1998;19(10):337–341

Vreeman RC. Managing vomiting: should I consider options besides rehydration? *Contemporary Pediatr.* 2011;28(8):53–59

CHAPTER 48

Acute Bleeding

Elizabeth H. Mack, MD, MS

Key Points

- Response to visible external bleeding should include application of direct pressure.

- Heart rate is a particularly sensitive indicator of intravascular status in children, as blood pressure may be preserved until 20% to 30% of blood volume is lost. Children do not typically develop bleeding with mild trauma until the platelet count is $<$50,000/mm^3 or spontaneous bleeding unless platelet count is $<$10,000/mm^3.

- Children exposed to multiple blood products may develop alloimmunization-induced thrombocytopenia, thereby not eliciting a 1 hour posttransfusion response to platelet administration unless ABO-type or HLA-matched platelets are administered.

- Classically, upper gastrointestinal bleeding, unless acute and massive, presents as hematemesis or melena, whereas lower gastrointestinal bleeding presents with bright red blood per rectum. Intussusception classically presents with currant jelly stools and can potentially be reduced with air contrast enema. Meckel's diverticulum often presents with massive rectal bleeding and requires surgical resection.

- Traumatic coagulopathy may precipitate further bleeding, and in addition to product replacement, physicians and other health care providers must manage the hypothermia, hypocalcemia, and acidosis.

Overview

Anemia can be caused by decreased red blood cell production, increased destruction, or blood loss. In addition to acute (or chronic) anemia, serious consequences of acute bleeding include hypoperfusion of important organs and shock due to hypovolemia and decreased oxygen and nutrient supply. Children can develop life-threatening bleeding for a wide variety of reasons. Bleeding due to malignancy, coagulopathy and nonmalignant hematologic disorders, gastrointestinal (GI) lesions, and traumatic hemorrhage can be particularly problematic for children and require quick and appropriate evaluation and management.

Pediatric oncology patients are at risk for hemorrhage for multiple reasons including associated chemotherapy-induced thrombocytopenia, mucosal injury, coagulopathy, alloimmunization-associated thrombocytopenia, and fibrinolytic disorders. Coagulopathy in cancer patients may be due to the primary disease, hepatic dysfunction, chemotherapy, sepsis, and vitamin K deficiency (Table 48-1). The most common sites of hemorrhage in oncology patients are intracranial, retinal, pulmonary, bladder, and gastrointestinal. Hemorrhage can be life threatening in these patients and must be managed aggressively. In fact, up to 10% of children with acute promyelocytic leukemia die of hemorrhage in the first 2 weeks of therapy.

Disorders of platelet and coagulation factor quantity and function also predispose children to bleeding. Children do not typically develop bleeding with mild trauma until the platelet count is less than 50,000/mm^3 and usually do not develop spontaneous bleeding unless the platelet count is less than 10,000/mm^3. Thrombocytopenia in children has many causes (Figure 48-1). Drugs and viruses are common causes of thrombocytopenia due to decreased production. Drugs are also a major cause of dysfunctional platelets, or thrombocytopathy (Box 48-1). The combination of thrombocytopenia with platelet dysfunction is a significant bleeding risk for children.

Causes

Causes of GI bleeding in children vary by location and age of the child (Box 48-2). Gastric and duodenal ulcers and varices are common causes of upper GI bleeding, and these are the most common causes of GI bleeding in older children. Meckel diverticulum, the most common congenital GI malformation, is due to persistence of the vitellointestinal duct and results in ectopic ileal or gastric mucosa prone to bleeding. The classic presentation in children of Meckel diverticulum–induced bleeding is massive, painless rectal bleeding. The "rule of 2," though certainly not universal in cases of Meckel diverticulum, indicates that it is present in 2% of the population, is often located 2 ft from the ileocecal valve, and is often 2 in in length. Henoch-Schönlein purpura (HSP), an IgA-mediated autoimmune vasculitis that typically presents in younger children, may present with hematochezia, but intussusception associated with HSP must be excluded as a cause of GI bleeding in this disorder. Hematemesis is less frequent, and frank GI hemorrhage is relatively rare (<2%) in HSP.

Trauma is a common cause of significant hemorrhage in children, and trauma is also often associated with traumatic coagulopathy, which can further worsen the hemorrhage and lead to shock and death due to exsanguination. Frequent assessment, intervention, and reassessment are the cornerstone of trauma resuscitation and management.

Table 48-1. Causes of Bleeding in Pediatric Cancer Patients

Cause	Diagnostic Test	Treatment	Monitoring
Local anatomic causes	Visual inspection Unexplained drop in hemoglobin	Surgical control and pressure dressings	Hemoglobin, dressing inspection
Thrombocytopenia: chemotherapy induced	Posttransfusion platelet increase	1 RDP unit/10 kg of body weight or 1 SDP unit/50 kg will increase platelets by 40,000.	Platelet count daily
Thrombocytopenia with alloimmunization	No increase with 1 hour posttransfusion platelet count	ABO-type specific or HLA-matched platelets	1 hour posttransfusion platelet count
Thrombocytopenia with sepsis	Drop in platelet count between 1 and 6 hours posttransfusion	1 RDP unit/10 kg of body weight as often as needed to maintain platelets > 20,000/mm^3	Platelet count 6 hours posttransfusion
Coagulopathy: DIC	Prolonged PT/INR Elevated D-dimer or FDPs Low fibrinogen	FFP to control bleeding. Cryoprecipitate for fibrinogen <100 ng/mL.	PT/INR, fibrinogen, D-dimer every 6 hours
Coagulopathy: hepatic dysfunction	Prolonged PT/INR Factors II, V, VII, IX, X are low. Factors VIII and fibrinogen are normal.	FFP to maintain INR <1.5	PT/INR 6 hours after FFP and daily
Coagulopathy: vitamin K deficiency	Prolonged PT/INR Factors II, VII, IX, X are low. Factors V and VIII are normal.	FFP if bleeding Vitamin K orally/SC	PT/INR 6 hours after vitamin K and daily
Fibrinolytic disorder	Consider if bleeding out of proportion to coagulopathy in appropriate clinical setting (APL, ALL). Diagnostic laboratory tests of limited utility: euglobulin lysis test TAT/ roTEG (research).	Consider antifibrinolytic therapy for life-threatening bleeding.	None

Abbreviations: ALL, acute lymphoblastic leukemia; APL, acute promyelocytic leukemia; DIC, disseminated intravascular coagulopathy; FDP, fibrin degradation product; FFP, fresh frozen plasma; HLA, human leukocyte antigen; PT/INR, prothrombin/international normalized ratio; RDP, random donor platelet; roTEG, rotational thromboelastography; SC, subcutaneously; SDP, single donor platelet; TAT, thrombin–antithrombin complex.

From Meija R, et al. Oncologic emergencies and complications. In: Nichols DG, ed. *Rogers' Textbook of Pediatric Intensive Care.* 4th ed. Philadelphia, PA: Lippincott Williams & Wilkins, 2008:1721, with permission.

Thrombocytopenia		
Decreased Production	**Increased Destruction**	**Sequestration**
Acquired • Bone marrow infiltration • Drug-toxin related • Folate or vitamin B12 deficiency • Renal failure • Viral infections (HIV, EBV, CMV) **Congenital** • Alport syndrome • Bernard-Soulier syndrome • Fanconi syndrome • Inherited metabolic disorders • May-Hegglin anomaly • Thrombocytopenia with absent radius • TORCH • Trisomy 13 & 18 • Wiskott-Aldrich syndrome	**Immunologic** • Drug-toxin related • Idiopathic thrombocytopenic purpura • Infection • Maternal idiopathic thrombocytopenic purpura • Neonatal (alloimmune) **Nonimmunologic** • Congenital heart disease • Disseminated intravascular coagulopathy • Massive transfusion • Hemolytic-uremic syndrome (HUS/TTP) • Heparin induced • Hypothermia • Microangiopathic (umbilical artery catheters, ECMO) • Nephritic syndrome • Neonatal (asphyxia/sepsis) • Primary pulmonary hypertension	• Cavernous hemangioma (Kasabach-Merritt syndrome) • Splenomegaly (hypersplenism)

Figure 48-1. Differential diagnosis of thrombocytopenia.
Note: "Pseudo-thrombocytopenia" occurs with platelet clumping, either spontaneously or from collection-tube preservatives (EDTA or citrate).

Abbreviations: CMV, cytomegalovirus; EBV, Epstein-Barr virus; ECMO, extracorporeal membrane oxygenation; HIV, human immunodeficiency virus; HUS, hemolytic-uremic syndrome; TORCH, toxoplasmosis, other infections, rubella, cytomegalovirus infection, and herpes simplex; TTP, thrombotic thrombocytopenic purpura.

From Sadowitz PD, Amanullah S, Souid AK. Hematologic emergencies in the pediatric emergency room. *Emerg Med Clin North Am.* 2002;20(1):177–198, vii, with permission.

Evaluation

Assessment of the child with bleeding involves evaluation of hemodynamics (eg, heart rate, blood pressure, perfusion) and an estimation of risk for further bleeding. Constant reassessment of vital signs, including pulse oximetry, is indicated. Heart rate is a particularly sensitive indicator of intravascular status in children, as blood pressure may be preserved until 20% to 30% of blood volume is lost, but physicians must note if children are on beta-blockers (as is often the case in portal hypertension) because these children may not manifest tachycardia. For patients undergoing transfusion, particularly massive transfusion, temperature must be closely monitored to assess for hypothermia (due to room temperature blood) or febrile transfusion reactions.

Children with platelet deficiency or dysfunction or von Willebrand disease often present with capillary-type bleeding, such as oozing, bruising, or mucous

Box 48-1. Drugs That Inhibit Platelet Function (Thrombocytopathy)

Nonsteroidal anti-inflammatory drugs

Aspirin, ibuprofen, indomethacin, naproxen, and others

Antibiotics

Penicillins, cephalosporins, nitrofurantoin

Cardiovascular drugs

Amrinone/milrinone, dipyridamole, diltiazem, propranolol, nitroprusside, nifedipine, nitroglycerin, procainamide, verapamil

Anticoagulants, fibrinolytics, and anti-fibrinolytics

Aprotinin, ϵ-aminocaproic acid, heparin, protamine, alteplase

Anesthetics

Propofol, ketamine, benzocaine, cocaine, lidocaine, procaine, tetracaine, halothane, heroin

Anticonvulsants/psychotropic drugs

Valproate, amitriptyline, haloperidol, imipramine, nortriptyline, chlorpromazine

Chemotherapy

Carmustine, daunorubicin, vincristine, L-asparaginase

Antihistamines

Chlorpheniramine, diphenhydramine, ranitidine, cimetidine

Herbal/alternative medicines

Garlic, ginseng, ginko biloba

Other dugs/toxins

Guaifenesin, dextran, pseudoephedrine, hetastarch, mustard gas

From Easley RB, Brady KM, Tobias JD. Hematologic emergencies. In: Nichols DG, ed. *Rogers' Textbook of Pediatric Intensive Care.* 4th ed. Philadelphia, PA: Lippincott Williams & Wilkins, 2008:1745, with permission.

membrane bleeding. Children with large-vessel bleeding, such as hemarthrosis or hematomas, are more likely to have coagulation factor deficiencies or inhibitors. Thrombocytopenia is caused by decreased platelet production, increased destruction, or sequestration (see Figure 48-1). Drugs and viruses are common causes of thrombocytopenia because of decreased production or function. Drugs can also affect factor function leading to coagulopathy. In cases of normal platelet count and factor levels, physicians should consider platelet function disorders that are typically caused by drugs (see Box 48-1). In cases of thrombocytopathy, platelet morphology is often unusual on the peripheral smear. Patients in pediatric oncology settings often are exposed to many blood products and therefore develop thrombocytopenia related to alloimmunization and antiplatelet antibodies.

Box 48-2. Causes of GI Bleeding in Children by Age and Location

Upper GI bleeding	Lower GI bleeding
Neonate/Infant	*Neonate/Infant*
Swallowed maternal blood	Swallowed maternal blood
Esophagitis	Anal fissures
Gastritis	Upper GI bleed
Ulcer/erosions—gastric/duodenal	Milk protein allergy
Vascular malformation	Necrotizing enterocolitis
Vitamin K deficiency	Hirschsprung enterocolitis
	Malrotation and volvulus
Child	Infectious enterocolitis
Esophagitis	
Mallory-Weiss syndrome	*Child*
Gastritis	Polyps
Ulcer—gastric/duodenal	Hereditary illness
Helicobacter pylori infection	Intussusception
Arteriovenous malformations	Infectious enterocolitis
Esophageal or gastric varices	Meckel diverticulum
Adverse drug reactions—NSAIDs	Hemolytic uremic syndrome
Portal hypertension	Henoch-Schönlein purpura
Swallowed epistaxis	Inflammatory bowel disease
Adolescent	*Adolescent*
Esophagitis	Infectious enterocolitis
Mallory-Weiss syndrome	Inflammatory bowel disease
Gastritis	Arteriovenous malformation
Ulcer—gastric/duodenal	Polyps
Helicobacter pylori infection	Hereditary illness
Arteriovenous malformations	Hemolytic uremic syndrome
Esophageal or gastric varices	
Adverse drug reactions—NSAIDs	
Portal hypertension	

Abbreviations: GI, gastrointestinal, NSAID, nonsteroidal anti-inflammatory drug

From Baltodano A, Cooper MK. Critical aspects of intestinal disorders. In: Nichols DG, ed. *Rogers' Textbook of Pediatric Intensive Care*. 4th ed. Philadelphia, PA: Lippincott Williams & Wilkins, 2008:1577, with permission.

Etiology of GI bleeding in children varies by age and source of bleeding (ie, upper or lower GI tract) (see Box 48-2). It is important to distinguish GI bleeding from blood of maternal origin, in the case of a neonate, and blood originating from the nose or lungs. The ligament of Treitz marks the division between upper and lower GI tracts. Classically, upper GI bleeding, unless acute and massive, presents as hematemesis or melena; whereas, lower GI bleeding presents with bright red blood per rectum. "Currant jelly" stools, classically seen with intussusception, are caused by ischemic bleeding. When bleeding is not massive, it is important to confirm the red or black material noted is actually blood with heme testing.

Massive upper GI bleeding in children is commonly caused by esophageal or gastric varices, vascular anomalies, and gastric or duodenal ulcers. Ulceration may be caused by medications, so it is important to get a complete prescription and over-the-counter medication history. Children with liver disease are at particularly high risk for upper GI bleeding due to portal hypertension. Variceal rupture may be the first sign of long-standing liver disease. Massive lower GI bleeding is often caused by ulcerative colitis, Crohn disease, infectious colitis, intussusception, Meckel diverticulum, HSP, vascular anomalies, and congenital intestinal duplication. Infectious gastroenteritis or colitis as well as inflammatory bowel disease often present with fever, elevated levels or rates of acute phase reactants (eg, C-reactive protein, erythrocyte sedimentation, procalcitonin), or both. Stool samples should be evaluated for infectious causes. Blood urea nitrogen level may be disproportionately elevated in cases of upper GI bleeding. Nasogastric lavage may help differentiate upper from lower GI bleeding.

Patients with evidence of GI bleeding may undergo endoscopic, radiological, or sonographic studies to determine the source of bleeding. However, particularly with lower GI endoscopy, blood may obscure the view through the camera and not lead to identification of the source. Wireless capsule endoscopy may be useful for less acute bleeding. Rectal examination should be performed when lower GI bleeding is suspected to rule out fissures and external hemorrhoids. Plain radiography is not likely to be useful except in cases of suspected necrotizing enterocolitis. Air contrast enema, ultrasound, or both may be useful in diagnosing intussusception. Contrast computed tomography scans may be useful in localizing lower GI bleeding, particularly if endoscopy does not reveal a source. Nuclear medicine studies such as ^{99m}Tc (technetium)-labeled red blood cell scan and technetium-99m pertechnetate scan (also called Meckel scan), may be helpful in localizing an otherwise unidentified source, particularly in the case of Meckel diverticulum. The technetium-99m pertechnetate scan is specific to ectopic gastric mucosa, not to Meckel diverticulum, and may be positive in gut duplication cysts or other cases of ectopic gastric mucosa.

Traumatic sites of hemorrhage involve large body cavities such as peritoneum, hemithorax, pelvic, and thigh compartments. Trauma resuscitation must include prevention and management of traumatic coagulopathy. Causes of traumatic coagulopathy include traumatic brain injury, dilution of factor and platelet levels during resuscitation, hypocalcemia, acidosis, and hypothermia.

Basic laboratory studies recommended in the case of a child with hemorrhage include complete blood count, prothrombin/international normalized ratio/partial thromboplastin time levels, and fibrinogen level. Thromboelastography has been specifically proposed as point-of-care testing for management of traumatic coagulopathy to direct transfusion of particular blood products in order to restore clotting homeostasis. Thrombin time and mixing studies may also be pursued in the evaluation.

Management

For significant acute bleeding, vascular access is essential and best obtained with 2 large-bore intravenous lines (or potentially central venous access) if possible. If vascular access is unable to be obtained in the patient in unstable condition, an intraosseous line should be placed in a non-fractured extremity, ideally medial to the tibial tuberosity. Direct pressure should be applied to any area of external hemorrhage. Dressings with topical thrombin or tissue sealants are available to address localized bleeding. Hemorrhagic shock can be treated with isotonic crystalloid solutions (0.9% sodium chloride or lactated Ringer solution) until blood products are available. In cases of thrombocytopenia, if bleeding is ongoing, or in cases with patients at high risk for bleeding, such as in the perioperative/postoperative period, the goal is to keep the platelet count greater than 100,000/mm^3. Otherwise, the goal platelet count may be lower (>20,000/mm^3 or 50,000/mm^3) depending on the circumstances. Platelet transfusions are given in doses of 6 units/kg for an adult or 0.1 units/kg for children (or platelet pheresis pack). Empiric administration of fresh frozen plasma and platelets is recommended when greater than 80 mL/kg of packed red blood cells has been transfused because of dilutional coagulopathy and thrombocytopenia. In cases of massive hemorrhage, massive transfusion protocols that quickly deliver blood products in physiologic ratios should be employed.

The approach to management of bleeding in the patient in a pediatric oncology setting depends on etiology of the bleeding (see Table 48-1). Children exposed to multiple blood products, particularly those with leukemia and aplastic anemia, often develop antibodies to platelets and therefore will not have a 1-hour posttransfusion response to platelet administration unless ABO-type or HLA-matched platelets are administered.

Management of GI bleeding, after basic resuscitative measures have been addressed, depends on the cause. Feeding should be discontinued when GI bleeding is noted. Acid suppression therapy is often indicated, with either H$_2$-receptor antagonists or proton pump inhibitors. Other more aggressive pharmacologic therapies may include octreotide and vasopressin, which decrease splanchnic flow. Invasive management, depending on the cause, may include cautery, banding, resection, sclerosis, embolization, and transjugular intrahepatic portosystemic shunt. Management of variceal bleeding due to portal hypertension depends on stability of the patient (Figure 48-2). Care must be taken not to over-resuscitate children with portal hypertension, so as not to precipitate further increased portal pressures and bleeding. Gastrointestinal hemorrhage due to HSP is rarely responsive to invasive interventions and may be treated with immunomodulating agents, such as methylprednisolone, cyclophosphamide, or rituximab. Meckel diverticulum must be surgically resected. Intussusception may potentially be reduced by air contrast enema, or it may require surgical reduction.

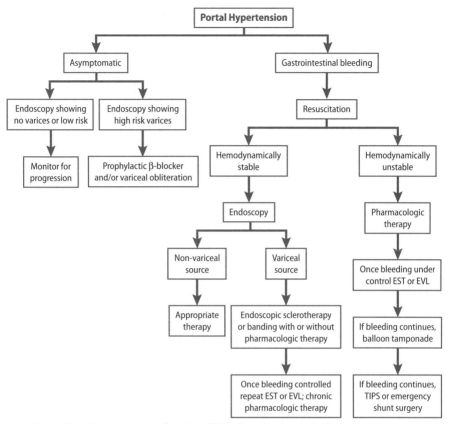

Figure 48-2. Management of variceal bleeding due to portal hypertension.

Abbreviations: EST, endoscopic sclerotherapy; EVL, endoscopic variceal band ligation; TIPS, transjugular intrahepatic portosystemic shunt.

From Gugig R, Rosenthal P. Management of portal hypertension in children. *World J Gastroenterol.* 2012;18(11):1179–1784, with permission.

Traumatic resuscitation must involve treatment of volume deficits, anemia, hypothermia, hypocalcemia, acidosis, and hemorrhagic shock. Hypotensive resuscitation in trauma has been proposed, so as not to propagate further bleeding with increased intravascular filling. Care must be taken, however, to avoid under-resuscitation in this effort.

Other non-blood product therapies sometimes used in the case of hemorrhage include aprotinin, aminocaproic acid, tranexamic acid, protamine (in cases of heparin-induced bleeding), vitamin K (in cases of warfarin-induced bleeding), and recombinant factor VIIa.

Suggested Reading

Avarello JT, Cantor RM. Pediatric major trauma: an approach to evaluation and management. *Emerg Med Clin N Am.* 2007;25(3):803–836

Baird JS, Cooper A. Multiple trauma. *Rogers' Textbook of Pediatric Intensive Care.* Philadelphia, PA: Lippincott Williams & Wilkins; 2008:384–405

Baltodano A, Cooper MK. Critical aspects of intestinal disorders. In: Nichols DG, ed. *Rogers' Textbook of Pediatric Intensive Care.* Philadelphia, PA: Lippincott Williams & Wilkins; 2008:1562–1583

Chang WL, Yang YH, Lin YT, Chiang BL. Gastrointestinal manifestations in Henoch-Schönlein purpura: a review of 261 patients. *Acta Pædiatr.* 2004;93(11):1427–1431

Chen SY, Kong MS. Gastrointestinal manifestations and complications of Henoch-Schönlein purpura. *Chang Gung Med.* 2004;27(3):175–181

Easley RB, Brady KM,Tobias JD. Hematologic emergencies. In: Nichols DG, ed. *Rogers' Textbook of Pediatric Intensive Care.* Philadelphia, PA: Lippincott Williams & Wilkins; 2008:1725–1758

Gugig R, Rosenthal P. Management of portal hypertension in children. *World J Gastroenterol.* 2012;18(11):1176–1184

Mejia R, Cortes JA, Brown DL, et al. Oncologic emergencies and complications. In: Nichols DG, ed. *Rogers' Textbook of Pediatric Intensive Care.* Philadelphia, PA: Lippincott Williams & Wilkins; 2008:1710–1724

Sagar J, Kumar V, Shah EK. Meckel's diverticulum: a systematic review. *J Royal Soc of Med.* 2006;99(10):501–505

Shamir R, Eliakim R. Capsule endoscopy in pediatric patients. *World J Gastroenterol.* 2008;14(26):4152–5155

Spinella PC, Holcomb JB. Resuscitation and transfusion principles of traumatic hemorrhagic shock. *Blood Rev.* 2009;23(6):231–240

Wright SS, Nogueira J, Thame K, et al; American Federation for Medical Research. Successful treatment of intractable gastrointestinal bleeding in Henoch-Schönlein purpura with rituximab: first reported case. http://www.afmr.org/abstracts/2009/SR2009_abstracts/20.cgi. Published 2009. Accessed January 12, 2015

CHAPTER 49

Anaphylaxis, Urticaria, and Angioedema

Vandana Kudva Patel, MD, and Douglas T. Johnston, DO

Key Points

- Food allergy accounts for 30% of fatal anaphylaxis and is most commonly associated with peanuts, tree nuts, and crustaceans.

- Early treatment of anaphylaxis with epinephrine is the greatest priority.

- Venom immunotherapy is successful in preventing subsequent anaphylaxis in up to 98% of patients with venom-mediated diseases.

- Upper respiratory tract infections and IgE-mediated allergic reactions account for most episodes of acute urticaria in children.

- Laboratory testing is not usually helpful in cases of chronic urticaria; only in the event of unresponsiveness to antihistamines or severe manifestations should studies be pursued.

Overview

Anaphylaxis is an acute, life-threatening systemic reaction that may cause death. Mechanisms of anaphylaxis may be IgE or non-IgE mediated and involve release of mediators from mast cells and basophils. Prompt recognition of signs and symptoms of anaphylaxis and early administration of epinephrine along with supportive care are the cornerstones of initial therapy. Subsequent care involves equipping the patient with an epinephrine autoinjector, educating the patient about avoidance of suspected triggers, and providing a written action plan.

Urticaria commonly presents in the pediatric practice, occurring in approximately 20% of the general population at least once during their lifetime. Urticaria is characterized by the swelling of the superficial skin surrounded by erythema associated with itching or burning sensation. Urticaria can occur rapidly and is transient with lesions resolving usually within 1 to 24 hours in a particular location.

Angioedema is defined as transient, non-pitting, localized swelling of the subcutaneous tissues, mucosal tissues, or both. Angioedema may be painful rather than itchy and tends to resolve more gradually than urticaria, up to 72 hours at times. Urticaria and angioedema are common in anaphylaxis.

Anaphylaxis

Causes

Across all age groups, including children, the most common triggers for anaphylaxis are ingested foods (33%), insect stings (19%), and medications (14%) (Evidence Level II-2). Other causes include exercise-induced and idiopathic anaphylaxis. Examples of conditions that may mimic anaphylaxis include vasovagal reactions, systemic mastocytosis, and urticarial pigmentosa (Box 49-1).

Box 49-1. Differential Diagnosis of Anaphylaxis

Reactions caused by excess endogenous production of histamine
    Systemic mastocytosis
    Urticaria pigmentosa
    Basophilic leukemia
    Acute promyelocytic leukemia with retinoic acid treatment
    Hydatid cyst
Vasovagal response
Forms of shock (eg, hemorrhagic, endotoxic, cardiogenic, hypoglycemic)
Flushing disorders
    Carcinoid
    Red man syndrome from vancomycin
    Autonomic epilepsy
    Vasointestinal peptide and other vasoactive peptide–secreting tumors
Ingestant-related reactions
    Monosodium glutamate
    Sulfites
    Scombroidosis
Miscellaneous
    C1 esterase inhibitor quantitative and qualitative defects
    Pheochromocytoma
    Neurologic (eg, seizure, stroke)
    Capillary leak syndrome
    Panic attack
    Vocal cord dysfunction syndrome

In children, the most common food allergens are cow's milk, peanuts, tree nuts, eggs, shellfish, and, finally, fruits and vegetables (Evidence Level I). Food accounts for 30% of fatal anaphylaxis, more commonly associated with certain foods such as peanuts, tree nuts, and crustaceans. Those affected are typically teenagers and young adults. They commonly have a prior diagnosis of food allergy and asthma, as well as a failure to promptly administer epinephrine.

Based on a US population study, approximately 150 deaths per year are due to food-induced anaphylaxis (Evidence Level II-3).

Venom-induced anaphylaxis from stinging insects has been well studied in Europe, North America, and Australia where flying hymenoptera are a well-documented cause. In North America, stings from the non-flying imported fire ant (*Solenopsis* species) are also implicated. Anaphylaxis occurs in 1% of children who are stung and may be fatal with the initial sting, though most children have systemic reactions confined to the skin with occasional respiratory symptoms. Skin tests of venom extract or fire ant whole-body extract are the most accurate, but in vitro testing may be used as well. A history suggestive of a systemic reaction is the indication to proceed to testing (Evidence Level III).

The most common drug allergies are to antimicrobials and nonsteroidal anti-inflammatory drugs. Penicillin is the most common antimicrobial implicated. Skin testing to penicillin with commercially available reagents has a 97% negative predictive value. The extent of cross-reactivity between penicillin and cephalosporins is not well defined but thought to be low. Diagnosis of non–β-lactam antimicrobial-induced reactions is limited, as no skin tests are standardized for these drugs.

The most common cause of pediatric perioperative anaphylaxis involves latex, neuromuscular blocking agents, and antibiotics (Evidence Level II-3). Other drugs that have been implicated as triggers of anaphylaxis include biologics, such as omalizumab and allergen immunotherapy.

Signs and Symptoms

The accurate diagnosis of anaphylaxis in children can be difficult. Children are often unable to report subjective symptoms, and cutaneous symptoms are lacking in about 18% of cases (Box 49-2). Although diagnosis of anaphylaxis usually depends on involvement of 2 organ systems (eg, skin plus respiratory, skin plus cardiovascular), anaphylaxis may present as an acute cardiac or respiratory event with only hypotension (Table 49-1) (Evidence Level 3).

Box 49-2. Clinical Scenarios of Anaphylaxis

1.	The acute onset of a reaction (minutes to hours) with involvement of the skin, mucosal tissue, or both and at least one of the following symptoms: (1) respiratory compromise or (2) reduced blood pressure with evidence of end-organ dysfunction
2.	Two or more of the following symptoms that occur rapidly after exposure to a likely allergen for that patient: involvement of the skin/mucosal tissue, respiratory compromise, reduced blood pressure or associated symptoms, persistent intestinal symptoms, or a combination thereof
3.	Reduced blood pressure after exposure to a known allergen

Derived from Lieberman P, Nicklas R, Oppenheimer J, et al. The diagnosis and management of anaphylaxis practice parameter: 2010 update. *J Allergy Clin Immunol.* 2010;126(3):477–480.

Table 49-1. Signs and Symptoms of Anaphylaxis

Clinical Features	Frequency
Swelling tongue	13%
Swelling/tightness in throat	11%
Difficulty talking/hoarse voice	13%
Urticaria	72%
Angioedema	55%
Pruritus	11%
Vomiting, diarrhea/abdominal cramps	29%
Hypotension, pale, impaired, loss of consciousness, collapse	17%

Adapted from de Silva IL, Mehr SS, Tey D, Tang ML. Pediatric anaphylaxis: a 5 year retrospective review. *Allergy.* 2008;63(8):1071–1076, with permission.

Evaluation

Clinical history is the most important tool for guiding further investigations. When obtaining the history, the onset of symptoms, setting in which it occurred, treatment given, and duration of episode can be useful information. A list of all foods and drugs taken within 6 hours of the episode should be noted. Other useful information may be any insect stings or bites, location of the episode (indoor vs outdoor), if the event occurred during exercise, and whether the event may have been related to physical factors such as temperature.

Management

Anaphylaxis is a continuum of events that can progress from mild symptoms to life-threatening issues quickly. The more rapidly anaphylaxis develops, the more likely it is to be severe. Once anaphylaxis is suspected, it is best to administer epinephrine. Treatment in order of importance is intramuscular epinephrine delivered in the anterolateral thigh, patient position, oxygen, intravenous fluids, nebulized therapy, vasopressors, antihistamines, corticosteroids, and other agents (Figure 49-1).

Anaphylaxis can be phasic, protracted, or biphasic, with symptoms recurring at least 1 hour after apparent resolution of initial symptoms. Hence, a prolonged period of medical observation is warranted in many cases. In one study, children who required more than one adrenaline dose, a fluid bolus, or both for treatment of the initial anaphylactic reaction were significantly more likely to develop biphasic reactions (Evidence Level 3).

Follow-up Care

Once the acute phase of anaphylaxis is over, the goal is to identify a trigger, if one can be found. At times, the trigger cannot be found or avoidance of the trigger cannot be accomplished. Avoidance management must be individualized, taking into account age, residential conditions, educational level, and level

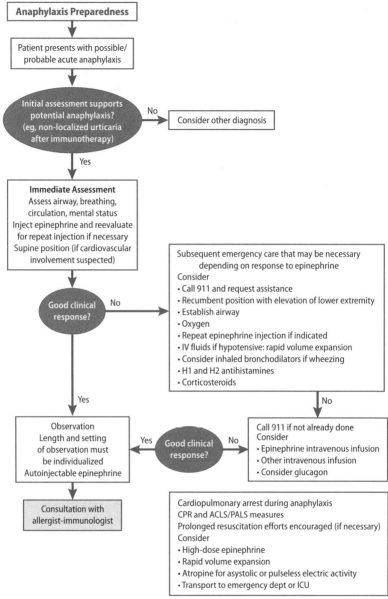

Figure 49-1. Algorithm for treatment of an anaphylactic event in the outpatient setting.

Abbreviations: ACLS, advanced cardiovascular life support; CPR, cardiopulmonary resuscitation; dept, department; ICU, intensive care unit; IV, intravenous; PALS, pediatric advance life support.

Adapted from Lieberman P, Nicklas R, Oppenheimer J, et al. The diagnosis and management of anaphylaxis practice parameter: 2010 update. *J Allergy Clin Immunol.* 2010;126(3):477–480, with permission.

of personal and parental anxiety. Identification of the allergen trigger followed by education on avoidance is part of management. Subsequent care involves educating the patient and family about self-management of anaphylaxis.

For venom-induced anaphylaxis, venom immunotherapy is successful in preventing subsequent episodes in up to 98% of patients. Pharmacologic prophylaxis (eg, antihistamines, corticosteroids) may be indicated in certain situations (anaphylaxis to radiocontrast materials and fluorescein or to prevent recurrent episodes in idiopathic cases). For patients with a history of anaphylaxis to a medication, desensitization to that drug may be indicated if ongoing use of the medication is required. For each subsequent course of that medication, the desensitization procedure must be repeated.

The most important part of subsequent management is educating the patient about effective prevention strategies. The patient should be able to identify high-risk situations, potential "hidden ingredients" in foods, crossreactivity of various drugs and foods, and how to administer epinephrine. A written "Anaphylaxis Action Plan" should be provided at discharge.

Urticaria and Angioedema

Acute Urticaria

Acute urticaria is defined as urticaria lasting fewer than 6 weeks. Upper respiratory tract infections and IgE-mediated allergic reactions make up most causes of acute urticaria (Table 49-2). Infections are thought to be most common cause of acute urticaria in children and symptoms resolve within 6 weeks. Acute urticaria can occur as part of a spectrum of symptoms in anaphylaxis and a careful history and physical examination should guide further studies and treatment. Antihistamines are the mainstay of treatment in children with acute urticaria. International guidelines encourage the use of second-generation non-sedating antihistamine, which have a more favorable side effect profile over first generation antihistamines (Evidence Level 1).

Chronic Urticaria

Unlike acute urticaria, chronic urticaria or chronic spontaneous urticaria is typically not due to IgE-mediated allergic reactions or infections. Chronic urticaria is defined as urticaria lasting more than 6 weeks. Although frequently reported by families, food allergy is rarely the etiology, occurring in less than 3% of children with chronic urticaria. Common causes of chronic urticaria are summarized in Box 36-3. Physical urticaria is a common cause of chronic urticaria in children, and history is often suggestive. Cryopyrin-associated periodic syndromes are a rare group of autoinflammatory diseases due to mutations in the gene *CIAS-1* that encodes cryopyrin. In these syndromes, urticaria often presents in the first several weeks of life.

Table 49-2. Common Causes of Acute and Chronic Urticaria

Acute	Chronic
Infections	Idiopathic
IgE-mediated allergic reaction (eg, food, drug, venom, aeroallergen contact, latex)	Physical urticaria (eg, solar, cold, delayed pressure, localized heat, dermatographic, vibratory, aquagenic)
Transfusion reactions/adverse drug reaction	Autoimmune urticaria
	Autoimmune/connective tissue disorder
	Chronic infection
	IgE mediated
	Cryopyrin-associated periodic syndromes (ie, familial cold autoinflammatory syndrome, Muckle-Wells syndrome, neonatal-onset multisystem inflammatory disorder)

Chronic autoimmune urticaria may represent up to 47% of children with chronic urticaria. The prognosis is generally good with remission in greater than 50% within 5 years. A thoughtful history and physical examination are the most important diagnostic tools, and these should guide laboratory testing. For patients unresponsive to antihistamines or with more severe disease, screening laboratory studies are warranted. These include complete blood count with differential, erythrocyte sedimentation rate, C-reactive protein level, thyroid function studies, thyroid autoantibody levels, and urinalysis. When history is not suggestive of a trigger or underlying etiology, laboratory studies are rarely helpful and additional studies should be guided by history and physical examination.

Treatment of chronic urticaria should aim to control symptoms and minimize oral corticosteroid use. Daily nonsedating antihistamines are used as first-line treatment. Antihistamine agents and typical doses are listed in Table 49-3 (Evidence Level I). International guidelines suggest titration of antihistamines up to 4 times the recommended dose followed by addition of a leukotriene antagonist prior to considering alternative therapies (Evidence Level III, for children). Several alternative therapies for chronic urticaria resistant to antihistamines and leukotriene antagonists have been suggested, but data in the pediatric population are limited. The use of cyclosporine has been reported to be efficacious in children (Evidence Level III, in children). Omalizumab is a promising therapy for chronic urticaria and is currently being studied.

Table 49-3. Common Pharmacologic Agents and Doses for Children With Acute and Chronic Urticaria

Agent	Typical Doses	Typical Doses
Antihistamine: First Generation		
Brompheniramine	2–5 y: 6 mg every 12 h 6–12 y: 12 mg every 12 h >12 y: 12–24 mg every 12 h	…
Chlorpheniramine	2–5 y: 2.5 mg every 4–6 h 6–12 y: 5 mg every 4–6 h >12 y: 10 mg every 4–6 h	0.1 mg/kg/dose every 4–6 h Max: 10 mg/kg/dose
Diphenhydramine	6–12 y: 25 mg every 4–6 h >12 y: 25–50 mg every 4–6 h	1.0 mg/kg/dose every 4–6 h Max: 50 mg/kg/dose
Hydroxyzine	6–12 y: 12.5–25 mg every 6–8 h >12 y: 25–100 mg every 6–8 h	0.5 mg/kg/dose Max: 50 mg/kg/dose
Antihistamine: Second Generation		
Cetirizine	<6 y: 2.5 mg every d >6 y: 5–10 mg every d	0.1 mg/kg/dose Max: 10 mg
Fexofenadine	6–12 y: 30 mg twice a d >12 y: 60 mg twice a d or 180 mg every d	1–3 mg/kg/dose Max: 180 mg
Loratadine	<6 y: 5 mg every d >6 y: 10 mg every d	0.1 mg/kg/dose Max: 10 mg
Levocetirizine	2–5 y: 1.25 mg every d 6–12 y: 2.5 mg every d >12 y and older: 5 mg every d	0.125 mg/kg/dose every d Max: 5 mg
Leukotriene Receptor Antagonists		
Montelukast	2–5 y: 4 mg every d 6–12 y: 5 mg every d >12 y: 10 mg every d	…
Zafirlukast	6–12 y: 10 mg every 12 h >12 y: 20 mg every 12 h	…
Glucocorticoids		
Prednisone	5–60 mg every 12–24 h (short course: 5–7 d)	0.5–1 mg/kg/dose Max: 60 mg

Abbreviations: d, day; h, hour; max, maximum; y, year.

Angioedema Without Urticaria

Urticaria and angioedema can occur together as part of a continuum in allergic and non-allergic conditions that lead to mast cell degranulation. At times, angioedema mediated by mast cell degranulation can occur without urticaria, such as in chronic autoimmune urticaria, adverse drug reaction, physical urticaria, exercised-induced anaphylaxis, and idiopathic angioedema. However, recurrent angioedema without urticaria deserves special attention.

Angioedema can occur in the absence of mast cell degranulation and histamine. Bradykinin, a product of the hematologic contact pathway, can induce severe angioedema in susceptible patients. Hereditary angioedema (HAE) is an autosomal dominant disease involving a defect in C1 inhibitor protein, which regulates contact system–mediated bradykinin. This results in increased bradykinin levels and periodic angioedema, often lasting 2 to 5 days. Symptoms often present during puberty and may include severe angioedema of the face, extremities, genitalia, larynx, and gastrointestinal tract (ie, recurrent unexplained abdominal pain). The swelling occurs without itching or urticaria, and laryngeal involvement can be fatal if untreated. The best screening test is a C4 level, which is low both during and in between swelling attacks. Testing to confirm the diagnosis in children includes C1 inhibitor protein level and function, which should be interpreted by a physician experienced in treating HAE. The US Food and Drug Administration–approved drugs for treatment of acute attacks of HAE are summarized in Table 49-4 (Evidence Level 1). It is important to recognize that antihistamines, corticosteroids, and epinephrine will not be effective in angioedema due to HAE. It is also important to note that 25% of patients have no family history of angioedema. Other examples of bradykinin-induced swelling include angiotensin-converting enzyme inhibitor-induced angioedema, which occurs in children.

Table 49-4. US FDA-Approved Treatment for Acute Attacks of Hereditary Angioedema

Therapies for Acute Attacks	Drug Class	Age Indicated (y)
Plasma-derived C1 inhibitor	C1 inhibitor	>12
Ecallantide	Kallikrein inhibitor	>16
Icatibant	Bradykinin β_2-adrenergic receptor	>18

Abbreviation: FDA, Food and Drug Administration.

Selected Reading

Gupta RS, Springston EE, Warrier MR, et al. The prevalence, severity, and distribution of childhood food allergy in the United States. *Pediatrics*. 2011;128(1):e9–e17

Hom KA, Hirch R, Ellura RG. Antihypertensive drug-induced angioedema causing upper airway obstruction in children. *Int J Pediatr Otorhinolaryngol*. 2012;76(1):14–19

Kaplan AP. Angioedema. *World Allergy Organ J.* 2008;1(6):103–113

Lieberman P, Nicklas RA, Oppenheimer J et al. The diagnosis and management of anaphylaxis practice parameter: 2010 Update. *J Allergy Clin Immunol.* 2010;126(3): 477–480

Marrouche N, Grattan C. Childhood urticaria. *Curr Opin Allergy Clin Immunol.* 2012;12(5):485–490

Mehr S, Liew WK, Tey D, Tang ML. Clinical predictors for biphasic reactions in young children presenting with anaphylaxis. *Clin Exp Allergy.* 2009;39(9):1390–1396

Ojeda IC, Cruz E, León R, et al. Chronic autoimmune urticaria in children. *Allergo et Immunopathol (Madr).* 2009;37(1):43–47

Sahiner UM, Civelek E, Tuncer A, et al. Chronic urticaria: etiology and natural course in children. *Int Arch Immunol.* 2011;156(2):224–230

Zitelli KB, Cordoro KM. Evidence-based evaluation and management of chronic urticaria in children. *Pediatr Dermatol.* 2011;28(6):629–639

Zuberbier T, Asero R, Bindslev-Jensen G, et al. EAACI/GA(2)LEN/EDF/WAO guideline: definition, classification and diagnosis of urticaria. *Allergy.* 2009;64(10): 1417–1426

CHAPTER 50

Animal Bites

Mary Jo Bowman, MD

Key Points

- Animal bites are a common pediatric injury with dogs and cats, accounting for most mammalian bites in the United States.

- Radiographs are important to consider for all types of animal bites; fractures may be detected, while foreign bodies and joint disruption may also be apparent and otherwise not diagnosed early without the radiographs.

- Types of injuries from mammalian bites typically differ by species. Dog bites tend to cause crush injuries, cat bites tend to cause puncture wounds and lacerations, and human bites tend to cause simple occlusion wounds.

- Types of pathogens from mammalian bites typically differ by species. Dog bites tend to involve *Pasteurella* species (*P canis*), staphylococci, streptococci, and anaerobes; cat bites may also introduce *Bartonella henselae* and *P multocida*; and human bites tend to involve healthy human mouth and skin flora (particularly *Eikenella corrodens*).

- Treatment for all bites consists of cleaning, debridement, and exploration when necessary.

- Amoxicillin-clavulanate is the most commonly recommended antibiotic for prevention and treatment of infection after animal bites. Most can be managed in an outpatient setting.

Overview

Animal bites are a common injury seen in the pediatric population. True incidence is unknown, as many bites are minor, not reported, or both. Dogs and cats account for most mammalian bites in this country (for snakebites, see Chapter 70). It has been estimated that about 5 million dog bites occur per year, with 800,000 requiring medical attention, comprising about 1% of emergency department visits. Dog bites usually cause a crushing-type wound because of the large amount of pounds per square inch (or psi) of pressure exerted. This may damage deeper structures such as bones, vessels, tendons, muscles, and nerves. The sharp pointed teeth of cats usually cause puncture wounds and lacerations, often inoculating bacteria deep into the tissue. Human bites may be simple occlusion wounds or more serious, as in the closed-fist injury.

Evaluation

· · · · · · · · · ·

Clinical

A number of important historical elements should be obtained when evaluating the child with an animal bite (Box 50-1).

Box 50-1. Important History to Obtain for a Child With an Animal Bite

- Type of animal
- Immunization status of animal
- General behavior of animal
- Circumstances surrounding bite
- Time of injury
- Location of animal now
- Sequence of events
- Prehospital care
- Patient immunization status
- Patient allergies

Additional concerns for human bites are transmission of human immuno-deficiency virus (HIV), hepatitis, and syphilis. Questions should focus on HIV risk factors of the perpetrator and any known diagnoses such as hepatitis B or C.

Major resuscitation is rarely indicated, but it is important to remember that infants, in particular, are at increased risk of severe injuries from bites. All children who experience an animal attack should be evaluated from head to toe to identify both penetrating and blunt trauma.

The physical examination is the most important aspect of the initial evaluation of bite wounds. Wounds should be assessed for location, depth, amount of devitalized tissue, and presence of foreign material. Assessment of neurovascular function as well as tendon and joint function are also needed, especially for wounds to hands and feet.

Diagnostic Tests

Few diagnostic tests will affect initial management of bite wounds, although checking the hemoglobin and hematocrit in the case of excessive blood loss is prudent. The white blood cell count is rarely helpful, even in the presence of infection. Erythrocyte sedimentation rate and C-reactive protein level are usually elevated in most clinically apparent infections. Cultures of grossly infected wounds may be useful in guiding antibiotic therapy. Some pathogens are slow growing, so cultures need to be held for 7 to 10 days. Obtaining wound cultures acutely has not been shown to be useful.

Radiographs play an important role in all types of animal bites. The force from a dog bite is sufficient to fracture a bone. Bites over joints may show air suggesting penetration of the joint space. Radiographs may also be useful if a foreign body is suspected. Up to 70% of radiographs taken to evaluate closed-fist injuries show foreign bodies, fractures or bony fragments, narrowing of the joint space, and air.

Other modalities, such as angiography and ultrasound, may be used to help in the evaluation of certain injuries. Head computed tomography may be needed if an infant has been bitten on the scalp, as the skull could be punctured.

Microbiology

The predominant pathogens in animal bite wounds are the oral flora of the biting animal and human skin flora. Most infections usually result from a mixture of organisms, with common pathogens including *P asteurella* species (*P canis* for dog and *P multocida* for cats), staphylococci, streptococci, and anaerobes. *Capnocytophaga canimorsus* can cause bacteremia and sepsis after animal bites, generally in immunocompromised hosts. Cat bites and scratches can transmit *Bartonella henselae*, the organism responsible for cat-scratch disease.

Pathogens found in human bite wound infections reflect healthy human mouth and skin flora. *Eikenella corrodens* is a common pathogen as well as viridians streptococci and staphylococci. Viruses such as hepatitis B, hepatitis C, and HIV can also be transmitted via human bites.

Management

Goals of wound management include optimal cosmesis, maintenance of function, and prevention of secondary infection. The surface of the wound should initially be cleansed with povidone-iodine, a skin wound cleanser, or other soap product to remove gross debris and bacteria. Copious irrigation with physiologic saline solution is recommended and helps reduce the risk of infection. Pressure irrigation can be accomplished using a 19-gauge needle and syringe, using at least 100 to 200 mL of saline or more, in heavily contaminated wounds. The wound should be anesthetized and explored (Evidence Level III).

Debridement is recommended to remove any devitalized tissue or clots that could act as a nidus of infection. Clean wound edges result in smaller scars and promote faster healing. One study showed debridement of dog bite wounds resulted in a 30-fold reduction in the rate of infection (Evidence Level III).

Primary closure of bite wounds varies with the location and type of bite. In general, low-risk wounds may be primarily closed. High-risk wounds (Box 50-2) should be left open or undergo delayed closure in about 72 hours.

Box 50-2. High-Risk Wounds

- Bites to hands and feet
- Human and cat bites to areas other than the face
- Bites in immunocompromised patients
- Crush injuries
- Puncture wounds
- Wounds older than 12 hours

Wounds of the face are usually closed primarily because good cosmesis is important and infection is less common, likely due to the good blood supply to the face and scalp. In general, subcutaneous sutures should be used sparingly. Sealing the wound with tissue adhesive should be avoided. Injured extremities should be properly immobilized.

Antibiotics

Once wound care is complete, a decision should be made regarding the use of empiric antibiotics for prevention of wound infection. Dog bites have the lowest rate of infection, and antibiotics are not warranted for most bites. Cat and human bites have higher rates of infection, and most should receive antibiotics. Indications for prophylactic antibiotics are listed in Box 50-3 (Evidence Level II-2 and III).

Box 50-3. Indications for Antibiotics

- Puncture wounds
- Wounds with associated crush injury
- Hand and foot wounds
- Cat and human bites
- Bites in immunocompromised hosts

Amoxicillin-clavulanate is the most commonly recommended antibiotic for prevention and treatment of infection after animal bites. This has excellent coverage against all common bite wound pathogens. The recommended dosage is 45 mg/kg/day divided into 2 doses. For patients allergic to penicillin, cephalosporins, or both, clindamycin plus trimethoprim-sulfamethoxazole are good alternatives in combination (other combinations are listed in Table 50-1).

Table 50-1. Recommended Antibiotics

Amoxicillin-clavulanate **OR** One of the following:	45 mg/kg/d (amoxicillin component) divided in 2 doses (max: 875 mg amoxicillin and 125 mg clavulanic acid per dose)
Trimethoprim-sulfamethoxazole	8–10 mg/kg/d (trimethoprim component) divided in 2 doses (max: 160 mg trimethoprim per dose)
Cefuroxime	20 mg/kg/d divided in 2 doses (max: 500 mg per dose)
Penicillin VK	50 mg/kg/d divided in 4 doses (max: 500 mg per dose)
Doxycycline **PLUS**	100 mg twice daily (not for use in children <8 y)
Clindamycin	30 mg/kg/d divided in 3 doses (max: 450 mg per dose)
Metronidazole	30 mg/kg/d divided in 3 doses (max: 500 mg per dose)

Abbreviations: d, day; max, maximum; y, year.

Adapted from Endom EE. Initial management of animal and human bites. In: Danzl DS, ed. *UpToDate*. Waltham, MA; 2011.

Antibiotics that are not recommended include cephalexin, dicloxacillin, and erythromycin, as these lack coverage against *P multocida* and *E corrodens*.

Tetanus Prophylaxis

Bite wounds are considered high risk for the transmission of *Clostridium tetani*, found in the teeth and saliva of many animals. The patient's tetanus immunization status should be determined for any bite that breaks the skin. If the wound is relatively minor with little devitalized or crushed tissue, tetanus immunization within the past 10 years is adequate. If the wound is heavily contaminated or involves crushed tissue or punctures, tetanus immunization should be given if it has been more than 5 years since the last dose. If immunization status is incomplete or unknown, both tetanus immune globulin and tetanus toxoid booster should be given (Evidence Level III).

Rabies Prophylaxis

Most reported rabies cases result from injuries caused by wild animals. Raccoons, skunks, bats, and foxes are the main sources of human rabies infection currently in the United States. Domesticated animals rarely transmit rabies. However, the Centers for Disease Control and Prevention recommends rabies post-exposure treatment in the setting of a suspicious bite, especially from a dog. Local health departments and animal control may be other good sources of information on rabies risk (Evidence Level III).

Long-term Monitoring

Most bite wounds can be treated in an outpatient setting. Close follow-up is recommended, and all wounds should be reevaluated within 24 to 48 hours. Indications for admission are included in Box 50-4.

Box 50-4. Indications for Admission of Bite Wounds

- Multisystem trauma
- Evidence of systemic infection
- Failure of outpatient therapy
- Infected human bite wound of the hand
- Immunocompromised patient
- Involvement of joints, tendons, or both

Suggested Reading

Bradford JE, Freer L. Bites and injuries inflicted by wild and domestic animals. In: Auerbach PS, ed. *Wilderness Medicine.* 6th ed. Philadelphia, PA: Mosby Elsevier; 2012:1102–1127

Fleisher GR. The management of bite wounds. *N Engl J Med.* 1999;340(2):138–140

Rempe B, Aloi M, Iskyan K. Evidence-based management of mammalian bite wounds. *Ped Emerg Med Practice.* 2009;6(9):1–20

Schalamon J, Ainoedhofer H, Singer G, et al. Analysis of dog bites in children who are younger than 17 years. *Pediatrics.* 2006;117(3):e374–e379

Stefanopoulos PK. Management of facial bite wounds. *Oral Max Surg Clin North Am.* 2009;21(2):247–257

Talan DA, Citron DM, Abrahamian FM, Moran GJ, Goldstein EJ. Bacteriologic analysis of infected dog and cat bites. *N Engl J Med.* 1999;340(2):85–92

CHAPTER 51

Burns and Thermal Injury

Laurie H. Johnson, MD

Key Points

- Most burn-related injuries in children are from heat sources and include scalds, sunburns, contact with hot objects, and flame or flash burns. Less common injuries include inhalation of smoke or vapors, as well as exposures to chemicals, cold temperatures, and electricity.

- The extent of the burn injury depends on the causative mechanism or agent, duration of exposure, size and location of the injury, and age and baseline medical condition of the patient.

- Cutaneous burns are classically described as first-, second-, third-, and fourth-degree and are characterized by the depth of the injured tissue. The estimation of the extent of a burn wound is based on total body surface area affected by partial- and full-thickness injuries.

- Inhalation injuries can be insidious initially and should be suspected in any fire exposure in a closed environment or in which the patient experienced a loss of consciousness.

Overview

Children have daily exposures to potential sources for burn-related injuries. Most burn-related injuries are from heat sources and include scalds, sunburns, contact with hot objects, and flame or flash burns. Less common injuries include inhalation of smoke or vapors, as well as exposures to chemicals, cold temperatures, and electricity. The extent of the burn injury depends on the causative mechanism or agent, duration of exposure, size and location of the injury, and age and baseline medical condition of the patient. Cutaneous wounds caused are classified according to the depth of injury to the skin and underlying tissues. Inhalation injuries can be insidious initially and should be suspected in any fire exposure in a closed environment or in which the patient experienced a loss of consciousness. Burn injuries can range from isolated skin findings, which are mild and require minimal treatment, to severe burns with associated sequelae, which require immediate fluid resuscitation, airway control, and operative intervention.

A detailed history and physical examination are necessary to determine if a patient can be managed closely as an outpatient or if he requires immediate referral to a burn center (Box 51-1). The most common injuries are mild and can therefore be effectively managed on an outpatient basis. Outpatient management of minor burn wounds focuses on meticulous wound care, infection prevention, pain control, maintenance of range of motion, and close follow-up. Specific referral criteria exist based on the percentage of the total body surface area affected by partial- and full-thickness burns and the type of injury.

Box 51-1. Historical Questions for Patients With Burn Exposure

General

How did the burn occur?

Are reported circumstances of the injury consistent with the characteristics of the wounds?

Flame Burns

Was the fire indoors or outdoors?

Was the patient found in a smoke-filled room?

How did the patient escape?

What injuries were sustained by others at the scene?

Did the clothes ignite? If so, how were they extinguished, and how long did it take?

Was gasoline or another fuel involved?

Was there an explosion?

Did the patient experience loss of consciousness at the scene?

If the circumstance of injury was a motor vehicle crash, what were details of the crash? (Include extrication time, damage to car, and mechanism of injury.)

Is a concomitant chemical burn evident?

Scalds

What were the type and volume of liquid?

What was the temperature of the liquid?

In what room or location did the burn occur?

What was the patient wearing at the time?

How quickly were the patient's clothes removed?

Was the burn cooled? If so, with what substance and for what duration?

Chemical Injuries

What was the agent?

Under what circumstances did the exposure occur (including possible ingestion or ocular exposure)?

What was the duration of contact?

What anatomic areas are involved?

Did any decontamination occur at the scene or en route?

Is a Material Safety Data Sheet available?

Is illegal activity evident?

Electrical Injuries

What kind of electricity was involved (eg, high or low voltage, AC or DC)?

What was the duration of contact?

Did the patient fall, or was the patient thrown?

Did the patient experience loss of consciousness?

What treatments were initiated at the scene?

Causes

Younger children most commonly suffer from scalds and contact with hot surfaces. Scalds occur because of splashes or spills from hot liquids or foods or because of contact with hot faucet water. Thermal injuries can also be sustained by touching hot surfaces, such as stove burners, ovens, room heaters, fireplace screens, irons, and other hot household items. Older children and adolescents often sustain injuries from exposure to sunlight, with less frequent but more serious injuries due to unsupervised use of gasoline, fireworks, and matches. Inhalation injury may be due to direct thermal injury to the upper airways or face, injury to the lower airways from noxious gases, or carbon monoxide or cyanide exposure. Any examination findings, history, or suspicion of flame exposure, especially in a patient who lost consciousness or was in an enclosed area, should alert the physician to the possibility of inhalation injury. Chemical burns result from contact with a caustic substance; in general, alkali burns cause more injury than acidic burns because of the liquefaction necrosis that occurs. Cold-induced injuries occur after failure of expected protective mechanisms against the thermal environment. Electrical injuries are described in detail in Chapter 57.

Physical and physiologic considerations must be taken into account when treating burn injuries in the pediatric patient. As with any injury in a child, the physician must maintain a high degree of suspicion for the possibility of intentional trauma or neglect. Children 6 years and younger have thinner skin than older children and adults, resulting in more extensive burns from a given mechanism (Table 51-1). Because of their large surface area to body mass ratio, children are more prone to hypothermia and increased fluid losses than adolescents or young adults. Pediatric body proportions vary with age, which can make accurate estimation of affected total body surface area (TBSA) a challenge to assess. This variation in body size also dictates that fluid resuscitation in pediatric burn victims must be based on body surface area calculated from height and weight, in order to avoid the complications of pulmonary edema, cerebral edema, and compartment syndrome associated with excessive fluid administration during resuscitation. Finally, the smaller airway of pediatric patients with inhalation exposure results in an increased risk of airway edema and obstruction. These considerations make early referral to a burn center for those with moderate to severe injuries even more critical.

Evaluation

Initial assessment of the patient with burn injury follows the systematic evaluation of any patient who has experienced a traumatic injury: the physician must first ensure that airway, breathing, and circulation are intact and that life-threatening conditions are definitively addressed. Once it has been determined that the airway is secure, the patient is oxygenating and ventilating

Table 51-1. Relationship of Hot Water Temperature and Burn Injury in Children

Water Temperature	Time for Third-degree Burn to Occur
120°F (48°C)	5 min
124°F (51°C)	3 min
127°F (52°C)	1 min
133°F (56°C)	15 s
140°F (60°C)	5 s
148°F (64°C)	2 s
155°F (68°C)	1 s

Abbreviations: min, minute; s, second.

appropriately, and adequate circulation with control of bleeding has been established, it is appropriate to proceed with identification and treatment of the burn wounds.

Burns to the skin are classically described as first-, second-, third-, and fourth-degree and are further characterized by the depth of the injured tissue. Superficial burns with involvement of only the epidermis are referred to as first-degree burns. These burns are red and painful with no blistering present and heal quickly within 2 to 3 days with no scarring (Figure 51-1). Second-degree burns extend into the dermal layer and are also known as partial-thickness burns. They are further categorized into superficial and deep partial–thickness burns. With superficial partial–thickness burns, the epidermis and less than half of the dermis are affected, while deep partial–thickness burns penetrate most of the dermis. Superficial second-degree burns are red and very painful, with blistering present, blanch easily, and may appear wet or weeping (Figure 51-2). These burns heal completely within 2 to 3 weeks without the need for surgical intervention, usually with no hypertrophic scarring or pigment changes. Deep second-degree burns have a mottled or waxy whitish appearance due to dermal blood vessel injury, and they may or may not blanch. These burns typically take longer than 2 to 3 weeks to heal and often require surgical intervention. Air currents moving over second-degree burns can cause extreme discomfort, so wounds should be kept covered with a clean dry sheet until definitive wound care is performed. Third-degree burns are full-thickness burns affecting the entire dermis and are painless because of destruction of dermal nerves. They are characterized by a dry, non-blanching appearance; may be leathery, translucent, mottled, or waxy; and are dark, black, or white in coloration (Figure 51-2). Fourth-degree burns are full-thickness burns that additionally include involvement of the underlying subcutaneous fat, fascia, muscle, and bone. Third- and fourth-degree burns often develop burn scar contractures despite surgical intervention with excision and grafting.

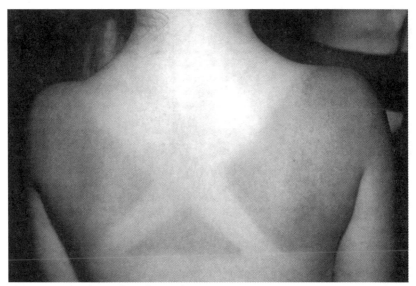

Figure 51-1. Sunburn (first-degree burn).
Courtesy of Richard J. Kagan, MD (Shriners Hospital for Children, Cincinnati, OH).

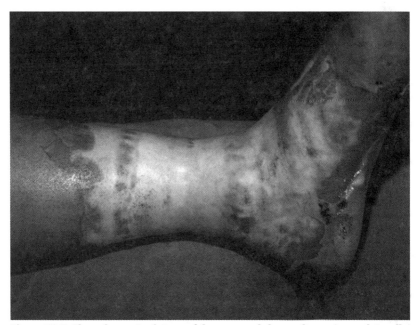

Figure 51-2. Flame burn. A mixture of deep second-degree burns (areas laterally) and third-degree burn (central region).
Courtesy of Richard J. Kagan, MD (Shriners Hospital for Children, Cincinnati, OH).

Table 51-2. Lund Browder Chart for Burn Wound Documentation

Area	Birth–1 year	1–4 years	5–9 years	10–14 years	15 years	Adult	2nd degree	3rd degree	% TBSA
Head	19	17	13	11	9	7			
Neck	2	2	2	2	2	2			
Anterior trunk	13	13	13	13	13	13			
Posterior trunk	13	13	13	13	13	13			
Right buttock	2.5	2.5	12.5	2.5	2.5	2.5			
Left buttock	2.5	2.5	2.5	2.5	2.5	2.5			
Genitalia	1	1	1	1	1	1			
Right upper arm	4	4	4	4	4	4			
Left upper arm	4	4	4	4	4	4			
Right lower arm	3	3	3	3	3	3			
Left lower arm	3	3	3	3	3	3			
Right hand	2.5	2.4	2.5	2.5	2.5	2.5			
Left hand	2.5	2.4	2.5	2.5	2.5	2.5			
Right thigh	5.5	6.5	8	8.5	9	9.5			
Left thigh	5.5	6.5	8	8.5	9	9.5			
Right lower leg	5	5	5.5	6	6.5	7			
Left lower leg	5	5	5.5	6	6.5	7			
Right foot	3.5	3.5	3.5	3.5	3.5	3.5			
Left foot	3.5	3.5	3.5	3.5	3.5	3.5			
						Totals			

Abbreviation: TBSA, total body surface area.

The estimation of the extent of a burn wound is based on the TBSA affected by partial- and full-thickness injuries. This may be challenging to assess during the initial presentation because of the dynamic nature of the wound during the immediate post-injury period. The burn wound evolves over the first 3 to 5 days and is comprised of 3 zones: zone of coagulation (the most deeply affected tissue), zone of stasis (initially uninjured tissue which may experience microvascular thrombosis and ischemia), and zone of hyperemia (which has compensatory increased blood flow and may be confused with cellulitis). The quickest but least precise method for categorizing the TBSA of the burn wound is commonly known as the Rule of Nines, which divides the regions of the body into multiples of 9% TBSA (Figure 51-3). The TBSA for large wounds is best calculated using a chart with designated proportions for body areas based on the patient's age group (Table 51-2). Smaller wounds can be estimated using the entire palmar surface of the hand as 1% of the TBSA.

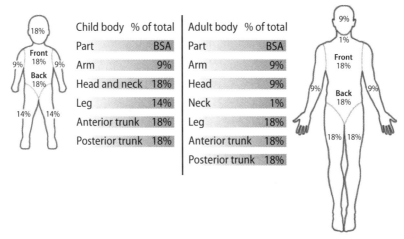

Figure 51-3. Rule of Nines diagrams.

Management

Treatment of a patient with burn injury first requires that airway, breathing, and circulation are intact and that all life-threatening injuries are immediately addressed. Patients with direct airway burns, possible inhalation injury, or exposure to cyanide or carbon monoxide should be placed on 100% oxygen via face mask; and careful airway protection maintained. Examination findings suspicious for inhalation or airway injury include singed eyebrows or nasal hairs, carbonaceous sputum, signs of respiratory compromise (eg, hoarseness, dyspnea, stridor), altered mental status, and facial or neck burns.

Burn-specific treatment should begin once the patient has been stabilized. Initiation of burn-specific care involves stopping the burning process and removal of affected clothing. Tepid sterile water or physiologic saline solution may be used to irrigate and soothe less extensive burns, but hypothermia should be avoided. Pain control for mild burns can often be managed with acetaminophen or ibuprofen. Narcotics are usually required for adequate analgesia for partial- and full-thickness burns. The patient's tetanus immunization status must be documented, and updated if necessary, in accordance with standard tetanus guidelines.

Emergent referral to a regional burn center should be made for patients with partial- or full-thickness burns to specific body regions (eg, face, hands, feet, joints, genitalia, perineum) or those greater than 10% of the TBSA. Referral should also occur if the patient experienced inhalation, chemical, or electrical injury or if the patient would benefit from the specialized treatment team available at such a center (Box 51-2). Extensive wounds (ie, superficial or deep partial–thickness burns greater than 10% of the TBSA and any full thickness) should not be debrided prior to transfer but should be treated conservatively until definitive treatment can be performed. Initial treatment of these wounds consists of removing all clothing and jewelry in anticipation of local and systemic edema and covering the wounds with a clean dry sheet. Clothing which has become adhered to the skin should be left in place until definitive treatment at a burn referral center to avoid further tissue damage. The decision to initiate intravenous fluids (unless immediately necessary because of hemodynamic instability) should be made in conjunction with the regional burn center, as fluid resuscitation must be calculated based on the patient's body surface area and carefully titrated to avoid under- or over-resuscitation.

Box 51-2. Burn Center Referral Criteria

- Partial-thickness burns of 10% or more total body surface area
- Burns with involvement of the face, hands, feet, major joints, genitalia, perineum
- Third-degree burns in any age group
- Electric burns, including lightning injury
- Chemical burns
- Inhalation injury
- A burn injury in a patient with preexisting medical conditions that could complicate management, prolong recovery, or affect mortality
- A patient with concomitant trauma where the burn injury poses the greatest risk of morbidity or mortality
- A burn injury in a pediatric patient admitted to a hospital without qualified personnel or equipment for pediatric care
- A burn injury in a patient with special social, emotional, or long-term rehabilitative support or a combination thereof

Adapted from American Burn Association. *Advanced Burn Life Support Provider Manual.* Chicago, IL: American Burn Association; 2011:25–27. Copyright © American Burn Association. Used with permission.

Most first-degree and smaller superficial second-degree burns can be managed on an outpatient basis. These wounds should be cleansed with room temperature sterile water or physiologic saline solution and a mild soap. First-degree wounds are managed with topical moisturizer therapy and rarely require hospitalization unless the burn involves a significant amount of body surface area in a very young child. Burns initially treated as first-degree burns that develop blisters should be reexamined and treated accordingly as superficial second-degree burns. Controversy exists on whether blisters should be left intact, aspirated, or debrided. As a general rule, blisters of less than 1 cm in diameter can be left intact. Blisters which are larger, non-intact, or occur over areas where range of motion would be limited should be debrided (Figure 51-4). Although initial treatment of deep partial–thickness burns is similar to that of superficial second-degree wounds, they heal similarly to third-degree burns and would benefit from treatment by a burn surgeon. Most deep second-degree and all full-thickness burns require surgical intervention, with excision and primary closure or excision with full- or split-thickness grafting. Early surgical treatment is associated with improved cosmesis and functional outcome.

The goal of burn wound care is to promote wound healing and prevent infection while minimizing patient discomfort. A variety of dressing materials

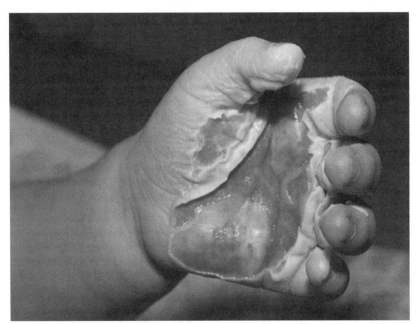

Figure 51-4. Contact burn after debridement (superficial second-degree burn from a curling iron).
Courtesy of Richard J. Kagan, MD (Shriners Hospital for Children, Cincinnati, OH).

are commercially available, including traditional gauze, films, foams, composites, sprays, gels, biological skin replacements, and bioengineered skin substitutes. The newer biosynthetic materials are associated with improved healing time and pain reduction during dressing changes, but they are more expensive than traditional non-adherent dressing pads (Evidence Level I). Topical antimicrobial agents are applied after irrigation and debridement to prevent desiccation and to slow bacterial growth. A commonly used topical agent with few to no side effects is an antibiotic ointment such as bacitracin, and it should be applied to nonstick porous gauze, which is covered with dry occlusive sterile gauze; evidence for effectiveness with this approach is limited (Evidence Level I). Topical agents such as silver sulfadiazine and mafenide are typically used in deep second-degree burns and in third-degree burns; outpatient treatment of such burns is usually best reserved for a specialist with burn wound experience. Regular twice daily wound cleansing and dressing changes with reevaluation of the burn wound every 1 to 2 days is of the utmost importance in outpatient management. Dressing changes may be discontinued once the wound has epithelialized. Patients who are not maintaining adequate hydration or who are unable to adhere to the wound care regimen may require hospitalization. Prophylaxis with systemic antibiotics is not recommended because of the potential for bacterial resistance; systemic antibiotics should be reserved for those with wound infection. Wounds that evolve to be more extensive or deeper than originally estimated may need referral to a burn center or surgeon with experience in burn care. Referrals should also be made for burn wounds that have not completely healed within 2 to 3 weeks.

Treatment of chemical burns is similar to that of thermal burns. With a cutaneous chemical exposure, care should be taken to avoid further tissue injury during the decontamination process, as well as to protect the health care professionals from injury. Dry powders should be brushed away, and copious irrigation with sterile water or physiologic saline solution should be initiated for at least 30 minutes; monitoring the pH of the effluent may be useful in determining duration of lavage. Neutralization agents are not recommended, as they may cause further tissue damage. Principles of wound care for chemical burns are similar for thermal burns, with early excision and grafting advocated for all nonviable tissue.

Cold-induced injuries of frostnip and frostbite are also managed similarly to thermal burns and most commonly affect the fingers, toes, ears, nose, and cheeks. The term *frostnip* is used for cutaneous areas that experience numbness and pallor after exposure to cold temperatures but which do not experience freezing of the dermis or underlying tissues. Frostnip resolves nearly completely with rewarming, with occasional hyperemia, swelling, or tingling to the affected region. In contrast, frostbite involves the freezing and subsequent destruction of the affected dermal and soft tissue. The frostbitten area seems numb initially but progresses to severe pain upon rewarming. Treatment for both conditions is passive rewarming in warm water (40–42°C [104–108°F]) for approximately 30 minutes. Rubbing or massaging the affected areas can cause further tissue damage and should be avoided (Evidence Level II-1 and Evidence Level II-2). Jewelry should be removed, and affected areas should be protected to avoid further injury due to lack of sensation. Cold-induced wounds are classified much like thermal burns, ranging from first degree to fourth degree, with first degree being the most superficial. The vesicles and blisters associated with second- and third-degree wounds form within 1 to 2 days of injury; those of third-degree wounds are often hemorrhagic, which evolve into a thick dark eschar within 1 to 2 weeks. While second-degree wounds typically have a favorable outcome with traditional burn wound management, third- and fourth- degree cold-induced wounds require the expertise of a burn surgeon.

Long-term Monitoring/Implications

Most burn wounds that heal within 2 to 3 weeks have no functional impairment, hypertrophic scarring, or hypopigmentation. Wounds that are discovered to be more extensive upon immediate follow-up or those taking longer than 3 weeks to heal should be evaluated by a surgeon with burn wound experience or referred to a regional burn center for further care.

Patients presenting with more severe wounds are at risk of the immediate complications of burn shock and burn edema due to local and systemic fluid shifts, wound infections, sepsis, contractures, and limitations of movement. Additional short-term complications include hypermetabolism, systemic inflammatory response syndrome, and sepsis. Inhalation injuries may accompany cutaneous burn wounds or may occur in isolation. Complications of inhalation injuries include airway edema and loss of airway patency, pneumonia, acute respiratory distress syndrome, and hemodynamic instability (due to impaired oxygen-carrying capacity from carbon monoxide or cyanide exposure). Hypopigmentation, contractures, and psychosocial limitations are among the long-term sequelae of extensive burn injuries.

Growing awareness of burn-injury prevention has resulted in decreased burn-related injuries in children. Child-safety devices and close supervision of children help minimize and eliminate potential sources of burn injury. Specific safety measures include strategic positioning of kitchen appliances, such as microwaves and coffee makers, out of reach of young children; maintaining "kid-free" zones near other dangerous areas (such as ovens, stovetops, and fireplace screens); adjusting the temperature setting of hot water heaters to 49°C/120°F; and practicing safe storage and proper handling of chemicals. Other measures include flame-resistant clothing and furniture as well as skin protection from sun exposure and cold temperatures. Physicians should encourage families to engage in fire-safety education, with fire detectors and carbon monoxide detectors on each floor of the home, fire escape plans, and the provision of safe practices regarding matches and other sources of flames. Resources for fire safety and burn prevention are available to the public at www.ameriburn.org/prevention.php.

Suggested Reading
· · · · · · · · · · · · · · · ·

American Burn Association. *Advanced Burn Life Support Course: Provider Manual.* Chicago, IL: American Burn Association; 2011

Aziz Z, Abu SF, Chong NJ. A systematic review of silver-containing dressings and topical silver agents (used with dressings) for burn wounds. *Burns.* 2012;38(3):307–318

D'Souza AL, Nelson NG, McKenzie LB. Pediatric burn injuries treated in US emergency departments between 1990 and 2006. *Pediatrics.* 2009;124(5):1424–1430

Fleisher GR, Ludwig S, eds. *Textbook of Pediatric Emergency Medicine.* 6th ed. Philadelphia, PA: Wolters Kluwer Health/Lippincott Williams & Wilkins; 2010

Gomez R, Cancio LC. Management of burn wounds in the emergency department. *Emerg Med Clin North Am.* 2007;25(1):135–146

Herndon DN, ed. *Total Burn Care.* 4th ed. Edinburgh, Scotland: Saunders Elsevier; 2012

Klein GL, Herndon DN. Burns. *Pediatr Rev.* 2004;25(12):411–417

Mikrogianakis A, Valani R, Cheng A; Hospital for Sick Children. *The Hospital for Sick Children: Manual of Pediatric Trauma.* Philadelphia, PA: Wolters Kluwer Health/ Lippincott Williams & Wilkins; 2008

Palmieri TL, Greenhalgh DG. Topical treatment of pediatric patients with burns. *Am J Clin Dermatol.* 2002;3(8):529–534

Sheridan RL, ed. *Burns: A Practical Approach to Immediate Treatment and Long-term Care.* London, England: Manson Publishing; 2012

Wasiak J, Cleland H, Campbell F. Dressings for superficial and partial thickness burns. *Cochrane Database Syst Rev.* 2008(4):CD002106

Zafren K. Frostbite: prevention and initial management. *High Alt Med Biol.* 2013;14(1):9–12

CHAPTER 52

Child Maltreatment

Patricia D. Morgan, MD

Key Points

- Child maltreatment is a complex, challenging, and significant issue in the United States and worldwide. Primary care physicians are on the front line of appropriate suspicion, detection, and referral to child abuse professionals and Children Protective Services.

- A thorough history, a complete physical examination, an ancillary evaluation, and an index of suspicion are critical in diagnosing child maltreatment.

- For an infant or child who presents with injuries, child physical abuse should be placed on the differential diagnosis list. Subsequent evaluations can adjust the differential list.

- Consider medical conditions that may mimic child abuse in evaluating unusual physical findings or physical findings that do not simply fit the history.

- The physical findings in sexual abuse will be "normal" in 95% of cases. Normal findings do not exclude or confirm the diagnosis of child sexual abuse.

Overview

The Centers for Disease Control and Prevention defines child maltreatment as any act or series of acts of commission or omission by a parent or caregiver that results in harm, potential for harm, or threat of harm to a child. A child is defined as an unemancipated minor 18 years and younger. Federal and state definitions of child maltreatment provide mandates for various child protective services (CPS) agencies. Broadly, child maltreatment consists of child abuse and child neglect. It is estimated that a little more than 3 million reports to CPS agencies are made in the United States each year. Sadly, the actual number of incidents of possible child maltreatment is thought to be 3 times higher. Each year, about one-third of those CPS agency referrals are substantiated to be some form of abuse, neglect, or other family concern. It is imperative that pediatricians and primary care physicians recognize and report concerns for child maltreatment.

About 5 children die each day in the United States because of child maltreatment. The most common form of child maltreatment is child neglect (Figure 52-1). The leading cause of death due to child maltreatment is abusive head trauma (AHT), also known as shaken baby syndrome in nonmedical fields.

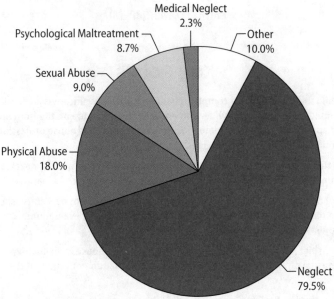

Figure 52-1. Types of child abuse.

From US Department of Health and Human Services, Administration for Children and Families, Administration on Children, Youth and Families, Children's Bureau. *Child Maltreatment 2013*. Washington, DC: US Department of Health and Human Services; 2015. Available at www.acf.hhs.gov/programs/cb/resource/child-maltreatment-2013. Accessed June 26, 2015.

Differential Diagnosis

Child abuse can occur across all socioeconomic, religious, cultural, and ethnic groups. However, certain characteristics of children, parents, and families, as well as risk factors, make child maltreatment more likely to occur (Box 52-1) (Evidence Level III).

Box 52-1. Risk Factors for Child Abuse

- Children with complex medical problems
- Children with developmental delays
- Children who are unwanted
- "Difficult" children with colic or hyperactivity
- Caregiver under significant life stressors
- Caregiver with unrealistic developmental expectations of children

Derived from Christian CW. Etiology and prevention of child abuse. In: Ludwig S. Kornberg AE, eds. *Child Abuse: A Medical Reference*. 2nd ed. New York: Churchill Livingstone; 1992:39–47.

As with any other clinical presentation, the physician should develop a differential diagnosis. Conditions that are dermatologic, hematologic, metabolic, infectious, or unintentional may mimic abuse (Table 52-1).

Table 52-1. Conditions in Children That May Mimic Abuse

Dermatologic	Bullous impetigo, dermal melanosis (ie, mongolian spots), phyto-photodermatitis, senna-containing laxative dermatitis
Hematologic	Von Willebrand disease, hematologic disease of the newborn, vasculitides
Metabolic	Osteogenesis imperfecta, rickets, metabolic bone disorders, glutaric aciduria type I
Infectious	Staphylococcal/streptococcal infections

Derived from Bays J. Conditions mistaken for child physical abuse. In: Reece RM, Ludwig S, eds. *Child Abuse: Medical Diagnosis and Management.* 2nd ed. Baltimore: Lippincott, Williams and Wilkins; 2001.

Identifying a medical condition does not preclude the existence of child maltreatment. Other mimickers of abuse include unintentional trauma, such as falls, straddle injuries, and cultural practices (such as cupping, coining, and moxibustion). Cultural practices that cause physical or emotional trauma may require referrals to CPS agencies. Numerous studies show that falls from distances fewer than 4 ft rarely result in significant injury.

Clinical Features

Child Neglect

Child neglect is failure to provide for a child's basic needs (such as physical, medical, emotional, or educational needs) or failure to protect a child from harm or potential harm. Five main types of neglect have been classified: physical, medical, educational, emotional, and psychological.

Other instances of neglect, depending on local statutes and customs, might include in utero drug exposure; failure to protect in cases of physical abuse, sexual abuse, or both; and exposure to domestic violence.

Physical Neglect

Physical neglect is failure to provide for a child's physical needs, such as food, clothing, shelter, and supervision. It is the most common form of child maltreatment. It differs from poverty but can severely affect a child's development by causing poor growth and development, poor self-esteem, possible serious illnesses, and physical harm in the form of cuts, bruises, and burns due to lack of supervision. Failure to thrive is a common presentation of physical neglect.

Medical Neglect

Medical neglect is failure to comply with or provide recommended medical treatment for a child, such as medications. It also includes not seeking medical care for an injury or illness. Immunization refusal does not constitute medical neglect. Lack of insurance should not affect whether treatment or immunizations are pursued. It is important to intervene if the condition could cause significant illness or possible death. Dental caries may represent dental neglect.

Educational Neglect

Educational neglect is failure to enroll a school-aged child in school or home school or failure to ensure school attendance if enrolled (ie, chronic truancy). This type of neglect can lead to school withdrawal, underachievement in acquiring necessary basic skills, and behavioral changes.

Emotional Neglect

Emotional neglect is failure to provide for the emotional needs of the child, which can cause significant behavioral issues or failure to thrive.

Psychological Neglect

Psychological neglect is failure to comply with or provide recommended mental health services. This can lead to serious emotional or behavioral disorders.

Child Abuse

Child abuse consists of physical, sexual, or emotional abuse of a child. The leading cause of death in children 4 years and younger continues to be physical abuse. Child physical abuse is the infliction of acts by a parent or caregiver that results in injury, serious harm, or death. It is usually the result of biting, burning, kicking, punching, shaking, or otherwise causing harm to a child. Injuries in infants younger than 6 months should be particularly scrutinized.

Abusive head trauma is the leading cause of death in children younger than 4 years. Crying is a common trigger in infants or children affected by this form of abuse. Findings include intracranial injury (eg, subdural hemorrhage), hypoxic-ischemic changes, edema, infarct, diffuse axonal injury, and contusions. Additional findings include fractures (commonly posterior rib and metaphyseal) and retinal hemorrhages.

Child Sexual Abuse

Child sexual abuse is defined as involvement of children in sexual activities of which (1) they cannot give informed consent (each state has an age of informed consent for sexual activity), (2) they do not fully comprehend (such as developmental delay), or (3) violate social taboos (such as incest). It is estimated that by 18 years of age, 1 in 4 girls and 1 in 6 boys will be sexually abused. Children younger than 12 years will know their perpetrators in cases of child sexual abuse more than 90% of the time.

Sexual abuse involvement ranges from no contact (such as sexual comments, exposing one's genitalia, or exposing the child to pornography or adult sexual activity) to physical contact (such as fondling of body parts like breasts and genitalia, oral contact, and vaginal or anal penetration). Exploitation and the use of technology to involve children in sexual abuse has also been on the rise. Expected sexual play occurs between children who are similar in age and development and are mutually curious. However, this behavior should not be imitative of adult sexual activity or involve coercion or force.

Emotional Abuse

Emotional abuse involves criticizing, threatening, or belittling a child and can include acts such as calling names or ridiculing the child.

Medical Child Abuse

Formerly referred to as Munchausen syndrome by proxy (and also referred to as pediatric condition falsification), medical child abuse involves a caregiver simulating or producing an illness in a child to enhance his or her role as caregiver.

Evaluation

History

A child will often be brought for medical attention because of concerns for abuse, neglect, or injuries by the unoffending caregiver. Behavioral indicators (such as aggression, withdrawal, or changes in sleep, appetite, or school performance) or physical indicators (such as pain, bleeding, and infection) may predominate. Children may also disclose being maltreated. These disclosures occur spontaneously or purposefully. An example of a spontaneous disclosure is the child who discloses being fondled during the physical examination of his well-child visit. With purposeful disclosures, children will seek a person to whom they share their disclosure, such as a teacher, family member, or friend.

The most essential part of evaluation in child maltreatment is medical history. The history, taken for the purpose of diagnosis and treatment, is admissible in court as an exception to the hearsay rule in some states. Health care providers should be nonjudgmental, unbiased, and culturally sensitive, and questions should be asked in an open-ended format to determine symptoms, timing of incident(s), and other pertinent information.

Eliciting information about when the infant or child was last well and the timeline of the preceding 24 to 48 hours can prove beneficial in determining timing of possible inflicted trauma. Physicians should explicitly ask about nonspecific symptoms (such as irritability and vomiting), common triggers (such as crying, toilet training, or illness), and family stressors (such as job loss and financial or marital problems). Obtaining a complete past medical history, including birth history, historical clues for an underlying illness, family history for genetic and metabolic conditions, bleeding disorders, patient's development, review of systems (see Table 52-2, Evidence Level III), and social history, is vital to assessing any case of suspected child maltreatment. Physicians should inquire about specific developmental milestones to determine if the history and injury are developmentally plausible.

Social history should include the household composition, usual caregivers, child's temperament, discipline, a HEADDSSS assessment (*home, employment and education, activities, diet, drugs, safety, sexual activity/sexuality, suicide/depression*) in adolescents, intimate partner violence, history of abuse, previous sexually transmitted illness (STI), pregnancy, and alcohol and substance abuse. During the evaluation, the parent-child interaction should also be closely observed. Often the parent who brings the infant or child for evaluation may be the unoffending parent or have no knowledge of abusive incidents.

Ideally, separate histories should be obtained from the parent and the verbal child. When obtaining a medical history from the child, anxiety is reduced by beginning and ending on non-abuse topics. When no history is provided, unexplained injuries should raise the index of suspicion.

A forensic interview is done by trained social workers or law enforcement personnel to gather specific details about possible child maltreatment. These interviews are forensic in nature and differ from a medical history.

Reviewing past medical records from primary care physicians, newborn screening, photographs, and documents of partner agencies (CPS and law enforcement) is also a crucial part of the evaluation and can provide additional details helpful to the final assessment.

Children who present with multiple injuries over time should raise a concern for neglect, inadequate supervision, or injurious environment.

Review of Systems

Key aspects of the systems review are listed in Table 52-2.

Table 52-2. Key Review of Systems Features in Suspected Abuse

System	Symptom
GI	Change in stooling pattern, encopresis
GU	Urinary problems, UTI, pain, discharge, bleeding
Behavior	Sleep disturbances, change in appetite, decline in school performance, aggressive, withdrawn, sexually acting out, excessive or inappropriate masturbation

Abbreviations: GI, gastrointestinal; GU, genito-urinary; UTI, urinary tract infection.
Derived from Reece RM, Ludwig S, eds. *Child Abuse: Medical Diagnosis and Management.* Baltimore, MA: Lippincott Williams & Wilkins; 2001.

Physicians should inquire about previous injuries such as fractures, lacerations, or burns and a thorough review of systems may also uncover psychosomatic concerns such as abdominal pain and headaches.

Physical Examination

Any child suspected of being abused or neglected should have a complete head-to-toe physical examination. The purpose of the examination is to identify injuries, medical conditions, or both, keeping in mind that children may be subjected to multiple types of maltreatment (Table 52-3). The child should have an appropriate support person present during the examination. However, CPS agencies and law enforcement should not be present. The child should be told what the examination will entail to reduce trauma and anxiety. She should be undressed and in a gown so that the skin can be closely inspected and examined. Her appearance should be noted. Growth parameters, weight, length/height, and head circumference (for children 3 years and younger), should be plotted on the appropriate age/sex growth chart. Previous growth charts are helpful in determining appropriate growth patterns.

Table 52-3. Physical Examination in Children Suspected of Abuse

Area	Examination Findings
General	Appearance, hygiene, demeanor
Growth parameters	Weight, length or height, head circumference (3 years and younger)
Skin, nails	Bruises, burns, pattern marks, concerning scars
Head, eyes, ears, nose	Scalp hematoma, alopecia, head or eye trauma, eye bruising, ophthalmological evaluation for retinal hemorrhages and intraocular trauma, ear and pinna bruising, hemotympanum, tympanic membrane perforation, clear nasal discharge, bleeding, septal deviation
Mouth	Lesions, torn frenulum, palatal petechiae, trauma to dentition, dental caries
Neck	Ligature marks, bruises
Chest	Deformity, tenderness, bruises
Back	Skin, costovertebral angle tenderness, bruises
Extremities	Crepitus, deformity, tenderness, soft-tissue swelling
Abdomen	Appearance, bowel sounds, percuss and palpate looking for tenderness, masses, bruising (uncommon)
Genitalia	Sexual maturity rating, position, pain, discharge
Anorectal	Lateral decubitus position helpful; sphincter tone, lesions
Neurologic	Mental status, neurologic changes, tone, seizures

Derived from Reece RM, Ludwig S, eds. *Child Abuse: Medical Diagnosis and Management.* Baltimore, MD: Lippincott Williams & Wilkins; 2001.

Careful attention should be placed on the head and scalp, oral cavity, ears, chest, abdominal, genital, and neurologic examinations (see Table 52-4, Evidence Level III). The skin is the largest and most frequently traumatized organ system in child physical abuse. The physician should carefully inspect all areas to identify bruises, pattern marks, scars, or other concerning areas.

Bruises

Different parts of the body are considered of high and low suspicion for inflicted versus non-inflicted injuries. Injuries to the upper arms, back of the body (including the back of the hands), trunk, front of the thighs, sides of the face, ears/pinnae, neck, genitalia, stomach, and buttocks are all more likely to be associated with inflicted injuries. Injuries to the shins, hips, lower arms, forehead, or bony prominences (ie, shins and knees) are more likely to signify non-inflicted injury.

As coined by Sugar et al, "If you don't cruise, you rarely bruise." If an infant does not have the gross motor ability or developmental skill to cruise, they will not typically have bruises. Therefore, bruising in infants younger than 6 months should be of concern. Do not attempt to date the bruise, but rather document the color, location, number, size, shape or pattern, and any associated tenderness.

Burns

Burns commonly occur in homes in an unintentional manner. However, certain characteristics are seen with intentional burns. Lines of demarcation and symmetry (seen with immersion burns), patterns (such as "stocking and glove" distribution), contact burn patterns (such as irons and curling irons), and cigarette burns are common burns seen in intentional scenarios. Scald burns, the most common type of both unintentional and abusive burn, may have splash-droplet or spill patterns due to the hot liquid. Location of the burn (high vs low suspicion parts of the body), burn classification (partial vs full thickness), areas of sparing (such as soles of feet), or areas of flexion should be noted. Scene investigations are usually necessary to assess temperature of the water heater and other aspects of water flow.

Pattern Marks

Classic pattern of bites, slap and grab marks, and looped cord can be well recognized. Bite marks are typically semicircular, and distances greater than 2.5 cm between canines (intercanine distance) and involving one arch most likely represent an adult bite.

Genitalia Examination

Examination of the genitalia, usually the last portion of the complete examination, should be done in a non-threatening and safe environment. The most qualified person should perform examination of the genital and anal areas. This may be the physician or mid-level professional such as a pediatric nurse practitioner or pediatric sexual assault nurse examiner. The child should be reassured, and all measures should be taken to keep the child comfortable during the examination. This may require having the child sit on his or her parent's lap or have the parent on the examination table with the child.

Good lighting and magnification are necessary to maximize effectiveness of the examination. Otoscopes, colposcopes, and digital cameras are appropriate methods. The use of digital cameras should be explained to parents and children because the use of technology and photographs is sometimes an important aspect of sexual abuse evaluation. The hymen is a thin membrane that surrounds the vaginal opening and comes in different shapes (such as annular and crescent) (Figure 52-2). All girls are born with a hymen, which normally has an opening, but many fallacies exist regarding the hymen. Activities such as gymnastics, cheerleading, and horseback riding and tampon use do not disrupt the integrity of the hymenal membrane. The hymenal edge should be assessed for disruption, which may be seen with penetrating trauma.

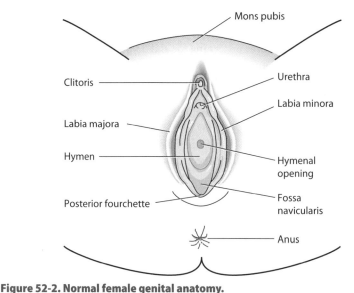

Figure 52-2. Normal female genital anatomy.
From Berkowitz CD, ed. *Berkowitz's Pediatrics: A Primary Care Approach.* 5th ed. Elk Grove Village, IL: American Academy of Pediatrics; 2014.

Speculum examinations are not usually necessary but may be needed if bleeding or concern for other trauma is present. Patients with significant trauma or significant anxiety with concern for trauma necessitate the use of sedation, especially in prepubertal girls. Prepubertal girls should be examined in the following positions: supine frog leg, supine, or prone knee-chest. Techniques used in these positions include labial traction, labial separation, and buttocks traction. It is useful to place the child in more than one position to verify any findings of concern.

Pubertal girls should be placed in the supine lithotomy position. Again, speculum examinations are not usually necessary. Estrogen changes the appearance of the hymen and causes it to become thickened and redundant. A moistened cotton swab can be used to trace the hymenal margin to identify any disruptions. In the Foley catheter technique, a catheter is inserted into the vagina and a balloon inflated; the slow withdrawal of the balloon allows the hymen to stretch, which aids in identification. Physicians not comfortable with these techniques should defer to the most skilled examiner.

Boys should have their mouths carefully examined. A thorough inspection of the genitalia and the anorectal examination should be performed with the boy supine, prone, or lateral decubitus. The external genitalia should be examined for redness, bruises, other signs of trauma, or labial adhesions. Findings should be identified using the face of a clock, typically with the urethra at 12 o'clock and the anus at 6 o'clock in the supine position. Findings below the 9 to 3 o'clock positions should be carefully assessed. Examiners should be familiar with findings which are normal, normal variants, and abnormal and those which are concerning for and definitive evidence of penetrating trauma. It is important to know that approximately 95% of examinations in sexual abuse will be normal.

Reasons why the examination may be normal include
1. Non-penetrative contact or incidents that did not cause trauma
2. False perception of *in* vs *on* (as in vulvar coitus)
3. Time from incident to disclosure delayed
4. Injuries that heal quickly (Mucosal injury heals in a matter of days.)
5. Use of lubricant
6. Effects of estrogen on the hymen, which causes thickening and elastic

In cases of fondling, physical injury is uncommon. There may be erythema or post-fondling dysuria. With the onset of puberty, evidence of injury can be obscured by changes in hymen tissue due to the effects of estrogen. The estrogenized hymen and anal sphincters stretch and therefore may not be injured. Reassurance is one of the most important aspects of the physical examination. The ability to have a child understand that they are well or that their body will heal is often invaluable.

Laboratory Testing

If a complete history and thorough physical examination do not provide the etiology for the child's presentation, it is helpful to obtain other diagnostic studies.

Depending on the type of child maltreatment being considered, testing may include a complete blood count; prothrombin and activate partial thromboplastin time; platelet function assay 100 (to assess for platelet activity); basic metabolic profile; testing for the level of liver enzymes (ie, aspartate transaminase and alanine transaminase) and pancreatic enzymes (ie, amylase and lipase); urine for urinalysis, urine culture with dysuria, and urine organic acids; and stool for occult blood. Serial hemoglobins may be helpful in determining ongoing blood loss. Additional laboratory work-up for child physical abuse based on evaluation may include toxicology; testing for the level of cardiac enzymes; evaluation for metabolic bone disorders (including calcium, phosphorous, alkaline phosphatase, parathyroid hormone, vitamin D levels); urine or serum pregnancy tests (or both); cultures from genital, pharynx, and rectal sites; and a urine nucleic acid amplification test (NAAT). Factor VIII deficiency should be considered in male infants with isolated intracranial bleeding and abnormal coagulation studies.

The need for testing for STIs, such as chlamydia and gonorrhea, should be assessed in cases of child sexual abuse. Some examiners test all children with suspected sexual abuse for STI, while others limit testing to those who may be at increased risk for infection, such as those with a history of previous STI, sexual activity, household members or reported perpetrator with a STI, vaginal or urethral symptoms such as discharge, pain, anogenital lesions, injuries, or evidence of penetration. In cases of acute sexual assault, it is important to remember that performing tests for gonorrhea, chlamydia, trichomonas, and bacterial vaginosis should occur within 2 weeks following the assault. Additional testing for syphilis, human immunodeficiency virus, and hepatitis B should be performed. Patients who test positive for one STI should be tested for all other STIs. Prepubertal girls are more likely to be symptomatic if they have chlamydia or gonorrhea, while pubertal girls often have no symptoms. Prepubertal children should have appropriate STI testing prior to any treatment.

Urine nucleic acid amplification tests have been increasingly used in STI testing because of their high sensitivity and high specificity and noninvasive testing method. There is an increase in literature that supports these tests as appropriate for medicolegal purposes versus cultures for *Neisseria gonorrhoeae* and *Chlamydia trachomatis,* which are sometimes still considered the "gold standard" for sexual abuse evaluations. Some physicians obtain NAAT and then confirm positive NAAT screening with a culture or repeat NAAT using alternate target sequence prior to treatment.

For incidents of sexual abuse or sexual assault that occur fewer than 72 hours from the child's presentation, a sex crimes kit may be obtained. The collection of the kit includes samples of hair, nail scraping, and swabbing for DNA evidence. In children, the highest DNA yield is from clothing, which should be stored in a paper bags.

Diagnostic Imaging

Skeletal survey should be obtained in all children 2 years and younger who present with a suspicious injury such as a fracture, burn, or other concerning symptom. A complete skeletal survey consists of 13 to 15 specific images and should not be a "babygram" when a single image is obtained to identify fractures of various body parts.

Images obtained during a skeletal survey include
- Appendicular skeleton: humeri (anteroposterior), forearms (anteroposterior), hands (oblique and posteroanterior), femurs (anteroposterior), lower legs, (anteroposterior), feet (anteroposterior)

- Axial skeleton: thorax (anteroposterior and lateral); ribs/thoracic spine, abdomen, lumbosacral spine, pelvis (anteroposterior); lumbar spine (lateral); cervical spine (lateral); skull (frontal and lateral)

Any abnormality seen should be viewed with at least 2 views. Oblique views of the ribs are helpful in identifying acute rib fractures. A repeat skeletal survey 2 weeks after the initial survey is helpful in identifying possible healing of fractures (ie, callous formation) or additional occult fractures. Skull fractures do not show typical signs of healing radiologically, making it challenging to date skull fractures.

Fractures that are highly specific for inflicted trauma include posterior rib fractures, metaphyseal fractures (eg, chip, corner, bucket handle fractures), scapula, spinous process, and sternum (Table 52-4, Evidence Level III).

Table 52-4. Fracture Types and Likelihood of Child Abuse (Specificity)

Low	Moderate	High
Clavicular fracture	Multiple fractures	Metaphyseal lesion
Long-bone shaft fracture	Epiphyseal separation	Posterior rib fracture
Linear skull fracture	Vertebral body fracture/ subluxation	Scapular fracture
	Digital fracture	Spinous process fracture
	Complex skull fracture	Sternal fracture

Adapted from Kleinman PK. *Diagnostic Imaging of Child Abuse.* 2nd ed. St Louis, MO: Mosby; 1998.

Plain radiographs are useful (see skeletal survey text), but additional modalities are often needed. Computed tomography is acute and fast, requires no sedation, and is better for certain intracranial injuries, such as hypoxic-ischemic changes. Magnetic resonance imaging is more sensitive in the identification of subtle injuries that may not be seen on computed tomography scans, such as diffuse axonal injury; of dating of injuries, especially with subacute or injuries; and of vascular conditions. Many child abuse diagnostic teams have begun to include evaluation for possible cervical injury as part of the evaluation. Magnetic resonance imaging of the cervical spine is considered in infants but is not presently a routine part of evaluation in child abuse, as cervical spine injuries are rare.

Ultrasound is useful because it is rapid and may be done at bedside to address concerns for intracranial findings (ie, younger infants with anterior fontanelle) and intra-abdominal concerns, such as injury to the liver, spleen, or pancreas, as well as presence of fluid or blood. Other imaging techniques to consider include bone scan and testing for osteogenesis imperfecta (involving skin biopsy or blood for DNA purposes). The best imaging technique should be discussed with the pediatric radiologist or, if not available, a radiologist with the most expertise of the body region.

Management

Primary and secondary resuscitative measures, stabilization, and prompt medical treatment are essential to improve outcomes in cases of child maltreatment. Medical treatment includes medications such as anticonvulsants, intravenous fluids, surgical intervention, C-spine immobilization, and wound and fracture care. Abdominal trauma is the second leading cause of death in child physical abuse. It requires a high index of suspicion, as there is often no external evidence.

Antimicrobial treatment may be offered in cases of sexual abuse but should not be given before cultures are obtained. Prepubertal patients should not be routinely given antibiotics prior to obtaining testing results. Pregnancy prophylaxis should be offered to adolescent girls. Human immunodeficiency virus prophylaxis, usually a 28-day regimen, should be considered based on the risk-benefit to the patient.

A consultation with a child abuse pediatrician is invaluable, especially early in the course of suspected child maltreatment. Other possible consultants include social work, trauma, surgery, orthopedics, neurosurgery, neurology, and forensic odontology. Child protection services agencies and law enforcement should serve as partners as well.

The emotional well-being of the child is paramount. Individual, family, or group psychotherapy is beneficial to the ultimate healing of the child and family.

Assessment

When assessing injuries, it is important to consider the following questions:
- Is the history consistent with the injury?
- Is there another condition or medical explanation for the cause of this injury?
- What is the developmental ability of the child?
- Does additional information support the assessment of child maltreatment?

Partnering agencies need the assistance of medical physicians to identify the cause of findings. Information from CPS agencies and law enforcement, such as pictures from the home or scene investigation, may be helpful in concluding the etiology of the child's presentations.

Documentation

Careful documentation of history, examination findings, diagnostic evaluation, assessment, and treatment/recommendations is important in any child maltreatment case. If pictures are taken, use the best technique and individual to take the picture (ie, good lighting, medical photographer). As the medical physician, you may also be called on to provide testimony regarding any portion of that documentation.

Key points to remember: use verbatim statements and quotation marks whenever possible; include drawings or photographs; document the size, location, and any possible patterns or shapes; and identify genital findings by noting the examination position and clock-face location.

Also, avoid terminology such as *within normal limits, hymen intact, alleged, no evidence of penetration,* and *rule out,* but rather describe the findings. Provide details of the findings and the likelihood of abuse based on the history (ie, the history being consistent with the findings, the physical examination, ancillary evaluation, and corroborative information). It is helpful to document pertinent positive and negative findings of trauma. Using the TEARS (*t*ears, *e*cchymoses, *a*brasions, *r*edness, *s*cars/swelling) or BARBS (*b*ruises, *a*brasions, *r*edness, *b*leeding, *s*welling or scars) classifications can be helpful. A normal physical examination does not exclude or confirm sexual abuse or sexual contact.

Mandated Reporter

Physicians and other health care providers who have a suspicion or concern for child maltreatment must report to their local CPS agencies. If a child discloses abuse or neglect, it is not necessary to investigate the report before referring to CPS agencies. Physicians and other health care providers who report in good faith have immunity from civil and criminal liability. In some states, failure to report child maltreatment may lead to penalties including fines and charges and possible suspension of medical licensure.

During the course of an investigation for possible child maltreatment, information may need to be shared with partner agencies. The parents or legal guardian should give permission to share medical information with nonmedical team members. The Health Insurance Portability and Accountability Act does not preclude sharing of medical information with CPS agencies during an active investigation. Law enforcement may obtain information from CPS agencies or medical institutions with the appropriate consent or court document.

Prevention

Home visits, parent education, appropriate discipline, and parenting skills can all aid in prevention. Well-established AHT prevention programs can be utilized. Parents and caregivers should be instructed to avoid physical discipline. Children should be taught body safety and that the parts under the bathing suit should not be touched.

Safety is of the utmost importance in determining the disposition of the patient suspected of being maltreated. Infants and children need to be in a home where there is no risk for future harm. The best environment is also one where the child feels supported so that the risk of recantation or retracting of the initial disclosure is minimized.

Long-term Implications

During the initial medical course, infants and children with AHT should be monitored for increased intracranial pressure, disseminated intravascular coagulation, and syndrome of inappropriate antidiuretic hormone. Injuries due to AHT may lead to significant long-term disabilities including seizures, visual abnormalities, spasticity, paralysis, behavioral problems, learning deficits, attention-deficit/hyperactivity disorder, and cognitive and developmental abnormalities. Other problems may include posttraumatic stress disorder, depression, substance use/abuse, and self-mutilation.

Suggested Reading

Christian CW, Block R; Committee on Child Abuse and Neglect. Abusive head trauma in infants and children. *Pediatrics.* 2009:123(5);1409–1411

Flaherty EG, Stirling J Jr; Committee on Child Abuse and Neglect. The pediatrician's role in child maltreatment prevention, *Pediatrics.* 2010:126(4);833–841

Kellogg ND; Committee on Child Abuse and Neglect. Evaluation of suspected child physical abuse. *Pediatrics.* 2007:119(6);1232–1241

Kleinman PK. Skeletal trauma: general considerations. In: Kleinman PK, ed. *Diagnostic Imaging of Child Abuse.* Baltimore, MD: Lippincott Williams & Wilkins; 1987:8–25

American College of Radiology. ACR–SPR Practice Parameter for Skeletal Surveys in Children. 2014. http://www.acr.org/,/media/ACR/Documents/PGTS/guidelines/Skeletal_Surveys.pdf. Accessed March 11, 2015

Pressel DM. Evaluation of physical abuse in children. *Am Fam Physician.* 2000:15;61(10):3057–3064

Reece RM, Hanson RF, Sargent J, eds. *Treatment of Child Abuse: Common Ground for Mental Health, Medical, and Legal Practitioners.* 2nd ed. Baltimore, MD: Johns Hopkins University Press; 2014

Reece RM, Ludwig S, eds. *Child Abuse: Medical Diagnosis and Management.* 3rd ed. Baltimore, MD: Lippincott Williams & Wilkins; 2009

Section on Radiology. Diagnostic imaging of child abuse. *Pediatrics.* 2009:123(5); 1430–1435

Stirling J Jr; Committee on Child Abuse and Neglect. Beyond Munchausen syndrome by proxy: identification and treatment of child abuse in a medical setting. *Pediatrics.* 2007:119(5);1026–1030

Sugar NF, Taylor JA, Feldman KW. Bruises in infants and toddlers: those who don't cruise rarely bruise. *Arch Pediatr Adolesc Med.* 1999;153(4):399–403

US Department of Health and Human Services; Administration for Children and Families; Administration on Children, Youth and Families; Children's Bureau. *Child Maltreatment, 2012.* Administration for Children and Families Web site. http://www.acf.hhs.gov/sites/default/files/cb/cm2012.pdf. Accessed January 14, 2015

CHAPTER 53

Determination of Brain Death

Dwight M. Bailey, DO

Key Points

- Brain death is recognized as the absence of all brainstem reflexes and verified apnea in a patient who is comatose.

- The determination of pediatric death is established based on the presence of all 3 of the following neurologic criteria: (1) identification of an untreatable and irreversible cause of coma; (2) correction of confounding factors that may interfere with the neurologic examination; and (3) completion of 2 independent physical examinations by 2 different practitioners and 2 apnea tests, all consistent with the absence of neurologic function.

- The foundation of the determination of brain death is the neurologic examination.

- To establish and assure the irreversibility of the brain death proclamation, the 2011 task force has proposed the use of 2 examinations, including apnea testing, separated by an age-related observation period.

- The diagnosis of brain death is intricately linked to the issue of organ donation. The potential for organ donation may offer comfort to some bereaving families; however, it should never be the impetus for the diagnosis of brain death.

Overview

The determination of brain death is the diagnosis of death by neurologic criteria. According to the Uniform Determination of Death Act, "An individual who has sustained either: (1) irreversible cessation of circulatory and respiratory functions, or (2) irreversible cessation of all functions of the entire brain, including the brainstem, is dead." The irreversible cessation of circulatory and respiratory functions is determined by standard methods of assessing cardiac and pulmonary function. The irreversible cessation of all functions of the entire brain involves a careful and detailed assessment of neurologic function.

The history of the determination of brain death has been fraught with controversy and challenge. Add to this equation the increasing complexity of understanding the neonatal and pediatric intracranial physiology, and the discussion becomes exponentially more difficult. In 1987, consensus-based guidelines for the determination of pediatric brain death were published because of the failure to adequately address pediatric criteria for the determination of brain death within the 1981 *Journal of the American Medical Association* report to the presidential commission. The 1987 guidelines highlighted the importance of history and clinical examination in determining the etiology of pediatric coma so that reversible or correctable conditions were eliminated. Additionally, age-related observation periods and the need for neurodiagnostic specific testing were recommended for children younger than 1 year. In children older than 1 year, recommendations for the diagnosis of brain death could be made solely on the basis of the clinical examination.

The determination of brain death within the pediatric population relied upon these guidelines despite their recognized limitations and inherent weaknesses. These limitations have resulted in the lack of a standardized approach in the determination of brain death in children. In 2011, the Society of Critical Care Medicine and the Section on Critical Care of the American Academy of Pediatrics, in conjunction with the Child Neurology Society, updated the 1987 task force recommendations for the determination of brain death in infants and children.

Death by Neurologic Criteria

The clinical diagnosis of brain death is recognized as the absence of all brainstem reflexes and verified apnea in a patient who is comatose. Upon the determination of brain death, death can be declared. The consensus-based 2011 updated pediatric brain death guidelines represent the most comprehensive and thorough review of the available literature to date and provide a well-documented grading of recommendations to guide the standardization of practice across practitioners and institutions.

The foundation of the determination of brain death is the neurologic examination. Qualified clinicians for the examination include pediatric intensivists, neonatologists, pediatric neurologists and neurosurgeons, pediatric trauma surgeons, and pediatric anesthesiologists with critical care training.

The determination of pediatric (ie, full-term newborns >37 weeks' gestational age–young adults 18 years of age) death is established based on the satisfaction of all 3 of the following neurologic criteria: (1) the identification of an untreatable and irreversible cause of coma; (2) the correction of confounding factors that may interfere with the neurologic examination; and (3) the completion of 2 independent physical examinations by 2 different practitioners and 2 apnea tests, all consistent with the absence of neurologic function. Because of insufficient data in the literature, recommendations for preterm newborns younger than 37 weeks' gestational age are not included in these recommendations.

Prerequisites to the Clinical Brain Death Examination

The identification of an untreatable and irreversible cause of coma should be the initial step to any determination of death by neurologic criteria process. These causes can include but are not limited to traumatic brain injury, inoperable intracranial tumor, anoxic brain injury, and refractory intracranial pressure consistently elevated above arterial blood pressure.

Determination of brain death by neurologic examination should be performed in the setting of establishing and maintaining reference range age-appropriate physiologic parameters and only after the correction of any abnormal contributing factors, if they exist, due to their likely interference with the examination.

Shock or persistent hypotension based on healthy systolic or mean arterial blood pressure values for the patient's age need to be corrected via fluid resuscitation, inotropic support, or both, as indicated. The measurement of invasive blood pressure via an indwelling arterial catheter is the recommendation of choice and will assist with accurate $Paco_2$ levels during the apnea testing portion of the examination.

A core body temperature greater than 35°C (95°F) is necessary during the neurologic criteria testing because of the likelihood that hypothermia can depress central nervous system function and may lead to a false diagnosis of brain death. Additionally, hypothermia can alter the rate of metabolism and clearance of medications that have the potential to interfere with neurologic testing.

Metabolic disturbances, including electrolyte and glucose abnormalities, severe pH imbalances, hepatic or renal dysfunction, or inborn errors of metabolism, may cause potentially reversible coma and are essential to identify and correct prior to neurologic testing.

Pharmaceutical intoxications, including but not limited to opioids, benzodiazepines, other sedatives, inhalation and intravenous anesthetics, barbiturates, other antiepileptics, and alcohols, can all cause severe central nervous system depression and mimic brain death, altering the ability to achieve an accurate neurologic examination. Testing for these drugs should be completed if recent ingestion or administration is evident or documented. In the scenario where neuromuscular-blocking agents have been used, they should be discontinued, and clearance from the system should be documented via the use of a nerve stimulator and the presence of twitch response.

Assessment of neurologic function may be unreliable immediately following cardiopulmonary arrest and subsequent resuscitation, or other acute brain injuries, and serial neurologic examinations are necessary to establish or refute the diagnosis of brain death. It is reasonable to defer the examination to determine brain death for 24 hours or longer if indicated and determined by the treating practitioner.

Clinical Brain Death Examination

The cardinal features of death by neurologic criteria are coma and the absence of brainstem reflexes, including apnea testing consistent with brain death.

The diagnosis of coma implies the loss of function of *both* cerebral hemispheres and the reticular activating system of the upper midbrain, pons, and thalamus. The patient must reveal the absence of all evidence of responsiveness; the absence of response to noxious stimuli, including the absence of movement of bulbar musculature, such as facial and oropharyngeal muscles; and the absence of deep muscular movements, with the exception of spinally mediated reflexes. A result consistent with brain death is the absence of all of the described movements *plus* the absence of autonomic responses (eg, papillary, heart rate, or blood pressure changes) when deep pressure is applied to the condyles at the level of the temporomandibular joints, the supraorbital ridge, or the nail beds of the toes and fingers. The clinical differentiation of spinal reflexes from motor responses associated with brain activity can be difficult and requires expertise. Documenting the absence of any form of repetitive, sustained purposeful activity is imperative, as is differentiating brain death from other states of unconsciousness, such as the vegetative state. Decerebrate and decorticate reflex posturing are not consistent with brain death.

The presence of function at different levels of the brainstem is tested through a series of reflex pathways. The pupillary reflex is tested by shining a light into each eye separately while observing for a response during both the application of light and its withdrawal. A response consistent with brain death reveals pupils that are fixed in mid-position or fully dilated (ie, 4–9 mm) and that show no reactivity or change in size bilaterally when exposed to light. Assurance that the pupillary responses, or lack thereof, occur in the absence of drugs influencing papillary activity is imperative. Additional pitfalls include the presence of preexisting pupillary abnormalities (anisocoria is present in approximately 10% of the population). Anisocoric pupils should remain responsive to light in the healthy patient population.

The corneal reflex is tested via the application of a cotton tip applicator, tissue paper, or squirts of water directly to the cornea, being careful not to do damage, as well as avoiding the sclera. A result consistent with brain death is the absence of eyelid movement, closure, and upward deviation of the eye (ie, Bell phenomenon).

The pharyngeal or gag reflex is tested via stimulation of the posterior pharynx with a tongue blade or suction device. The tracheal reflex is most reliably tested by examining the cough response to tracheal suctioning by inserting the catheter into the trachea and advancing to the level of the carina, followed by 1 to 2 suction passes. A result consistent with brain death is the absence of palatal, lingual, and pharyngeal movement with the appropriate stimulation.

The oculocephalic reflex (ie, doll's eye reflex) remains a part of the updated adult recommendations for brain death criteria but has been eliminated from the updated 2011 pediatric guidelines. The primary concern of the oculoce-phalic reflex is the risk to the cervical spine given suspected or documented spinal fracture or instability in patients with head trauma, neck trauma, or both. It is likely this risk, combined with the ability to complete an accurate and thorough assessment of brain death in the pediatric population in the absence of oculocephalic testing, has led the committee to omit it from the 2011 guidelines. Unlike the oculocephalic test, oculovestibular (ie, cold caloric) reflex testing remains a necessary portion of the pediatric brain death examination. Cold caloric testing is completed by elevation of the head to 30 degrees, confirmation of patency of the external auditory canal, and irrigation of each canal separately (an interval of several minutes between each is recommended) with 10 to 50 mL of ice water. A test consistent with brain death reveals the absence of eye movement for up to 1 minute following irrigation. Tympanic membrane rupture does not interfere with the ability to perform or the validity of the test.

The apnea test is designed to evaluate the ability of the respiratory center to respond to elevated levels of CO_2 and stimulate respiratory effort. Apnea testing is an essential part of the examination must be done in conjunction with the clinical examination to determine brain death based on clinical criteria unless a medical contraindication exists. Contraindications include conditions that invalidate the apnea test (eg, high cervical spine injury) or cause concern for patient safety (eg, high oxygen requirements or high ventilator settings). If apnea testing cannot be safely completed, ancillary testing needs to be per-formed to assist with the determination of death by neurologic criteria.

Apnea testing in full-term newborns, infants, and children is conducted similar to adults. Prior to beginning the test, the ventilator should be titrated to achieve normalization of the pH and $Paco_2$. Maintaining oxygenation during the apnea test requires a technique known as "apneic oxygenation." This requires preoxygenation of the patient via exposure to 100% Fio_2 for 5 to 10 minutes, followed by delivery of a continuous flow of oxygen. Continuous oxygen delivery during the test can be provided by placing the patient on mechanical ventilation with continuous positive airway pressure only (no set respiratory rate on the ventilator). Be aware of ventilators that automatically convert to a backup ventilatory mode in the event of apnea, as this setup will not allow for the apnea test to be completed. Continuous flow of oxygen can also be provided by placing the patient on a Mapleson circuit (or "anesthesia bag") with an adequate flow of oxygen. The practitioner(s) performing the apnea test need to continuously monitor and maintain age-appropriate reference range values for the patient's heart rate and blood pressure, and oxygen saturations greater than 85%, while observing for the presence of spontaneous respiratory effort throughout the entire procedure. An apnea test consistent with the diagnosis of brain death requires the absence of *any* respiratory effort in the presence of an adequate stimulus for respiratory drive, defined as a $Paco_2$, measured by arterial blood gas (ABG) analysis, greater than or equal to 20 mm Hg above the measured baseline $Paco_2$ level *and* greater

than or equal to 60 mm Hg. At this time, the patient is placed back on ventilatory support and medical management is continued until a second neurologic
exam and apnea test are confirmatory for death by neurologic criteria.

The apnea test is terminated under any of the following circumstances:

- If any respiratory effort is seen, the test is over, and the patient is not
  brain dead. The patient should immediately be mechanically ventilated to
  restore the $Paco_2$ to reference range levels. Complex spinal reflexes may
  occur during the apnea test, which do not rule out the diagnosis of brain
  death. Differentiating spinal reflexes from true respiratory effort is
  difficult and requires expertise.
- If the patient begins to desaturate, the patient should be observed until
  the oxygen saturation is less than 85%, at which time an ABG should be
  drawn and the patient immediately returned to mechanical ventilation to
  restore reference range levels of oxygen saturation, Pao_2, and $Paco_2$.
- If the patient begins to become hypotensive, efforts should be made to
  maintain blood pressure. If these are ineffective, an ABG should be drawn
  when the blood pressure reaches the lower limit of the reference range for
  the patient's age, ventilatory support is restored, and efforts to maintain
  the blood pressure are continued.

Observation Periods and Age-Specific Requirements

By definition, all patients who are declared brain dead are comatose and apneic
and lack brainstem reflexes. These criteria may not be present on admission in
most children, usually evolving during the initial days of hospitalization.
Therefore, serial examinations are an essential part of the neurologic brain
death assessment process. Additionally, the wide breadth of age ranges and the
resultant variations of physiology present within pediatrics suggest that the time
of observation between examinations may need to vary between extremes of
age. To establish and assure the irreversibility of the brain death proclamation,
the 2011 task force has proposed the use of 2 examinations, including apnea
testing, separated by an age-related observation period. They recommend that
2 different attending physicians perform the examinations; however, the same
physician may perform apnea testing. The guidelines recommend an observation period of 24 hours for full-term newborns (>37 weeks' gestation) to
infants aged 30 days. For infants and children older than 30 days up to 18 years,
the guidelines call for a 12-hour observation period. The first examination
determines whether the child has met the accepted neurologic examination
criteria for brain death. The second confirms brain death based on an un-
changed and irreversible condition.

Ancillary Testing and Shortening of the Inter-examination Observation Period

Accurate and comprehensive serial clinical neurologic examinations are sufficient in determining brain death. The task force guidelines state that ancillary studies (ie, electroencephalogram and radionuclide cerebral blood flow) are not required to establish brain death and are not a substitute for the neurologic examination. These studies may be used when components of the examination or apnea testing cannot be completed safely because of the underlying medical condition. They can also be considered if the results of the neurologic examination are uncertain, if a medication effect may be present, or to reduce the inter-examination observation period. When ancillary studies are used, a second clinical examination and apnea test should continue to be performed, and components that can be completed must remain consistent with brain death.

With the possible exception of a 4-vessel cerebral angiography test showing no cerebral blood flow (CBF), no test is absolutely confirmatory of brain death and can only be consistent with the diagnosis and, therefore, used to supplement the clinical impression, not to make the diagnosis. Four-vessel cerebral angiography is the criterion standard among cerebral blood flow tests for brain death. However, the test is invasive; requires transportation to the angiography suite, increasing the likelihood of further destabilization of the patient outside the walls of the intensive care unit; and is difficult to perform in small infants and children.

Electroencephalographic (EEG) documentation of electrocerebral silence and the measurement of the absence of CBF via radionuclide CBF analysis remain the most widely available and useful methods to assist in the diagnosis of brain death. Electroencephalographic testing and radionuclide CBF testing need to be completed in accordance with the 1994 guidelines for brain death recordings developed by the American Electroencephalographic Society. The data suggest that both of these modalities have similar confirmatory value and remain acceptable tests to assist with the determination of brain death in infants and children.

If an ancillary study supports the first neurologic examination diagnosis of brain death, the inter-observation interval may be reduced and the second examination and apnea testing, performed at any time thereafter for children of all ages.

In the event that an ancillary study is not consistent with brain death (eg, the evidence of blood flow or cellular uptake on a CBF study or the presence of electrical activity on EEG), the patient cannot be pronounced dead. In this scenario, medical support should be continued and the patient observed until (1) brain death can be declared via the appropriate clinical neurologic examination, and apnea testing can be based upon the previously discussed criteria and observation periods; (2) repeat ancillary testing is used in conjunction with clinical testing, and together they are consistent with brain death; or (3) the decision to withdrawal life support is made, independent of neurologic testing for brain death. Should the use of repeat ancillary testing be needed or used, a waiting period of 24 hours is recommended. The task force states that waiting for a period of 24 hours prior to repeat EEG is reasonable and recommended; the same time frame prior to repeat radionuclide CBF resting is necessary for adequate clearance of the radiolabeled contrast Tc 99m.

Organ System Failure, Brain Death, and Organ Donation

Brain ischemia leads to sympathetic nervous system collapse with vasodilation and cardiac dysfunction. Pulmonary edema, hypothalamic-pituitary-adrenal axis impairment, and neuroendocrine dysfunction, such as diabetes insipidus and syndrome of inappropriate antidiuretic hormone, are all common early consequences of brain death and may precipitate cardiopulmonary failure.

Once the diagnosis of brain death is confirmed, the information should be communicated to the family. Care of the grieving family is one of the most vital services a physician can provide. Some families have beliefs that oppose the equivalence of brain death with death, and the perception that death has occurred often differs from one person to another. The diagnosis of brain death is intricately linked to the issue of organ donation and may influence a family member's decision-making. Family members approached to donate the organs of their brain-dead relative need to have a clear understanding of what the diagnosis means. The differences between cardiopulmonary versus brain death criteria of death need to be explained. The potential for organ donation may offer comfort to some bereaving families; however, it should never be the impetus for the diagnosis of brain death. The responsibilities of the physician involved in the declaration of brain death must always be clearly demarcated from those physicians interested and involved in organ procurement.

Summary

Although the diagnosis of brain death in pediatric patients is based on the same principles as it is in adults, the variabilities of physiology between the newborn, toddler, adolescent, and adult make an all-inclusive, one-size-fits-all approach, not only impossible, but inappropriate. A standardized checklist for documentation of brain death in infants and children was developed by the 2011 task force and should be referenced to help ensure all components of the examination are carried out.

Suggested Reading

American Academy of Pediatrics Task Force on Brain Death in Children. Report of the special task force: guidelines for the determination of brain death in children. *Pediatrics.* 1987;80(2):298–300

Ashwal S, Schneider S. Brain death in children: part I. *Pediatr Neurol.* 1987;3(1):5–11

Ashwal S, Schneider S. Brain death in children: part II. *Pediatr Neurol.* 1987;3(2):69–77

Chang MY, McBride LA, Ferguson MA. Variability in brain death declaration practices in pediatric head trauma patients. *Pediatr Neurosurg.* 2003;39(1):7–9

Choi EK, Fredland V, Zachodni C, Lammers JE, Bledsoe P, Helft PR. Brain death revisited: the case for a national standard. *J Law Med Ethics.* 2008;36(4):824–836

Goh AY, Mok Q. Clinical course and determination of brainstem death in a children's hospital. *Acta Paediatr.* 2004;93(1):47–52

Nakagawa TA, Ashwal S, Mathur M, et al. Guidelines for the determination of brain death in infants and children: an update of the 1987 Task Force recommendations. *Crit Care Med.* 2011;39(9):2139–2155

Wijdicks EF, Varelas PN, Gronseth GS, Greer DM. Determining brain death in adults: report of the Quality Standards Subcommittee of the American Academy of Neurology. *Neurology.* 2010;74(23):1911–1918

CHAPTER 54

Diabetic Ketoacidosis

Mark J. McDonald, MD

Key Points

- Despite its low occurrence rate, the most common cause of mortality in children with diabetic ketoacidosis (DKA) is cerebral edema.

- The degree of dehydration is often overestimated in DKA; assume most patients are less than 10% dehydrated.

- Correct the patient's deficit over the course of 48 hours. Despite slower rehydration, most patients resolve their acidosis within 24 hours.

- Give insulin as a continuous infusion, avoiding insulin boluses and acute glucose drops, which may predispose a patient to cerebral edema.

- Do not use bolus sodium bicarbonate to treat metabolic acidosis. A bicarbonate bolus should only be *considered* if cardiovascular collapse has occurred, which is very rare.

- If the sodium level falls during treatment, the patient needs close observation for evidence of cerebral edema.

Overview

Diabetic ketoacidosis (DKA) is frequently encountered in pediatric emergency departments and critical care units and may occasionally present to the pediatric office. Causes of DKA are multiple, including new onset diabetes mellitus, omission of home insulin, insulin pump failure, and conditions increasing insulin requirements. Each treating physician must evaluate varying degrees of acidosis, hyperglycemia, and dehydration while trying to ensure proper treatment to prevent DKA-associated morbidity and mortality. The most common cause of death in children with insulin-dependent diabetes mellitus is DKA and the complication of cerebral edema accounts for nearly all of the mortality despite the literature suggesting a less than 1% occurrence rate.

Historically, the low incidence of cerebral edema has made randomized, prospective trials evaluating treatment and prevention of cerebral edema difficult, if not impossible, to perform. Therefore, much of the data to date are based on case series and retrospective analyses. Generally, management of pediatric DKA has not only varied from hospital to hospital but according to specialty training. Controversies continue to exist over the definitive cause of cerebral edema and the appropriate therapeutic interventions to prevent this complication. This chapter will discuss current evidence related to DKA management and suggest a rational approach toward cerebral edema prevention during DKA therapy.

Definition and Pathophysiology

The consensus definition for DKA in children is listed in Table 54-1 and includes hyperglycemia, ketosis, and metabolic acidosis. All patients in DKA are insulin deficient with increased counterregulatory hormones including glucagon, epinephrine, cortisol, and growth hormone. These hormones promote lipolysis and proteolysis and increase serum glucose through glycogenolysis and gluconeogenesis. After the serum glucose exceeds the renal glucose threshold, glucosuria ensues, causing an osmotic diuresis, electrolyte loss, and subsequent dehydration.

Table 54-1. Diabetic Ketoacidosis Definition

Hyperglycemia	Plasma glucose >250 mg/dL
Acidosis	Plasma bicarbonate <15 mmol/L and/or venous pH <7.3
Presence of ketones	Elevated urine ketones and/or blood acetone

Lipolysis contributes to DKA through a breakdown of triglycerides into free fatty acids, which undergo hepatic mitochondrial oxidation to ketoacids. The ketoacids produced are acetoacetate, β-hydroxybutyrate, and acetone, which are responsible for the metabolic acidosis in DKA. Acetoacetate can be broken down to acetone, which can be partly excreted from the body in the breath, causing the characteristic "fruity breath" associated with DKA. Acetoacetate is also converted to β-hydroxybutyrate. Under normal circumstances, the ratio of acetoacetate to β-hydroxybutyrate is 1:3, but it may increase greatly in severe DKA. The net metabolic effect of ketone formation is an acidosis from the accumulation of keto anions and the formation of 3 hydrogen ions for every triglyceride molecule metabolized.

Clinical Features

The triad of polyuria, polydipsia, and polyphagia are classically uncovered during the patient history. Commonly, dehydration and weight loss are present and manifested by decreased skin turgor, dry mucous membranes, sunken eyes, delayed capillary refill, poor perfusion, and tachycardia. However, hypotensive shock is rare in DKA. Pediatric literature suggests the degree of dehydration in DKA to be less than 10%, with most physicians overestimating this. To avoid misjudging DKA dehydration, physicians should assume that most DKA patients are less than 10% dehydrated and treat accordingly. Respiratory examination may show tachypnea, hyperpnea, and a fruity odor from the patient's breath. Kussmaul respirations are representative of DKA and characterized as deep, regular, and sigh-like. Patients frequently have vomiting and may complain of varying degrees of abdominal pain. Neurologic assessment is extremely important and examinations may vary from normal to suggesting symptomatic cerebral edema (Box 54-1). Cerebral edema carries a high risk of morbidity and mortality and may occur at any time during treatment, including prior to initiation of therapy.

Box 54-1. Signs of Cerebral Edema

- Headache
- Vomiting
- Bradycardia
- Hypertension
- Altered mental status
- Incontinence
- Posturing
- Focal neurologic deficits
  - Fixed and dilated pupil(s)
  - Extraocular muscle palsies
- Respiratory decompensation
  - Agonal breathing
  - Cheyne-Stokes respirations

Evaluation

Initial Laboratory and Clinical Tests

Confirmation of DKA by laboratory tests should occur when the diagnosis is suspected through history and clinical examination. Essential and optional tests are listed in Table 54-2. A 12-lead electrocardiogram may be obtained if there is concern about initial hyperkalemia. Arterial blood gases may be avoided because blood gases will not alter treatment, as acidosis can be followed with bicarbonate levels. An anion gap can be calculated from the chemistry (Table 54-3). Serum osmolality, a measured value including osmotic serum ketoacids, is an essential test and can be followed serially (see Table 54-3). Serum osmolarity is calculated at the bedside, does not account for serum ketoacids, and is less informative.

Table 54-2. Laboratory and Clinical Tests

Essential	Optional
Chemistry: Na, K, Cl, HCO_3, BUN, creatinine, glucose, phosphorous	Hemoglobin A_{1c}
Bedside glucose	ABG
Urine for ketones	Serum acetone
Serum osmolality	CBC
	Mg, Ca
	ECG
	Lipase
	Cultures
	Head CT

Abbreviations: ABG, arterial blood gas; BUN, blood urea nitrogen; CBC, complete blood cell count; CT, computed typography; ECG, electrocardiogram.

Table 54-3. Calculations

Measure	Equation	Range
Anion gap	$Na - (Cl + HCO_3)$	Normal 12 ±2 mmol/L
Serum osmolarity calculated	$(2 [Na]) + (BUN/2.8) + (glucose/18)$	Normal 275–295 mmol/L
Osmolal gap	Measured osmolality – calculated osmolarity	Range +10 to −10 mOsm/kg
"Corrected" serum sodium	Corrected Na = measured Na + $\left(\dfrac{[serum\ glucose - 100] \times 1.6}{100}\right)$	

Abbreviation: BUN, blood urea nitrogen.

Acetoacetate, not β-hydroxybutyrate, is the ketone detected in the urine. The accumulation of β-hydroxybutyrate in DKA will lead to the persistence of ketones in the urine during and following correction as the ratio of β-hydroxybutyrate to acetoacetate returns to normal. Literature suggests lipase elevation may occur in DKA patients; however, this is rarely clinically significant and evaluation should be reserved for patients with persistent abdominal pain. The most common imaging done in DKA patients is a computed tomography (CT) scan of the head. This is usually ordered to evaluate for possible cerebral edema. If symptomatic cerebral edema is present, treatment should occur prior to evaluation by CT scan. Routine head CT scans are not necessary unless symptoms of cerebral edema exist (see Box 54-1).

Electrolyte Abnormalities

Initial electrolyte levels, including sodium, potassium, and phosphorus, may be quite abnormal in DKA. Hyponatremia was long ago recognized to occur with hyperglycemia, although presenting DKA sodium levels may be low or high. As the DKA patient becomes more dehydrated, low sodium levels will eventually increase and the patient may become hypernatremic, indicating a more dehydrated hyperosmolar state. A "corrected" sodium can be calculated using a correction factor of 1.6 (see Table 54-3). However, this calculation only addresses the effect glucose elevation has on serum sodium. More important is the measured serum osmolality, which takes into account sodium, glucose, and all other osmolal serum components. Increased serum vasopressin may also contribute to the hyponatremia seen in DKA patients, presumed secondary to dehydration or central nervous system pathology.

Prior to renal hypoperfusion from dehydration, potassium in the serum is lost via the kidneys through an osmotic diuresis, creating a total-body potassium deficit. However, initial serum potassium is usually high secondary to potassium being drawn out of cells by a serum hyperosmolar gradient and electrical hydrogen–potassium exchange associated with the metabolic acidosis. The physician should be cognizant of the total body potassium depletion and need for potassium replacement during treatment. Insulin therapy and the correction of the acidosis will lower the potassium, often to hypokalemic levels. A similar extracellular shift occurs with phosphorus during DKA with a subsequent loss in the urine leading to a total-body phosphorus deficit. Again, initial serum levels may be high, but intracellular phosphorus shifts during acidosis correction and insulin infusion will lead to hypophosphatemia. Therefore, phosphate replacement in DKA fluid therapy should be strongly considered.

Cerebral Edema Etiology

Cerebral edema remains the major cause of DKA morbidity and mortality. At one time, cerebral edema was thought to occur only in children; however, adults can also be affected. Symptomatic cerebral edema may occur at any time from prior to hospital presentation to more than 24 hours following DKA treatment. To understand how to prevent and treat DKA cerebral edema, research has tried to understand how and why it occurs. Many concepts associated with DKA cerebral edema include the presence of subclinical cerebral edema, edema secondary to osmolal fluid shifts, vasogenic edema from increased perfusion and blood-brain barrier (BBB) permeability, vasopressin secretion, and brain infarction.

Literature exists verifying the presence of subclinical cerebral edema in asymptomatic DKA patients. The importance of subclinical cerebral edema and why only a few patients go on to develop symptomatic cerebral edema are unknown. Historically, the most widely held belief for DKA cerebral edema has been a rapid change in serum osmolality during treatment. More recent innovative studies have used multiple techniques to show vasogenic edema to be present in DKA. This has suggested vasogenic edema and not cellular swelling as a mechanism of cerebral edema. Related to this may be altered BBB permeability during DKA. Endogenous vasopressin may also be involved in cerebral edema development. The hypothesis of vasopressin's role in cerebral edema stems from the development of hyponatremia during treatment prior to DKA-associated cerebral edema. Brain infarcts have been found on some postmortem examinations of expired DKA patients. Diabetic ketoacidosis may predispose patients to thrombosis from cerebral vasoconstriction associated with hypocapnia, dehydration, and hyperosmolality. This raises the possibility of cerebral edema being a response to previous infarction, rather than a result of therapy. At this point, DKA cerebral edema is best explained as multifactorial.

Cerebral Edema Risk Factors

Because the pathophysiology behind DKA cerebral edema is not clear, retrospective studies have sought to find risk factors associated with the development of cerebral edema. Younger and newly diagnosed patients are more likely to develop cerebral edema, although it can still occur in any DKA patient. Literature suggests lower initial levels of $Paco_2$ and higher initial blood urea nitrogen (BUN) concentrations to be significant risk factors for cerebral edema. Similarly, literature examining mannitol recipients with DKA cerebral edema found significantly lower $Paco_2$ levels, higher BUN concentrations, higher glucose levels, and lower bicarbonate values when compared with controls. It is possible that hypocapnia secondary to severe metabolic acidosis may compromise cerebral perfusion. These studies would imply the DKA patient with greatest risk for cerebral edema to be severely acidotic, hyperventilating, and severely dehydrated.

Data are conflicting concerning the amount of fluid that should be administered to patients with DKA. Historically, it was felt that administration of large amounts of fluid contributed to cerebral edema. However, literature examining cohorts of DKA patients spanning 5.5 years encompassing 865 patients on separate DKA protocols showed total intravenous fluid (IVF) administration rates decreasing from 5.3 to 4.1 $L/m^2/24$ hours, but the incidence of cerebral edema did not change. Recent articles on the amount of dehydration actually present in DKA patients imply that earlier studies may have overestimated the fluid needs of patients with cerebral edema. Limiting the majority of DKA patients to a fluid deficit of less than 10% would be most consistent with the current literature.

The rate of rehydration of DKA patients has generally varied between 36 and 48 hours. However, rate of rehydration has not been found to be a risk factor for cerebral edema in current literature. Similarly, rate of change of serum glucose, presence of an insulin bolus, and tonicity of replacement fluids have not been found to be risk factors for cerebral edema. Conversely, treatment with bicarbonate is a risk factor for DKA cerebral edema. The proposed mechanism behind this is a paradoxical cerebral spinal fluid (CSF) drop in pH and CSF oxygen tension created by the bicarbonate infusion.

Finally, and possibly most important, is the association of DKA cerebral edema with a decrease or minimal increase in serum sodium during therapy. Sodium is the principal factor in serum osmolality. Ideally, sodium will rise to offset the decreasing BUN, glucose, and ketoacid levels in the serum osmolality. A decreasing serum sodium during treatment may be an early warning sign for cerebral edema. The cause of this is not yet defined; hypotonic fluids, cerebral salt wasting, and elevated serum vasopressin have all been suggested as possible etiologies. In an attempt to avoid a decrease in serum sodium during treatment, higher sodium solutions are used as replacement fluids to try to ensure an increase in sodium during treatment. No matter the etiology, treating physicians need to be cautious and mindful of this warning sign during DKA treatment.

Management

Patients with DKA are all at risk for the development of cerebral edema and treatment has centered on preventing this complication. A rational approach to the management of DKA is shown in Figure 54-1 and includes the following key concepts:

1. Assume patients to be less than 10% dehydrated.
2. Correct the patient's deficit over 48 hours; despite slower rehydration, acidosis usually resolves within 24 hours.
3. Give insulin as a continuous infusion and avoid insulin boluses; dropping glucose acutely with insulin may drop osmolality acutely and can potentially lead to cerebral edema.
4. Do not use bolus sodium bicarbonate. A bicarbonate bolus should only be *considered* in a patient with cardiovascular collapse, which is extremely rare.
5. Use a high-sodium solution for rehydration and maintenance fluids; IVF sodium concentrations should contain at least 115 mEq/L. Sodium in the IVF may be decreased later in therapy if needed.
6. Central venous lines should be avoided in the hyper-viscous DKA patient at risk for thrombosis.

All patients should receive continuous cardiac monitoring and hourly neurologic examinations. Complaints of headache should be investigated with a detailed neurologic assessment and monitored closely. A bedside glucose should be performed hourly while on an insulin drip. Electrolytes and serum osmolality should be checked routinely.

Initial laboratory tests should be performed to confirm the diagnosis, and the patient should receive a 10 to 20 mL/kg infusion of isotonic fluid over 1 hour. There likely will be a drop in serum glucose with volume expansion; this is the result of increased renal perfusion and subsequent glucosuria, not serum

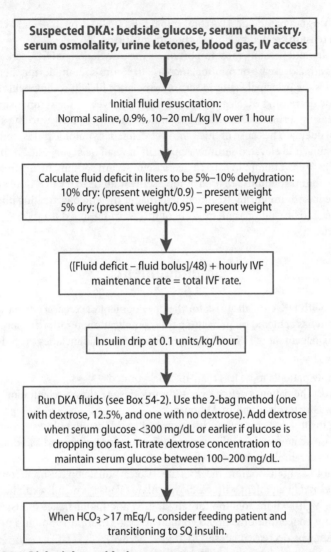

Figure 54-1. Diabetic ketoacidosis management.
Abbreviations: DKA, diabetic ketoacidosis; IV, intravenous; IVF, intravenous fluids; SQ, subcutaneous.

glucose dilution. After confirmation of the correct diagnosis, treatment will include administration of insulin as well as maintenance and deficit IVFs. Most patients with DKA will be less than 10% dehydrated. Dehydration deficit should be calculated using 5% to 7% for moderate dehydration and 10% for severe dehydration DKA. After subtracting the initial fluid bolus, the remaining deficit should be given evenly over 48 hours in addition to an hourly maintenance IVF rate. Most patients correct their acidosis much faster despite the slow rehydration. Initial insulin and bicarbonate boluses should be avoided. Drops in serum sodium and osmolality during DKA treatment should serve as warning signs to the possibility of the development of cerebral edema. A rise in serum sodium does not imply there is no risk of cerebral edema. The author recommends the patient maintain nothing by mouth status during DKA treatment. Allowing clear liquids to a thirsty DKA patient has the potential to be deleterious through the ingestion of large amounts of hypotonic fluid.

A continuous regular insulin infusion at 0.1 units/kg/hour should be administered with IVFs and continued until metabolic acidosis is resolved (HCO_3 >17 mEq/L). It is important to continue the insulin infusion at this rate because the cause of DKA is insulin deficiency. Dextrose concentration can be easily titrated using the 2-bag method, which decreases cost and the time to change IVF dextrose concentrations. This is best accomplished using 2 IVF bags with the same electrolyte concentrations—one bag with 12.5% dextrose (D12.5) and one bag dextrose free. Occasionally, even with all D12.5 IVF running, the patient will not receive enough substrate to prevent hypoglycemia. In this case, the insulin drip may be decreased by 10% to 20% to avoid further hypoglycemia. Historically, glucose has been added to fluids when the serum glucose decreases below 300 mg/dL, although tighter control of the decreasing glucose level may be achieved by earlier addition of dextrose. A goal blood glucose level of 100 to 200 mg/dL should be maintained until acidosis resolves (HCO_3 >17 mEq/L).

The ideal IVF electrolyte composition for treating DKA is unknown. Evidence points to using a high-sodium solution with at least 115 mEq/L. Other reasonable electrolyte additions are potassium and phosphorus to treat total body deficits. Using all chloride as the IVF anion will further drive down bicarbonate values secondary to hyperchloremia. Therefore, phosphate and acetate may be used to avoid worsening the acidosis with excess chloride. Different DKA IVF electrolyte prescriptions are listed in Box 54-2.

Box 54-2. Diabetic Ketoacidosis Intravenous Fluid Electrolyte Prescriptions

½ NS with 40 mEq/L of sodium acetate, 20 mEq/L of potassium chloride, 20 mEq of potassium acetate
¾ NS with 20 mEq/L of potassium acetate, 20 mEq of potassium acetate
NS with 40 mEq/L of potassium acetate
NS with 20 mEq/L of potassium acetate, 20 mEq of potassium acetate

Abbreviation: NS, normal saline.

If symptomatic cerebral edema does develop (see Box 54-1), it should be treated aggressively, as the patient is at great risk for morbidity and mortality. Head CT scan is usually the fastest way to confirm cerebral edema, although treatment should occur prior to a CT scan if clinical symptoms warrant. Mannitol and hypertonic saline are options that will increase serum osmolality and can decrease cerebral edema. A mannitol dose of 1 g/kg would be a reasonable initial treatment dose. If hypertonic saline is used, the author recommends 5 mL/kg of 3% saline for initial DKA cerebral edema treatment and then repeating as needed if there is no improvement in symptoms. Intracranial pressure monitoring may be considered in patients with DKA cerebral edema. To have a chance to prevent the morbidity and mortality associated with DKA cerebral edema, symptomatic cerebral edema must be recognized early and treated immediately.

When metabolic acidosis has been corrected ($HCO_3 >17$ mEq/L), plans for transitioning to subcutaneous (SQ) insulin may occur. There are many acceptable insulin regimens with different dosing and types of insulin. For patients with new onset diabetes mellitus, plans may be discussed with an endocrinologist or physician, who will care for the patient outside the intensive care unit, to determine the preference of an acceptable insulin regimen. Patients known to have diabetes mellitus may resume their home regimen. After SQ insulin, patients may be allowed to eat and the insulin drip and IVFs may be turned off 30 to 60 minutes later. Laboratory tests and intensive care monitoring may also be deescalated.

Suggested Reading

Felner EI, White PC. Improving management of diabetic ketoacidosis in children. *Pediatrics*. 2001;108(3):735–740

Fiordalisi I, Novotny WE, Holbert D, Finberg L, Harris GD; Critical Care Management Group. An 18-yr prospective study of pediatric diabetic ketoacidosis: an approach to minimizing the risk of brain herniation during treatment. *Pediatr Diabetes*. 2007;8(3):142–149

Glaser N, Barnett P, McCaslin I, et al. Risk factors for cerebral edema in children with diabetic ketoacidosis. The Pediatric Emergency Medicine Collaborative Research Committee of the American Academy of Pediatrics. *N Engl J Med*. 2001;344(4): 264–269

Glaser NS, Kuppermann N, Yee CK, Schwartz DL, Styne DM. Variation in the management of pediatric diabetic ketoacidosis by specialty training. *Arch Pediatr Adolesc Med*. 1997;151(11):1125–1132

Glaser NS, Wootton-Gorges SL, Marcin JP, et al. Mechanism of cerebral edema in children with diabetic ketoacidosis. *J Pediatr*. 2004;145(2):164–171

Harris GD, Fiordalisi I. Physiologic management of diabetic ketoacidemia. A 5-year prospective pediatric experience in 231 episodes. *Arch Pediatr Adolesc Med*. 1994;148(10):1046–1052

Katz MA. Hyperglycemia-induced hyponatremia—calculation of expected serum sodium depression. *N Engl J Med*. 1973;289(16):843–844

Levitsky LL. Symptomatic cerebral edema in diabetic ketoacidosis: the mechanism is clarified but still far from clear. *J Pediatr*. 2004;145(2):149–150

Menon R, Sperling MA. Diabetic ketoacidosis. In: *Pediatric Critical Care*. Fuhrman B, Zimmerman JJ, eds. St. Louis, MO: Mosby-Year Book; 1998:844–852

Poirier MP, Greer D, Satin-Smith M. A prospective study of the "two-bag system" in diabetic ketoacidosis management. *Clin Pediatr (Phila).* 2004;43(9):809–813

Roe TF, Crawford TO, Huff KR, Costin G, Kaufman FR, Nelson MD Jr. Brain infarction in children with diabetic ketoacidosis. *J Diabetes Complications.* 1996;10(2):100–108

Wolfsdorf J, Glaser N, Sperling MA; American Diabetes Association. Diabetic ketoacidosis in infants, children, and adolescents: a consensus statement from the American Diabetes Association. *Diabetes Care.* 2006;29(5):1150–1159

CHAPTER 55

Disseminated Intravascular Coagulation and Acute Hemolysis

Ada T. Lin, MD

Key Points

- Diagnosis of disseminated intravascular coagulation (DIC) depends on clinical findings of hemorrhage and microthrombi in patients with predisposing underlying conditions and abnormal coagulation tests. No single test is used to confirm diagnosis.

- Clinical differential diagnosis for DIC is broad and includes a number of diseases that present with bleeding. Laboratory evaluation is key in diagnosis.

- Treatment of the underlying primary disease is of central importance in controlling DIC.

- A hemolytic process can be measured directly by determining erythrocyte survival or indirectly via the presence of increased levels of the metabolic products of hemolysis.

- Patients with hereditary spherocytosis are at risk of an acute exacerbation of their anemia due to an aplastic, hemolytic, or megaloblastic crisis typically triggered by drugs or infections.

- Glucose-6-phosphate dehydrogenase deficiency is a common condition manifested by acute hemolytic episodes induced by infection or certain oxidant drugs.

Overview

Disseminated intravascular coagulation (DIC) and acute hemolysis are uncommon but serious, potentially life-threatening findings in children normally related to infection or malignancy. Disseminated intravascular coagulation is characterized by a consumptive coagulopathy, leading to easy bleeding and hemorrhage, as well as microvascular thrombosis that causes end-organ injury. Acute hemolysis is a rapid drop in red blood cells (RBCs) due to intravascular or extravascular destruction. Often an underlying abnormality is in the RBCs that predisposes them to destruction when stressed by disease. Both DIC and acute hemolysis require rapid investigation and specific treatment. Therapies range from supportive care to blood products and immuno-suppression, depending on the cause.

Causes

Because the causes of DIC and hemolytic anemias are diverse (Boxes 55-1 and 55-2), the evaluation for these entities must include a detailed patient and family history, physical examination, and confirmatory laboratory studies. Not only do these aspects help discern identifiable causes, they also help exclude other diagnoses that might present as acute bleeding, thrombocytopenia, or anemia.

Box 55-1. Causes of Disseminated Intravascular Coagulopathy in Children

Infection
- Bacteria, especially with sepsis, meningococcemia, RMSF
- Virus: HIV, VZV, CMV, Dengue fever, Ebola disease
- Fungal: *Candida* species, *Aspergillus* species
- Malaria

Malignancy
- Acute promyelocytic leukemia
- Acute lymphoblastic leukemia

Trauma
- Brain injury
- Crush injury
- Massive burns
- Extensive surgery

Microangiopathic disorders
- Giant hemangioma known as Kasabach-Merritt syndrome

Gastrointestinal disease
- Liver disease
- Reye syndrome

Neonatal
- Birth asphyxia
- Respiratory distress syndrome
- Meconium aspiration
- Amniotic fluid aspiration
- NEC
- Congenital such as TORCH

Congenital thrombotic disorders
- Homozygous deficiencies of proteins C and S
- Antithrombin III deficiency

Abbreviations: CMV, cytomegalovirus; HIV, human immunodeficiency virus; NEC, necrotizing enterocolitis; RMSF, rocky mountain spotted fever; TORCH, toxoplasmosis, other agents, rubella, cytomegalovirus, herpes simplex; VZV, varicella zoster virus.

Box 55-2. Causes of Hemolytic Anemias

Intrinsic red blood cell defects[a]

Enzyme deficiencies (eg, glucose-6-phosphate dehydrogenase or pyruvate kinase deficiencies)

Hemoglobinopathies (eg, sickle cell disease, thalassemias, unstable hemoglobins)

Membrane defects (eg, hereditary spherocytosis, elliptocytosis)

Extrinsic red blood cell defects

Autoimmune hemolytic anemia (antibodies to patient's own RBCs)

- Warm reactive[b]
- Cold reactive (paroxysmal cold hemoglobinuria/cold agglutinin disease)[c]

Liver disease (cirrhosis, hypersplenism, acquired disorders of RBC membrane)

Hypersplenism

Oxidant agents (dapsone, nitrites, aniline dyes)

Microangiopathies

- Hemolytic uremic syndrome
- Disseminated intravascular coagulation
- Artificial heart valves
- Kasabach-Merritt phenomena

Paroxysmal cold hemoglobinuria[d]

Paroxysmal nocturnal hemoglobinuria[e]

Use of anti-D immune globulin

---

[a] Typically, the intrinsic red blood cell defects require a stressor (drug or infection) to cause an acute hemolytic response. The extrinsic causes typically present as acute hemolysis and associated symptomatic anemia.

[b] Occurs after viral respiratory infections.

[c] Associated with mycoplasma and some viral infections (Epstein-Barr virus).

[d] Congenital or acquired syphilis in past, now with viral infections.

[e] Morning hemoglobinuria, worse with viral illnesses and more chronic than acute.

The clinical manifestations for DIC and acute hemolysis are unique. For DIC, the examination is notable for an unwell patient with bleeding at venipuncture sites, or even severe hemorrhage, as well as thrombosis manifesting as end-organ damage to the kidneys, liver, lungs, and brain and spine. Physical examination can also demonstrate skin manifestations of purpura and acral gangrene (ie, purpura fulminans). Acute hemolysis, because of the acute drop in hemoglobin, typically presents as symptomatic anemia (eg, pallor, hypoxia, tachycardia, dyspnea) and is often associated with splenomegaly, hemoglobinuria, or jaundice. Intravascular hemolysis is more commonly associated with hemoglobinemia and hemoglobinuria (characterized by dark urine), while extravascular hemolysis is more often associated with splenomegaly, jaundice, and anemia.

Evaluation

Laboratory evaluations including serial levels of coagulation parameters (eg, prothrombin time, partial thromboplastin time, fibrinogen, platelet count) aid in monitoring the evolution and resolution of DIC (Table 55-1). Low anti-thrombin and protein C and S levels may also be present but do not affect management.

Table 55-1. Laboratory Evaluation of DIC

Item	Result
Platelet count and peripheral smear	Low numbers, large platelets
PT	Elevated (prolonged)
PTT	Elevated (prolonged)
Fibrinogen	Low
Factor V and VII	Low
FDPs	High
D-dimer assay	High

Abbreviations: DIC, disseminated intravascular coagulation; FDP, fibrin/fibrinogen degradation products; PT, prothrombin time; PTT, partial thromboplastin time.

The differential diagnoses for DIC includes other diseases that present with bleeding, but the laboratory evaluation helps make the final identification. Idiopathic thrombocytopenic purpura also presents with low platelet counts, easy bruising, and slow clotting, but children with it otherwise appear healthy and produce expected findings during coagulation studies.

Hemolytic uremic syndrome also has thrombocytopenia and a microangio-pathic hemolytic anemia, but the prothrombin time and partial thromboplastin time are usually within reference range, and the history and clinical settings are usually very different (Table 55-2). Abnormal coagulation values with a platelet count that is within range is more consistent with other bleeding disorders such as hemophilia or even vitamin K deficiency. Bleeding with coagulation values that are within range and platelet counts indicate platelet dysfunction disorders such as Glanzmann thrombasthenia or fibrinogen activation defects.

Table 55-2. Laboratory Evaluation of Acute Hemolysis

Item	Result
Blood smear	Schistocytes, bite cells, Heinz bodies; if auto-immune mediated (could see rouleaux formation or agglutination of RBCs)
Hemoglobin/hematocrit test	Low (Hgb can drop as low as 2–5 g/dL.)
Haptoglobin test[a]	Low or absent
LDH test	High
UA for blood	Positive (with few or no RBC/high power field)
Direct antiglobulin test (Coombs test)	Positive in autoimmune hemolytic anemia

Abbreviations: Hgb, hemoglobin; LDH, lactate dehydrogenase; RBC, red blood cell; UA, urinalysis.
[a] Not measurable before 2 to 3 months of age. Rule out congenital haptoglobin deficiency.

Management

Both disease processes require immediate identification and treatment of any triggers such as infection, malignancy, or drugs.

Management of DIC

The top priority in managing DIC is to identify and treat whatever is triggering the coagulation cascade. In the interim, issues related to secondary hemorrhage/thrombosis may arise. Listed therapies are scant and when studied are supported by Evidence Levels II-3 or III.

Therapy can be divided into 3 groups: coagulation factor replacement, anticoagulation, and, most recently, anticoagulation factor replacement.

▶ Coagulation factor replacement therapy
  • Use fresh frozen plasma (FFP), cryoprecipitate, and platelets to treat significant bleeding (causing hemodynamic instability) secondary to platelet loss and clotting factor consumption (Evidence Levels II-3 and III).
  • Replace those at high risk because of impending procedures. Replace with goal to reduce or stop significant bleeding by keeping platelet counts above 50 and fibrinogen levels above 100 (Evidence Levels II-3 and III). Replace coagulation factors with cryoprecipitate or FFP. Fresh frozen plasma has both procoagulant and anticoagulant proteins. Replace every 12 to 24 hours at 10 to 15 mL/kg). Cryoprecipitate has higher levels of factor VII and fibrinogen and should be given every 6 hours at 10 mL/kg (Evidence Levels II-3 and III).
  • Published cases so far have not confirmed the theory that transfusing these products results in worsening DIC (Evidence Level III).

▶ Anticoagulation therapy
  • Heparin is contraindicated in central nervous system injury or liver failure, and no controlled trials demonstrate beneficial effects in adults or children with DIC. Even in cases of clinically overt thrombosis and potential end-organ failure, little evidence supports that a heparin infusion improved organ function or prevented subsequent injury.
  • New guidelines recommend that patients critically ill from DIC but without bleeding receive prophylaxis with heparin or low-molecular-weight heparin (Evidence Levels II-1 to III).

▶ Anticoagulant factor replacement: antithrombin and protein C (decreased in DIC)
  • Protein C concentrate has been used to treat purpura fulminans in children with congenital homozygous protein C deficiency and has decreased mortality compared to placebo used in other children. The same is true for some patients with purpura fulminans and meningococcemia (including some children), with reduction in morbidity and

mortality including fewer amputations (Evidence Level II-2). Antithrombin infusion has very limited data in children (Evidence Level II-3). No benefit has been shown in adults with severe sepsis or shock, and the infusion should not be used until safety demonstrated.

- Recombinant human soluble thrombomodulin is a new investigative drug that inactivates coagulation, by binding to thrombin, and activates protein C. It is currently in phase III clinical trials in Japanese patients older than 15 years with DIC from infection or malignancy and shows promise when compared with heparin therapy (Evidence Level II-3).

Management of Acute Hemolysis/Acute Hemolytic Anemia

If the hemolytic episode is infection related, it is most important to treat the infection; if drug related, stop the offending agent (Box 55-3 and Table 55-3).

Box 55-3. Drugs That Can Cause Acute Hemolysis in Patients With G6PD Deficiency, Partial List

- Acetanilid
- Dapsone
- Furazolidone
- Methylene Blue
- Nalidixic acid
- Naphthalene
- Niridazole
- Nitrofurantoin
- Phenazopyridine
- Phenylhydrazine
- Primaquine
- Sulfacetamide
- Sulfamethoxazole
- Sulfanilamide
- Sulfapyridine
- Thiazolsulfone
- Toluidine Blue
- Trinitrotoluene
- Uricase (rasburicase, pegloticase)

Abbreviation: G6PD, glucose-6-phosphate dehydrogenase.

Table 55-3. Laboratory Characteristics and Therapy for Primary Autoimmune Hemolytic Anemia (Acute Forms)

Parameter	Warm-Reactive	Cold Agglutinin	Paroxysmal Cold Hemoglobinuria
Autoantibody isotype	IgG	IgM	IgG
Positive DAT (Coombs)	IgG, ± C3	C3	C3, ± IgG
Type of hemolysis	Extravascular	Both	Intravascular
First-line therapy (Evidence is Level II-2, at best.)	Corticosteroids	Avoidance of cold	Avoidance of cold
Second-line therapy (Level II-3–Level III)	Splenectomy, rituximab (off-label)	Plasmapheresis	Corticosteroids

Transfusion may be required if the affected child is hemodynamically unstable or hypoxic but only provides transient relief. In the case of the autoimmune hemolytic anemias, completely compatible blood is challenging to find, and often incomplete matched units must be given.

In both DIC and acute hemolysis, once the underlying cause is removed and the patient is stabilized with the appropriate therapies, these patients can make a complete recovery. The outcome is generally more driven by the underlying cause and effectiveness of the specific therapy.

Suggested Reading

Bick RL. Disseminated intravascular coagulation current concepts of etiology, pathophysiology, diagnosis and treatment. *Hematol Oncol Clin North Am.* 2003;17(1): 149–176

Franchini M, Manzato F. Update on the treatment of disseminated intravascular coagulation. *Hematology.* 2004;9(2):81–85

Levi M. Disseminated intravascular coagulation. *Crit Care Med.* 2007;35(9):2191–2195

Levi M, Toh CH, Thachil J, Watson HG. Guidelines for the diagnosis and management of disseminated intravascular coagulation. British Committee for Standards in Haematology. *Br J Haematol.* 2009;145(1):24–33

Oski FA, Brugnara C, Nathan DG. A diagnostic approach to the anemic patient. In: *Nathan and Oski's Hematology of Infancy and Childhood.* 6th ed. Nathan DG, Orkin SH, Ginsberg D, Look AT, eds. Philadelphia, PA: WB Saunders; 2003:409

Recht M, Pearson H. The hemolytic anemias. In: *Oski's Pediatrics.* McMillan JA, Deangelis CD, Feigin RD, Warshaw JB, eds. Philadelphia, PA: Lippincott Williams & Wilkins; 1999:1453

Williams M, Chalmers EA, Gibson BE, et al. The investigation and management of neonatal haemostasis and thrombosis. *Br J Haematol.* 2002;119(2):295–309

CHAPTER 56

Drowning

Nicole O'Brien, MD

Key Points

- Nearly all patients who demonstrate significant problems with oxygenation or ventilation will do so within 4 to 6 hours of the incident. Patients who remain asymptomatic after this time period can be safely discharged.

- Pneumonia is often misdiagnosed initially because of the radiographic appearance of water in the lungs. Prophylactic antibiotic therapy has not been proven to have any benefit.

- The major determinant of morbidity and mortality following drowning in the pediatric patient is the degree of neurologic injury sustained.

- Up to 80% of drowning episodes in pediatric patients are preventable. Adult supervision of infants and children around toilets, bathtubs, and bodies of water is imperative. Appropriate barriers, such as pool fencing with a latching, self-closing gate, are recommended. Swimming lessons have not been shown to decrease the risk of drowning and may not be developmentally appropriate for children younger than 4 years.

Overview

Exact definitions of drowning have varied widely over the years. At the World Congress on Drowning in 2002, a new consensus definition was reached in an attempt to allow for more accurate reporting of the disease as well as analysis and comparison of studies. Drowning is defined as respiratory impairment from submersion/immersion in a liquid, the outcome of which can be no morbidity, morbidity, or mortality (Evidence Level III). Any incident of submersion/immersion without evidence of respiratory impairment should be termed a *water rescue* rather than a *drowning*. Terms such as *near drowning, dry or wet drowning*, and *active or passing drowning* should not be used in modern clinical medicine.

Differential Diagnosis

In very young children, the possibility of unintentional injury should be considered. In adolescents, alcohol/drug intoxication, the possibility of a suicide attempt, or both should be entertained. Seizures occurring during swimming can lead to drowning and should be considered and evaluated for in the absence of other precipitating factors for drowning. Similarly, fatal arrhythmias can be triggered by water-related activities in children with long-QT (particularly type I) or catecholaminergic polymorphic ventricular tachycardia and should be evaluated for in cases of drowning without significant risk factors. Of note, head or spine trauma occurs in less than 0.5% of persons who drown, and immobilization is required only in cases when head or neck injury is strongly suspected (eg, diving accidents).

Clinical Features

A wide spectrum of clinical features can be seen following a drowning episode. Patients may be completely asymptomatic or may have multiple organ systems affected because of significant systemic hypoxemia and acidosis.

Pulmonary

Aspiration of freshwater results in denaturation of alveolar surfactant with subsequent atelectasis, marked ventilation/perfusion mismatching, and systemic hypoxia. Aspiration of saltwater results in the creation of a large osmotic gradient with fluid pulled into the alveoli and subsequent dilution of surfactant. The result is similar to that of freshwater aspiration with subsequent atelectasis, ventilation/perfusion mismatching, and systemic hypoxia. The severity of respiratory impairment following drowning varies widely. Children rescued after a brief period of submersion will often have a limited period of hypoxia that resolves during initial resuscitative efforts. These patients will often present with no or few respiratory concerns. Children who have been submerged for longer periods of time will often have more significant hypoxia. Rapid progression to acute respiratory distress syndrome with severe refractory hypoxemia is not uncommon following drowning. Furthermore, aspiration of vomit or other debris may result in further problems with gas exchange or severe bronchospasm with clinically evident wheezing.

Cardiovascular

Cardiovascular instability is often encountered following drowning. Hypoxia and acidosis may lead to ventricular dysrhythmias, pulseless electrical activity, or asystole. Increased pulmonary artery pressures often occur because of release of pulmonary inflammatory mediators. Pulmonary hypertension leads to increased right ventricular afterload, decreased left ventricular preload, and subsequent decreased cardiac output. Additionally, prolonged hypoxia can lead to myocardial ischemia and dysfunction with resultant further decreased cardiac output and cardiogenic shock. Clinical evidence of shock includes tachycardia, poor peripheral perfusion and pulses, and hypotension.

Neurologic

Variable degrees of hypoxic ischemic encephalopathy can be seen following drowning. Patients may be awake and alert on presentation, blunted to stuporous but with expected pupillary and pain responses, or comatose with abnormal pupillary responses and decorticate/decerebrate movements. Seizures, myoclonic jerking, or both may occur because of diffuse cerebral hypoxia.

Other Organ Systems

Prolonged systemic hypoxia can result in acute tubular necrosis with subsequent renal dysfunction, as evidenced by oliguria or anuria and elevated creatinine. Hepatic injury may result in elevated transaminase levels, decreased albumin concentrations, and prolonged clotting times. Disseminated intravascular coagulation is also frequently encountered. Of note, most patients experiencing an episode of drowning do not develop blood volume alterations with subsequent anemia or electrolyte disturbances such as hyponatremia or hypernatremia. While most patients aspirate an average of 3 mL/kg, aspiration of greater than 11 mL/kg is required for blood volume alterations, and greater than 22 mL/kg is required for electrolyte alterations (Evidence Level II-3).

Evaluation

Pediatric patients who are asymptomatic following submersion injury require no specific evaluation. They should have basic vital signs, including oxygen saturation, checked. Routine measurement of hematocrit or serum electrolyte levels is not necessary. Blood gases are only indicated for children with significant respiratory insufficiency and concern for impending respiratory failure or following intubation for ongoing respiratory failure. Chest radiographs can be obtained in individuals who are symptomatic and can be as expected, show patchy peripheral infiltrates, or have evidence of frank pulmonary edema.

Management

Pre-hospital Management

Once rescued, the child who has drowned should undergo standard checks for responsiveness, breathing, and pulse. If necessary, emergency medical services should be called and cardiopulmonary resuscitation (CPR) with rescue breaths and chest compressions should be initiated. Cardiopulmonary resuscitations with chest compressions only is not advised for drowning persons (Evidence Level III). The main goal of pre-hospital care should be to improve oxygenation and ventilation as rapidly as possible to improve long-term neurologic outcome.

In-hospital Management

The 4 most important management issues involve the respiratory system, the cardiovascular system, infectious diseases, and neurologic support and treatments.

Respiratory

Patients who are asymptomatic can be observed. Nearly all patients who demonstrate significant problems with gas exchange will do so within 4 to 6 hours of the incident. Therefore, patients remaining asymptomatic after this period of observation can be safely discharged. Patients with mild hypoxia can receive supplemental oxygen via nasal cannula or face mask. Some patients will have continued hypoxemia despite supplemental oxygen and will also require bilevel or continuous positive airway pressure. Positive airway pressure improves atelectasis and pulmonary edema, reduces intrapulmonary shunting, and can improve moderate hypoxemia following drowning. Children will often require supplemental oxygen or noninvasive ventilation for 48 to 72 hours, as this is the amount of time it takes for pulmonary surfactant to reconstitute. Patients with significant respiratory distress not responding to noninvasive ventilation or with decreased mental status and inability to protect their airway require intubation and mechanical ventilation. Current management of severe respiratory failure resembles management of patients with acute respiratory distress syndrome. Avoidance of ventilator-induced lung injury is important, and an open-lung approach allowing tidal volumes of 5 to 6 mL/kg while using positive end-expiratory pressure to support oxygenation should be the mainstays of management. Inhaled nitric oxide, artificial surfactant, liquid ventilation, and extracorporeal membrane oxygenation have been used with some success for refractory hypoxemia (Evidence Level II-2).

Cardiovascular

Dysrhythmias are frequently encountered early in resuscitation following drowning. Rapid correction of hypoxia and acidosis should be undertaken. Additionally, standard pediatric advanced live support techniques with appropriate medication administration should be undertaken. Isotonic fluids should be used to correct hypovolemia. Inotropic support with dobutamine or epinephrine may be required for ongoing poor perfusion, lactic acidosis, or hypotension following appropriate fluid resuscitation.

Infectious Diseases

Pneumonia is often initially misdiagnosed because of the radiographic appearance of water in the lungs. Prophylactic antibiotic therapy has not proven to have any benefit (Evidence Level II-2). However, these patients are at risk of pulmonary infection with waterborne or oropharyngeal organisms as well as nosocomial pathogens. Patients should be monitored closely for fever, sustained leukocytosis, or persistent/new pulmonary infiltrates on chest radiography. If any of these are present, broad-spectrum empiric antibiotics are appropriate. Tracheal cultures with sensitivity testing may be useful to narrow antibiotic treatment when results are available.

Neurologic

The degree of central nervous system hypoxic ischemic injury is currently the major determinant of morbidity and mortality following pediatric drowning. Historical factors that may correlate with poor neurologic outcome following drowning include duration of submersion less than 4 to 5 minutes, warm water temperature ($>70°F$ [$21°C$]), need for CPR in the field, and continued apnea, asystole, or coma after arrival to the emergency department. Initial laboratory values such as pH less than 7.1 and elevated serum glucose levels have also been found to correlate with worse neurologic outcome (Evidence Level II-3). Children without purposeful movements on neurologic examination less than 24 hours from the drowning incident have dismal long-term neurologic outcomes (Evidence Level II-2). Lastly, pediatric patients with evidence of hypoxic ischemic injury, such as loss of gray-white differentiation, low density lesions in basal ganglia and thalami, or effacement of cisterns on initial or subsequent head computed tomography scan, routinely have poor neurologic outcomes (Evidence Level II-2). Therefore, historical features of the drowning event should be noted, basic laboratory values obtained, and serial neurologic examinations performed. Additionally, head computed tomography should be performed in children with altered mental status to help prognosticate neurologic outcome for family members.

The treatment goal is to avoid instances where hypoxic ischemic brain injury is worsened. Therefore, seizures with subsequent increased cerebral metabolic demand should be avoided. Additionally, hypoglycemia should be avoided and a normal partial pressure of carbon dioxide (35–45 mm Hg) should be maintained. Various interventions such as intracranial pressure monitoring, hyperventilation, and pharmacologic therapy have not been shown to improve outcomes in children sustaining hypoxic ischemic injury, and routine use should not be undertaken (Evidence Level I). Cerebral oxygen consumption is reduced by 5% to 7% for each 1°C (1.8°F) reduction in body temperature below 37°C (98.6°F). As such, induced hypothermia to 32 to 34°C (89.6–93.2°F) for 24 hours may reduce the degree of hypoxic ischemic injury sustained by these patients and can be considered as part of the management strategy for children who remain comatose following initial resuscitation (Evidence Level III).

Other Organ Systems

Typically, both renal and hepatic injuries are self-limited and resolve with supportive care alone.

Long-term Implications

Most children experiencing a drowning episode will be asymptomatic at the time of discharge from the hospital. Provided the child is at his or her baseline, routine follow-up with a primary care physician is appropriate for these children. Children with significant neurologic injury may require occupational or physical therapy and rehabilitation evaluation and treatment.

About up to 80% of drowning episodes in pediatric patients are preventable. Adult supervision of infants and children around toilets, bathtubs, and bodies of water is imperative. Appropriate barriers, such as pool fencing with a latching, self-closing gate, are recommended. It should be noted that swimming lessons have not been shown to decrease the risk of drowning and may not be developmentally appropriate for children younger than 4 years.

Suggested Reading

Bowman SM, Aitken ME, Robbins JM, Baker SP. Trends in US pediatric drowning hospitalizations, 1993-2008. *Pediatrics*. 2012;129(2):275–281

Meyer RJ, Theodorous AA, Berg RA. Childhood drowning. *Pediatr Rev*. 2006;27(5): 163–169

Rafaat TK, Spear RM, Kuelbs C, Parsapour K, Peterson B. Cranial computed tomographic findings of children with drowning. *Pediatr Crit Care Med*. 2008;9(6): 567–572

Suominen PK, Vahatalo R, Sintonen H, Haverinen A, Roine RP. Health-related quality of life after a drowning incident as a child. *Resuscitation*. 2011;82(26):1318–1322

Szpilman D, Bierens JLM, Handley AJ, Orlowski JP. Drowning. *N Engl J Med*. 2012;366(22):2102–2110

Vanden Hoek TL, Morrison LJ, Shuster M, et al. Part 12: cardiac arrest in special situations: drowning: 2010 American Heart Association Guidelines for Cardiopulmonary Resuscitation and Emergency Cardiovascular Care. *Circulation*. 2010;122(18 Suppl 3):S847–S848

Warner D, Knape J. Recommendations and consensus brain resuscitation in the drowning victim. In: Bierens JJLM, ed. *Handbook on Drowning: Prevention, Rescue, and Treatment*. Berlin, Germany: Springer-Verlag; 2006:436–439

CHAPTER 57

Electrical Injury

Mary Jo Bowman, MD

Key Points

- Electrical injuries are relatively common, generally unintentional, and typically preventable in children.

- The 3 major types of electrical injuries are those due to direct effect of the current; those due to conversion of electrical to thermal energy, resulting in burns; and those due to blunt mechanical trauma.

- Electrical injuries often cause multiorgan injury and dysfunction as well as thermal burns and traumatic injuries. Cardiac, renal, neurologic, eye, musculoskeletal, and dermal injuries are particularly important concerns.

- Evaluation of a child with an electrical injury should include an electrocardiogram; testing of serum chemistries, creatine phosphokinase level, complete blood count, and unstable angina; and radiographs of any suspected injuries.

- Children with high voltage electrical injury or lightning strike should be treated like any major trauma patient; continuous cardiac monitoring, aggressive fluid resuscitation, and continued monitoring for evidence of organ system dysfunction are important priorities.

Overview

Electrical injuries in children are relatively common, generally unintentional, and typically preventable. Three major types of injuries occur: those due to direct effect of the current; those due to conversion of electrical to thermal energy, resulting in burns; and those due to blunt mechanical trauma. All mechanisms can lead to tissue destruction and organ dysfunction.

Classifications of electrical injuries usually focus on the power source (ie, electrical or lightning), voltage (ie, high or low), and type of current (ie, alternating or direct). Each of these classifications is associated with certain patterns of injury. Knowing these patterns will assist in diagnosis and management of the injuries (Table 57-1).

Table 57-1. Comparison Among Lightning, High Voltage, and Low Voltage Electrical Injuries

	Lightning	High Voltage	Low Voltage
Voltage, V	>30 × 10	>1,000	<600
Current, A	>200,000	<1,000	<240
Duration	Instantaneous	Brief	Prolonged
Type of current	DC	DC or AC	Mostly AC
Cardiac arrest	Asystole	Ventricular fibrillation	Ventricular fibrillation
Respiratory arrest	Direct CNS injury	Indirect trauma or tetanic contraction of respiratory muscles	Tetanic contractions of respiratory muscles
Muscles	Single	Single (DC); Tetanic (AC)	Tetanic
Burns	Rare, superficial	Common, deep	Usually superficial
Rhabdomyolysis	Uncommon	Very common	Common
Blunt injury (cause)	Blast effect	Fall (muscle contraction)	Fall (uncommon)
Acute mortality	Very high	Moderate	Low

From Koumbourlis AC. Electrical injuries. *Crit Care Med.* 2002; 30(11 Suppl):S424–S430, with permission.

Young children (<6 y) often are injured when biting into electrical cords or coming into contact with electrical outlets. These are low voltage injuries. Older children and adolescents generally sustain high voltage injuries from coming in contact with power lines while climbing trees or utility poles.

Lightning injuries are a subset of electrical injury and can occur in any age group. These are extremely high voltage injuries. A new source of electrical injury is from an electrical weapon, such as a stun gun or a Taser, a conducted electrical weapon. These devices deliver short bursts of high voltage, with low amperage current.

Clinical Features

Electrical injuries often cause multiorgan dysfunction as well as thermal burns and traumatic injuries.

Cardiac

Approximately 15% of patients have arrhythmia due to electrical injury. Most of these are benign and occur within the first few hours. However, cardiac arrest can occur because of asystole (usually lightning or DC current) or ventricular fibrillation (AC current). Ventricular fibrillation is the most common fatal arrhythmia, occurring in a large percentage of patients in whom the current flows from one hand to another. The most common electrocardiogram (ECG) abnormalities are sinus tachycardia and nonspecific ST-T wave changes.

Renal

Renal injury may occur from rhabdomyolysis (ie, massive tissue necrosis), which causes myoglobin release from damaged muscle. Hypovolemia may worsen and complicate the process of renal tubular cell damage from the myoglobin.

Neurologic

Damage can occur to both the central and peripheral nervous systems. This may manifest as loss of consciousness, weakness or paralysis, amnesia, and autonomic dysfunction. Sensory and motor deficits are common. Kerauno-paralysis is paralysis specific to lightning injury and is characterized by blue, mottled, and pulseless extremities. These findings are thought to be secondary to vascular spasm and generally resolve.

Eyes

Cataracts are the most common injury seen in electrical and lightning injury, developing immediately or later in the course. Hyphema and vitreous hemorrhage may also occur, especially following lightning injury.

Musculoskeletal

Bones can fracture because of falls, blast injury, or repetitive tetanic muscular contractions. In addition, acute compartment syndrome can develop because of tissue necrosis and edema from deep injury.

Skin

All types of burns can be seen, from superficial to deep full-thickness burns. They are most common at the site of electrical contact and at places in contact with the ground at the time of injury. The most common entry points are the hands and skull, with feet having the most common exit wounds. The degree of internal damage cannot be determined by the degree of external injury. Oral burns can occur in young children who chew or suck on electrical cords, resulting in injuries that are often full thickness and involve the lips and oral commissure. Initially, these burns may be painless and bloodless. When the eschar separates, usually in 1 to 2 weeks, severe hemorrhage can occur from the labial artery (Figure 57-1). Deep burns are unusual in lightning injury because of the short duration of contact. Feathering superficial branching burns (known as Lichtenburg figures) are pathognomonic of lightning injury and occur from the flashover effect of the lightning.

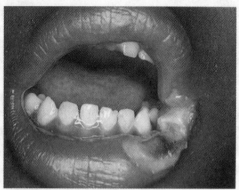

Figure 57-1. Oral commissure burn in toddler.

From Martin B, Baumhardt H, D'Alesio A, et al. Oral disorders. In: Zitelli BJ, McIntire SC, Nowalk AJ, eds. *Zitelli and Davis' Atlas of Pediatric Physical Diagnosis*. 6th ed. Philadelphia, PA: Elsevier Saunders; 2012:796, with permission.

Other

Ruptured tympanic membranes are very common in lightning injury. Damage to internal organs is uncommon, unless the victim falls or is thrown.

Evaluation

Diagnostic studies should be obtained on a case-by-case basis, determined by results of the physical examination and type of injury. Knowing the patterns of injury and their sequelae will help guide the work-up. In general, however, most patients sustaining electrical injury should have the following diagnostic studies performed (Evidence Level III):

- ▶ ECG
- ▶ Serum electrolyte levels, including those of potassium and calcium
- ▶ Creatine phosphokinase level
- ▶ Renal function studies (of blood urea nitrogen and creatinine)
- ▶ Complete blood count
- ▶ Urinalysis
- ▶ Radiographic studies of any suspected injuries

Management

Patients who sustain high voltage electrical injury or lightning strike should be treated like any major trauma patient. Attention to airway, breathing, and circulation (commonly referred to as the ABCs), including cervical spine immobilization, is important. Prolonged cardiopulmonary resuscitation should be undertaken, even in the case of asystole, as good outcomes have been reported. Paralysis of respiratory muscles may occur, and endotracheal intubation may be needed. Arrhythmias are treated as per Pediatric Advanced Life Support guidelines. Cardiac monitoring is a must if loss of consciousness occurred, arrhythmia is in the field, or the initial ECG findings are abnormal. Fluid resuscitation should be aggressive. Use of the Parkland or similar formulas for fluid resuscitation should be avoided, as they often underestimate the extent of the burn injury. Monitoring urine output is more reliable in this instance. Avoid use of potassium initially in fluids because of the risk of severe hyperkalemia. A patient in a coma or having a neurologic deficit should undergo appropriate brain imaging, spine imaging, or both (Evidence Level III).

Once the patient has been stabilized, it is important to complete a secondary assessment to identify other injuries. Skin burns should be treated per usual protocol. Tetanus prophylaxis should be given if indicated. If other injuries are identified, appropriate management and consultation should be obtained. These may include orthopedic, ophthalmologic, or otolaryngologic injuries.

Monitoring should be ongoing for acute compartment syndrome and rhabdomyolysis with resultant renal injury. Urine may need to be alkalinized with fluids containing bicarbonate. Adequate urine output of 1 to 2 mL/kg per hour should be maintained. Mannitol or furosemide may be used to promote good urine output and can be used if the patient is hemodynamically stable (Evidence Level III).

Children who sustain lip or oral commissure burns (or both) should be seen by a pediatric burn surgeon. Consultation or follow-up with a plastic surgeon or pediatric oral surgeon may be needed. It is important that families are counseled on the risk of delayed severe hemorrhage when the eschar separates and to seek prompt medical care. Oral appliances are sometimes used to help decrease scarring and improve function (Evidence Level III).

Disposition

Severely injured patients and those experiencing cardiopulmonary arrest are admitted to the hospital, generally to an intensive care unit. Transfer to a burn center is warranted in the case of severe electrical burns.

Patients sustaining a high voltage exposure or lightning strike should be admitted for cardiac monitoring and observation. Any patient who lost consciousness, who has an arrhythmia, or whose findings on the ECG or laboratory are abnormal should also be admitted for further monitoring.

Patients who sustain a low voltage exposure, who are asymptomatic, and whose findings on the physical examination are within reference range do not require ancillary testing and can be discharged safely. Patients with mild symptoms or minor burns whose findings on the ECG and test for unstable angina are within reference range can be observed for a few hours and discharged with close follow-up.

Patients who come in contact with electrical weapons are rarely injured by the device itself. The most common injuries are due to the fall after being "stunned." No evidence suggests delayed arrhythmia or cardiac damage, especially if exposure is less than 15 seconds. Deaths have been rarely reported due to fatal arrhythmia. These were felt to be due to concurrent intoxication with cocaine, phencyclidine, methamphetamine, or other stimulants. Patients who are asymptomatic and alert after exposure do not need prolonged observation or diagnostic testing.

Suggested Reading

Cooper MA, Holle RL, Andrews CJ, et al. Lightning injuries. In: Auerbach PS, ed. *Wilderness Medicine.* 6th ed. St Louis, MO: Mosby; 2012

Gardner AR, Hauda WE II, Bozeman WP. Conducted electrical weapon (TASER) use against minors: a shocking analysis. *Pediatr Emer Care.* 2012;28(9):873–877

Koumbourlis AC. Electrical injuries. *Crit Care Med.* 2002;30(11 Suppl):S424–S430

Rabban JT, Blair JA, Rosen CL, Adler JN, Sheridan RL. Mechanisms of pediatric electrical injury. New implications for product safety and injury prevention. *Arch Pediatr Adolesc Med.* 1997;151(7):696–700

Rosen CL, Adler JN, Rabban JT, et al. Early predictors of myoglobinuria and acute renal failure following electrical injury. *J Emerg Med.* 1999;17(5):783–789

Spies C, Trohman RG. Narrative review: electrocution and life-threatening electrical injuries. *Ann Intern Med.* 2006;145(7):531–537

CHAPTER 58

Epistaxis

Delia L. Gold, MD, and Leslie Mihalov, MD

Key Points

- Most pediatric epistaxises are from anterior sources. These bleeds frequently stop with simple compression of the nares against the anterior septum.

- Epistaxis is rarely the only manifestation of systemic illness. Laboratory evaluation is rarely indicated in pediatric epistaxis. If there is clinical suspicion of a bleeding disorder, a complete blood count with differential and peripheral smear, prothrombin time, partial thromboplastin time, and screening test for von Willebrand disease should be obtained. A positive family history of abnormal bleeding and a prolonged partial thromboplastin time are predictive of a coagulopathy.

- Vaseline does not confer any therapeutic benefit over simple observation in treatment for epistaxis. Antibiotic ointment is effective in decreasing recurrent epistaxis in the short-term but has not been proven to confer long-term benefit.

- The patient should be referred to an otolaryngologist (ie, ear, throat, and nose specialist) if epistaxis does not respond to ointments or chemical cautery, if the bleed requires anterior packing, or if there is suspicion of a nasal mass.

- The patient should be referred to the emergency department for an emergent ear, nose, and throat evaluation if there is a posterior bleed, if the bleed is severe, or if hemodynamic instability is noted.

Overview

Epistaxis, or nasal bleeding, is a common condition in childhood and one of the most common reasons for referral of children to an otolaryngologist (ie, ear, nose, and throat specialist). Although this is often a benign self-limited condition, epistaxis can be alarming to parents and children alike. Diagnosis and treatment depend on defining the etiology, location, and intensity of bleeding and implementing the most effective treatment strategies related to the defining features.

Causes and Differential Diagnosis

Epistaxis is often described as either anterior or posterior bleeding, depending on the location of the source. The most common site of bleeding is known as *Kiesselbach plexus,* an area of the anterior septum of the nose where vessels from the ethmoid branches of the internal carotid arteries and the facial and internal maxillary divisions of the external carotid arteries anastomose (Figure 58-1). The anterior location and thin mucosal covering make this area especially prone to trauma, and anterior nosebleeds account for roughly 90% of cases in children. Posterior epistaxis generally arises from the posterior nasal cavity via branches of the sphenopalatine arteries and may be more difficult to diagnose, as it is often harder to visualize the actual site of bleeding.

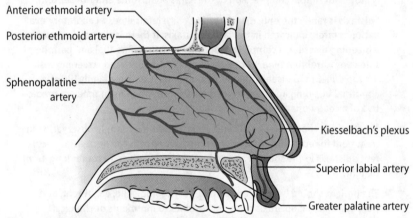

Anterior ethmoid artery

Posterior ethmoid artery

Sphenopalatine artery

Kiesselbach's plexus

Superior labial artery

Greater palatine artery

Figure 58-1. Vascular anatomy of nasal septal blood supply.

The etiologies of epistaxis can be divided into 2 general categories, local or systemic causes (Box 58-1). The most common causes of nosebleeds in children include digital trauma, mucosal dryness, rhinitis, and foreign body. Self-inflicted digital trauma is particularly common in children, but other more potentially serious forms of trauma such as nasal fracture, vascular injury to the carotid artery, or intentional trauma should also be considered. Intentional trauma may also be a cause of epistaxis, especially in a baby younger than 1 year, as epistaxis in this age group is exceedingly rare and often associated with injury or serious illness (Evidence Level III). Any cause of acute inflammation or irritation will predispose the nose to bleeding, including changes in humidity, allergies or rhinitis, infection, use of nasal sprays, or exposure to inhalants or substances of abuse. Viral and bacterial upper respiratory tract infections in particular cause inflammation of the nasal mucosa, which leads to more friable tissue that is prone to bleeding. Nasal colonization with *Staphylococcus aureus* may be associated with an increased risk of epistaxis, with a recent prospective study demonstrating that *S aureus* was 33% more prevalent in the patient group with epistaxis as compared to control groups (Evidence Level II-2). Neoplasms of the nasal cavity are a rare but important potential cause of epistaxis in children. Benign localized neoplasms include juvenile nasopharyngeal angio-fibroma, hemangiomas, and telangiectasias, as seen in Osler-Weber-Rendu disease, pyogenic granulomas, and nasal papillomas. Malignant neoplasms compose a very small portion of pediatric head and neck cancers, with rhabdomyosarcoma being the most common nasal malignancy (Evidence Level III).

Box 58-1. Differential Diagnosis of Epistaxis

Local Predisposing Factors
- Trauma
  - Direct vascular or mucosal
  - Picking
  - Intentional trauma
  - Foreign body
  - Post-procedure (eg, surgery, nasogastric tube, nasotracheal intubation)
- Local inflammation
  - Acute viral upper respiratory tract infection
  - Bacterial rhinitis/sinusitis
  - Allergic rhinitis
  - Dry air (eg, *rhinitis sicca*)
  - Inhaled irritants/drugs
  - Localized skin or mucosa infection
  - Nasal polyps (cystic fibrosis, allergic, generalized)
- Vascular malformations (eg, telangiectasias, hemangiomas)
- Juvenile angiofibroma
- Tumors (eg, pyogenic granuloma, rhabdomyosarcoma, nasopharyngeal carcinoma)

Systemic Predisposing Factors
- Hematologic diseases
  - Platelet disorders
    - Quantitative: idiopathic thrombocytopenic purpura, leukemia, aplastic anemia
    - Qualitative: von Willebrand disease, Glanzmann disease, uremia
  - Hemophilias
  - Clotting disorders associated with severe hepatic disease, disseminated intravascular coagulation, vitamin K deficiency
  - Drugs: aspirin, NSAIDs, warfarin, valproic acid, rodenticide
- Granulomatous disease (eg, Wegener granulomatosis, sarcoidosis, tuberculosis)
- Vicarious menstruation
- Hypertension
  - Arterial (unusual in children)
  - Venous: superior vena cava syndrome, increased venous pressure (eg, secondary to paroxysmal coughing, exertion)

Abbreviation: NSAID, nonsteroidal anti-inflammatory drug.

Epistaxis is rarely the only manifestation of systemic disease. Systemic disease is more likely if the nosebleeds are severe or recurrent, there is a family history of bleeding disorders, constitutional signs or symptoms are present, screening laboratory results are abnormal, or all other local causes have been excluded. Bleeding disorders such von Willebrand disease or other platelet dysfunction, as well as others such as leukemia, hemophilia, or idiopathic thrombocytopenic purpura, can cause epistaxis. Medications that affect the coagulation cascade may lead to epistaxis, as well as arterial hypertension, increased venous congestion in the nose, or inflammatory disorders such as polyangiitis with granulomatosis (Wegener granulomatosis). A rare condition known as *vicarious menstruation* should be considered in a young woman who has monthly epistaxis in association with her menses. This is thought to be due to increased capillary permeability secondary to changes in hormone levels associated with menstruation.

Clinical Features

Epistaxis usually occurs suddenly from one nostril, but occasionally it can stem from both. As most nosebleeds are anterior in origin, one may be able to visualize the source of bleeding immediately and attempt to apply pressure there by pinching the nose. If the bleeding occurs at night only, or is posterior in origin, the blood may be swallowed and cause stomach upset, vomiting, hematemesis, or melena. Blood seen in the oropharynx, blood seen in both nares, difficulty controlling the bleeding despite appropriate anterior pressure, and no direct visualization of the bleeding site are features more often seen in posterior bleeds.

Evaluation

Although epistaxis is rarely life threatening, the initial step of evaluation is to ensure that the patient is medically stable. A rapid assessment of general appearance, vital signs, airway protection, and mental status will ensure that the patient does not have hemodynamic or respiratory instability that necessitates transfer to an emergency department. Once that is determined, the history and physical examination can be performed. In the history, special care should be taken to establish the duration of symptoms, perceived amount of bleeding, history of previous treatment modalities and their effectiveness, and if history includes trauma to the area. Evaluation for associated or systemic symptoms will also help determine etiology of the epistaxis. For instance, extensive gastrointestinal tract symptoms, such as abdominal pain or vomiting, may suggest a posterior nasal bleed. History positive for nasal congestion, discharge, or obstruction may indicate allergic rhinitis, a foreign body, or possibly a mass. Last, investigation into allergies, medications, or illicit drug use, as well as a family history of easy bruising or bleeding problems in the patient or family, will help guide further evaluation and management.

Physical examination is an integral part of evaluation. The immediate goal is to identify the source of bleeding and control it. Examination of the nose and nasopharynx of a young child may be difficult and may be facilitated by application of a topical anesthetic combined with a vasoconstricting agent. The area of Kiesselbach's plexus should be examined first, as this is the source of most nosebleeds. A foreign body or nasal mass may also be visualized if it is located in the nares.

Laboratory evaluation is not indicated in most children with self-limited epistaxis. If the bleeding is from an anterior source, resolves spontaneously or with minimal intervention, and is not significant, blood work will likely be within reference range. On the other hand, if a bleeding disorder, severe epistaxis, recurrent epistaxis, or a nasal mass is suspected or evident, additional studies are warranted (Evidence Level III). Recommended laboratory studies are listed in Box 58-2. If any of these labs are abnormal, referral to a pediatric hematologist is reasonable. A retrospective study of children referred to a pediatric hematologist for recurrent epistaxis found that 33% of the study population had a bleeding disorder, and that von Willebrand disease was the most common diagnosis in their series. Additionally, a family history of abnormal bleeding and a prolonged partial thromboplastin time were variables that if positive were predictive of diagnosing a coagulopathy (Evidence Level III). Imaging of the nasal cavity should be performed in children with epistaxis if a mass is suspected or directly visualized. Contrast-enhanced computed tomography or magnetic resonance imaging may delineate the mass, but the work-up of a nasal mass should not be undertaken without consultation with an ears, nose, and throat (ENT) specialist. Other indications for consultation include bleeds that are severe or posterior in origin, recurrent epistaxis that is distressing to the patient or family, or epistaxis that requires extensive emergency department management such as nasal packing or cautery.

Box 58-2. Laboratory Studies in Evaluation of Severe or Recurrent Epistaxis or Concern for a Coagulation Disorder

- Complete blood count with a peripheral smear
- Prothrombin time
- Activated partial thromboplastin time
- Screening tests for von Willebrand disease (usually VWF antigen, VWF activity [ristocetin cofactor] and factor VIII activity)
- Blood type and screen for patients who may require transfusion

Abbreviation: VWF, von Willebrand factor.

Management

Simple bleeding often responds to direct compression, which involves pinching the cartilaginous segment of the nares together for at least 5 full minutes. The correct position of the child during nasal compression is sitting up, leaning forward at the waist to decrease blood flow to the mouth and throat. If the child is cooperative, a segment of rolled cotton gauze may be placed below the upper lip and pushed upward toward the nose to compress the superior labial artery. If the bleeding does not abate with compression, and medications were not already used to facilitate examination, local vasoconstriction will help decrease blood flow. Oxymetazoline hydrochloride, 0.05% (eg, Afrin), or phenylephrine, 0.25% (eg, Neo-Synephrine), are common vasoconstricting agents and can either be applied directly to the nose or by cotton pledget soaked in the medication and placed in the nose with removal after 5 minutes. Oxymetazoline is preferred if available, as it has no effects on systemic blood pressure. If no anterior source of bleeding is located, examine the oropharynx for signs of blood. This may indicate posterior bleeding, which likely will require a more extensive examination by an otolaryngologist with a flexible or rigid nasal endoscope. The rest of the general examination should focus on signs of hematologic abnormalities, such as pallor, petechiae, bruising, or gingival bleeding. Inspection for organomegaly or enlarged lymph nodes may also indicate a coagulopathy or malignancy. The patient's skin should be inspected for telangiectasias, hemangiomas, or icterus, which could signal a genetic disease or liver dysfunction that is causing the nosebleed.

An anterior bleed that is not responsive to compression or vasoconstrictors may benefit from either chemical or electrical cautery (Figure 58-2). Cauterization is also often used as treatment for recurrent benign epistaxis in the ENT outpatient setting. Chemical cautery with silver nitrate can be performed in a general pediatrician's office depending on comfort level and available equipment, but electrical cautery is best reserved for an ENT specialist. The patient will need to be cooperative with the procedure, and topical anesthetic is recommended to promote successful cauterization. Local anesthetic such as lidocaine, 2% to 4% (maximum dose of 3–5 mg/kg); cocaine hydrochloride, 4% or 10%; or tetracaine, 0.4%, can be used. After adequate anesthesia and hemostasis, a silver nitrate stick should be applied to the affected area in concentric circles, starting at the outer limits of the area and working toward the center. Petroleum jelly, a water-based jelly, or antibiotic ointment smeared over the unaffected areas of mucosa may protect against unintended exposure to the chemical (Evidence Level III). The physician should perform only unilateral cauterization, even if both nares are bleeding, as bilateral cauterization increases the risk of septal perforation. Silver nitrate is manufactured in different concentrations, but evidence suggests that silver nitrate, 75%, is more effective in the short-term and less painful than the 95% formulation (Evidence Level I). After cauterization, petroleum jelly, water-based jelly, or antibiotic ointment should be applied at least daily to promote adequate hydration and healing of the affected tissue.

If epistaxis continues despite local compression, vasoconstriction, and cautery, anterior nasal packing is indicated to tamponade bleeding (Figure 58-3). If nasal packing is required, ENT consultation is recommended to help treat the bleeding, determine its cause, and evaluate if further medical work-up is needed. Nasal packing should be preceded by the application of topical anesthesia and nasal decongestant. It is most easily accomplished with a

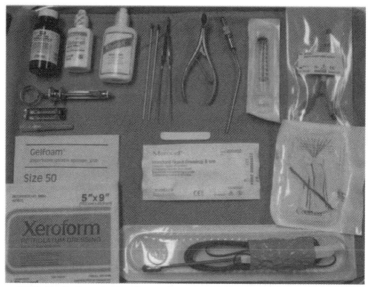

Figure 58-2. Typical contents of an epistaxis tray.
Top row: nasal decongestant sprays and local anesthetic, silver nitrate cautery sticks, bayonet forceps, nasal speculum, Frazier suction tip, posterior double balloon system, and syringe for balloon inflation. *Bottom row:* packing materials, including nonadherent gauze impregnated with petroleum jelly and 3 percent bismuth tribromophenate (Xeroform), Merocel, Gelfoam, and suction cautery.
From Kucik CJ, Clenny, T. Management of epistaxis. *Am Fam Physician.* 2005;71(2):305–311, with permission.

commercial prefabricated nasal tampon (eg, Merocel, Rhino Rocket), which is inserted with bayonet forceps along the floor of the nose. Coating the tampon with lubricant or antibiotic ointment will help with insertion and later removal. The nasal tampon will expand once in the nasal cavity, as the material expands on contact with fluid, but additional fluid may need to be applied to fully expand the material. With the development of these easy-to-use commercial sponge products, the traditional method of layered gauze packing is rarely used but sufficient if needed.

If anterior packing failed to stop a visualized anterior bleeding source, consider bilateral packing to increase the compression of the nasal septum. If an anterior bleeding source was never visualized and bleeding continues despite adequate packing, a posterior source should be suspected. Because nasal packs are foreign bodies in a bacteria-rich environment, risk of infection theoretically increases. The role of prophylactic antibiotics is not well established in acute epistaxis, with wide variations in practice. Oral anti-staphylococcal antibiotics should be considered in all patients that are going to be discharged home with nasal packing in place. Ideally, the patient should be reevaluated in an outpatient ENT setting 24 to 48 hours after the pack is placed. Bleeds that do not cease with appropriate anterior nasal packing, require a hemostatic compound

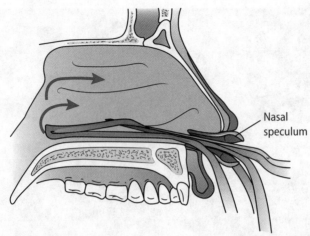

Figure 58-3. Traditional method of placing an anterior nasal pack using Vaseline gauze.
A bayonet forceps is used to insert the gauze straight back along the floor of the nasal cavity. The speculum is removed after each layer is applied and then reinserted to gently pack the gauze down. The gauze is layered in accordion fashion until the nasal cavity is filled.

(eg, FloSeal, Surgicel, Gelfoam), or stem from the posterior nasopharynx require emergent ENT consultation and are beyond the scope of this chapter.

Long-term Management of Recurrent Epistaxis

The preceding sections describe the evaluation and management of acute epistaxis. In children, however, recurrent episodes of benign epistaxis are more common than severe epistaxis that cannot be controlled. Although these nosebleeds rarely signify a more serious condition, recurrent epistaxis can be very distressing to patients and parents alike. The first step is to ensure that no foreign body, nasal mass, or hematologic disease is evident on physical examination, as all can cause recurrent bleeds. The most common etiology of recurrent epistaxis is likely a combination of dry mucosa due to weather, allergies, or medications with mild trauma. Humidification of the nasal mucosa with a humidifier in the child's room at night may help, unless the patient has allergies that are worsened with humidification. Saline nose spray can also be used if tolerated by the patient, and nasal corticosteroids should be discontinued during periods of frequent epistaxis. Petroleum jelly has been suggested in the past as a possible treatment for recurrent nosebleeds but has been demonstrated to confer no benefit over simple observation (Evidence Level I).

Antibiotic ointment has also been evaluated for efficacy. Nasal colonization with *Staphylococcal aureus* is thought to play a role in inflammation and vessel injury in the nasal mucosa, and the presumed mechanism of antibiotic ointment is that it reduces the amount of crusting and vestibulitis that predisposes to epistaxis. In patients without active bleeding, application of antibiotic ointment to areas of ulcerations, crusting, or prominent blood vessels is as effective as cautery (Evidence Level I). In a more recent single-blind, randomized, controlled trial of antiseptic cream versus no intervention for 4 weeks preceding a specialist evaluation, the treatment arm demonstrated improvement in the epistaxis with a relative risk reduction of 47% (Evidence Level I), but at a 5-year follow-up, 65% of the original treatment group had ongoing epistaxis requiring further treatment (Evidence Level II-3). A recent Cochrane review on interventions of recurrent idiopathic epistaxis supports that there is not enough evidence to determine the optimal management of children with recurrent epistaxis. Despite this conclusion, there does not seem to be any harm in using antibiotic ointment to aid in epistaxis prevention, as significant evidence has demonstrated short-term efficacy.

Suggested Reading

Benoit MM, Bhattacharyya N, Faquin W, Cunningham M. Cancer of the nasal cavity in the pediatric population. *Pediatrics.* 2008;121(1):e141–e145

Kubba H, MacAndie C, Botma M, et al. A prospective, single-blind, randomized controlled trial of antiseptic cream for recurrent epistaxis in childhood. *Clin Otolaryngol.* 2001;26(6):465–468

Loughran S, Spinou E, Clement WA, Cathcart R, Kubba H, Geddes NK. A prospective, single-blind, randomized controlled trial of petroleum jelly/Vaseline for recurrent paediatric epistaxis. *Clin Otolaryngol.* 2004;29(3):266–269

McIntosh N, Mok JY, Margerison A. Epidemiology of oronasal hemorrhage in the first 2 years of life: implications of child protection. *Pediatrics.* 2007;120(5):1075–1078

Nadel F, Henretig FM. Epistaxis. In: Fleischer GR, Ludwig S, eds. *Textbook of Pediatric Emergency Medicine.* 6th ed. Philadelphia, PA: Lippincott Williams & Wilkins; 2010:236–239

Patel PB, Kost SI. Management of epistaxis. In: King C, Henetrig FM, eds. *Textbook of Pediatric Emergency Procedures.* 2nd ed. Philadelphia, PA: Lippincott Williams & Wilkins; 2008:604–615

Qureishi A, Burton MJ. Interventions for recurrent idiopathic epistaxis (nosebleeds) in children. *Cochrane Database Syst Rev.* 2012;9:CD004461

Robertson S, Kubba H. Long-term effectiveness of antiseptic cream for recurrent epistaxis in childhood: five-year follow up of a randomized, controlled trial. *J Laryngol Otol.* 2008;122(10):1084–1087

Ruddy J, Proops DW, Pearman K, Ruddy H. Management of epistaxis in children. *Int J Pediatr Otorhi.* 1991;21(2):139–142

Sandoval C, Dong S, Visintainer P, Ozkaynak MF, Jayabose S. Clinical and laboratory features of 178 children with recurrent epistaxis. *J Pediatr Hematol Oncol.* 2002;24(1):47–49

Whymark AD, Crampsey DP, Fraser L, Moore P, Williams C, Kubba H, et al. Childhood epistaxis and nasal colonization with *Staphylococcus aureus. Otolaryngol Head Neck Surg.* 2008;138(3):308–310

CHAPTER 59

Heart Failure

Andrew R. Yates, MD, and Philip T. Thrush, MD

Key Points

- Heart failure can be defined as insufficient cardiac output to meet the metabolic demands of the body, with clinical features that often include respiratory symptoms (eg, tachypnea, respiratory distress), failure to thrive/poor growth, and exercise intolerance, and it may also manifest as poor feeding in infants.

- Evaluation for an etiology of heart failure should include clinical examination, chest radiograph, electrocardiogram, echocardiogram, and laboratory assessment for treatable conditions.

- Treatment modalities are aimed at the underlying etiology (when applicable), and pharmacologic agents tailored to support cardiac dysfunction in an effort to maximize cardiac output, relieve symptoms, maintain euvolemic status, and ensure reasonable quality of life and development for the child.

Overview

Adult heart failure (HF) is a significant public health epidemic, with an incidence rate of 3 persons per 1,000 per years. Although considerably smaller numbers of pediatric patients have HF, these patients see further-reaching ramifications than adults, with HF being a significant cause of morbidity and mortality. Additionally, complex medical care affects the family, including increased risk of divorce for parents of children with congenital heart disease (CHD) and financial stresses due to lost days of productivity while caring for their children. The cost of treating HF in children may be higher because of the frequent need for surgical or cardiac catheterization–based interventions. There can also be societal effects when a child's death is secondary to HF, such as the loss of possible productive years as an adult in the workforce. As such, it is important to thoroughly evaluate for various etiologies of HF in pediatrics and to treat them aggressively.

Definition
· · · · · · · · · ·

Heart failure in children, although easily recognized, can be difficult to define. The clinical manifestations can include failure to thrive, peripheral edema, activity intolerance, respiratory distress, and other findings, but the pathophysiology that leads to these symptoms has been found to be multifactorial. Pediatric HF is not merely pump failure or excessive pulmonary blood flow. Simply put, HF can be defined as insufficient cardiac output to meet the metabolic demands of the body. In actuality, we know that HF pathophysiology is a result of complex interaction between circulatory, neurohormonal, and molecular abnormalities. While the pathophysiology is beyond the scope of this chapter, Hsu et al pose an excellent working definition: "HF in children is a progressive clinical and pathophysiological syndrome caused by cardiovascular and non-cardiovascular abnormalities that results in characteristic signs and symptoms including edema, respiratory distress, growth failure, and exercise intolerance, and accompanied by circulatory, neuro-hormonal, and molecular derangements."

Heart failure in adults has historically been classified by the New York Heart Association Functional Classification; however, this classification does not lend itself well to the pediatric population, especially infants and small children. The Ross classification was developed to overcome the limitations of the New York Heart Association classification and provide an objective grading scale for pediatric patients with HF. This has subsequently been revised to the modified Ross classification and includes age-based classification of HF. The most current revision incorporates feeding, weight percentile/growth, breathing, respiratory rate, heart rate, perfusion, nausea/vomiting, hepatomegaly, N-terminal pro-B-type natriuretic peptide, ejection fraction (by echocardiography), atrioventricular valve insufficiency, and maximum percentage of $\dot{V}o_2$ (in older children) in order to assess HF. This age-base classification has separate criteria for those patients 0 to 3 months, 4 to 12 months, 1 to 3 years, 4 to 8 years, and 9 to 18 years of age.

Causes
· · · · · · ·

The causes of pediatric HF are markedly different than those of adults. For example, myocardial ischemia is exceptionally rare in infants and children, except perhaps for those with coronary anomalies or prior Kawasaki disease, whereas CHD and metabolic abnormalities are uncommon causes of HF in adults.

The causes of HF in children can be grouped in several different ways based on age of presentation, underlying pathophysiology (eg, pressure overload vs volume overload), or by right-sided vs. left-sided etiologies (Table 59-1).

Table 59-1. Common Causes of Pediatric Heart Failure

Right-Sided HF	Left-Sided HF

Congenital heart disease
Volume overload
    Left-to-right shunts (ASD, PAPVR, AVM)
    Pulmonary regurgitation
Right-sided obstructive lesions
    Severe pulmonary stenosis
Impaired left-sided heart filling
    Mitral stenosis
    Pulmonary vein stenosis
    Left ventricular dysfunction
	Congenital heart disease
	Volume overload
	    Left-to-right shunts (VSD, PDA, AP window)
	    Aortic regurgitation
	    Mitral regurgitation
	Left-sided obstructive lesions
	    Severe aortic stenosis
	    Coarctation
	Hypoplastic left-sided heart syndrome
	Unbalanced AVSD
	Systemic right ventricle (I-TGA)

Arrhythmias Ectopic atrial tachycardia AV/AV nodal reentrant tachycardia PJRT Ventricular tachycardia	*Arrhythmias* Ectopic atrial tachycardia AV/AV nodal reentrant tachycardia PJRT Ventricular tachycardia

Cardiomyopathy
Dilated
Restrictive
Neuromuscular disorders
	Cardiomyopathy
	Dilated
	Hypertrophic
	Restrictive
	Neuromuscular disorders
	    Dystrophinopathies
	    Freidrich ataxia
	    Emory-Dreifuss dystrophy
	Mitochondrial
	Metabolic disorders
	    Glycogen storage disorders

Acquired lesions
Coronary disease (Kawasaki disease)
Myocarditis
    Enterovirus
    Parvovirus B19
    Adenovirus
    Human herpesvirus 6
    Epstein-Barr virus
Sepsis
Toxins
    Anthracyclines
    Daunorubicin/doxorubicin
    Other chemotherapeutics
	Acquired lesions
	Coronary disease (Kawasaki disease)
	Myocarditis
	    Enterovirus
	    Parvovirus B19
	    Adenovirus
	    Human herpesvirus 6
	    Epstein-Barr virus
	Rheumatic heart disease (aortic or mitral valve regurgitation)
	Hypertension
	Sepsis
	Toxins
	    Anthracyclines
	    Daunorubicin/doxorubicin
	    Other chemotherapeutics

Table 59-1 *(cont)*

Right-Sided HF	Left-Sided HF

Pulmonary causes
  Parenchymal disease (CF, IPF)
  Bronchopulmonary dysplasia
  Pulmonary hypoplasia
  Hyaline membrane disease
	Other noncardiac causes
	  Anemia
	  DKA
	  Hypothyroidism
	  Renal failure

Extrinsic causes
  Thoracic deformities
  Upper airway obstruction	

Pulmonary hypertension
  Pulmonary thromboembolic disease
  Pulmonary veno-occlusive disease
  PPHN
  Alveolar capillary dysplasia
  Primary idiopathic PAH	

Abbreviations: ASD, atrial septal defect; AP, aortopulmonary; AV, atrioventricular; AVM, arteriovenous malformation; AVSD, atrioventricular septal defect; CF, cystic fibrosis; DKA, diabetic ketoacidosis; HF, heart failure; IPF, idiopathic pulmonary fibrosis; PAH, pulmonary arterial hypertension; PAPVR, partial anomalous pulmonary venous return; PDA, patent ductus arteriosus; PJRT, persistent junctional reentrant tachycardia; PPHN, persistent pulmonary hypertension of the newborn; TGA, transposition of the great arteries; VSD, ventricular septal defect.

Clinical Features

While the etiologies of HF in children are varied, some characteristic signs and symptoms are irrespective of the specific cause. These often include respiratory symptoms (eg, tachypnea, respiratory distress), failure to thrive/poor growth, and exercise intolerance, which may manifest as poor feeding in infants. These manifestations are included, along with other findings such as echocardiography, in staging schemes of pediatric HF, such as the age-stratified modified Ross classification. Specific features and findings in pediatric HF depend on underlying etiology and are ultimately driven by whether the patient has right- or left-sided HF.

The timing of onset of HF is often determined by the underlying lesion and can be quite variable. For example, volume loading of the right ventricle, as seen in patients with a large atrial septal defect (ASD) or partial anomalous pulmonary venous return (PAPVR), is far better tolerated than volume loading of the left ventricle with a large ventricular septal defect (VSD). This is because the right ventricle is more compliant than the left ventricle, which allows it to accommodate to a higher blood volume without increasing filling pressure. While a large VSD may result in HF symptoms within 3 to 4 months postnatally, a large ASD may remain asymptomatic for years. Onset can also vary depending on the type of lesion affecting the right or left ventricle; for example, acute onset of severe pulmonary hypertension may result in rapid failure of the right ventricle, while in patients with ductal dependent obstructive lesions, such as severe aortic stenosis and coarctation, symptoms present in infancy.

Right-sided HF manifests predominantly as signs of venous congestion. Patients often present with peripheral edema, hepatomegaly or splenomegaly (or both), and ascites due to elevated venous pressures and congestion. Patients with right-sided HF may also experience dyspnea on exertion and syncope, both due to inability to augment blood flow through the pulmonary vascular bed and inability to augment the cardiac output. Infants with HF can also present with diaphoresis, tachypnea, and poor growth.

In addition to these general HF symptoms in the setting of elevated right ventricular diastolic pressure or significant tricuspid regurgitation, right-sided HF can also lead to right atrial dilation, as well as subsequent right atrial arrhythmias. These patients may present with palpitations, shortness of breath, chest pain, dizziness, or, rarely, syncope.

Left-sided HF manifests as signs of inadequate systemic perfusion, pulmonary edema, or both. In patients who have obstructed or inadequate systemic output, symptoms may include abdominal pain or feeding intolerance due to inadequate mesenteric perfusion, chest pain or arrhythmia due to inadequate coronary perfusion, and syncope due to inadequate cerebral perfusion. In some, these symptoms are absent at rest and can be provoked with exercise and exercise testing. Lesions resulting in these symptoms include congenital heart disease, such as aortic stenosis, hypoplastic left heart syndrome, cardiomyopathy with resultant left ventricular systolic dysfunction, or severe mitral regurgitation. Lesions that result in elevated left ventricular diastolic pressure (eg, restrictive cardiomyopathy, aortic regurgitation, and mitral regurgitation) or impaired left ventricular filling (eg, mitral stenosis, cor triatriatum, or pulmonary vein stenosis) result in symptoms related to pulmonary edema. These symptoms include shortness of breath, exertional dyspnea, cough, and cardiac wheezing.

As left-sided HF progresses, left atrial pressure increases, resulting in increased pulmonary pressures and, ultimately, increased right ventricular diastolic pressure. With increased afterload on the right ventricle and increased diastolic or filling pressure of the right ventricle, symptoms of right-sided HF can also develop. As such, right-sided symptoms also require a careful evaluation for causes of left-sided HF.

Arrhythmias can also be an important presenting feature of left-sided HF. These can include atrial arrhythmias, such as ectopic atrial tachycardia and atrial flutter, due to left atrial dilation and ventricular arrhythmias due to the primary disease process or secondary to underlying cardiomyopathy. In patients with cardiomyopathy, sudden cardiac death may be the first presenting symptom and is more commonly associated with hypertrophic cardiomyopathy (HCM). The 5-year incidence of sudden cardiac death in dilated cardiomyopathy has been reported as 3%. In patients with HCM, the risk of sudden cardiac death has been reported as high as 20% at 10 years and 40% at 20 years after initial evaluation for those with severe spectrum of disease (maximal wall thickness >30 mm).

Multiple studies have demonstrated that initial presentation is not predictive of outcomes in pediatric HF. As such, all patients with symptoms of HF, regardless of severity of symptoms, require not only aggressive treatment but also a thorough evaluation for definable etiologies.

Evaluation

The evaluation of pediatric HF must be multifaceted. When patients present with new-onset ventricular dysfunction, a thorough and complete evaluation is important to identify conditions with known treatments and conditions with defined outcomes (Evidence Level III).

Clinical Examination

A thorough physical examination, including a full cardiac examination, remains an integral part of the evaluation of the patient with HF. It is important to assess the overall appearance of the patient, as many younger patients demonstrate failure to thrive and poor weight gain. Evaluation of general appearance, dysmorphic features, and neuromuscular weakness or deformities (or both) may suggest a syndromic diagnosis. Rales or wheezing may be a sign of pulmonary interstitial edema secondary to left atrial hypertension. The abdominal examination may demonstrate hepatomegaly or hepatosplenomegaly secondary to venous congestion and elevated right-sided heart pressures.

During cardiac examination, one should observe, palpate, and auscultate for abnormalities. Patients with right ventricular dilation and elevated pulmonary pressures may have a visible precordial heave, and a hyperdynamic precordium can result from cardiomegaly. A displaced point of maximal impulse may be noted when the left ventricle is dilated. In patients with HF, it is common to find tachycardia, as this may be the only mechanism the patient has to increase his cardiac output secondary to a fixed stroke volume. Tachycardia may also indicate tachycardia-induced cardiomyopathy. While an S3 gallop may be an expected finding, S3 and S4 gallops are common in patients with dilated cardiomyopathy and restricted cardiomyopathy, respectively. Systolic murmurs are present in semilunar valve stenosis and atrioventricular valve regurgitation, and diastolic murmurs may be audible with semilunar valve regurgitation. Diastolic flow rumbles are low-frequency sounds associated with increased antegrade flow across atrioventricular valves often noted in large left-to-right shunts. Of course, specific cardiac findings will depend on the underlying lesions.

Chest Radiograph

The chest radiograph in patients with HF can detect cardiomegaly and pulmonary edema, resulting in increased pulmonary vascular markings and Kerley lines. Left atrial dilation may be evident by elevation and compression of the left main bronchus. Pleural effusions may also be noted. Characteristic mediastinal silhouettes may indicate specific forms of CHD. Examples include the "egg on a string" in transposition of the great arteries, "snowman sign" in total anomalous pulmonary venous return, and a "wall-to-wall" heart in Ebstein anomaly.

Electrocardiogram

The electrocardiogram (ECG) is of primary importance in determining if an associated arrhythmia is present, either as the primary problem or secondary to the HF. The most common finding on ECG is sinus tachycardia, as many of these patients have limited ability to augment cardiac output via increased stroke volume. In the setting of dilated cardiomyopathy or HCM, it is not uncommon to have voltage criteria for ventricular hypertrophy, and it is especially important to evaluate the ST segments and T waves for ischemic changes in patients with HCM.

Echocardiography

Echocardiography remains the primary imaging modality of children with HF. This is typically accomplished transthoracically, but transesophageal imaging is occasionally necessary if the transthoracic images are inadequate. Echocardiography allows full evaluation of the heart for CHD and structural defects, chamber sizes, valve abnormalities, proximal coronary abnormalities, and estimation of both systolic and diastolic function. For severely depressed ventricular function or severely dilated atria, echocardiography is also important to assess for thrombus formation. While assessment of the left ventricle, using shortening fraction and ejection fraction, is technically easier than assessment of right ventricular function because of its more uniform shape, advanced echocardiographic techniques, such as tissue Doppler and myocardial performance index, may be helpful in some populations.

Cardiac Catheterization

Cardiac catheterization allows for direct measurement of oxygen saturations and pressures in the various chambers of the heart. Specifically, catheterization permits measurement of ventricular end-diastolic pressure, permits pressure gradients across valves or septal defects, and allows for shunt calculation of CHD. Angiography is occasionally performed to assess for vascular stenosis, coronary anatomy/lesions, and ventricular function. Interventional cardiac catheterization is also critical for some forms of congenital heart disease, including balloon valvuloplasty for severe or critical aortic or pulmonary stenosis.

Advanced Imaging

Advanced imaging, including cardiac magnetic resonance imaging (CMR) and computed tomography, can be useful in some patients. Both imaging modalities offer the ability to delineate coronary anatomy without more invasive cardiac catheterization. Computed tomography is generally faster than CMR but exposes patients to radiation. Cardiac magnetic resonance imaging, on the other hand, often requires general anesthesia in small children and patients with claustrophobia. It offers excellent resolution of the endomyocardial border, and, as such, provides very accurate data regarding ventricular function, even for the asymmetric right ventricle. Appropriateness criteria have been developed to aid physicians in determining the most appropriate advanced imaging.

Laboratory Assessment

In the absence of anatomic etiologies for HF in pediatrics, laboratory assessment can be crucial to identifying the etiology of HF. In patients with suspected myocarditis, it is important to fully evaluate for viral pathogens (Box 59-1).

Box 59-1. Common Viral Etiologies of Myocarditis

- Adenovirus
- Cytomegalovirus
- Enterovirus
  - Coxsackieviruses A and B
  - Echovirus
  - Poliovirus
- Epstein-Barr virus
- Hepatitis C
- Herpes simplex virus
- Human immunodeficiency virus
- Influenza A and B
- Parvovirus B19
- Respiratory syncytial virus
- Rubella
- Varicella

In addition to viral causes, other potentially testable causes for myocarditis include bacterial infections, notably meningococcal, *Klebsiella* species, *Salmonella* species, and tuberculosis, and protozoal infections, such as *Trypanosoma cruzii* and fungi/yeast infections. Studies directed towards systemic diseases, such as sarcoidosis, scleroderma, systemic lupus erythematosus, and rheumatic fever, may be pursued as causes of myocarditis. Various drugs, including sulfonamides, other antibiotics and antifungals, and phenytoin, can also result in myocarditis.

Inflammatory markers, such as C-reactive protein level and erythrocyte sedimentation rate, may be beneficial in the evaluation of myocarditis, as well as other systemic inflammatory disease processes. C-reactive protein level has also been shown to correlate with poorer outcomes in adults with HF, but this has not been replicated in pediatric studies.

Cardiac troponin level elevation can be a marker of cardiac myocyte injury, useful in the assessment of children with coronary anomalies or myocarditis. This study has not been shown to be beneficial in the assessment of children and adolescents with chest pain without constitutional symptoms (ie, fever or an abnormal ECG). Similarly, it is not prognostic in patients with myopericarditis.

Finally, B-type natriuretic peptide (BNP) and N-terminal pro-B-type natriuretic peptide (NT-proBNP) levels may be used in the management of patients with HF. These biomarkers are produced by ventricular myocytes in response to increased wall tension due to pressure and volume overload. These biomarkers have been found to be useful in screening and risk stratifying adults. Also, BNP and NT-proBNP have been found to be useful prognostic indicators for children with symptomatic HF, not only in aiding the assessment for mechanical circulatory support of children with acute HF, but also in monitoring pulmonary pressures after rejection in pediatric heart transplant patients.

Management

Management of pediatric HF involves acute stabilization of the patient in decompensated HF, assessment for potential treatments and recovery, and chronic management of compensated HF. Included in acute management of HF are those patients who require primary surgical or interventional catheter-based treatments to address a primary structural, repairable etiology. The International Society for Heart and Lung Transplantation has developed practice guidelines for pediatric HF, but none of these recommendations are based on Evidence Level I, and only 7 of 49 are based on Evidence Levels II-1 or II-2 (Table 59-2). The remainders of the recommendations are Evidence Level III.

Acute Care

The primary goal in acute management of a pediatric patient with acute decompensated HF/cardiogenic shock is first to medically stabilize the patient hemodynamically and then to treat underlying causes, whether these are structural defects/CHD or systemic disease processes. Initial management often includes inotropic support using milrinone, dopamine, epinephrine, dobutamine, or a combination thereof. Milrinone is a phosphodiesterase-3 inhibitor and has become a drug of choice, as it increases contractility, improves lusitropy (ie, relaxation of the ventricles), and has some vasodilatory effects resulting in decreased afterload. Patients may require blood pressure support with epinephrine, norepinephrine, or vasopressin to maintain adequate organ perfusion pressures. Additionally, diuretic therapy may be utilized if the initial presentation includes fluid overload. Respiratory support, either intubation/mechanical ventilation or noninvasive measures such as bilevel positive airway pressure or continuous positive airway pressure, may be necessary to decrease the metabolic demand placed on the heart due to work of breathing and to provide relief from interstitial pulmonary edema. Positive pressure ventilation (invasive or noninvasive) results in decreased left ventricular transmural pressure and,

Table 59-2. Therapeutic Recommendations From ISHLT Guidelines for Management of HF in Children (Evidence Levels II-1 or II-2)

Category	Recommendation
No structural disease	Digoxin is employed for ventricular dysfunction and symptoms of HF for relief of symptoms.
	For the treatment of moderate/severe degrees of left ventricular dysfunction with/without symptoms, ACE inhibitors are routinely used unless a specific contraindication is present.
	With limited information available concerning efficacy and safety of beta-blockers in infants and children with HF, no recommendation is available concerning use for left ventricular dysfunction.
Left ventricular diastolic dysfunction	Diastolic dysfunction refractory to optimal medical or surgical management should be evaluated for heart transplantation because the patient is at high risk for developing secondary pulmonary hypertension and sudden death.
Systemic right ventricle	With right ventricle in systemic position, the patient is at risk of developing systemic ventricular dysfunction, so periodic evaluation of ventricular function is required.
Acute HF	Mechanical cardiac support is considered in patients with or without structural congenital heart disease who have acute decompensation of HF as a bridge to cardiac transplantation.
	Mechanical cardiac support is considered in patients who have experienced cardiac arrest, hypoxia with pulmonary hypertension, or severe ventricular dysfunction with low cardiac output after surgery for congenital heart disease, including "rescue" of patients who are unable to wean from cardiopulmonary bypass or who have myocarditis.

Abbreviations: ACE, angiotensin-converting enzyme; HF, heart failure; ISHLT, International Society for Heart and Lung Transplantation.

ultimately, decreased afterload. Finally, some patients may require mechanical circulatory support, either extracorporeal membrane oxygenation or ventricular assist devices (VADs), because of inadequate cardiac output. Currently, few VADs are available for use in pediatric patients, and they have been used for bridge to recovery, bridge to orthotopic heart transplantation, and destination therapy. Despite maximal medical therapy, some patients' health may continue to decline or never compensate, leading to evaluation for orthotopic heart transplantation. Other patients' health will stabilize, and they may be transitioned to a chronic medical regimen.

Chronic Care

Chronic therapy for systolic dysfunction is based on continued treatment of the underlying etiology of failure, if identified. Treatment, specifically for diastolic dysfunction, is beyond the scope of this text, and we will focus on primarily systolic dysfunction in patients with biventricular failure. In the setting of volume- or pressure-overloaded HF secondary to congenital heart lesions, treatment of the underlying lesion should be undertaken via surgical or transcatheter interventions to improve long-term outcomes.

Chronic medical management consists of several therapies, mainly based on adult studies of HF that provide the foundation for pediatric HF guidelines. Chronic diuretic therapy is employed to maintain euvolemic status (Evidence Level III). Digoxin therapy has been advocated for in patients with symptomatic HF (Evidence Level II-1) but not for patients with asymptomatic HF associated with left ventricular dysfunction (Evidence Level III). The optimal methodology for modulation of the renin-angiotensin-aldosterone system has not been fully elucidated but remains a target for pharmacotherapy with spironolactone- (historically) or angiotensin-converting enzyme inhibitors. Current pediatric guidelines recommend "up-titration" of angiotensin-converting enzyme inhibitors to a maximally tolerated dosage (Evidence Level II-1) except for in children with a pressure-overloaded left ventricle (Evidence Level III) or in the setting of acute decompensated HF (Evidence Level III). Beta-blocker therapy in pediatric patients has not demonstrated the favorable benefit in survival seen in adult trials. The most recent guidelines by the International Society for Heart and Lung Transplantation from 2004 recommend against the use of beta-blocker therapy in pediatrics (Evidence Level III). However, in 2007, a multicenter, randomized, placebo-controlled study of carvedilol in 161 pediatric patients with systolic HF demonstrated an improvement in ejection fraction (EF) without improvement in outcomes (Evidence Level I). However, the study may have been underpowered and had a high placebo affect, further complicating the interpretation of findings.

Alternative chronic therapies for HF are less well defined than pharmacotherapy in pediatric patients. Optimal antiarrhythmic medication choices and the role of implantable defibrillators and cardiac resynchronization with biventricular pacing remain unclear in pediatric patients with HF (Evidence Level III). Additionally, the use of VADs as destination therapy in pediatrics has been limited to rare case reports (Evidence Level III).

Long-term Monitoring/Implications

Long-term monitoring of these patients requires frequent outpatient evaluations, including physical examination, echocardiography, ECGs, Holter monitoring, and intermittent laboratory assessments. Outcomes generally depend on the underlying etiology and its natural history, quality of surgical repair when applicable, medication adherence, and comorbidities. Some patients may eventually be discharged from follow-up (eg, the patient with an ASD or VSD that closes spontaneously or the patient with myocarditis that fully recovers), but many require lifelong cardiac care. While some ultimately improve, others remain in a chronic state of compensated HF or continue to develop progressive HF, requiring further medical and possibly mechanical intervention, ultimately leading to heart transplantation.

Suggested Reading

Hendel RC, Patel MR, Kramer CM, et al. ACCF/ACR/SCCT/SCMR/ASNC/NASCI/SCAI/SIR 2006 appropriateness criteria for cardiac computed tomography and cardiac magnetic resonance imaging. *J Am Coll Cardiol.* 2006;48(7):1475–1497

Hsu D, Pearson GD. Heart failure in children: part I: history, etiology, and pathophysiology. *Circ Heart Fail.* 2009;2(1):63–70

Jefferies JL, Morales DL. Mechanical circulatory support in children: bridge to transplant versus recovery. *Curr Heart Fail Rep.* 2012;9(3):236–243

Liesemer K, Casper TC, Korgenski K, Menon SC. Use and misuse of serum troponin assays in pediatric practice. *Am J Cardiol.* 2012;110(2):284–289

Pahl E, Sleeper LA, Canter CE, et al. Incidence of and risk factors for sudden cardiac death in children with dilated cardiomyopathy: a report from the pediatric cardiomyopathy registry. *J Am Coll Cardiol.* 2012;59(6):607–615

Rosenthal D, Chrisant MR, Edens E, et al. International society for heart and lung transplantation: practice guidelines for management of heart failure in children. *J Heart Lung Transplant.* 2004;23(12):1313–1333

Ross RD. The Ross classification for heart failure in children after 25 years: a review and an age-stratified revision. *Pediatr Cardiol.* 2012;33(8):1295–1300

Shaddy RE, Boucek MM, Hsu DT, et al. Carvedilol for children and adolescents with heart failure: a randomized controlled trial. *JAMA.* 2007;298(10):1171–1179

Spirito P, Bellone P, Harris KM, Bernabo P, Bruzzi P, Maron BJ. Magnitude of left ventricular hypertrophy and risk of sudden death in hypertrophic cardiomyopathy. *New Engl J Med.* 2000;342(24):1778–1785

Tang WH, Francis GS, Morrow DA, et al. National Academy of Clinical Biochemistry Laboratory Medicine practice guidelines: clinical utilization of cardiac biomarker testing in heart failure. *Circulation.* 2007;116(5):e99–e109

CHAPTER 60

Infantile Botulism

Elizabeth H. Mack, MD, MS

Key Points

- Infantile botulism is characterized by a descending paralysis caused by the ingestion of *Clostridium botulinum* spores followed by germination and intestinal colonization of the organism.

- Infantile botulism is caused by formation of toxin in vivo, as opposed to foodborne botulism, which is caused by ingestion of preformed botulinum toxin.

- Infantile botulism symptoms range from mild weakness and constipation to sudden fatal respiratory arrest. The binding of the toxin to the neuromuscular junction explains the anticholinergic symptoms of botulism, including mydriasis and constipation. Classically, botulism involves an acute, descending, afebrile, symmetric, flaccid paralysis. Altered mental status and sensory changes are not seen in botulism.

- Preliminary diagnosis involves isolating the organism or the toxin from the feces, but confirmatory diagnosis is made by the mouse inoculation test at the state laboratory or the Centers for Disease Control and Prevention.

- Treatment is supportive (eg, mechanical ventilation and supplemental nutrition, if needed) and specific (eg, administration of antitoxin). Antitoxin has been shown to decrease the severity of illness as well as cost and length of stay for patients with either type A or B toxin.

Overview

Infantile botulism (IB) is characterized by a descending paralysis caused by the ingestion of *Clostridium botulinum* spores followed by germination and intestinal colonization of the organism. Colonization leads to production of the most potent and lethal toxin known. This toxin is then absorbed into the bloodstream from the gut and carried to the neuromuscular junction where it binds irreversibly to the presynaptic cholinergic receptors and blocks acetylcholine release (Figure 60-1). Infantile botulism is caused by formation of toxin in vivo, as opposed to foodborne botulism, which is caused by ingestion of preformed botulinum toxin.

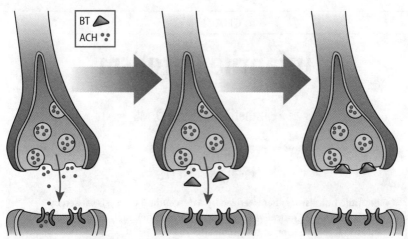

Figure 60-1. Schematic representation of the action of botulinum toxin on a neuromuscular junction.

Abbreviation: ACH, acetylcholine; BT, botulinum toxin.

Differential Diagnosis

Differential diagnosis should include sepsis, tick paralysis, Guillain Barré syndrome, polio, magnesium toxicity, myasthenia gravis, and Eaton-Lambert syndrome.

The first two cases of IB were reported in 1976. The average incidence rate in the United States from 2001–2005 according to the California Department of Health Services was 2.34 per 100,000 live births. In 2005, 96 cases were reported in the United States. Incidence rate does not appear to be affected by sex, race, or seasonality. *C botulinum* spores are ubiquitous; they are found in soil and dust around the world. Toxin type A is predominantly found in IB cases in the western United States, whereas type B is more common in the eastern United States. Interestingly, this parallels the pattern of spores found naturally in the soil. Exposure to honey is the only known avoidable source of *C botulinum* spores. Most babies with a history of honey ingestion will not develop IB, and most patients with IB do not have a history of honey ingestion. In fact, a recent outbreak in the United Kingdom linked to powdered formula contaminated with *C botulinum* spores, and the finding of spores in powdered formula in the United States highlights this potential exposure for infants. Thus, honey ingestion is neither necessary nor sufficient for the diagnosis of IB.

Signs and Symptoms

Symptoms range from mild weakness and constipation to sudden fatal respiratory arrest. The binding of the toxin to the neuromuscular junction explains the anticholinergic symptoms of botulism, including mydriasis and constipation. Classically, botulism involves an acute, descending, afebrile, symmetric, flaccid paralysis. Altered mental status and sensory changes are not seen in botulism.

Evaluation

Preliminary diagnosis involves isolating the organism or the toxin from the feces, but confirmatory diagnosis is made by the mouse inoculation test at the state laboratory or the Centers for Disease Control and Prevention (CDC). The CDC becomes aware of cases through mandatory reporting by physicians and state laboratories and by providing the confirmatory diagnostic test. This toxin neutralization bioassay involves intraperitoneal injection of the mice with stool from the affected patient. Symptoms of botulism and death occur in the mouse that does not receive subsequent type-specific antitoxin, and survival of the mouse that receives type-specific antitoxin to neutralize the toxin will confirm the diagnosis. The following studies should be within reference range: cerebrospinal fluid indices, blood cultures, electroencephalogram findings, and neuroimaging findings. Standard precautions should be taken in the hospital setting; no other isolation is required.

Management

Management is directed to providing supportive care and antitoxin; close monitoring and appropriate supportive care diminishes chances of significant complications in these children. Complications of botulism include hyponatremia due to antidiuretic hormone release, which is caused by decreased preload from venous pooling; toxic megacolon; iatrogenic infections; and aspiration pneumonia.

Treatment involves supportive therapies (ie, mechanical ventilation and supplemental nutrition, if needed) and administration of antitoxin. The antitoxin human botulism immune globulin (licensed as BabyBIG, available as a public-service orphan drug in the United States) has been shown to decrease the severity of illness as well as cost and length of stay for patients with either type A or B toxin (Evidence Level I). The dose is 1 mL/kg (50 mg/kg) given as a single intravenous infusion. If the patient experiences flushing, slow down the rate of administration. If the patient experiences anaphylaxis, stop the infusion immediately and institute the usual measures for the treatment of anaphylaxis. Treatment should be given as soon as possible and should not be delayed for confirmatory testing. Information may be obtained at www.infantbotulism.org and by phone from the Infant Botulism Treatment and Prevention Program at 510/231-7600.

Long-term Implications

The prognosis for IB is generally excellent if no hypoxic event occurs prior to recognition, as infants are not left with residual neurologic deficits. Infants should be monitored initially in an intensive care setting. Enteral nutrition is recommended, and is often tolerated, even in the absence of bowel sounds. Typically the disease progresses over 1 to 2 weeks followed by recovery over 3 to 4 weeks. Recovery is due to regeneration of nerve terminals. Patients often need rehabilitative services.

Determination of the causative agent has led to a primary prevention strategy that is universal and relatively inexpensive. Case definition is consistent, as the criterion standard is the mouse neutralization assay performed by the CDC. Unfortunately, IB is still likely a disease that is poorly recognized, particularly outside the United States, and therefore underreported. Pediatric organizations, public health agencies, and honey manufacturers recommend against feeding honey to children younger than 12 months, as it is nutritionally nonessential.

Suggested Reading

Arnon SS, Schechter R, Maslanka SE, Jewell NP, Hatheway CL. Human botulism immune globulin for the treatment of infant botulism. *N Engl J Med.* 2006;354(5):462–471

Barash JR, Hsia, Arnon SS. Presence of soil-dwelling clostridia in commercial powdered infant formulas. *J Pediatr.* 2010;156(3):402–408

Pickett J, Berg B, Chaplin E, Brunstetter-Shafer MA. Syndrome of botulism in infancy: clinical and electrophysiologic study. *N Engl J Med.* 1976;295(14):770–772

Smith LD. The occurrence of *Clostridium botulinum* and *Clostridium tetani* in the soil of the United States. *Health Lab Sci.* 1978;15(2):74–80

CHAPTER 61

Malignant Hyperthermia

Deanna Todd Tzanetos, MD, MSCI, and Scottie B. Day, MD

Key Points

- Malignant hyperthermia (MH) is an inherited susceptibility to muscle hypermetabolism on exposure to triggering agents, such as inhalational anesthetics and succinylcholine.

- Previous uneventful anesthesia with triggering agents does not exclude the possibility of developing MH on subsequent anesthetic exposure.

- All family members of patients with MH should be treated as genetically susceptible to MH until a diagnosis is confirmed. Patients with central core disease, King-Denborough syndrome, and Duchenne muscular dystrophy are at increased risk of MH.

- The definitive treatment for MH is dantrolene; management of complications of MH (eg, hypoxia, hyperthermia, and dysrhythmias) are important priorities, as is close monitoring during the course of the episode and for 48 hours after the last observed sign of MH.

Overview

Malignant hyperthermia (MH) is an inherited predisposition to skeletal muscle hypermetabolism when exposed to halogenated inhalational anesthetics (such as halothane) or depolarizing neuromuscular-blocking agents (such as succinylcholine). Children compose more than half of all persons with MH. Several mutations have been identified that can cause the disorder. Approximately 50% of families with a history of MH demonstrate a mutation in the gene that encodes the ryanodine receptor (ie, *RYR1*). The ryanodine receptor protein forms the calcium release channel of the sarcoplasmic reticulum in skeletal muscle. An *RYR1* mutation allows uncontrolled release of calcium from the sarcoplasmic reticulum after exposure to triggering agents. The mutation is typically inherited in an autosomal dominant pattern.

Clinical Features

There are several *RYR1* variants that are associated with a variety of clinical MH phenotypes. In fact, the first sign can range from myoglobinuria to cardiac arrest. Signs and symptoms of MH include masseter spasm, respiratory acidosis, metabolic acidosis, tachycardia, generalized muscle rigidity, myoglobinuria, and elevated temperature. A prior history of uneventful anesthesia with exposure to triggering agents does not exclude the disease. Because of the variability in presentation, a clinical grading scale to predict MH susceptibility has been created (Table 61-1). If MH is suspected, the patient should be treated immediately as described next. The scoring system is used to determine the likelihood that the patient had MH in retrospect. The list of clinical indicators is reviewed, and points are assigned for each indicator present. If more than one indicator represents a single process, only the indicator with the highest score is counted. The exceptions to this are arterial pH and base excess, which are counted regardless of points assigned elsewhere for acidosis. The raw score range is then assigned an MH rank, which provides a qualitative likelihood that the episode was or was not MH (Table 61-2). The onset of MH is variable after anesthetic agent exposure, and the maximal latency period between the end of anesthesia and the onset of symptoms is unknown. Most often the onset of MH occurs in the operating room during the administration of a triggering agent; however, delayed presentations in the early postoperative period have been reported.

Evaluation

The criterion standard for diagnosis of MH in genetically susceptible patients is a muscle contracture test. The in vitro muscle contracture test is performed in Europe, and the caffeine-halothane contracture test is performed in the United States and Canada. Both tests are typically performed on a biopsy of muscle from the vastus medialis. The specimen is exposed to halothane and caffeine. Three diagnostic groups are in the in vitro muscle contracture test. The patient is diagnosed as being MH susceptible if a pathologic contracture occurs after exposure to halothane and after exposure to caffeine. The patient is diagnosed as being MH equivocal if a pathologic contracture occurs after exposure to one agent but not the other. The patient is deemed MH negative if no pathologic contracture occurs after exposure to either agent. Clinically, patients with an MH equivocal diagnosis should be treated as though they were MH susceptible, though their scientific status is considered unknown. Two diagnostic groups are in the caffeine-halothane contracture test: those who have a pathologic contracture in any of the muscle strips exposed to halothane or those who have all of the strips exposed to caffeine are labeled MH susceptible. Otherwise, the test results are negative. Patients designated as MH susceptible should never be exposed to triggering agents in the future.

Table 61-1. Clinical Indicators for Use in Determining the MH Raw Score (Evidence Level III)

Process	Indicator	Points
Process I: Rigidity	Generalized muscle rigidity	15
	Masseter spasm after succinylcholine administration	15
Process II: Muscle Breakdown	Creatinine kinase level >20,000 IU after anesthesia with succinylcholine	15
	Creatinine kinase level >10,000 IU after anesthesia without succinylcholine	15
	Cola-colored urine in perioperative period	10
	Urine myoglobin level >60 mcg/L	5
	Serum myoglobin level >170 mcg/L	5
	Serum potassium level >6 mEq/L	5
Process III: Respiratory Acidosis	P_{ETCO_2} >55 mm Hg with appropriate ventilation	15
	Pa_{CO_2} >60 mm Hg with appropriate ventilation	15
	P_{ETCO_2} >60 mm Hg with spontaneous ventilation	15
	Inappropriate hypercarbia	15
	Inappropriate tachypnea	10
Process IV: Temperature Increase	Rapid rise in temperature	15
	Temperature >38.8°C (101.8°F), which is inappropriate in anesthesiologist's judgment	10
Process V: Cardiac Involvement	Inappropriate sinus tachycardia	3
	Ventricular tachycardia or fibrillation	3
Other Indicators That Are Not Part of a Single Process	Arterial base excess more negative than − 8 mEq/L	10
	Arterial pH <7.25	10
	Rapid reversal of MH symptoms with IV dantrolene	5

Abbreviations: IV, intravenous; MH, malignant hyperthermia.
Adapted from Larach MG, Localio AR, Allen GC, et al. A clinical grading scale to predict malignant hyperthermia susceptibility. *Anesthesiology.* 1994;80(4):771–779, with permission.

Muscle contracture testing is recommended for anyone who has a high MH clinical grade or first-degree relatives of patients with a history suspicious for MH who have not been tested. Genetic testing is recommended for individuals who have a family member with positive genetic test results for MH or for patients with positive contracture test results. Unfortunately, considering that not all genetic mutations for MH are known, genetic screening is imperfect and likely to miss approximately 50% of patients genetically susceptible to MH.

Patients with certain neuromuscular diseases should be treated as though they are MH susceptible. One disease in particular, central core disease, is likely

Table 61-2. Likelihood of MH as Determined by Raw MH Clinical Grading Score (Evidence Level III)

Raw Score Range	MH Rank	Description of Likelihood
0	1	Almost never
3–9	2	Unlikely
10–19	3	Somewhat less than likely
20–34	4	Somewhat greater than likely
35–49	5	Very likely
≥50	6	Almost certain

Abbreviation: MH, malignant hyperthermia.

Adapted from Larach MG, Localio AR, Allen GC, et al. A clinical grading scale to predict malignant hyperthermia susceptibility. *Anesthesiology*. 1994;80(4):771–779, with permission.

related to MH. Central core disease is a myopathy characterized by "cores" seen in muscle fibers on biopsy specimens. There is association with MH seen by clinical and laboratory evidence in several families with large pedigrees.

The association of MH in patients with King-Denborough syndrome (KDS) and Duchenne muscular dystrophy (DMD) warrants mentioning. KDS is characterized by progressive myopathy, abnormal facies, short stature, pectus carinatum, kyphoscoliosis, and cryptorchidism. It is still unclear whether the association between KDS and MH is sporadic or whether MH is part of the clinical syndrome. Either way, these patients should be treated as MH susceptible. Duchenne muscular dystrophy is an x-linked muscular dystrophy. Sudden cardiac death and clinical episodes that may represent MH in patients with DMD have been reported. Furthermore, some but not all patients with DMD have positive results from muscle contracture tests. It is unknown whether this association is independent or genetically associated with DMD; therefore, all patients with DMD should be treated as MH susceptible.

Management

Once a diagnosis of MH is suspected, treatment should begin immediately. The Malignant Hyperthermia Association of the United States (www.mhaus.org) has a 24-hour hotline for MH emergencies and a recommended treatment protocol. In the acute phase, it is recommended to stop all volatile agents and succinylcholine. The anesthesiologist should call for additional assistance and begin rapid administration of intravenous dantrolene (2.5 mg/kg) (Evidence Level II-2). Dantrolene is a direct-acting skeletal muscle relaxant that dissociates excitation-contraction coupling in the muscle by inhibiting release of calcium from the sarcoplasmic reticulum. The patient should be placed on 100% inspired oxygen, and minute ventilation should be maximized to aid in the clearance of CO_2. Metabolic acidosis can be treated with sodium bicarbonate. If hyperthermia is present, cooling to less than 38°C (100.4°F) with ice packs should be pursued. Hyperkalemia should be treated with glucose, insulin, and calcium. Calcium channel blockers are to be avoided for treatment of dysrhythmias, as they may cause hyperkalemia and cardiac arrest. Because 25% of patients may have return of symptoms after an episode of MH, it is recommended that maintenance doses of dantrolene are given for 48 hours after the last observed sign of acute MH. Prior to the availability of dantrolene, mortality of MH was as high as 70%. It is now reported to be between 1.4% and 6%. Mortality in patients younger than 18 years is reported to be less than 1%.

Suggested Reading

Denborough M. Malignant hyperthermia. *Lancet.* 1998;352(9134):1131–1136

Islander G, Twetman ER. Comparison between European and North American protocols for diagnosis of malignant hyperthermia susceptibility in humans. *Anesth Analog.* 1999;88(5):1155–1160

Kolb ME, Horne ML, Martz R. Dantrolene in malignant hyperthermia. *Anesthesiology.* 1982;56(4):254–262

Larach MG, Gronert GA, Allen GC, Brandom BW, Lehman EB. Clinical presentation, treatment, and complications of malignant hyperthermia in North America from 1987 to 2006. *Anesth Analog.* 2010;110(2):498–507

Larach MG, Localio AR, Allen GC, et al. A clinical grading scale to predict malignant hyperthermia susceptibility. *Anesthesiology.* 1994;80(4):771–779

O'Flynn RP, Shutack JG, Rosenberg H, Fletcher JE. Masseter muscle rigidity and malignant hyperthermia susceptibility in pediatric patients. *Anesthesiology.* 1994;80(6):1228–1233

Rosero EB, Adesanya AO, Timaran CH, Joshi GP. Trends and outcomes of malignant hyperthermia in the United States, 2000 to 2005. *Anesthesiology.* 2009;110(1):89–94

Wedel DJ. Malignant hyperthermia and neuromuscular disease. *Neuromuscul Disord.* 1992;2(3):157–164

CHAPTER 62

Pleural Effusion

William T. Tsai, MD

Key Points

- Pleural effusion most often occurs in the setting of pneumonia, with *Streptococcus pneumoniae* and *Staphylococcus aureus* being the most commonly identified causative agents.

- In equivocal cases, pleural fluid analysis may help elucidate the etiology of the effusion. In all patients with fluid aspiration, drainage, or both, laboratory analysis and culture of the fluid should be pursued.

- Not all pleural effusions require drainage. The decision to drain the pleural effusion is based on the patient's clinical picture and the need for a definitive diagnosis.

- To manage complicated pneumonia with empyema, video-assisted thoracoscopy should be considered early in the disease course to assist in obtaining diagnostic studies of the fluid and to provide symptomatic relief.

Overview

Pleural effusion is a relatively common finding in children. Its incidence is underreported because in many cases the volumes are not easily discernible and sensitivity is lacking in the standard diagnostic test (ie, chest radiograph). Pleural effusion occurs when fluid accumulates in the potential space bounded by the parietal and visceral pleura of the lung. Normally, a small amount of fluid in this potential space serves as a lubricating fluid; however, when homeostatic mechanisms become deranged secondary to infectious processes and changes in hydrostatic or oncotic pressure, fluid may accumulate. This accumulation may range from the clinically insignificant to volumes that can cause respiratory distress or acute cardiovascular collapse. Infection is by far the most common cause of detectable and symptomatic pleural effusion.

Causes and Differential Diagnosis

The type of fluid recovered from the pleural space may help identify the etiology of the effusion. Fluid may be exudative, transudative, or chylous as defined by diagnostic testing of the fluid (Table 62-1 and Box 62-1). Hemor-rhagic effusion may occur in the setting of trauma. Most cases of pleural effusion occur in the setting of an infectious disorder, such as a complicated pneumonia. Accumulation of fluid in the pleural space may embarrass respiratory function but may also become secondarily infected, leading to empyema. The quality of the fluid in infectious processes is exudative.

Table 62-1. Types of Pleural Effusion

Diagnostic Test	Exudative	Transudative	Chylous
pH	<7.20	>7.20	Variable
Protein[a]	>0.5	<0.5	Variable
LDH[b]	>0.6	<0.6	Variable
WBC	>10,000 PMN	<10,000 PMN	Lymphocytes
Triglycerides	Negative	Negative	Elevated
Glucose	<40 mg/dL	>40 mg/dL	Variable
RBC	>5,000 mm³	<5,000 mm³	Variable
Chylomicrons	Negative	Negative	Positive

Abbreviations: LDH, lactate dehydrongenase; PMN, polymorphonuclear; RBC, red blood cell; WBC, white blood cell.
[a] Pleural fluid protein to serum protein ratio (mg/dL).
[b] Pleural fluid LDH to serum LDH ratio (mg/dL).

Box 62-1. Causes of Pleural Effusion

Exudative
   Bacterial infection (eg, *Streptococcus pneumoniae, Staphylococcus aureus*)
   Viral infections
   Mycobacteria
   Fungal
   Systemic lupus erythematosus and other autoimmune processes
   Pancreatitis
   Malignancy
   Uremia
   Acute respiratory distress syndrome
   Post-cardiac injury syndrome

Transudative
   Congestive heart failure
   Nephrotic syndrome
   Fontan procedure
   Hypoalbuminemia
   Cirrhosis
   Superior vena cava obstruction

Chylous
   Thoracic duct injury

Transudative effusions occur from processes that alter capillary hydrostatics, capillary oncotic pressure, or lymphatic drainage.

Chylous effusions occur in the setting of recent cardiothoracic surgery or trauma and require a different management strategy.

Clinical Features

Pleural effusions may present asymptomatically, cause significant dyspnea, or progress to significant cardiovascular compromise. In the setting of pneumonia, pleural effusion may present as chest pain, pleurisy, dyspnea, or tachypnea and may range from small accumulations of fluid to large volume effusions that may become loculated. In general, children with significant effusions demonstrate decreased unilateral lung sounds or decreased bilateral lung sounds in the setting of bilateral effusions. Tachypnea and retractions may be noted with larger fluid accumulations. Hypoxia can result from significant ventilation/perfusion mismatch. More specific manifestations such as the presence of fever, cough, edema, recent surgery, poor feeding, and weight gain may help narrow the differential diagnosis.

Pleural fluid may become infected, creating a fibrinous, parapneumonic effusion of exudative fluid that may progress to empyema. Empyema, or pus in the pleural space, may be encased in a fibrous shell, leading to poor antibiotic penetration, persistently collapsed lung segments, and poor response to standard antibiotic treatments.

Transudative effusion may become symptomatic in the setting of congestive heart failure. The combination of extra lung water and pleural effusion secondary to increased left atrial pressure may result in the classic signs of orthopnea and paroxysmal nocturnal dyspnea. In infants, this may present as difficulty feeding and poor weight gain. Hypoalbuminemic states, such as nephrotic syndrome, may cause pleural effusions but rarely serve as the initial presenting symptom in these patients. Body edema is more likely to be the initial presentation in hypoalbuminemic states than respiratory symptoms secondary to pleural effusion.

Chylous effusions occur most commonly after cardiac surgery as increased chest tube output or persistent pleural effusions after removal of chest tubes. The appearance of this fluid may be opalescent and milky. Trauma may also cause chylothorax.

Evaluation

Standard chest radiograph will frequently identify pleural effusions (Figure 62-1). Findings on chest radiograph include blunting of the costophrenic angle, a pleural stripe, a meniscus sign, or complete opacity of the hemithorax. In supine patients, pleural fluid may cast a hazy appearance on the involved hemithorax. In cases with an opacified hemithorax, ultrasonography or computed tomography may help elucidate between atelectatic lung and pleural effusion.

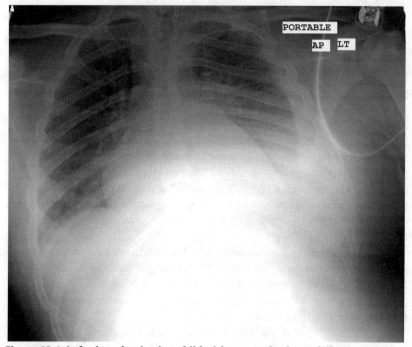

Figure 62-1. Left pleural stripe in a child with congestive heart failure.

Ultrasonography is useful in determining the quality of the fluid in the pleural space. It is also an effective method to quantify pleural effusion volume. Exudative fluid tends to be echogenic, while transudates are echolucent. Fibrinous material, blood, and loculations may all be identified by ultrasonography. While computed tomography of the chest provides a more comprehensive picture of the extent of the fluid and has the ability to map loculations better, its use must be tempered because of the amount of radiation and intravenous contrast required.

If pleural fluid is obtained, it should be sent for chemical and microbiologic analysis. Laboratory tests to help differentiate the type of fluid are listed in Table 62-1. Analysis of the pleural fluid may help in identifying the etiology of the pleural effusion and help guide therapy (Evidence Level III).

Management

The decision to drain a pleural effusion should rest on the need to improve the patient's clinical symptoms and the necessity for a definitive diagnosis. Most pleural effusions do not need drainage. In patients with complicated pneumonia, thoracentesis may help provide not only a microbiologic diagnosis but therapeutic benefit. In parapneumonic effusions, video-assisted thoracoscopy or the use of intrapleural fibrinolytic agents should be considered over use of simple chest tube because of faster resolution of symptoms and less need for re-intervention (Evidence Level II-2).

Transudative effusions are amenable to simple chest tubes and may be removed with small-bore tubes that are more comfortable for the patient. In many cases, diuretics alone or methods to treat underlying causes such as hypoalbuminemia may be enough to eliminate effusions.

Chylothorax may be treated with a simple chest tube. Re-expansion of the lung followed by time often results in spontaneous resolution. Frequently, chylous effusions are also treated with a fat-restricted diet that is supplemented with medium-chain triglycerides. Medium-chain fatty acids are not transported via the thoracic duct and may lessen chylous effusion. Somatostatin may be used to lessen the production of chyle. In refractory cases, thoracic duct ligation or pleurodesis may be necessary to prevent chronic, large chylous effusions.

Suggested Reading

Calder A, Owens CM. Imaging of parapneumonic pleural effusions and empyema in children. *Pediatr Radiol.* 2009;39(6):527–537

Doski J, Lou D, Hicks B, et al. Management of parapneumonic collections in infants and children. *J Pediatr Surg.* 2000;35(2):265–270

Givan DC, Eigen H. Common pleural effusions in children. *Clin Chest Med.* 1998;19(2):363–371

Hawkins JA, Scaife ES, Hillman ND, et al. Current treatment of pediatric empyema. *Semin Thorac Cardiovasc Surg.* 2004;16(3):196–200

Kercher K, Attorri R, Hoover J, Morton D Jr. Thoracoscopic decortication as first-line therapy for pediatric parapneumonic empyema. A case series. *Chest.* 2000;118:24–27

Light RW, Macgregor MI, Luchsinger PC, et al. Pleural effusions: the diagnostic separation of transudates and exudates. *Ann Intern Med.* 1972;77(4):507–513

Maldonado F, Finn JH, Daniels CE, Doerr CH, Decker PA, Ryu JH. Pleural fluid characteristics of chylothorax. *Mayo Clin Proc.* 2009;84(2):129–133

Scarci M, Zahid I, Bille A, Routledge T. Is video-assisted thoracoscopic surgery the best treatment for paediatric pleural empyema? *Interact Cardiovasc Thorac Surg.* 2011;13(1):70–76

Shoseyov D, Bibi H, Shatzberg G, Klar A, Akerman J, Hurvitz H, Maayan C. Short-term course and outcome of treatments of pleural empyema in pediatric patients vs repeated ultrasound-guided needle thoracocentesis vs chest tube drainage. *Chest.* 2002;121(3):836–840

Thompson A, Hull J, Kumar M, Wallis C, Balfour Lynn IM. Randomized trial of intrapleural urokinase in the treatment of childhood empyema. *Thorax.* 2002;57(4):343–347

CHAPTER 63

Poisoning

Kristin Stukus, MD

Key Points

- Prevention of poisonings is of utmost importance. Families should be instructed on appropriate storage of medications and household poisons. Families should also be reminded to contact Poison Control at 1-800-222-1222 with concerns. Adolescents should be screened for depression and self-harming behaviors.

- Several household substances and medications can be harmful or deadly at very small doses. These include beta-blockers, calcium channel blockers, clonidine, oral hypoglycemic, tricyclic antidepressants, benzocaine, camphor, and methyl salicylates.

- Button battery ingestions should be referred for immediate imaging and removal.

Overview

Accidental or intentional ingestion of a toxic agent is common in the pediatric population. Ingestions have a bimodal population distribution, with the first peak in those aged 1 to 5 years, typically associated with exploratory behaviors and ingestion of a single agent. Children younger than 6 account for half of all calls to poison centers. The second peek occurs during adolescence, is associated with intent to produce altered mental state or intent to harm/suicidal intent, and often involves more than one agent. There is a male predominance within the younger age group, which reverses in the older population. Nearly 65% of the ingestions in those younger than 5 were characterized as unintentional, while 24% of the ingestions in the 13-to-19-years-of-age group were classified as intentional.

Management of acute poisonings will vary greatly depending on the agent and amount taken. Consultation with the local Poison Center, available nationally at 1-800-222-1222, will be immensely helpful in determining the course of action necessary for the treatment of the acutely poisoned child.

Administration of activated charcoal may be considered in an alert, hemodynamic stable patient who presents within 1 hour of ingestion. Activated charcoal is not effective in treating ingestions of heavy metals, such as iron or lithium, or toxic alcohols. Specific antidotes are available for some toxins and will be discussed in further detail in following sections. Other nonspecific treatment options for critically ill patients include gastric lavage or whole bowel irrigation.

Prevention of unintentional ingestions is of utmost importance in the primary care setting. Anticipatory guidance should be provided to families regarding safe storage of medications, household cleaners, and access to poison control. Syrup of ipecac is no longer recommended to be kept in the home for treatment of household ingestions. Parents should be instructed to keep all medications out of the reach of children. When no longer in use or after expiration, medications should be discarded safely. Household poisons should be in locked cabinets and should never be transferred to unmarked containers. Parents should be reminded not to refer to medications as "candy." Care should be taken when visiting with grandparents or other family members, to ensure that medications are handled appropriately. Often, older adults will forgo childproof caps for ease of use. They are also more likely to have dangerous medications for blood pressure or blood sugar management in the home. Parents should be encouraged to keep the national poison center phone number next to their phone, as well as programmed into their cell phone. Adolescents should be screened for symptoms of depression or thoughts of self-harm. The patient's medications as well as medications in the home should be documented.

Differential Diagnosis

Differential diagnosis will vary widely depending on the drug ingested. A high index of suspicion for ingestion should be maintained at all times. Children should be screened for access to medications and other poisons, and all medications in the home should be documented. Box 63-1 lists the most common types of poisonings seen in children and adolescents. Specific evaluation principles and management approaches follow.

Evaluation and Management

Nonsteroidal Analgesics

Most ingestions involving nonsteroidal anti-inflammatory drugs are asymptomatic and without long-term sequelae. Ingestions of ibuprofen less than 150 mg/kg may be observed at home. With larger ingestions, typical signs and symptoms primarily affect the gastrointestinal (GI) tract. Within a few hours of ingestion, patients will often complain of GI tract upset and nausea. With acute or chronic exposure, erosions can occur within the lining of the stomach, leading to GI tract bleeding, hematemesis, and in rare circumstances perfora-

Box 63-1. Most Common Types of Poisoning in Children and Adolescents

- Acetaminophen
- Acids/alkalis
- Anticholinergics
- Antihypertensives
- Button batteries
- Carbon monoxide
- Coins
- Cough and cold medications
- Ethanol
- Ethylene glycol (toxic alcohols)
- Iron
- Hydrocarbons
- Nonsteroidal analgesics
- Opiates
- Organophosphates
- Plants
- Salicylates
- Tricyclic antidepressants

tion. Nonsteroidal anti-inflammatory drug ingestion may also lead to renal injury, especially in those with diabetes or hypertension.

Acetaminophen

Acetaminophen is the most commonly administered pediatric antipyretic and analgesic. It is also one of the 10 most common drugs ingested by adolescents and adults with intentional ingestion. The patient may not reveal or be aware of the acetaminophen ingestion, as it is a common co-ingredient in many cough and cold preparations. All patients with an unknown ingestion and all adolescents with a known ingestion should be screened for acetaminophen co-ingestion as well.

Symptoms of acute acetaminophen poisoning are vague, including nausea, vomiting, and anorexia. These symptoms typically last 12 to 24 hours after the ingestion and then resolve. If the ingestion is unrecognized and untreated, liver damage begins to occur, with elevation of transaminases. However, the patient will remain asymptomatic until hepatic disease becomes clinically evident 3 to 5 days after the ingestion.

Patients should have an acetaminophen level drawn at 4 hours after the ingestion. The decision of whether to treat should be based on the level and the acetaminophen nomogram (Figure 63-1).

The treatment of acetaminophen overdose is with N-acetylcysteine. This causes acetaminophen metabolism in the liver to change to a nontoxic form, which is then excreted. N-acetylcysteine can be administered in either oral or

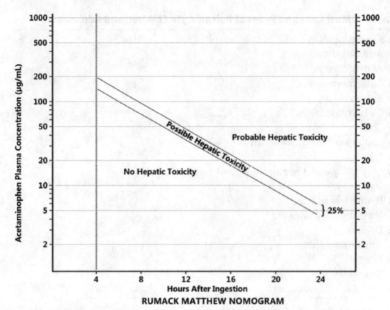

Figure 63-1. Plasma or serum acetaminophen concentration versus time post-acetaminophen ingestion.

Adapted from Rumack BH, Matthew H. Acetaminophen poisoning and toxicity. *Pediatrics*. 1975;55(6):871–876 and Rumack BH. Acetaminophen hepatoxicity: the first 35 years. *J Toxicol Clin Toxicol*. 2002;40(1):3–20.

intravenous (IV) forms. Patients with elevated acetaminophen levels require hospitalization for multiple doses of N-acetylcysteine administration, as well as monitoring of hepatic and renal functioning.

Opiates

Opiate ingestion leads to a toxidrome characterized by miosis, depressed mental status, respiratory depression, nausea, and vomiting. Suspected opiate intoxication is treated with naloxone. It is important to remember, however, that the length of action of the opiate may be longer than the duration of action of the dose of naloxone, so all patients should be referred to a center comfortable with the treatment and monitoring of pediatric ingestions.

Anticholinergics

Many medications (including over-the-counter), plants, and mushrooms have an anticholinergic effect (Box 63-2).

Ingestion of anticholinergic agents leads to a toxidrome, the associated behavior and appearance of which is often remembered by the mnemonic "dry

Box 63-2. Drugs and Chemicals That May Produce the Central Anticholinergic Syndrome

- **Antidepressants:** amitriptyline (Elavil), imipramine (Tofranil), doxepin (Sinequan, Adopin)

- **Antihistamines:** chlorpheniramine (Ornade, Teldrin), diphenhydramine (Benadryl), orphenadrine (Norflex)

- **Ophthalmologic preparations:** cyclopentolate (Cyclogyl), tropicamide (Mydriacyl)

- **Antispasmodic agents:** propantheline (Pro-Banthine), clidinium bromide (Librax)

- **Antiparkinson agents:** trihexyphenidyl (Artane), benztropine (Cogentin), procyclidine (Kemadrin)

- **Proprietary drugs:** Sleep-Eze (scopolamine, methapyrilene), Sominex (scopolamine, methapyrilene), Asthmador (belladonna alkaloids), Excedrin PM (methapyrilene)

- **Belladonna alkaloids:** atropine, homatropine, hyscine, hyoscyamus, scopolamine

- **Toxic plants:** mushroom (*Amanita muscaria*), bitter-sweet (*Solanum dulcamara*), Jimson weed (*Datura stramonium*), potato leaves and sprouts (*Solanum tuberosum*), deadly nightshade (*Atropa belladonna*)

From Osterhoudt KC, Burns Ewald M, Shannon M, Henretig FM. Toxicologic emergencies. In: Fleisher GR, Ludwig S, eds. *Textbook of Pediatric Emergency Medicine.* 6th ed. 2010; Philadelphia, PA: Lippincott Williams & Wilkins; 2010: 1218, with permission.

as a bone, red as a beet, mad as a hatter, blind as a bat, hot as a hare." Typically, patients will develop mydriasis, decreased salivation, and decreased sweat production, with facial flushing, fevers, tachycardia, and tremors. Patients often are agitated with altered mental status and may experience hallucinations. Because anticholinergic drugs slow GI tract motility, activated charcoal may be considered for a longer period after the ingestion. Treatment of anticholinergic ingestions is primarily symptomatic, with benzodiazepines typically used to treat the agitation. Another treatment option for anticholinergic symptoms is physostigmine. However, administration of physostigmine may result in seizures or asystole and may cause cardiac conduction abnormalities when given in the presence of other co-ingestants. For this reason, it should be given only in controlled environments, with resuscitation equipment prepared.

Salicylates

Acute aspirin intoxication causes a hallmark pattern of mixed metabolic acidosis and respiratory alkalosis. In addition to aspirin, salicylates may also be present in some household compounds as oil of wintergreen. Salicylates act on the respiratory center of the medulla, causing tachypnea. Other signs of acute intoxication include fever, nausea and vomiting, depressed mental status, and seizures. Concern of tinnitus or hearing changes should raise high suspicion of salicylate poisoning, either acute or chronic. Chronic salicylism may present with similar symptoms at lower blood salicylate levels. Chronic salicylate poisoning may be difficult to diagnosis because of vague symptoms. Treatment of salicylate ingestion is aimed at increasing the excretion of salicylic acid in the urine with the administration of IV fluids with sodium bicarbonate and potassium. Hemodialysis may be indicated in those with elevated drug levels, severe acidosis, renal failure, or neurologic dysfunction.

Antihypertensives

Multiple classes of medications fall under the umbrella of antihypertensives, with different mechanisms of action. Beta-blockers and calcium channel blockers may both cause profound cardiovascular and neurologic symptoms, with bradycardia, hypotension, seizures, or coma. Both are potentially fatal with the ingestion of 1 or 2 pills in a small child. Ingestion of beta-blockers may be accompanied by hypoglycemia, while calcium channel blocker ingestion may be associated with hyperglycemia and metabolic acidosis. Treatment is supportive, with atropine, IV fluids, and vasopressor agents if necessary. In addition, those with known calcium channel blocker ingestion should be treated with calcium infusion.

Clonidine is an antihypertensive that is frequently prescribed to pediatric patients for treatment of attention-deficit/hyperactivity disorder. Small doses of medication may cause profound symptoms in children, including hypothermia, lethargy, and coma. Treatment includes IV fluids and vasopressor support as needed. Some data suggest that naloxone in large doses may reverse the neurologic and cardiovascular symptoms of clonidine ingestion.

Tricyclic Antidepressants

Tricyclic antidepressants (TCAs) are present in many households and present a significant danger when ingested. Although these medications may have profound anticholinergic and sedating effects, the most common cause of death is from cardiac conduction abnormalities. The most common TCAs and their predominant adverse effects are listed in Table 63-1. Tricyclic antidepressants commonly cause prolongation of the QRS interval but may also cause sinus tachycardia and premature ventricular contractions. Large overdoses may lead to complete heart block and asystole. In small children, 1 or 2 tablets may be fatal.

Management of TCA overdose consists of GI tract contamination if possible. Like other anticholinergics, TCAs delay gastric emptying. Thus, GI tract decontamination with activated charcoal may be effective beyond the initial hour after ingestion. Initial 12-lead electrocardiogram and continuous cardiac monitoring is indicated in TCA ingestions. Sodium bicarbonate is indicated to stabilize the cardiac membranes and should be continued in the event of widened QRS complexes.

Ethanol

Ethanol is a substance commonly found in most households. In addition to being present in alcoholic beverages, ethanol is present in some mouthwashes

Table 63-1. Tricyclic Antidepressants and Related Compounds

Drug	Adverse Effects					
	ACh	Drowsiness	Orthostatic Hypotension	Conduction Abnormalities	GI Distress	Weight Gain
Amitriptyline	4+	4+	3+	3+	1+	4+
Amoxapine	2+	2+	2+	2+	0	2+
Clomipramine (Anafranil®)	4+	4+	2+	3+	1+	4+
Desipramine (Norpramin®)	1+	2+	2+	2+	0	1+
Doxepin	3+	4+	2+	2+	0	4+
Imipramine (Tofranil, Tofranil PM)	3+	3+	4+	3+	1+	4+
Maprotiline	2+	3+	2+	2+	0	2+
Nortriptyline (Pamelor)	2+	2+	1+	2+	0	1+
Protriptyline (Vivactil)	2+	1+	2+	3+	1+	1+
Trimipramine (Surmontil)	4+	4+	3+	3+	0	4+

Abbreviations: ACh, acetylcholine; GI, gastrointestinal.
Adapted from Taketomo CK, Hodding JH, Kraus DM, eds. *Pediatric and Neonatal Dosage Handbook*. 21st ed. Hudson, OH: Lexicomp; 2014.

and perfumes, as well as hand sanitizers. Children with ethanol ingestion may develop nausea, vomiting, ataxia, and altered mental status, including coma. Young children are particularly sensitive to alcohol and develop a triad of coma, hypothermia, and hypoglycemia. This may occur at blood ethanol levels between 50 to 100 mg/dL. Treatment of ethanol ingestion is primarily supportive.

Hydrocarbons

Hydrocarbons are carbon-containing compounds that are liquid at room temperature and have low viscosity. They are present in many households in substances such as lamp oil, gasoline, kerosene, and furniture polish. Hydrocarbons are generally safe if ingested but may cause respiratory distress and even death if aspirated. Their low viscosity allows them to spread over large surface areas within the lungs, disrupting the surfactant and gas exchange within the alveoli. Vomiting should never be induced after hydrocarbon ingestion. Any child with vomiting after hydrocarbon ingestion or history of choking and coughing at the time of the ingestion should undergo a chest x-ray and be referred for observation. If the initial chest radiograph is clear, it should be repeated 4 to 6 hours after the ingestion to look for signs of pneumonitis. Any patient with tachypnea, hypoxia, or respiratory distress should be referred to a pediatric center with critical care capabilities.

Organophosphates

Poisoning from organophosphates may occur by ingestion, inhalation, or penetration through skin. Most commonly found in some commercial pesticides, organophosphates prevent the enzyme acetylcholinesterase from working at the neuromuscular junction, allowing buildup of acetylcholine. This leads to a predictable toxidrome characterized by the mnemonic SLUDGE (salivation, lacrimation, urination, defecation, gastrointestinal cramping, and emesis) from its effects on the autonomic nervous system, as well as tremors, twitches, weakness, and paralysis from its effects on skeletal muscles. Patients may also develop bronchorrhea and wheezing, which may progress to pulmonary edema. Organophosphate poisoning may also lead to profound central nervous system effects, with dizziness, headaches, ataxia, seizures, and coma.

The first step after identification of an organophosphate poisoning is decontamination. As the poison may continue to be absorbed from the skin, the patient's clothes should be removed and placed in a plastic bag to prevent others from being harmed. The affected areas of skin should be washed thoroughly. Decontamination with activated charcoal or gastric lavage may be considered. Patients should be treated with atropine, with doses repeated every 10 to 30 minutes until bronchial secretions resolve. Patients should also be treated with pralidoxime, or 2-PAM, which binds to the organophosphate and allows acetylcholinesterase to function at the neuromuscular junction of skeletal muscles. Patients with organophosphate poisoning should be admitted to the hospital for repeated doses of both atropine and pralidoxime.

Carbon Monoxide

Carbon monoxide is produced from burning of carbon-based fuel, including its production during house fires. Symptoms from low levels of exposure are vague, including headache, nausea, vomiting, and fatigue. With higher levels of exposure, syncope, seizures, cardiac arrhythmias, and altered mental status may develop. It is necessary to have a high index of suspicion to diagnose carbon monoxide poisoning. Highest risk for exposure is during winter months when kerosene and space heaters are in use and infectious agents causing similar symptoms are at their peak.

Management of carbon monoxide poisoning depends on the level of exposure and symptoms. At room air, the half-life of carbon monoxide is about 4 hours. At 100% O_2, the half-life decreases to 90 minutes, and with hyperbaric treatment, it decreases further to less than 30 minutes. Hyperbaric oxygen therapy is recommended in pregnant patients and those with neurologic symptoms (eg, altered mental status, seizures, or coma) and should be considered in those with cardiac sequelae or with carboxyhemoglobin levels of 25 to 40%. Rapid screening may be done with bedside detectors, which are noninvasive, although blood testing is also recommended if the reading is elevated. Survivors of house fires should also be considered for treatment for cyanide poisoning.

Acids/Alkali

Many household cleaning products are either acidic or alkali and may produce burns to the GI tract if ingested. Acidic products act by causing coagulation necrosis and superficial burns, whereas alkalis cause deep burns by liquefaction necrosis. Ingestion of alkalis may lead to esophageal perforation and potentially mediastinitis. Alkali ingestions also cause deep scarring and stricture formation. After ingestion of a household cleaning product, poison control should be contacted to assist in the identification of the agent and to determine the need for further treatment. Vomiting should not be induced, and patients should not be given anything to drink, both because of the risk of esophageal perforation and the potential need for endoscopy. Any patients with identified corrosive ingestion should be referred to a pediatric center for further management.

Button Batteries

The incidence of button or disc battery ingestion has increased in recent years with their increasing frequency of usage. The danger of button battery ingestion lies in batteries' caustic breakdown when contact with the mucosa occurs. This should prompt immediate removal of the foreign body if the ears or nose are involved. If a button battery has been ingested, a chest radiograph should be obtained immediately to determine its position. If the battery has lodged in the esophagus, the patient should be referred to a pediatric facility for immediate removal. If the battery has passed into the stomach, a period of watchful waiting can occur, with parents straining the stool for the battery. If the battery has not passed in a week, a repeat abdominal radiograph should be obtained. Rarely do button batteries within the lower GI tract require removal.

Coins

Coins are frequently found and ingested by young children. Although nontoxic, they may get stuck within the upper respiratory tract or gastrointestinal tract and cause significant symptoms. In a patient with sudden episode of choking, coughing, or gagging, a series of radiographs should be obtained to rule out foreign body. This includes radiographs of the lateral neck to visualize the upper airway and hypopharynx, a chest radiograph, and an abdominal radiograph. A coin is most likely to lodge in the upper esophagus at the thoracic outlet, in the mid-esophagus at the aortic notch, or at the lower gastroesophageal junction. Coins that are ingested and reside below the diaphragm need no treatment or further evaluation.

Iron

Iron ingestion is typically from iron-containing vitamins found in the home. The incidence of iron ingestions has decreased over the last 2 decades after the initiation of blister packages for iron tablets and child-resistant caps for vitamins.

Iron poisoning is typically characterized by 4 separate phases. The initial phase is caused by direct mucosal injury within the stomach, which causes nausea, vomiting, and occasionally GI tract blood loss. This phase typically lasts about 6 hours after the ingestion and is followed by a relatively asymptomatic period from 6 to 24 hours. Depending on the amount ingested and the initial management, the patient may progress to full recovery. In large ingestions, the patient may progress to metabolic acidosis, seizures, coma, and shock from hepatic injury. Laboratory studies performed in this period may show elevated bilirubin and transaminases. Phase 4 occurs after recovery from these injuries and is characterized by pyloric stenosis and gastric outlet obstruction.

Treatment of iron ingestion consists of early recognition and quantification of the amount ingested. Iron levels may be drawn at 3 to 5 hours after the ingestion and correlate with severity of illness. Typically, levels less than 350 mcg/dL have a benign or asymptomatic course. Levels between 350 to 500 typically manifest phase 1 symptoms but do not generally progress to shock. Levels above 500 are at significant risk for phase 3 manifestations.

The type of treatment approach to iron ingestion depends on the presenting symptoms. Asymptomatic patients may be monitored for 6 hours, with an iron level drawn. An abdominal radiograph may also be obtained to look for radiopaque iron tablets. If the iron level is reassuring, the abdominal radiograph findings negative, and the patient asymptomatic, they may be discharged after a 6-hour observation period. In patients with severe symptoms, large reported ingestion, positive abdominal radiograph findings, or serum iron level above 500 mcg/dL, treatment should be initiated with whole bowel irrigation, laboratory studies, and IV deferoxamine. Activated charcoal is not indicated in iron ingestions, as it does not bind to heavy metals. Whole bowel irrigation with polyethylene glycol may minimize necrosis from direct contact with iron and may break up iron concretions. A follow-up abdominal radiograph should be obtained to ensure that no concretions persist. Chelation therapy with IV deferoxamine enhances excretion of the iron. It should be administered by continuous IV infusion until the metabolic acidosis resolves and the iron levels return to normal.

Ethylene Glycol (Toxic Alcohols)

Several toxic alcohols may be present in the home and pose a significant health threat if ingested. Ethylene glycol is most commonly found in antifreeze. Ethylene glycol is metabolized within the body to glycoaldehyde, glycolic acid, and oxalate. The result is metabolic acidosis and calcium oxalate deposition within the tissues. The timeline of ethylene glycol poisoning includes central nervous system changes within a few hours of ingestion, with nausea, vomiting, seizures, progression to coma, and cardiopulmonary failure. Within 24 to 72 hours of ingestion, renal failure may occur. Laboratory findings are significant for profound hypocalcemia, metabolic acidosis with large anion gap, osmolar gap, and crystals in the urine. In addition, if antifreeze is the source of the ethylene glycol, the urine may fluoresce with Wood lamp examination. Treatment of ethylene glycol intoxication consists of sodium bicarbonate to treat the acidosis; calcium to treat the hypocalcemia; pyridoxine and thiamine, which change the metabolism of ethylene glycol to nontoxic metabolites; and ethanol or fomepizole, which competitively inhibit the metabolism of ethylene glycol.

Isopropyl alcohol may be ingested or may be absorbed through the skin. Parents should be instructed to never give alcohol baths to children with fevers. Symptoms of intoxication are similar to that of ethanol, with severe gastritis. Unlike the other toxic alcohols, isopropyl alcohol is converted to acetone when it is metabolized and does not lead to metabolic acidosis. Isopropyl alcohol ingestion can be identified by ketones in the urine without acidosis.

Methanol is a toxic alcohol that may be present in the home in fuels, paint removers, and antifreeze. It is metabolized to formic acid and formaldehyde, which cause toxicity. The toxic effects are slow to appear, generally 8 to 24 hours after ingestion. The presentation of methanol ingestion includes visual disturbances, which, if left untreated, may progress to blindness, metabolic acidosis, and central nervous system depression. Metabolic acidosis leads to multiorgan dysfunction, including cardiac arrhythmias, seizures, and pancreatitis. Treatment of known methanol ingestion includes sodium bicarbonate for treatment of the acidosis, folate to increase the elimination of formic acid, and ethanol or fomepizole to competitively inhibit the metabolism of methanol.

Plants

Most household and garden plants are nontoxic when ingested. Ingestions of toxic plants should be treated supportively, with specific remedies as indicated

(Box 63-3). Patients ingesting plants with digitalis effects may be treated with digitalis-specific antibody. Ingestion of plants with atropinic effects may be treated with physostigmine as described previously. Plants with cyanogenetic effects may cause symptoms similar to that seen with the cellular hypoxia of cyanide poisoning, with headache, nausea and vomiting, tachypnea, hypertension, anxiety, and excitation that may progress to seizures. Patients should be treated with 100% O_2, cardiopulmonary resuscitation, and cyanide antidote, consisting of inhaled amyl nitrate or IV sodium nitrite, followed by sodium thiosulfate. A newer treatment option is the administration of hydroxocobalamin, which binds with cyanide to form vitamin B12 (cyanocobalamin).

Box 63-3. Common Plant Toxidromes

- **Gastrointestinal irritants.** *Philodendron, Dieffenbachia,* pokeweed, *Wisteria,* spurge laurel, buttercup, daffodil, rosary pea, castor bean
- **Digitalis effects:** lily-of-the-valley, foxglove, oleander, yew
- **Nicotinic effects:** wild tobacco, golden chain tree, poison hemlock
- **Atropinic effects:** jimsonweed (thorn apple), deadly nightshade
- **Epileptogenic effects:** water hemlock
- **Cyanogenetic effects:** *Prunus* species (chokecherry, wild black cherry, plum, peach, apricot, bitter almond), pear (seeds), apple (seeds), crab apple (seeds), *Hydrangea,* elderberry

From Osterhoudt KC, Burns Ewald M, Shannon M, Henretig FM. Toxicologic emergencies. In: Fleisher GR, Ludwig S, eds. *Textbook of Pediatric Emergency Medicine.* 6th ed. 2010; Philadelphia, PA: Lippincott Williams & Wilkins; 2010: 1206, with permission.

Ingestion of poisonous mushrooms is responsible for roughly half of all plant-related deaths. Toxicity can be determined by the timing of symptom onset. Development of symptoms within 6 hours of ingestion confers a benign prognosis. These ingestions are characterized by GI tract upset, and some may have muscarinic or anticholinergic effects. Symptom onset more than 6 hours after ingestion is concerning for *Amanita* species poisoning. Initial GI tract upset is followed by hepatic dysfunction within 24 hours of ingestion, often leading to liver failure and death without transplantation. Treatment of mushroom poisonings is primarily supportive, although repeated doses of activated charcoal may offer some benefit.

Over-the-counter Cough and Cold Medications

Cough and cold medications are commonly available in many households and often contain multiple ingredients. It is essential to identify the components ingested to treat the patient appropriately. Cough and cold preparations often contain acetaminophen or ibuprofen. They may also contain antihistamines, causing anticholinergic symptoms. Pseudoephedrine is a stimulant medication and may cause anxiety, tachycardia, hypertension, and agitation. Cough preparations often contain dextromethorphan, which is commonly abused by adolescents in attempts to achieve altered mental status rather than in an attempt at self-harm. However, these patients should also be assessed for co-ingestants.

Suggested Reading

American Academy of Pediatics Committe of Injury, Violence, and Poison Prevention. Poison treatment in the home. *Pediatrics*. 2003;112(5):1182–1185

Bronstein AE, Spyker DA, Cantilena LR Jr, Green JL, Rumack BH, Dart RC. 2010 Annual Report of the American Association of Poison Control Centers' National Poison Data System (NPDS): 28th Annual Report. *Clin Toxicol (Phil)*. 2011;49(10):910–941

Erickson TB, Ahrens WR, Aks SE, Baum CR, Ling LJ, eds. *Pediatric Toxicology*. New York, NY: McGraw Hill; 2005

Fleisher GR, Ludwig S, eds. *Textbook of Pediatric Emergency Medicine*. 6th ed. Philadelphia, PA: Lippincott Williams & Wilkins; 2010

Nelson LS, Lewin NA, Howland MA, et al. *Goldfrank's Toxicologic Emergencies*. 9th ed. New York, NY: McGraw Hill; 2010

CHAPTER 64

Respiratory Distress and Apnea

Ryan A. Nofziger, MD, and Margaret A. Chase, MD

Key Points

- Respiratory distress is the final common pathway for a variety of illnesses.

- Establishing the diagnosis requires investigation of historical clues and physical examination findings and can be aided through radiograph and blood gas analysis.

- Timely support of the patient is imperative and can be provided through oxygen, adjunctive airways, heliox, and noninvasive ventilation support, as well as bag-valve-mask and intubation/mechanical ventilation depending on the patient's needs.

- Management of the child in severe respiratory distress and failure requires a multisystem approach and is best guided by a pediatric critical care specialist.

Overview

Respiratory distress is one of the most common reasons children are brought in for urgent evaluation. It is also one of the most common causes for hospitalization and admission to the pediatric intensive care unit. Clinically, respiratory distress is a combination of signs and symptoms that develop as the body attempts to improve minute ventilation or respond to alterations in respiratory mechanics or as a consequence of disordered control of breathing. Respiratory failure is defined as the inability of the respiratory system to meet the gas exchange needs of the body. Apnea, or the complete cessation of airflow, is one manifestation of respiratory failure. Respiratory distress or failure may not always result from pulmonary processes but can also be a consequence of a disease process in organ systems other than the lungs.

Differential Diagnosis

A careful history and physical examination can guide a practitioner from a broad differential to the correct diagnosis and appropriate therapies (Table 64-1).

Table 64-1. Causes and Differential Diagnosis of Respiratory Distress

Location	Potential Sounds	Differential Diagnosis	
Upper Airway	Stridor Stertor	*Structural* Airway edema Foreign body Laryngeal web/cyst Laryngomalacia Subglottic stenosis Tonsillar hypertrophy Vascular ring Vocal cord dysfunction	*Infectious* Croup Epiglottitis Retropharyngeal abscess *Central* Obstructive sleep apnea Postictal Sedation
Lower Airway	Wheezes Rales Grunting	ARDS Asthma Bronchiolitis BPD Foreign body	Interstitial lung disease Pneumonia Pulmonary edema Tracheomalacia
Extrapulmonary and Trauma	Normal	*Extrapulmonary* Abdominal distension Pleural effusion Restrictive chest wall	*Trauma* Diaphragmatic hernia Flail chest Pneumothorax Pneumomediastinum
Neuromuscular	Normal Stertor	Botulism Diaphragm paralysis Guillain-Barré syndrome Ingestion Myasthenia gravis	Muscular dystrophy Phrenic nerve injury Spinal muscular atrophy Transverse myelitis
Central	Normal Stertor	Central apnea Head bleed/trauma Increased ICP Meningitis/encephalitis	Ondine's curse Sedation/medication Seizure/postictal
Apnea	Absence of sound	ALTE Bronchiolitis Central apnea Croup Epiglottitis Foreign body Increased ICP	Medication/ingestion Meningitis Obstructive sleep apnea Prematurity Pertussis Seizure Sepsis
Cardiac	Normal Rales Wheezes	Cardiac shunt Congestive heart failure Myocarditis	Pericardial effusion Pulmonary embolism
Systemic	Normal	Diabetic ketoacidosis Ingestion Metabolic acidosis	Sepsis Shock

Abbreviations: ALTE, apparent life-threatening event; ARDS, acute respiratory distress syndrome; BPD, bronchopulmonary dysplasia; ICP, intracranial pressure.

Clinical Features and Evaluation

The initial assessment of a child with respiratory distress should include a search for characteristic clinical signs and symptoms. Vital signs, including high or low heart rate, respiratory rate, blood pressure, or decreased oxygen saturations, may be initial clues as to the degree of illness. Features, such as the presence of increased effort with retractions and accessory muscle use, abnormal color, perfusion or energy level, may further indicate the severity of distress. The presence of adventitious noises on physical examination, such as stridor, stertor, wheezing, grunting, or rales, can help direct your differential diagnosis and initial therapies.

Stridor

The presence of stridor indicates an upper airway or extrathoracic process. Stridor is typically appreciated during inspiration but can be biphasic in the setting of more severe airway narrowing. While assessing the child with stridor and obtaining a history, a quick assessment of the child's stability is imperative. In the high-risk patient with stridor, such as the patient with epiglottitis or severe airway edema, the priority in management becomes keeping the child calm, with minimal airway manipulation, while awaiting an urgent evaluation by an otolaryngologist (ears, nose, and throat specialist), anesthesia, or both. These patients may distinguish themselves by their toxic appearance or inability to handle oral secretions. In the patient with acute but not critical stridor, obtaining a neck radiograph to assess for airway narrowing may be beneficial. Children with stridor resulting from suspected croup or mild airway edema may improve with trial of nebulized racemic epinephrine, followed by the initiation of dexamethasone. For children with inadequate response to nebulized racemic epinephrine, initiation of heliox (a helium-oxygen gas mixture) to improve laminar flow through the narrowed airway may dramatically decrease work of breathing and distress (Evidence Level I). Alternately, placement on noninvasive ventilation (NIV) support may also improve air exchange and work of breathing in distressed patients (Evidence Level III). For more detailed descriptions of heliox and NIV and their uses, see the Management section of this chapter.

Stertor

An additional sound produced through upper airway dysfunction is stertor. These sonorous respirations are associated with upper airway laxity or obstruction and are most commonly found in the setting of obstructive sleep apnea or in a patient in the sedated or postictal state. Acutely, these patients may show improvement in airflow and decrease in stertor with repositioning on the side or prone. The use of jaw thrust or placement of a nasal or oral airway may also be beneficial as a temporizing measure.

A nasopharyngeal airway, also known as a nasal trumpet, is a soft and flexible airway adjunct that may be used in both responsive and unresponsive patients to aid in stenting open the airway. The correct size is measured from nares to the tragus of the ear (Figure 64-1). It should not be used in patients with basilar skull or nasal fractures, as placement of the nasopharyngeal airway may cause more damage.

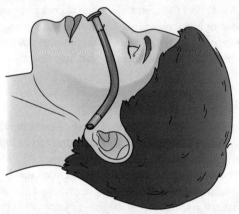

Figure 64-1. Sizing of a nasopharyngeal airway.

An oropharyngeal airway is a hard plastic device that should only to be used in an unresponsive patient who lacks a gag reflex. Placement of an oropharyngeal airway in a responsive patient may induce emesis and cause aspiration, potentially worsening respiratory distress. Correct size is measured from corner of mouth to tragus of the ear (Figure 64-2). Sizing is important, as too large of an oral airway may displace the tongue and worsen obstruction. Oral airways should be avoided in patients with oral or facial trauma.

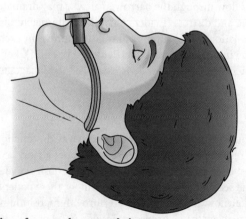

Figure 64-2. Sizing of an oropharyngeal airway.

For the patient with chronic or persistent obstruction, sleep apnea, or neuromuscular laxity, the use of NIV support may be beneficial (Evidence Level II-2).

Wheezing

The presence of wheezing signifies a lower or intrathoracic airway process including the bronchi, bronchioles, or both. Asthma is a likely culprit when the predominant symptom is wheezing. It is, however, important to consider other diagnosis such as bronchiolitis or viral-induced wheezing, pulmonary edema, cardiac dysfunction, or the presence of a foreign body. A chest radiograph may aid in narrowing the differential diagnosis. In the setting of suspected foreign body, the addition of an expiratory radiograph or lateral decubitus radiograph may be helpful in demonstrating hyperinflation or unilateral air trapping. In patients with suspected viral induced wheezing, a trial of beta agonists is often utilized with variable effectiveness. Recent evidence, however, suggests that the use of nebulized hypertonic saline (5%) decreases length of stay and risk of hospitalization in preschool-aged patients with viral induced wheezing (Evidence Level I). When asthma is suspected, initial management should include the administration of albuterol and early delivery of steroids. Evidence suggests that the early administration of systemic steroids reduces hospitalization rates, improves symptom scores, and reduces relapse and beta agonist use in asthmatics (Evidence Level I). However, there is lack of consensus as to the dose, frequency, and route of administration. In the emergency department setting, use of a metered-dose inhaler with spacer may be as efficacious as a nebulized delivery of albuterol (Evidence Level I). During the acute inpatient and intensive care unit (ICU) setting, however, nebulized treatments may be preferred because of suggestions of shortened hospital stay and decreased therapist time.

In patients who do not respond adequately to this first tier of therapy, escalation of support may proceed stepwise according to severity and clinical response. Box 64-1 describes some common therapies used in status asthmaticus. For the patient with severe distress secondary to status asthmaticus, an aggressive approach utilizing medications from multiple tiers of therapies may be appropriate and should be guided by a critical care–trained physician.

Rales

An adventitious rattling or crackling noise, known as rales or crackles, may be appreciated in parenchymal lung processes. Commonly pneumonia, whether viral or bacterial, will have areas of decreased aeration or rales appreciated as alveoli open and close. Additionally, bronchiolitis, pulmonary edema, interstitial lung disease, pneumonitis, cystic fibrosis, bronchopulmonary dysplasia, and acute respiratory distress syndrome may all manifest with rales. The diagnosis in this setting will depend on the full clinical picture and may be aided by chest radiograph and blood gas analysis. Depending on the degree of respiratory

Box 64-1. Tiered Approach to Status Asthmaticus

Tier 1
  Supplemental O_2
  Inhaled beta agonists—repeated or continuous administration[a]
  Systemic steroids[a]
  Systemic beta agonists (IM epinephrine or subcutaneous terbutaline—often used
    when air movement is poor and systemic beta agonists have no proven advantage
    over inhaled beta agonists)

Tier 2
  IV magnesium (1-Data is mixed; meta-analysis favors use.)
  Heliox[a]
  Noninvasive bilevel ventilatory support[a]

Tier 3
  Increased adverse effects with lower quality or conflicting evidence for use
  IV terbutaline infusion
  IV aminophylline infusion
  IV ketamine

Tier 4
  Intubation and mechanical ventilation
  Inhaled anesthetics
  ECMO

[a] Evidence Level I
Abbreviations: ECMO, extracorporeal membrane oxygenation; IM, intramuscular; IV, intravenous.

distress in these settings, the patient may benefit from placement on NIV or invasive ventilation.

Grunting

Grunting is a sound produced by exhalation against a closed glottis. It is an attempt by the child to maintain positive end-expiratory pressure. Any process that leads to premature closing of alveoli will induce grunting. This is most predominant in the younger child/infant and often associated with bronchiolitis, pulmonary edema, pneumonia, and atelectasis. Managing the underlying disease and often providing support with positive pressure, such as continuous positive airway pressure (CPAP), can greatly decrease distress in these patients.

Bronchiolitis

Bronchiolitis deserves special mention, as it comprises a large volume of pediatric hospitalizations during the busy winter months. Children with it may manifest a cacophony of adventitious noises, including rales, wheezing, and grunting. Management of the patient with bronchiolitis is primarily supportive, with airway clearance and supplemental oxygen as needed. The use of additional measures is highly physician dependent due to lack of clear evidence and guidelines and is often tailored to the individual patient's examination and response to therapy. Multiple studies have investigated the benefits of additional therapies commonly used for bronchiolitis. Table 64-2 below summarizes these findings based on data from several Cochrane reviews (Evidence Level I).

Table 64-2. Therapies for Bronchiolitis

Humidified air	Did not lead to a significant decrease in respiratory clinical scores.
Nebulized albuterol	Did not improve oxygen saturation or reduce hospital admission or hospital LOS. Caused short-term improvement in respiratory scores.
Nebulized racemic epinephrine	Did not cause differences for inpatient LOS but may be effective for reducing hospital admissions.
Nebulized saline	As 3% saline (when compared to 0.9% saline), significantly reduced hospital LOS among infants.
Glucocorticoids	Did not significantly reduce admissions at days 1 and 7 when compared to placebo. As a combined treatment of nebulized epinephrine and systemic dexamethasone, may significantly reduce admissions.
Chest physiotherapy	Showed no additional benefit.
Antibiotics	Has no evidence to support it for bronchiolitis. May be justified in critically ill children because of high rate of secondary bacterial infections.

Abbreviation: LOS, length of stay.

A small percentage of hospitalized patients with bronchiolitis will require escalation of respiratory support and ICU care. For these patients, the use of heliox (Evidence Level I), high flow nasal cannula (Evidence Level III), and NIV support (lower quality, but Evidence Level I) may be especially helpful in ameliorating distress, improving hypercarbia, and possibly averting invasive ventilation.

Normal Lung Sounds

Respiratory distress in the absence of lung findings often creates a diagnostic challenge. In this setting, it is important to consider the lungs as part of the acid clearing system of the body. In processes in which metabolic acidosis develops, increased ventilation may serve to temporarily balance the system. Examples of this include diabetic ketoacidosis, with its characteristic Kussmaul respirations, or sepsis, in which the development of worsening perfusion and lactic acidosis may manifest as respiratory distress. For these processes, blood gas analysis is indicated and may be very helpful in clarifying the diagnosis.

The presence of cardiac dysfunction, whether through an obstruction to the outflow of blood from the heart or pump failure, can also lead to respiratory distress, often through the development of pulmonary edema or acidosis. Signs of cardiac dysfunction may be appreciated clinically through the presence of wheezes or crackles on pulmonary examination or the presence of extra heart sounds on cardiac examination. A chest radiograph may be a useful starting point, followed by echocardiography for a more detailed evaluation. With cardiology or ICU input, the initiation of gentle diuresis, inotropic support, or both may be indicated. In this setting, the use of respiratory support with NIV or invasive ventilation may also be appropriate so as to decrease afterload and cardiac demand.

Other considerations in the child with an atypical respiratory distress pattern or presentation include neurologic dysfunction. Examples of this might be a child with spinal muscular atrophy or spinal cord injury. Importantly, these children may not manifest the expected pattern of distress, as they may lack the muscular function to demonstrate retractions. This may be acute or chronic in nature and requires a high index of suspicion by the physician, and a blood gas may be very useful to detect retention of carbon dioxide.

Apnea

Respiratory distress in its extreme may present with frank apnea or cessation of airflow. Infants, however, with little energy reserves may present with apnea in response to many different etiologies. The presence of apnea in an infant is termed an *apparent life-threatening event* and often leads to a broad search for the underlying cause. In only an estimated 50% of cases, an underlying diagnosis is identified.

Although no guidelines or algorithms have been established for management of an apparent life-threatening event, experts agree that the most pivotal step in the work-up is obtaining a careful and directed history. Specific inquiries into the condition of the child, his or her location or activity during the event, and any breathing efforts, color change, abnormal movements, or change in tone, as well as duration of the event and what interventions were required, may be helpful. Additionally, information regarding birth history, past medical and family history, and any history of present illness should be sought. The differential diagnosis is broad, and a good summary of approach to this type of patient can be found in the 2005 Hall and Zalman article (see Suggested Reading).

Persistent apnea, requiring escalation of respiratory support with NIV or invasive mechanical ventilation, should increase the level of suspicion for an infectious process. Common culprits in this setting include pertussis and respiratory viral pathogens, such as respiratory syncytial virus; however, bacteremia, meningitis, or both should also be excluded.

The use of caffeine for apnea of prematurity is a well-supported therapy (Evidence Level I). It has also been employed in management of apnea secondary to respiratory infections in very young or formerly premature infants; however, at this time, no evidence for its use has been definitive.

Management

When evaluating a child with respiratory distress, timely diagnosis and intervention may mitigate progression to respiratory failure, sparing intubation.

As with all emergent situations, the ABCs (ie, airway, breathing, circulation) of pediatric advanced life support should be followed. Described next are additional respiratory support modalities.

Oxygen

A child manifesting respiratory distress or hypoxia should be placed on supplemental oxygen while a search for etiology is underway. While for most children support should be titrated to provide oxygen saturations greater than 94%, children with chronic hypoxia or with underlying uncorrected cardiac lesions may need a modified saturation goal. The O_2 delivery device, usually a nasal cannula versus mask, is often dictated by the comfort and tolerance of the patient. Humidified high-flow nasal cannula can be used to provide more flow and potentially provide some positive airway pressure. High-flow nasal cannula can be used with better patient tolerance than CPAP and can often prevent the need for sedation. Table 64-3 describes concentrations of oxygen provided by different delivery systems.

Table 64-3. Oxygen Delivery Systems

O_2 Delivery Device	F_{IO_2} Delivery	Considerations
Nasal cannula	1 L ≈ 24% 2 L ≈ 28% 3 L ≈ 32% 4 L ≈ 36%	Nasal mucosa can become dry and bleed.
Simple mask	30%–60%	Delivery depends on size and fit of mask. Is helpful in children who are mouth breathers.
Venturi mask	30%–50%	Each adapter entrains air differently to achieve air-O_2 admixture.
Non-rebreather	60%–95%	Delivery depends on fit of mask.
Humidified high-flow nasal cannula	1–8 L/min 21%–75% on blender	Higher flows can achieve pressures close to 6 cm H_2O. Adults have flow rates of 20–40 L/min.

Heliox

In disease processes with airway obstruction, such as croup, subglottic stenosis, or status asthmaticus, the addition of heliox, a helium-oxygen mixture, can be useful in improving ventilation through increased laminar flow. Heliox should be administered in highest helium concentration tolerated to be most efficacious, but hypoxia is often the limiting factor. Mixtures ranging from an 80:20 helium-to-oxygen ratio to a 50:50 helium-to-oxygen ratio can be used. Mixtures below a 60:40 helium-to-oxygen ratio probably do not provide any benefit over regular nitrogen-filled air. Heliox is most commonly and successfully utilized in the setting of upper airway edema and stridor associated with croup or airway manipulation (Evidence Level I). In the initial treatment of status asthmaticus, heliox has not been beneficial. However, studies show that its effects may be beneficial in patients who are asthmatic with more severe obstruction (Evidence Level I). In infants with respiratory syncytial virus bronchiolitis, evidence suggests that heliox may significantly reduce respiratory distress in the first hour after initiating treatment, but it does not result in reduction in the rate of intubation, in the need for mechanical ventilation, or in the length of pediatric ICU stay (Evidence Level I).

Continuous Positive Airway Pressure

In patients with significant lung or airway disease, the use of NIV may lead to marked improvement in respiratory distress. In choosing the type of NIV support, it is helpful to consider whether the goal is improvement in oxygenation, ventilation, or both. Continuous positive airway pressure provides a single level of pressure that helps stent open alveoli and improve oxygenation. It is most beneficial in the setting of pulmonary or airway edema, atelectasis, or isolated hypoxemia. Depending on the capabilities of the machine, CPAP is often initiated at 4 to 6 cm H_2O and titrated up to a relative maximum pressure of 10 to 12 cm H_2O.

Bilevel Positive Airway Pressure

In patients for whom ventilation is a problem, the use of bilevel support or both an inspiratory and expiratory pressure may be more helpful. This serves to augment the depth of respirations, off-loading the work of breathing while also providing positive pressure at exhalation. Bilevel NIV support (often referred to as BiPAP®) has been used successfully in patients with chronic respiratory insufficiency, neuromuscular disorders, and sleep apnea. In multiple recent studies, bilevel support has been shown to improve tachypnea, tachycardia, and hypoxemia, as well as to decrease the need for intubation and invasive ventilatory support in patients with acute respiratory distress (Evidence Level I). Bilevel support is often initiated with approximate inspiratory pressures of 10 to 12 cm H_2O and approximate expiratory pressures of 4 to 6 cm H_2O. Pressures are then titrated to achieve goals of decreased work of breathing, CO_2 elimination, and improved oxygenation. Maximum pressures for bilevel support are often practitioner dependent, but in general pressures exceeding 18 to 20 cm H_2O for inspiratory pressure and 10 to 12 cm H_2O for expiratory pressure are not well tolerated and may put the patient at increased risk of complications. The use of NIV continues to expand, and many patients with impending respiratory failure have been spared intubation with its use. However, to avoid complications and delayed intubation, it is important to select the appropriate patient for NIV and recognize early signs of NIV failure. Those characteristics predictive of NIV failure suggested by retrospective or prospective uncontrolled evaluation (Evidence Level II-3) include persistent acidosis, mean airway pressure or F_{IO_2} requirements of greater than 11.5 cm H_2O and greater than 60%, respectively, as well as the degree of organ failure.

Intubation and Mechanical Ventilation

Ultimately, for some patients, respiratory distress or apnea progresses to respiratory failure because of the inability of the lungs to provide adequate oxygen or removal of carbon dioxide to meet the metabolic demands of the body. These patients require intubation and mechanical ventilatory support (Box 64-2).

Box 64-2. Relative Indications for Intubation

- Respiratory failure (Pao_2 <60 mm Hg or $Paco_2$ >50 mm Hg)
- Shock or hemodynamic instability
- Increased intracranial pressure management
- Pulmonary clearance and suctioning
- Emergency medication delivery (of lidocaine, epinephrine, atropine, or naloxone)
- Airway protection
- Neuromuscular weakness (ie, negative inspiratory force <−20 cm H_2O or vital capacity <15 mL/kg)

One of the most crucial skills in treating a child with respiratory failure is the ability to provide bag-valve mask (BVM) respirations. This ensures adequate ventilation and oxygenation while preparing for intubation. The key to success of this maneuver is proper positioning of the child and hold of the mask on the face. If no contraindication such as trauma or cervical instability is apparent, optimal position for assisted ventilation is the "sniffing position," which is slight extension of the neck. The proper "E-C" hold and seal of the mask is paramount to effective BVM (Figure 64-3).

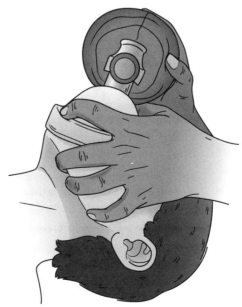

Figure 64-3. Proper "E-C" hold of bag-valve mask.

When faced with a child with respiratory failure, it is important to assess for the presence of a difficult airway, which might complicate the successful placement of an endotracheal tube. Use of the LEMON mnemonic may be a helpful tool (Table 64-4).

Table 64-4. LEMON Mnemonic for Assessing a Difficult Airway

L	Look externally	Facial or neck abnormalities (eg, Treacher Collins, Pierre Robin, trisomy 21), facial trauma, obesity
E	Examine for difficult airway	Mouth opening, hyomental distance, thyroid cartilage-mandibular distance
M	Mallampati score	Class I = soft palate, uvula, anterior and posterior pillars visible Class II = soft palate and uvula visible Class III = soft palate and only base of the uvula visible Class IV = soft palate and uvula not visible at all
O	Evidence of obstruction	Epiglottitis, peritonsillar abscess, retropharyngeal abscess, tonsillar hypertrophy, macroglossia, neck masses
N	Neck mobility	Cervical fusion, atlanto-occipital joint instability, surgical halo, spondylosis

For children with concerns for difficult airway, use of anesthesia resources may be warranted before attempting intubation. It is also prudent to have an appropriately sized laryngeal mask airway immediately available if there is an inability to intubate or BVM ventilate. Consultation of personnel trained in the management and placement of an emergent cricothyrotomy or tracheostomy, such as ears, nose, and throat or general surgery, should also be considered if a difficult airway is anticipated. In intubating a child with respiratory failure, preparation is key. Table 64-5 describes SOAP'EM, a mnemonic to prepare for the intubation process.

Table 64-5. SOAP'EM Mnemonic to Prepare for Intubation

S	Suction	Suction should be set up and ready to use.
O	Oxygen	Preoxygenate prior to intubation. Have an appropriately sized face mask for BVM support.
A	Airway equipment	Check laryngoscope light and ETT cuff. Have a ½ size smaller ETT or an LMA ready. Have an NP/OP airway available if needed.
P	Positioning	Sniffing position is preferred if possible. For infants, a pillow under the shoulders may better align the airway; for adolescents, a pillow under the head.
'E	End-tidal CO_2 detector	Use color change CO_2 detector or capnography.
M	Medications and Monitor	Make sure monitor is on and working and intubation medications are prepared.

Abbreviations: BVM, bag-valve mask; ETT, endotracheal tube; LMA, laryngeal mask airway; NP, nasopharyngeal; OP, oropharyngeal.

By convention, most people have used un-cuffed endotracheal tubes (ETTs) for pediatrics; however, with the advent of low-pressure cuffs, the use of cuffed endotracheal tubes has become more widespread and accepted. In selecting ETT size, the following calculation is used:

For un-cuffed endotracheal tube: $\dfrac{Age\ in\ Years}{4} + 4$

For cuffed endotracheal tube: $\dfrac{Age\ in\ Years}{4} + 5$

Endotracheal tube insertion depth: Endotracheal tube size $\times$ 3

When cuff pressure is monitored and ETT size is selected appropriately, there are no increased risks of complications with use of a cuffed ETT. Additionally, a cuffed ETT may provide a more appropriate selection of ETT size, subsequently decreasing the need for re-intubation, may decrease the risk of aspiration, and may be preferred in patients with air leak, poor lung compliance, and high ventilatory support needs (Evidence Level II-2).

There are two general approaches to medication administration prior to intubation. They are standard sequence and rapid sequence intubation. Standard sequence involves giving an analgesic medication first, followed by the induction agent. Once the patient is sedated and able to be ventilated by BVM, a dose of paralytic medication is given. Rapid sequence is often performed when a secured advanced airway is needed emergently or when a patient may have a full stomach and is at risk of aspiration. It is typically done without assisted ventilation, if possible, to avoid aspiration by gastric distension. The technique involves giving the induction and paralytic medications simultaneously to allow for rapid placement of the ETT.

When selecting medications for intubation, it is important to recognize the effects of these medications on the patient. Most analgesic and induction agents will lead to decreased blood pressure with administration, and practitioners must be prepared for the need for additional fluids/volume expansion. Medications commonly used in intubation are described in Table 64-6.

To ensure appropriate placement of the ETT, an end-tidal CO_2 detector or capnography should be used throughout the procedure, followed by a chest radiograph to confirm positioning. Once ETT placement has been confirmed and the ETT is secured, the child should be transitioned to ventilator support. In choosing initial ventilator settings, it is helpful to assess the overall lung compliance, which can be guided by the pressures needed to move the chest with bagging. No evidence supports superiority of one mode of ventilation over another. Regardless of the mode of ventilatory support chosen, settings should reflect goals of providing adequate support of ventilation and oxygenation while minimizing ventilator-associated lung trauma. Strategies to achieve these goals have been defined in the adult population through the Acute Respiratory Distress Syndrome Network guidelines and are extrapolated to children, though we lack clear evidence for their use. These "lung protective strategies" include the concepts of use of positive end-expiratory pressure to minimize

Table 64-6. Medication Options for Intubation

Intubation Medications	Dose	Notes
Analgesics		
Morphine	0.1 mg/kg IV, IM	Repeat as needed.
Fentanyl	1–2 mcg/kg IV, IM	Give slowly over 3–5 min to avoid rigid chest syndrome!
Induction Agents		
Lorazepam	0.05 mg/kg IV	Repeat as needed.
Midazolam	0.05–0.2 mg/kg IV	Repeat as needed.
	0.2 mg/kg intranasal, IM	
Ketamine	1–3 mg/kg IV	Is a good choice for hypotension.
	3 mg/kg IM	Possesses analgesic effects.
		Increases secretions, HR, and BP.
Etomidate	0.2–0.6 mg/kg IV	Has minimal cardiovascular effect.
		Does not have analgesic activity.
		Avoid in sepsis. Causes adrenal insufficiency!
Propofol	1–2 mg/kg IV	Is short acting.
		Is a good choice for a difficult airway.
Paralytics		
Vecuronium	0.1–0.2 mg/kg IV	
Rocuronium	0.6–1.2 mg/kg IV	
Pancuronium	0.1–0.15 mg/kg IV	
Succinylcholine	1–2 mg/kg IV	Is short acting.
	3–4 mg/kg IM	Causes risk for hyperkalemia and malignant hyperthermia.
		Do *not* use in burns or trauma.
Cisatracurium	0.1–0.2 mg/kg IV	Cleared via rapid nonenzymatic degradation (ie, Hofmann elimination). Is good for hepatic and renal failure.
Additional Agents		
Atropine	0.02 mg/kg IV	Used to blunt oral secretions as well as vagal response in infants.
	Min: 0.1 mg; max: 2 mg	
Glycopyrrolate	Min: 4 mcg/kg IV; max: 100 mcg	Used to blunt oral secretions.
Lidocaine	1 mg/kg	To be used if concerned for increased ICP.

Abbreviations: BP, blood pressure; HR, heart rate; ICP, intracranial pressure; IM, intramuscular; IV, intravenous; max, maximum; min, minimum.

atelectrauma, minimization of oxygen toxicity, and permissive hypercapnia and minimization of plateau pressures and tidal volumes to decrease barotrauma and volutrauma. A detailed description of ventilator strategies is beyond the scope of this chapter but can be investigated further in the 2010 Jauncey-Cooke article (see Suggested Reading).

In some patients, conventional ventilation is inadequate or suboptimal, and different ventilation modalities are required. These include but are not limited to high-frequency oscillation, airway pressure–release ventilation, and the ultimate therapy for respiratory failure, extracorporeal membrane oxygenation.

Suggested Reading

Ater D, Shai H, Bar BE, et al. Hypertonic saline and acute wheezing in preschool children. *Pediatrics.* 2012;129(6):e1397–e1403

Deis JN, Abramo TJ, Crawley Ll. Noninvasive respiratory support. *Pediatr Emerg Care.* 2008;24(5):331–338

Gupta VK, Cheifetz IM. Heliox administration in the pediatric intensive care unit: an evidence-based review. *Pediatr Crit Care Med.* 2005;6(2):204–211

Hall KL, Zalman B. Evaluation and management of apparent life-threatening events in children. *Am Fam Physician.* 2005;71(12):2301–2308

Jauncey-Cooke JI, Bogossian F, East CE. Lung protective ventilation strategies in paediatrics-a review. *Aust Crit Care.* 2010;23(2):81–88

Kleinman ME, Chameides L, Schexnayder SM, et al. Pediatric advanced life support: 2010 American Heart Association Guidelines for Cardiopulmonary Resuscitation and Emergency Cardiovascular Care. *Pediatrics.* 2010;126(5):e1361–e1399

Nagakumar P, Doull I. Current therapy for bronchiolitis. *Arch Dis Child.* 2012;97(9): 827–830

Najaf-Zadeh A, Leclerc F. Noninvasive positive pressure ventilation for acute respiratory failure in children: a concise review. *Ann Intensive Care.* 2011;1(1):15

National Asthma Education and Prevention Program. Expert Panel Report 3 (EPR-3): Guidelines for the Daignosis and Management of Asthma-Summary Report 2007. *J Allergy Clin Immunol.* 2007;120(5 Suppl):S94–S138

Schramm CM, Carroll CL. Advances in treating acute asthma exacerbations in children. *Curr Opin Pediatr.* 2009;21(3):326–332

CHAPTER 65

Rhabdomyolysis

Edward E. Conway, Jr, MD, MS

Key Points

- The most common causes of pediatric rhabdomyolysis are viral myositis (38%), trauma (26%), and connective tissue diseases (eg, dermatomyositis, polymyositis) contrasted with adults, in which trauma and drug-related toxicity are most common.

- The most significant injury that may occur following rhabdomyolysis is acute kidney injury, which is rare in pediatric patients.

- Although the exact mechanism of rhabdomyolysis-induced acute kidney injury is not known, mechanisms most commonly cited include vasoconstriction/hypoperfusion/hypovolemia, renal tubular dysfunction/cast formation, myoglobin-induced tubular cytotoxicity, or a combination thereof.

- The mainstay of therapy is critical monitoring and aggressive intravenous fluid resuscitation with isotonic normal saline in the first 24 hours.

Overview

Rhabdomyolysis is a clinical and biochemical syndrome characterized by muscle necrosis, which results in the release of large quantities of toxic muscle cell components, including myoglobin, creatine kinase (CK), serum aminotransferases, lactate dehydrogenase, aldoase, potassium, and phosphate into the extracellular fluid and circulation. Other associated metabolic abnormalities may include metabolic acidosis, hyperuricemia, hypocalcemia (early), and hypercalcemia (late). The classic triad (although not always observed) consists of skeletal muscle injury, pigmented urine, and some aspect of renal dysfunction. Acute kidney injury (AKI) is the most serious complication of both traumatic and nontraumatic rhabdomyolysis. Rhabdomyolysis was first described in 1941 in 4 patients who sustained crush injuries during the bombing of London during World War II. All developed acute renal failure and died within 1 week, and postmortem they demonstrated pigmented casts in the renal tubules.

Causes
· · · · · · ·

The cause of muscle injury may be excessive muscle stress or ischemia (eg, marathons, seizures, asthma, heat stroke), possible genetic defects (eg, malignant hyperthermia, disorders of glycogenolysis, glycolysis, lipid and purine metabolism), infection (usually viral), direct toxic damage (both prescribed and illicit drugs), or physical damage (ie, trauma). Drug-induced effects may occur by either a primary effect on the myocyte or via an indirect secondary effect that predisposes the myocyte to injury. Clinical features range from muscle weakness and tenderness (myositis) to fulminant life-threatening AKI, requiring dialysis. The leading causes of pediatric rhabdomyolysis are summarized in Figure 65-1.

Adult rhabdomyolysis is commonly caused by drugs (legal and illegal) and trauma (eg, crush injury), whereas the leading cause in pediatrics is viral myositis. The most common viral cause includes influenza A and B, enterovi-

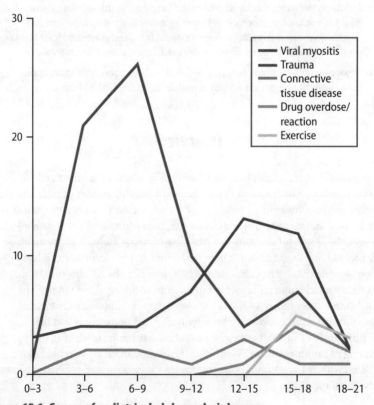

Figure 65-1. Causes of pediatric rhabdomyolysis by age.
From Mannix R, Tan ML, Wright R, Baskin M. Acute pediatric rhabdomyolysis: causes and rates of renal failure. *Pediatrics*. 2006;118(5);2119–2125.

ruses, and human immunodeficiency virus. Although many bacteria may cause rhabdomyolysis, it is more commonly associated with gram-positive organisms. In the adult population, a significant association exists between psychiatric medications and development of neuroleptic malignant syndrome, which may cause rhabdomyolysis. Although not used commonly in pediatric patients, statins have been implicated as a cause of rhabdomyolysis. The risk is increased when statins are co-administered with other medications that inhibit the P450 enzyme systems and thus prevent the metabolism of the statin. Propofol, a drug used frequently for pediatric procedural anesthesia, has been associated with the propofol infusion syndrome, which is a potentially fatal complication of prolonged or high dosage administration and is associated with rhabdomyolysis. Illicit drugs, such as cocaine, methamphetamines, amphetamines, and bath salts (ie, mephedrone, methylenedioxypyrovalerone) can increase activity to harmful levels and may precipitate seizures or hyperthermia and even contribute to ischemia from arterial vasoconstriction. Ethanol has been shown to cause direct toxicity to skeletal muscle. Subclinical myoglobinemia, myoglobinuria, and elevation of CK are common following physical exertion and have been demonstrated in long-distance runners. Massive rhabdomyolysis may occur with marked physical exertion (eg, military recruits, football players), particularly in physically untrained individuals; in extreme exercise in hot, humid conditions; or if normal heat loss through sweating is impaired.

Clinical Features

The hallmark of rhabdomyolysis is an elevation of CK to levels of more than 1,000 U/L, which may ultimately increase to greater than 100,000 U/L. A definitive diagnosis requires an elevation of CK concentrations to greater than 5 times normal in the absence of significant elevations of brain or cardiac CK fractions. The risk of AKI is usually low when CK levels on admission are less than 15,000 to 20,000 U/L. Although AKI has been described with CK values as low as 5000 U/L, this usually occurs when coexisting conditions such as sepsis, dehydration, and acidosis are present. The absolute CK level does not correlate with the onset or degree of renal dysfunction.

The role of CK is to convert myocyte creatine phosphate into high-energy phosphate groups (eg, adenosine triphosphate), which is used as energy by the muscle cells. Myoglobin is a heme protein found in skeletal muscle where it functions as an oxygen carrier. Once it is released into the serum following muscle injury, it is filtered into the urine, causing a red color. A urine dipstick for heme (known as an orthotolidine test) will cross-react with myoglobin and produce a false-positive test for heme, and microscopy should reveal the absence of red blood cells. This pseudohematuria occurs because the dipstick test is unable to differentiate between myoglobin and hemoglobin. The test has a sensitivity of 80%. Serum CK begins to increase 2 to 12 hours following the injury, peaking at 3 to 5 days. Myoglobin is eliminated from the bloodstream more quickly than CK, which explains why myoglobinuria resolves prior to the maximal CK elevation, and serum CK values may be within reference range in the early phase of rhabdomyolysis. Measurement of serum myoglobin has a low sensitivity and thus is not usually clinically helpful.

Evaluation

The cause of rhabdomyolysis is usually evident from the history or immediate circumstances preceding the disorder (eg, prolonged surgical procedure, status epilepticus, crush injury). On occasion the cause may not be immediately obvious, such as in patients with heritable muscle disorders, electrolyte abnormalities, infections, toxins, or endocrinopathies. Muscle injury may manifest as pain, swelling, tenderness, or weakness, but these signs may not always be present. The goal of management is to recognize and treat or remove the underlying cause and to prevent renal failure resulting from the myoglobinuria. The exact mechanism of rhabdomyolysis-induced AKI is not known but may be attributable to renal vasoconstriction/hypoperfusion/hypovolemia, renal tubular dysfunction/cast formation, or myoglobin-induced tubular cytotoxicity. Fluid is sequestered in injured muscle and activates the sympathetic nervous system, antidiuretic hormone, and renin-angiotensin system, all of which casue vasoconstriction and renal salt and water retention. Myoglobin-induced oxidative stress increases vasoconstrictors and decreases vasodilators. Acute kidney injury results from a combination of ischemia due to vasoconstriction and direct tubular toxicity of myoglobin coupled with the obstruction of distal tubules due to precipitation of Tamm-Horsfall protein-myoglobin complex causing casts. Endothelial injury and local inflammation further contribute to cellular injury and organ dysfunction (Figure 65-2).

Evaluation requires an assessment of risk factors for rhabdomyolysis, a thorough history and physical examination, and laboratory testing. The history should elicit information on prior exertional activities; environmental exposures; prolonged immobilization; trauma; prescription and over-the-counter medication and dietary supplement use; illicit drug or alcohol use; symptoms of infection, rash, or arthralgias; and any change in color or quantity of urine. Physicians need to be aware that patients who are intoxicated, psychotic (medication related), agitated, or comatose are at high risk for rhabdomyolysis. Baseline laboratory work should include (in addition to a dipstick and microscopic urinalysis) a basic metabolic panel that includes electrolytes (specifically, potassium, calcium, phosphorus) and renal function. An elevated creatinine level with a blood urea nitrogen-to-creatinine ratio less than 10:1 is often noted on presentation. The disproportionate increase of creatinine early in rhabdomyolysis may be due to the metabolism of released muscle creatine. An electrocardiogram should be obtained to look for evidence of hyperkalemia (ie, P-R prolongation, peaked t waves, wide QRS). Approximately 150 g of muscle necrosis releases 15 mmol of potassium and thus the patient may be at risk for

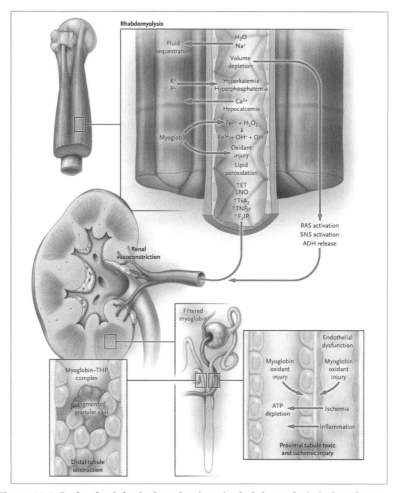

Figure 65-2. Pathophysiological mechanisms in rhabdomyolysis-induced acute kidney injury.

Fluid sequestration in injured muscle induces volume depletion and consequent activation of thesympathetic nervous system, antidiuretic hormone, and the renin-angiotensin system, all of which favor vasoconstriction and renal salt and water conservation. In addition, myoglobin-induced oxidative injury increases vasoconstrictors and decreases vasodilators. Kidney injury results from a combination of ischemia due to renal vasoconstriction, direct tubular toxicity mediated by myoglobin-associated oxidative injury (inset, lower right), tubular damage due to ischemia, and distal tubule obstruction due to precipitation of the Tamm–Horsfall protein-myoglobin complex (inset, lower left) in addition to sloughed tubular cells forming cellular cast. As in acute kidney injury due to other causes, endothelial dysfunction and local inflammation contribute to tissue damage and organ dysfunction.

Abbreviations: ET, endothelin; F_2 IP, F_2 isoprostanes; NO, nitric oxide; THP, Tamm-Horsfall protein; TNF-α, tumor necrosis factor α; TxA_2, thromboxane A_2; VC, vasoconstriction.

From Bosch X, Poch E, Grau JM. Rhabdomyolysis and acute kidney injury. *N Engl J Med.* 2009;361(1):62–72, with permission.

cardiac arrhythmias. A coagulation profile should also be obtained, as disseminated intravascular coagulation may be associated with severe rhabdomyolysis.

Management

As a result of fluid shifts into tissues and cells, hypovolemia is frequently present and may cause or exacerbate AKI. No randomized, controlled studies of rhabdomyolysis offer definitive guidance on the management of rhabdomyolysis. Most recommendations are based on retrospective observational studies with small numbers of patients, animal models, case reports, or series and opinion. The mainstay of therapy is aggressive hydration (Evidence Level II-1). There is a consensus that administration of intravenous (IV) isotonic fluid dilutes nephrotoxins and promotes renal tubular flow, which may prevent the accumulation of myoglobin and toxic products in the renal parenchyma. Intravenous fluid should be administered initially as a bolus (20 mL/kg of isotonic normal saline), and the patient should continue to receive IV hydration at a rate to maintain a good urinary output of 2 to 3 mL/kg/hour (which may require administration of 2–3 times the normal maintenance rate). Debate exists about which type of fluid to use (again, little data supports a firm recommendation), but it appears that isotonic fluid is prudent, as most of these patients are hypovolemic on presentation. Large amounts of IV fluids within the first 24 hours are associated with improved outcomes (Evidence Levels II-1 and II-2). In the pediatric intensive care unit, diuresis should be continued until the urine is clear of myoglobin, the plasma CK levels are less than 1,000 U/L, or signs of fluid overload are evident. Any medications that have the potential for nephrotoxicity (eg, nonsteroidal anti-inflammatory medications) should be avoided.

Another common intervention for which little adult and no pediatric data exists is that of alkalinizing the urine. Proponents of its use argue that myoglobin precipitates in an acidic milieu and therefore alkalization of the urine to maintain the urinary pH greater than 6.5 could theoretically decrease the deposition of myoglobin in the tubules. A current consensus statement recommends that sodium bicarbonate therapy (to alkalinize the urine) is neither necessary nor superior to normal saline diuresis in increasing urine pH. It must be remembered that alkalization will lead to a reduction in ionized calcium, which may exacerbate the symptoms on the early hypocalcemic phase of rhabdomyolysis.

One must continuously monitor patients for the development of metabolic acidosis, hyperkalemia, hyperphosphatemia, and hypocalcemia (early) and hypercalcemia (late). Several series have advocated the use of forced diuresis with mannitol and loop diuretics to promote urine output and to prevent the accumulation of renal debris in the tubules. Once again, data are lacking and the routine use of mannitol is not recommended for rhabdomyolysis, and it definitely should not be administered to hypovolemic or anuric patients. The use of loop diuretics has been advocated by some (Evidence Level II-3) to convert oliguria or anuria to nonoliguria, again with very little supportive data. In the event AKI does develop or fails to improve despite aggressive fluid management, renal replacement therapy should be considered. Indications for hemodialysis include hyperkalemia, intractable metabolic acidosis, volume overload, and azotemia.

Prognosis and Outcome

The outcome of rhabdomyolysis is usually good provided that there is no renal failure. Adult data suggest the long-term survival among patients with rhabdomyolysis and AKI is close to 80%. Although pediatric data is scant one of the larger series published to date (210 patients) demonstrated that the risk of renal failure in children is much less that the risk reported for adults. The authors found that no single symptom, sign, or laboratory value was highly predictive of developing AKI; urinary heme dipstick results of greater than 2+ seem to indicate a much reduced risk of developing AKI.

Suggested Reading

Bosch K, Poch E, Grau JM. Rhabdomyolysis and acute kidney injury. *N Engl J Med.* 2009;361(1):62–72

Bywaters EG, Beall D. Crush injuries with impairment of renal function. *Br Med J.* 1941;1(4185):427–432

Coco TJ, Klasner AE. Drug-induced rhabdomyolysis. *Curr Opin Pediatr.* 2004;16(2):206–210

Dalaksa MC. Toxic and drug-induced myopathies. *J Neurol Neurosurg Psychiatry.* 2008;80(8):832–838

Luck RP, Verbin S. Rhabdomyolysis: a review of clinical presentation, etiology, diagnosis, and management. *Pediatr Emerg Care.* 2008;24(4):262–268

Mannix R, Tan ML, Wright R, Baskin M. Acute pediatric rhabdomyolysis: causes and rates of renal failure. *Pediatrics.* 2006;118(5):2119–2125

Stucka KR, Mycyk MB, Leikin JB, Pallasch EM. Rhabdomyolysis associated with unintentional antihistamine overdose in a child. *Pediatr Emerg Care.* 2003;19(1):25–26

Zimmerman JL, Shen MC. Rhabdomyolysis. *Chest.* 2013;144(3):1058–1065

CHAPTER 66

Scrotal Pain, Acute

Renee P. Quarrie, MBBS, and Daniel M. Cohen, MD

Key Points

- The differential diagnosis of acute scrotal pain primarily includes testicular torsion, torsion of the appendix testis, and epididymitis; the child with acute scrotal pain should be presumed to have testicular torsion until history, physical examination, and possibly imaging rule this diagnosis out.

- A diagnosis of testicular torsion can be strongly suggested by history and physical examination findings, and as such surgical scrotal exploration should not be delayed by ultrasonography. The optimal time for testicular salvage is within 6 hours of symptom onset with virtually no salvage after 24 hours.

- Testicular torsion is *not* the most common cause of acute scrotal pain, if history and physical examination findings do not suggest this as a cause; ultrasonography can assist in making a diagnosis. Patients with scrotal trauma and significant swelling and pain will require ultrasound to evaluate the injury.

- Other possible causes of acute scrotal pain include incarcerated inguinal hernia, trauma, idiopathic scrotal edema, retrocecal appendicitis, orchitis, and vasculitides (as seen in Kawasaki disease and Henoch-Schönlein purpura).

Overview

The acute scrotum is defined as the sudden onset of scrotal pain, often accompanied by swelling and redness or discoloration, and can often generate fear and anxiety for patients, family members, and physicians. A large overlap can be found in the clinical presentations of the 3 most common causes of the acute scrotum: testicular torsion, torsion of the appendix testis, and acute epididymitis. Although it accounts for less than 1% of emergency department cases, the identification of the patient with testicular torsion is the single most important concern of the physician, as early intervention is key in preserving testicular viability. Because of the sensitive nature of the concern, there is frequently a delay in seeking care, making expeditious evaluation essential. Clear documentation of the time of symptom onset is crucial, especially in light of the medicolegal implications specifically related to the risk of testicular loss/salvageability for testicular torsion. The diagnosis of the acute scrotum is largely based on the history and physical examination findings, but in today's environment consultants may request diagnostic imaging. Any diagnostic testing that delays definitive care of testicular torsion for a potentially salvageable testis by a qualified pediatric urologist or surgeon is problematic. Ultrasound imaging with assessment of flow by Doppler is the most useful single imaging modality but should be performed in consultation with the surgical subspecialist to enhance diagnostic accuracy. Critically, physicians should recognize that this modality has limitations. Having a clear and open discussion with the family from the beginning of the encounter is key to a successful outcome and positive perceptions by the patient and family.

Causes

The most common causes of the acute scrotum in the pediatric patient are testicular torsion, torsion of the appendix testis, and epididymitis; however, the most likely cause varies by age of the patient. In the neonate, the principal diagnoses are testicular torsion (which may be prenatal or postnatal), inguinal hernias, and hydroceles. In the older child, typical diagnoses include torsion on the appendix testis, epididymitis, and testicular torsion (Table 66-1). Other less common causes include trauma, varicoceles, idiopathic scrotal edema, Henoch-Schönlein purpura (HSP), inguinal hernias, and Kawasaki disease, but these do not usually require emergent management. Key clinical features often assist in tailoring the evaluation process (Table 66-2).

Table 66-1. Most Common Etiologies of Acute Scrotal Pain in Children and Adolescents

Etiology	Features
Testicular torsion	• Is a medical/urological emergency. Can lead to permanent ischemic injury of testis. • Occurs when spermatic cord twists on itself, compromising blood supply to testicle. • Occurs at any age. Has bimodal age distribution (one peak perinatal other puberty). • Annual incidence is 1 in 4,000 males <25 y. • Intravaginal torsion occurs in 90% of cases (tunica vaginalis covers not only testicle and epididymis but also spermatic cord). Creates bell-clapper deformity that allows testis to rotate freely within tunica vaginalis (Figure 66-1). Is bilateral in 80% of cases. • Extravaginal torsion is usually seen in prenatal/neonatal period (usually in large newborns with birth weight >3 kg).

Table 66-1 (cont)

Etiology	Features
Torsion of spermatic cord	• Usually occurs without precipitating event; 4%–8% occur in context of trauma. • Venous return to testicle is obstructed and leads to compromise of arterial flow and testicular ischemia. Occurs within as little as 4 h and always by 24 h.
Torsion of the appendix testis	• Is most common cause of acute scrotal pain in males prior to puberty. • Peak occurrence is between 8–14 y. • Has 4 testicular and paratesticular embryological remnants. Torsion of the appendix testis or hydatid of Morgagni is the most common cause.
Epididymitis	• Acute epididymitis is the most common cause of acute scrotal pain in male adults. • In pediatric population, is most common in pubertal boys >12 y (accounts for up to 25% of acute scrotal pain cases in childhood). • Is rare in prepubertal boys; may occur with congenital anomaly of lower urinary tract, such as ectopic ureter, hypospadias, or neuropathic bladder, or after recent instrumentation of the urethra, such as catheterization. • In prepubertal patients, is most often idiopathic and bacterial pathogen is not found. • In sexually active boys, *Neisseria gonorrhoeae* and *Chlamydia trachomatis* are the most common causes.
Orchitis	• Is usually secondary to spread of inflammation from adjacent epididymitis. • May be seen in primary infections such as mumps and rarely from bacterial causes such as *Staphylococcus aureus* and *Streptococcus pyogenes*.

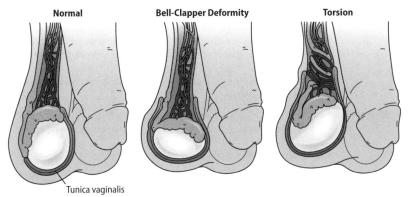

Figure 66-1. Normal testicular anatomy, bell-clapper deformity, and torsion of the spermatic cord.

Table 66-2. Findings in Most Common Etiologies of Acute Scrotal Pain and Masses in Children and Adolescents

Cause	Features That Aid in Evaluation and Diagnosis
Testicular torsion	• Typically present with acute and excruciating scrotal pain (usually no urinary symptoms). • Has the most rapid onset of pain of all causes of acute scrotal pain (often pain lasts <12 h). • Pain may refer to lower abdomen; nausea and vomiting occurs in 96% of cases. • Pain is usually unilateral with left testicle more commonly affected than right. • Some patients may have intermittent testicular torsion (acute and intermittent testicular pain/scrotal swelling with rapid resolution and long intervals without symptoms) • Swelling of testis with erythema of overlying skin is common (may not be present early). • Exhibits exquisite tenderness to palpation of testis. • Because of the torsion, there is shortening of spermatic cord and abnormal transverse lie of testis within the scrotum; affected testicle usually appears higher than unaffected one. • Normally posteriorly located epididymis may be located medially, anteriorly, or laterally depending on the degree of torsion. • Due to venous congestion, the affected testis may also appear larger. • Prehn sign (ie, relief of pain with testicular elevation) is not present. • Most sensitive physical finding is absence of cremasteric reflex (elicited by stroking medial thigh, causing contraction of cremaster muscle, which elevates testis [normally present in all neurologically intact boys >30 mo); loss of cremasteric reflex is 98% sensitive for testicular torsion.
Torsion of the appendix testis	• Symptoms mimic those of testicular torsion; however, pain is milder, more gradual, and often described as dull ache. • Pain may occur in lower abdomen/inguinal region; systemic symptoms are usually absent. • Pain may be more focal and not generalized to the entire testicle. • Scrotal edema is minimal; localized tenderness occurs over superior pole of testis. • A hard, tender nodule 2–3 mm in diameter may be palpable on upper lobe of the testicle; with gentle traction on scrotal skin, a small bluish discoloration may be observed in this area and is referred to as the "blue dot sign." • Epididymis usually remains in normal posterior orientation; affected testis is normal sized.
Epididymitis	• Scrotal pain develops gradually over hours to days. • May have dysuria and urethral discharge (most common in postpubertal males). • Constitutional symptoms are uncommon, but patients may have fever. • Findings are highly variable (ie, range from mild scrotal tenderness without other findings to severe scrotal edema and tenderness). • Prehn sign is often positive.

Table 66-2 (cont)

Cause	Features That Aid in Evaluation and Diagnosis
Orchitis	• Causes scrotal pain with systemic symptoms such as fever, malaise, myalgias, nausea, and headache. • Mumps orchitis follows the development of parotitis by 4–7 d. • With orchitis, there is testicular enlargement, with induration and tenderness as well as scrotal erythema and edema. The prostate may feel soft and boggy (prostatitis), and the parotid gland may be enlarged in patients with mumps orchitis.
Scrotal trauma	• Trauma is most frequently blunt but may also involve avulsion or penetration. • Scrotum may be quite swollen and tender (may also have testicular torsion associated with trauma, testicular hematoma, or rupture of the testicle). • Ecchymosis, significant tenderness, and swelling are often present.
Varicoceles	• Are usually idiopathic, resulting from incompetent valves in a testicular vein, leading to dilatation of the spermatic cord pampiniform venous plexus. • Varicoceles are more commonly located on left side. • Are usually present with more chronic concerns of dull scrotal pain or feeling of heaviness, although symptoms may be more acute. • Testis is most often non-tender with a twisted mass along the spermatic cord; this is often likened to feeling a "bag of worms." • When supine, gravity may drain pampiniform plexus, making mass less obvious.
Inguinal hernias	• Is most common scrotal mass in young patients, almost always indirect hernias resulting from patent processus vaginalis. • Indirect hernias are more common on the right because right processus vaginalis closes after left during development. • May present with either chronic or acute concerns of swelling and groin pain. • Abdominal pain/vomiting may indicate incarceration or strangulation of hernia contents; it is important to examine genitalia in all patients with abdominal pain, vomiting, or both. • Has scrotal swelling that extends along the inguinal canal. • Often, hernias are reducible with gentle upward pressure, relieving symptoms and confirming diagnosis. • If unable to be reduced, hernia incarceration should be considered (surgical emergency).
Hydroceles	• Are a common cause of scrotal swelling. • Are usually painless; may occasionally present with pain or diffuse discomfort. • In infants and young children, are almost always due to peritoneal fluid extending through a patent processus vaginalis. • In older patients, may result from inflammatory processes, testicular or appendiceal torsion, trauma, or tumors (degree of pain depends on coexisting abnormality). • Transillumination of scrotum may help confirm their presence but will not assist in evaluating for any associated pathology.

Table 66-2 (cont)

Cause	Features That Aid in Evaluation and Diagnosis
Idiopathic scrotal edema	• Is thought to be an allergic process. • Usually occurs in younger boys (mean age of 6 y). • Presents as bright-red erythema, edema, and swelling of scrotum, usually without tenderness. • Scrotal contents are normal on palpation. Usually subsides without intervention in 2–3 d.
Henoch-Schönlein purpura	• Is a small vessel vasculitis involving multiple organ systems, especially the skin (purpura), gastrointestinal tract (abdominal pain), joints (arthritis), and kidneys (hematuria). • A manifestation can be acute, painful swelling of the scrotum in prepubertal boys; occurs in 15%–38% of cases. • May precede the characteristic purpuric rash.

Evaluation

In the patient with an acute scrotum, the most critical determination that the physician must make is whether or not the patient has testicular torsion (Figure 66-2). Testicular survival is directly related to the time from onset of symptoms. The optimal time for testicular salvage is within 6 hours of symptom onset with virtually no salvage after 24 hours. The diagnosis of testicular torsion can be made from the history and physical examination findings in a significant number of patients, and if this diagnosis is strongly suggested by the clinical findings, surgical intervention should occur rapidly and should not be delayed by diagnostic studies.

If ultrasound is immediately available and will not delay operative intervention, it can be a valuable adjunct for the surgeon. Imaging should also be used for patients with unclear diagnoses, in patients with trauma, and in those with symptoms for longer than 24 hours, as, even if torsion is present, the chance of testicular salvage is remote and emergency surgery may not be required. Most cases of acute scrotal pain are not due to testicular torsion, and the physical examination may be difficult to perform on the ill child in the setting of scrotal trauma. As a result, imaging may be necessary. However, the physician must remember that while scrotal pain imaging has high sensitivity and specificity, it is not perfect, and if the results do not correlate with the clinical assessment, the clinical assessment must supercede in decisions regarding patient care and disposition. Other tests that the physician may consider in the patient with the acute scrotum are urinalysis, complete blood count, cultures, and other assessing inflammatory markers such as C-reactive protein level.

Imaging

Historically, the choice for imaging the acute scrotum was nuclear scintigraphy, but in the United States the current imaging of choice is color Doppler

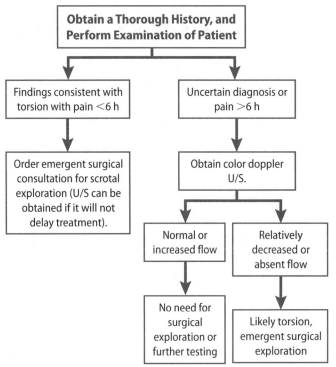

Figure 66-2. Algorithm for approach to evaluation of the acute scrotum (Evidence Level II-3 and Evidence Level III).
Abbreviation: U/S, ultrasound.

ultrasonography. Ultrasonography provides information about anatomy and blood flow and as such is invaluable in the overall assessment of the acute scrotum.

Testicular Torsion

On ultrasound, the acutely torsed testicle is more hypoechoic than normal, with an abnormal transverse lie of the testicle and a paratesticular mass that is composed of swollen edematous epididymis and spermatic cord. There may also be a reactive hydrocele (Figure 66-3) and scrotal skin thickening, especially in patients with later presentation. On Doppler, there is reduced or absent blood flow to the symptomatic testis (Figure 66-4). Doppler examination performed by someone with adequate technical expertise has a sensitivity of 90% to 100% for detecting testicular torsion in children and a specificity of 100%. Patients with intermittent or partial torsion of the spermatic cord may have normal ultrasound examination findings, which underscores the importance of a thorough history and physical examination. Nuclear medicine scan will reveal a central photon-deficient area in the ischemic hemi-scrotum.

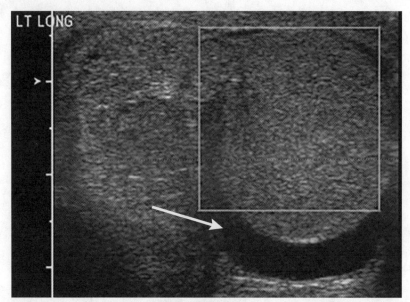

Figure 66-3. Ultrasounds of scrotum with reactive hydrocele surrounding left testicle (arrow).

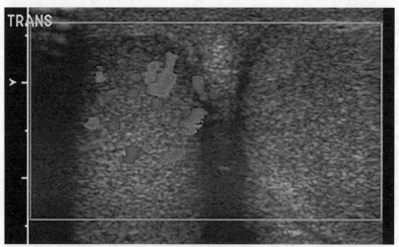

Figure 66-4. Doppler ultrasound assessing flow with normal flow to the right testicle and absent flow to the left testicle.

Torsion of the Appendix Testis

On ultrasound, torsion of the appendix will appear as a small hyperechoic or hypoechoic mass adjacent to the superior aspect of the testis or epididymis. Most are greater than 5 mm in size. The appendage in torsion has no flow, but it incites an intense inflammatory response in the adjacent tissues (Figure 66-5). Color Doppler imaging will therefore demonstrate marked hyperemia, either focally around the area of torsion or diffusely through the entire testis and epididymis. There may be severe swelling and edema of the testicle with a reactive hydrocele.

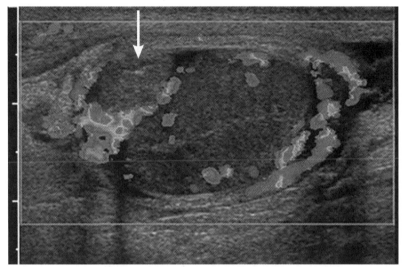

Figure 66-5. Doppler ultrasound showing a hypoechoic lesion representing the testicular appendage (arrow) with surrounding hyperemia.

Epididymitis and Orchitis (Figure 66-6)

In epididymitis or orchitis, there is increased flow on Doppler to the epididymis and testis compared with the asymptomatic side. Imaging also reveals epididymal enlargement that may be diffuse or localized to one portion of the epididymis (Figure 66-7). The swollen epididymis is usually hypoechoic, but subsequent hemorrhage or edema can produce variation in echogenicity. In patients who present later in the course of their illness, sonography may reveal abscess or pyocele. Nuclear medicine scan will show increased perfusion of the affected testis and hemiscrotum.

Trauma and Other Less Common Causes

Sonography can be extremely helpful when used to evaluate the acute scrotum or in cases of unclear diagnoses. Ecchymosis, significant tenderness, and swelling after trauma to the scrotum must prompt the clinician to carry out diagnostic imaging, such as ultrasonography, for evaluation, especially since the physical examination findings may be unreliable because of extreme pain and swelling. This imaging modality can reliably diagnose testicular fracture, hematoma, hematocele, hydrocele, ischemia or infarction, tumors and other masses, hernias, and varicoceles.

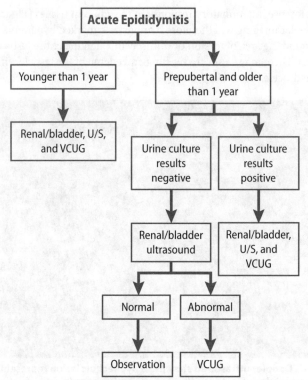

Figure 66-6. Algorithm for radiologic evaluation of acute epididymitis (Evidence Level II-3 and Evidence Level III).
Abbreviations: U/S, ultrasound; VCUG, voiding cystourethrogram.

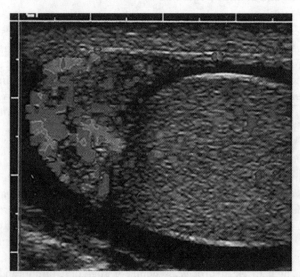

Figure 66-7. Doppler ultrasound showing epididymal enlargement and hyper-emia suggestive of epididymitis.

Other Studies

Urinalysis is often performed in the work-up of the child with acute scrotum. If a diagnosis of testicular torsion is suggested by history and physical examination findings, there is no need to delay surgical intervention by awaiting the results of urinalysis, but in cases in which the cause is not as clear, urinalysis can at times provide useful information. The finding of pyuria is linked to a diagnosis of epididymitis, but in studies of children with epididymitis, pyuria was found in only 7% to 24% of the patients. Hematuria and proteinuria may suggest nephritis associated with HSP. Hematuria may also suggest the presence of kidney stones, which can present with scrotal or penile pain and urinary symptoms.

Urine culture should also be performed in children with the acute scrotum, as it can guide treatment for epididymitis. In sexually active adolescents, urethral cultures for *Neisseria gonorrheae* and *Chlamydia trachomatis* should be performed. Many centers now offer DNA probe testing of urine for chlamydia and gonorrhea, and this can be used instead of cultures if available.

Serum studies do not clearly help with the diagnosis of the pediatric acute scrotum, but acute phase reactants such as white blood cell count and C-reactive protein have been found to be elevated more often in patients with epididymitis. They may also be elevated in other inflammatory conditions such as Kawasaki disease.

Management

Testicular Torsion

The current gold standard for treatment of testicular torsion is emergent scrotal exploration (Table 66-3). As such, the importance of early consultation to the urologist or surgeon cannot be overemphasized. Exploration should not be delayed by attempts at imaging if the history and physical examination findings strongly suggest torsion, as **TIME = TESTICLE**. The goal of surgery is twofold; first, it reestablishes circulation to the ischemic testicle, and second, it affords the opportunity for bilateral orchiopexy to be performed to prevent further episodes. The contralateral hemiscrotum must be explored at the time of surgery, as the bell-clapper deformity is usually bilateral.

If the testicle is deemed nonviable at the time of surgery, orchiectomy is performed. The most common current practice is to perform orchiectomy and offer testicular prosthesis placement at a later date, but some recent studies have suggested that orchiectomy and prosthesis exchange can be performed in the same surgery. Surgery should never be delayed by the assumption of nonviability based on a clinical estimate of the duration of torsion, as patients with a prolonged period of symptoms may have had intermittent torsion or a partial torsion, and the testicle may still be salvageable.

Table 66-3. Most Common Causes of the Acute Scrotum: Clinical Findings and Treatment

	Testicular Torsion	Appendix Testis Torsion	Epididymitis
Peak Incidence	Perinatal and Puberty	Prepubertal	<2 y and Postpubertal
Symptoms	• Acute onset of sharp, severe pain • Usually <12 h duration	• More gradual onset of dull less severe testicular pain, localized to the anterior-superior region	• Gradual onset of pain
Associated symptoms	• Nausea and vomiting	• Usually none	• Fever • Dysuria • Urethral discharge • Recent viral infection
Physical examination findings	• Testicular tenderness • Absent cremasteric reflex • High-riding testicle • Horizontal lie • Negative Prehn sign • Bell-clapper deformity	• Tenderness localized to superior pole of testicle • "Blue dot sign" • Normal testicular lie • Negative Prehn sign	• Tender and swollen spermatic cord and epididymis • Scrotal erythema and edema • Normal testicular lie • Positive Prehn sign
Ultrasound findings	• Decreased or absent flow to affected testicle • Spermatic cord knot	• Appendage in torsion with no flow but around it, an increase in flow	• Increased flow to affected testicle • Possible abscess and pyocele
Management	• Immediate scrotal exploration with orchiopexy (if salvageable) of both affected and unaffected testicles • If not salvageable, then orchiectomy with orchiopexy of unaffected side; subsequent prosthesis if desired	• Analgesics • Rest	• Analgesics, rest, and scrotal support • If pyuria or positive culture, then antibiotic course against coliforms • If sexually active: empiric antibiotics against chlamydia and gonorrhea

In select situations, manual detorsion of the testicle can be attempted by the emergency physician. However, this attempt should not delay surgical consultation or management, as it is merely a temporizing measure. It is rarely performed, as the time to arrange sedation and post-reduction Doppler ultrasonography would only delay the patient's scrotal exploration. Manual detorsion, if indicated, should be performed by a physician who is comfortable and experienced in the technique and only after sedation and analgesia have been administered. Surgical exploration should follow soon after. In certain extenuating cases detorsion may have to be attempted prior to obtaining surgical consult, as definitive care may be hours away. In most (but not all) cases of testicular torsion, the testis twists towards the midline. Initial attempts should therefore be made with lateral rotation of the affected testicle or away from the midline (ie, counterclockwise on the right and clockwise on the left when facing the patient). An initial rotation of 180 degrees is followed by a further 180 degrees and more if it is bringing relief to the patient. If it causes more pain, the direction must be reversed. Signs of successful detorsion include relief of pain and lengthening of the cord with the testis, assuming a more normal position in the scrotum. Scrotal exploration should then be undertaken immediately. The pitfall of manual detorsion is that the torsion could actually be made worse if attempts are made to detorse in the same direction of the torsion.

Torsion of the Appendix Testis

Management is supportive in these patients and includes analgesics, bed rest, and scrotal support to help to alleviate the swelling and discomfort (see Table 66-3). The pain usually resolves in 5 to 10 days. Surgical removal of the testicular appendix is reserved for patients with persistent pain, and the contralateral hemiscrotum does not need to be explored.

Epididymitis

Treatment of epididymitis varies according to the severity of symptoms at presentation and suspected etiology based on age and sexual history of patient (see Table 66-3). When sexually transmitted epididymitis is suspected, treatment includes antibiotics, analgesics, scrotal support, and bed rest in the early stages. It must also be ensured that the sexual partner is treated as well. The patient should also be tested for other sexually transmitted diseases, such as syphilis and human immunodeficiency virus.

The first-line treatment regimen recommended by the Centers for Disease Control and Prevention includes intramuscular ceftriaxone at 250 mg (single dose) plus doxycycline at 100 mg orally twice a day for 10 days. Quinolones are no longer recommended for treatment of epididymitis if *N gonorrhoeae* is suspected because of increasing resistance to these agents. If the patient is engaging in anal sex, coverage against coliforms must be added. The diagnosis and treatment regimen should be reconsidered if symptoms do not improve after 3 days of therapy.

In prepubertal boys, treatment will be guided by the presence of a concomitant urinary tract infection. Coliform bacteria are a common source of epididymitis in boys and men who have congenitally abnormal urinary tracts. In boys who have pyuria, positive urine cultures, and underlying risk factors for urinary tract infection, empiric antibiotics therapy should be started with trimethoprim-sulfamethoxazole (6–12 mg of the trimethoprim component per kilogram per day divided every 12 hours) or cephalexin (25–50 mg/kg per day divided every 6–8 hours). Most boys will have a non-bacterial cause, and as such antibiotics are not needed, but as the results of urine cultures are not immediately available, empiric antibiotics are often prescribed.

Trauma and Other Causes

Other causes of the acute scrotum warrant brief mention. Incarcerated inguinoscrotal hernias are a surgical emergency, and patients with them must be taken to the operating room as soon as possible to preserve the viability of the incarcerated bowel. In patients with penetrating scrotal injury, surgical exploration is needed so that conservative debridement of nonviable tissue can be performed. Extended lacerations of scrotal skin require surgical closure. Blunt trauma to the scrotum can cause significant hematocele without testicular rupture. Delayed surgical intervention has been shown to lead to increased risk of orchiectomy, and as such early surgical intervention is advised. Patients with hydroceles that persist past 1 year of age will require elective surgical repair; if they have significant symptoms such as skin breakdown, this can be scheduled sooner. Varicoceles are usually managed conservatively unless they cause significant discomfort. Patients with scrotal pain and swelling due to vasculitides such as Kawasaki disease and HSP are usually treated supportively and according to their underlying disease process.

Long-term Monitoring, Complications, and Considerations

Though controversial, some authors report decreased fertility due to impaired spermatogenesis in patients with unilateral testicular torsion when the testicle is left in situ. This is thought to be due to immune mediated damage to the contralateral testis. Parents and patients must be counseled on this possibility. Patients also need to be followed by the urologist, as an increased risk of testicular atrophy is on the affected side in the future. Some patients who undergo orchiectomy due to nonviability of the affected testicle desire the placement of a testicular prosthesis, and this is often scheduled as an elective surgery later on. Orchiectomy can have a great psychologic effect on the patient and his family.

Epididymitis, though most commonly idiopathic in prepubertal boys, can also be associated with urinary tract abnormalities. Unfortunately, there are no distinctive clinical findings in patients with urinary tract abnormalities. As such, prepubertal boys diagnosed with epididymitis must be referred for urologic follow-up and imaging (see Figure 66-6).

Suggested Reading
· · · · · · · · · · · · · · · · · · ·

Al-Taheini KM, Pike J, Leonard M. Acute epididymitis in children: the role of radiologic studies. *Urology.* 2008;71(5):826–829

Boettcher M, Bergholz R, Krebs TF, Wenke K, Aronson DC. Clinical predictors of testicular torsion in children. *Urology.* 2012;79(3):670–674

Guiney EJ. Emergency room problems. In: O'Donnell B, Koff SA, eds. *Pediatric Urology.* London, United Kingdom: CRC Press; 1997:281–285

Kadish HA, Bolte RG. A retrospective review of pediatric patients with epididymitis, testicular torsion, and torsion of the testicular appendages. *Pediatrics.* 1998;102 (1 Pt 1):73–76

Lewis AG, Bukowski TP, Jarvis PD, Wacksman J, Sheldon CA. Evaluation of the acute scrotum in the emergency department. *J Pediatr Surg.* 1995;30(2):277–282

Perron CE. Pain-scrotal. In: Fleisher GR, Ludwig S, eds. *Textbook of Pediatric Emergency Medicine.* Philadelphia, PA: Lippincott Williams & Wilkins; 2010:474–482

Ringdahl E, Teague L. Testicular torsion. *Am Fam Physician.* 2006;74(10):1740–1743

Yang C Jr, Song B, Liu X, Wei GH, Lin T, He DW. Acute scrotum in children: an 18-year retrospective study. *Pediatr Emerg Care.* 2011;27(4):270–274

CHAPTER 67

Seizures and Status Epilepticus

Scottie B. Day, MD, and Kristi S. Day, MD

Key Points

- Status epilepticus (SE) is a medical emergency that carries a high risk of mortality and morbidity. While earlier definitions included a seizure duration of greater than 30 minutes, more investigators now consider seizures of greater than 5 minutes as indicative of SE that requires intervention.

- Prompt, goal-directed therapy, with special attention to respiratory and hemodynamic support, as well as cessation of seizure activity and treatment of the underlying cause is indicated in the child with SE.

- The first-line agent for most pediatric SE is intravenous lorazepam (which has less seizure recurrence than diazepam), while phenobarbital is the preferred agent in neonates.

- Refractory status epilepticus is defined as a seizure that lasts for more than 1 hour (a very concerning condition with high morbidity and mortality); thus, pharmacologic coma is indicated in refractory status epilepticus.

- Prognosis following SE depends on several factors, including etiology, as well as length and duration of seizures before cessation.

Overview

Seizures are defined as a clinical expression of excessive, abnormal synchronous neuronal discharges from the cerebral cortex. Status epilepticus (SE), defined as seizures lasting 30 minutes or longer, is a life-threatening medical emergency based on the theory that neuronal damage may begin after 30 minutes of continuous seizures. Some references suggest a period of time as short as 5 minutes can cause damage; however, the consensus is that continuous or prolonged seizures require urgent intervention. Mortality and morbidity associated with SE largely depends on etiology and seizure duration, with worsening outcomes associated with increasing length of seizures. Early identification and prompt effective treatment of underlying etiology, as well as interventions that decrease seizure length, may improve outcomes. These interventions may occur in the prehospital setting, emergency department, or pediatric intensive care unit.

Status epilepticus is classified similarly as seizures. The International League Against Epilepsy Task Force on Classification and Terminology separates seizures into two major categories. *Generalized seizures* involve both cerebral hemispheres, and consciousness is impaired. These may be seizures with motor movements, nonconvulsive, or absence seizures. Focal or partial seizures indicate electrical discharges from a single hemisphere. Complex focal seizures are associated with impaired consciousness, while simple focal seizures have no impairment. A more frequently utilized classification system in critical care categorizes SE based on *presence or absence of motor symptoms*. Convulsive status epilepticus (CSE) consists of continuous clonic or tonic motor activity with bilateral epileptiform discharges on electroencephalography (EEG). Nonconvulsive SE consists of continuous EEG seizures without motor movements. Febrile SE can also occur and represents a complex febrile convulsion (see Chapter 23).

Causes

Almost any insult to the cerebral cortex can cause a seizure. It is important to address the causation of SE when considering prognosis and planning treatment. The most common presentation for a child with SE is a new-onset seizure. The 3 major causes of SE in children are infection with fever, remote symptomatic cause, and low anticonvulsant drug levels. The cause of SE is age dependent, with infection playing a greater role in the cause of SE in children than in adults. The cause also differs among younger and older children, with febrile and acute symptomatic SE being more common in children younger than 2 years, whereas idiopathic and remote symptomatic causes are more common in children older than 4 years. Prolonged febrile seizures are the most common type of SE overall in childhood, but this diagnosis is conditional on the absence of central nervous system (CNS) infection. The most common causes of acute symptomatic CSE in childhood include CNS infections, acute metabolic disturbances, head injury, drug use, hypoxia/anoxia, and cerebrovascular injuries. In children with idiopathic epilepsy, CSE consideration must be made for metabolic disturbances or pyridoxal phosphate-dependent epilepsy.

Clinical Features

Clinical signs and symptoms of seizures vary based on the cause. Seizures typically mirror previous episodes, are random in occurrence, and are rarely precipitated by environmental or psychological events. Although some individuals may have varying types of seizures, most children have one type that expresses itself most of the time. However, there are always exceptions to seizure patterns. In the early stage of acute seizures or SE, a large release of catecholamines results in tachycardia, arrhythmias, high systemic pressure, and pulmonary pressure. Lactic acid often results as well. In some instances, renal failure can ensue secondary to rhabdomyolysis and myoglobinuria. Cerebral blood flow increases initially with SE to meet elevated metabolic demands, which results in increased intracranial pressure, and later, cerebral edema may occur. The transition for these physiologic changes occurs after 30 to 60 minutes of continuous seizures.

Evaluation

The search for the etiology of SE should not take precedence over interventions to abolish the seizures. Anticonvulsant therapy in SE is indicated regardless of etiology and should not be postponed for diagnostic testing. All such patients, however, should have serum electrolytes (including calcium and phosphorus), liver function, and glucose testing, which according to the American Academy of Neurology is abnormal in 6% of cases and may guide further diagnostic testing (Evidence Level III). An EEG is recommended for those with suspected yet undiagnosed seizures or epilepsy. An EEG can provide prognostic information, be used to assess treatment response, and provide evidence that SE has ended. Physical examination is important, with particular attention to the eye examination, fever, or signs of infection; cardiac examination with electrocardiogram to evaluate for possible prolonged QT syndrome or pulmonary hypertension; and skin examination. For the febrile patient, blood and urine cultures should be obtained, with consideration for lumbar puncture (CNS infection is responsible for nearly 13% of cases according to the American Academy of Neurology) once an intracranial mass and cerebral edema have been excluded with the guidance of a non-contrasted head computed tomography scan (Evidence Level III). A head computed tomography scan is indicated in those felt at risk for brain occupying lesion or with new-onset seizure. If increased intracranial pressure is suspected, a lumbar puncture should not be performed because of the risk of herniation. However, magnetic resonance imaging is the preferred modality because of increased sensitivity for the most common abnormalities, such as mass lesions, neurocutaneous syndromes, trauma in the critical care setting, infection, or hypoxic-ischemic injury. For the child younger than 2 years with recurrent intractable seizures yet initially normal findings on a magnetic resonance imaging scan, a follow-up study after 30 months of age is recommended to better visualize the possibility of cortical dysplasia. The patient receiving chronic anticonvulsant therapy should have drug levels tested, as studies have shown levels to be low or subtherapeutic greater than 30% of the time (Evidence Level II-2). Urine and serum toxicology should also be tested in the setting of a possible ingestion, as this is the etiology in approximately 3% to 6% of children according to the American Academy of Neurology (Evidence Level III). Further selected laboratory testing may include serum ammonia, lactate, serum/cerebrospinal fluid amino, and urine organic acids, with consideration for genetic consultation with chromosomal karyotype in the non-urgent setting.

Management
· · · · · · · · · · · ·

Status epilepticus is a medical emergency, and prompt cessation is important, as seizure duration is inversely associated with ease of treatment response. Evidence suggests that SE becomes more difficult to control as the duration increases. Management of the child is directed toward cessation of seizures and supportive care for associated derangements and underlying conditions.

Initial Stabilization

As with any life-threatening emergency, SE management should always focus on airway, breathing, and circulation. Much of the morbidity and mortality associated with SE is related to hypoxia and its complications. Most children do not have underlying respiratory or cardiac abnormalities; thus, most cardiorespiratory compromise seen during SE is usually a result rather than an etiology. Therefore, it is imperative to investigate etiologies in parallel with efforts to abort seizures. Patients should be positioned on their side with the head below the body to minimize aspiration. Early intubation may be required in some cases, and short-acting sedatives and neuromuscular-blocking agents should be used to avoid compromising the neurologic examination. Rapid glucose testing should be obtained; hypoglycemia, treated appropriately.

Antiepileptic Drugs

During or after the initial resuscitative efforts, specific therapy aimed at aborting and preventing seizure activity should be initiated. The paucity of randomized clinical trials evaluating anticonvulsant efficacy in the pediatric population means our anticonvulsant choice is usually guided by clinician experience or expert opinion. The recommendations in this chapter coincide with the preferred treatments based on survey, the National Institute for Clinical Excellence efforts, and the Scottish Intercollegiate Guidelines Network efforts.

The first-line agent in the acute management of all seizures is benzodiazepines with the exception of neonatal seizures when phenobarbital is the preferred first-line agent (Evidence Level III). The first- and second-line agent can vary based on the classification of the seizure as detailed in Table 67-1. In addition, typical dosing for commonly used antiepileptic drugs (AEDs) for SE is included in Table 67-2.

Benzodiazepines

Benzodiazepines are the first-line drugs for the treatment of SE. With a rapid onset of action, they are very effective. All benzodiazepines will cause some degree of respiratory depression, which can be lessened with slower infusion rates and more time between doses. Both lorazepam and diazepam are highly effective, although seizure recurrence is higher with diazepam, making lorazepam the preferred agent. Intravenous administration is the preferred

Table 67-1. Preferred AEDs Based on Classification

Convulsive SE				
	GCSE	**Focal Motor**	**Myoclonic**	**Neonatal**
First-line	Lorazepam	Lorazepam	Lorazepam	Phenobarbital
Second-line	Fosphenytoin	Fosphenytoin	Fosphenytoin Valproate	Fosphenytoin Lorazepam

Nonconvulsive SE			
	Absence	**Complex Partial**	**NCSE with Coma**
First-line	Lorazepam	Lorazepam	Lorazepam
Second-line	Valproate	Fosphenytoin	Fosphenytoin Pharmacologic coma

Abbreviations: ADE, antiepileptic drug; GCSE, generalized convulsive status epilepticus; NCSE, nonconvulsive status epilepticus; SE, status epilepticus.

Derived from Wheless JW, Clarke DF, Carpenter D. Treatment of pediatric epilepsy: expert opinion, 2005. *J Child Neurol.* 2005;20(Suppl 1):S1–S6.

Table 67-2. Typical Dosing for SE

Medication	Dose	Re-dosing
Lorazepam	0.05–0.15 mg/kg/dose IV (max: 4 mg)	Repeat in 5 min.
Phenobarbital	15–20 mg/kg IV	Repeat in 5 mg/kg/dose.
Fosphenytoin	15–20 mg phenytoin equivalents per kg IV	Repeat in 10 mg/kg doses.
Valproate	15–20 mg/kg	

Abbreviations: SE, status epilepticus; max, maximum; IV, intravenous.

route, but alternatives include buccal or rectal administration. Diazepam may be rectally administered; it is available as a gel preparation and is often prescribed for families for emergencies in the prehospital setting (Evidence Level II).

Fosphenytoin

Fosphenytoin is the second-line agent for many classifications of SE. It is a pro-drug that is dephosphorylated to phenytoin. Fosphenytoin has similar efficacy to phenytoin with fewer adverse effects including less local injection site irritation and arrhythmias. Fosphenytoin administration will achieve peak levels of phenytoin roughly 20 minutes after intravenous infusion. Therapeutic levels of 20 mg/dL are typically targeted, although patients on concomitant valproate therapy or who have hypoalbuminemia or renal insufficiency may have total levels that cause much higher free plasma concentrations than is seen in children without these conditions.

Phenobarbital

Phenobarbital is the first-line agent for neonatal seizures as well as a second-line agent in other forms of SE when benzodiazepines may not be effective. Although phenobarbital is advantageous in a broad spectrum of seizure types, its associated drawbacks of sedation, respiratory depression, and hypotension make it less favorable in many clinical situations.

Valproate

As a second-line agent for absence and myoclonic SE, valproate is becoming more used in the critical care setting. It has been shown to be effective not only in nonconvulsive SE but also in controlling acute repetitive seizures. It has been shown that rapid intravenous loading of 25 mg/kg stopped seizures within 20 minutes of completion of the infusion, and children remained seizure free up to 12 hours after treatment with no adverse cardiovascular or respiratory effects. Further study will help clarify its position in the emergency setting.

Treatment of Refractory Status Epilepticus

Refractory SE refers to SE that persists beyond 1 hour despite AED therapy. As before, urgent treatment of refractory SE is warranted because of the ongoing risk of seizure-induced cerebral injury. Conventional AEDs should be continued during this phase. although they have little efficacy. Regardless of the agent chosen for pharmacologic coma, effective vital sign monitoring is necessary to preserve hemodynamics and effective ventilation. Because of the confounding sedative properties of AEDs, clinicians are often guided by continuous EEG monitoring, as the clinical expression of seizures may be subtle. Insufficient evidence exists to conclude which high-dose AED, either alone or in combination, has superior efficacy in refractory SE.

Midazolam infusions have been used to treat neonatal and pediatric refractory SE. Adverse effects are minimal and include transient mild hypotension. Barbiturates including pentobarbital, thiopental, and phenobarbital are widely used for refractory SE and may have neuroprotective effects. The main drawbacks to barbituates include the high risk of cardiovascular depression and hypotension. Furthermore, the time to regain consciousness is also greater. Finally, high dose, prolonged barbiturate therapy may have immunosuppressive properties.

Other medications such as propofol, ketamine, topiramate, and volatile anesthetics have been used as adjuncts in refractory SE. Propofol is most commonly used in this venue, especially in older adolescents and adults. However, propofol has been associated with "propofol infusion syndrome" and as such should be used with caution in children. Valproic acid has been shown effective in partial and generalized epilepsy syndromes in pediatrics. It is less sedating and has less respiratory depression and hemodynamic instability. The newest drug in the armamentarium for refractory SE is levetiracetam. It has been shown to be neuroprotective and not only stops seizures but also reduces seizure-induced brain damage (Evidence Level II-2). The preferential pharmacologic profile often makes it a preferred agent in transplant patients.

Finally, refractory SE that fails to respond to high-dose therapy has high morbidity and mortality. In these situations, surgical treatment modalities can be considered but are beyond the scope of this chapter.

Long-term Implications

The prognosis of patients with SE largely depends on the patient's age and the etiology of seizures. Children with febrile etiologies tend to fare better than those with acute symptomatic or progressive encephalopathic etiologies. Adverse outcomes are particularly high in infants with perinatal problems or neurologic abnormalities not identified prior to the onset of SE. Anoxia and acute bacterial meningitis with associated SE carries a very high risk.

The risk of developing epilepsy is higher in children who present with SE. Intractable epilepsy is associated with young age at the first SE episode and remote symptomatic SE.

Cognitive or motor disabilities are not uncommon following SE in children. Risk factors for poor outcomes include neuroimaging abnormalities, patients younger than 1 year, or acute symptomatic, remote symptomatic, or progressive encephalopathy etiology.

Suggested Reading

Barnard C, Wirrell E. Does status epilepticus in children cause developmental deterioration and exacerbation of epilepsy? *J Child Neurol.* 1999;14(12):787–794

Berg AT, Scheffer IE. New concepts in classification of the epilepsies: entering the 21st century. *Epilepsia.* 2011;52(6):1058–1062

DeLorenzo RJ, Hauser WA, Towne AR, et al. A prospective, population-based epidemiologic study of status epilepticus in Richmond, Virginia. *Neurology.* 1996;46(4):1029

Kumar MA, Urrutia V, Thomas CE, Abou-Khaled KJ, Schwartzman RJ. The syndrome of irreversible acidosis after prolonged propofol infusion. *Neurocrit Care.* 2005;3(3): 257–259

Riviello JJ, Ashwal S, Hirtz T, et al. Practice parameter: diagnostic assessment of the child with status epilepticus (an evidence-based review): report of the quality standards subcommittee of the American Academy of Neurology and the Practice Committee of the Child Neurology Society. *Neurology.* 2006;67(9):1542–1550

Sagduyu A, Tarlaci S, Sirin H. Generalized tonic-clonic status epilepticus: causes, treatment, complications, and predictors of case fatality. *J Neurol.* 1998;245(10):640–646

Wheless JW, Clarke DF, Carpenter D. Treatment of pediatric epilepsy: expert opinion. *J Child Neurol.* 2005;20(Suppl 1):S1–S6

Yu KT, Thompson N, Cunana C. Safety and efficacy of intravenous valproate in pediatric status epilepticus and acute repetitive seizures. *Epilepsia.* 2003;44(5):724–726

CHAPTER 68

Sepsis

Lauren Piper, MD, MS

Key Points

- Sepsis is a clinical syndrome defined as a systemic inflammatory response syndrome (SIRS) from a suspected or confirmed infectious cause, the hallmark an inflammatory cascade that leads to systemic inflammation and tissue injury.

- The International Pediatric Sepsis Consensus Conference (2005) defined the criteria for SIRS to include at least 2 of the following 4 features: core temperature greater than 38.5°C (101.3°F) or less than 36°C (96.8°F); white blood count elevated or depressed for the patient's age *or* greater than 10% immature neutrophils; tachycardia (or bradycardia if age <1 y); and tachypnea.

- Sepsis criteria include evidence of SIRS plus suspected or proven infection, the emphasis being on heightened suspicion and early detection to improve appropriate evaluation and management.

- The earliest signs of sepsis are characterized by the triad of fever (or hypothermia), tachycardia, and tachypnea.

- Management priorities include improving volume and perfusion, oxygenation, and aggressive treatment of the underlying infection. Children with septic shock relative to adults require larger volumes of fluid resuscitation, more inotropic and vasoactive agent support, hydrocortisone for relative adrenal insufficiency, and some may require extracorporeal membrane oxygenation support for refractory shock.

Overview

Sepsis is a clinical syndrome defined as a systemic inflammatory response syndrome (SIRS) from a suspected or confirmed infectious cause. The inflammatory cascade causing systemic inflammation and tissue injury may be triggered by bacterial, viral, fungal, or parasitic infections.

The International Pediatric Sepsis Consensus Conference in 2005 developed definitions for SIRS and the continuum of the sepsis spectrum, including sepsis, severe sepsis, and septic shock in infants and children (Table 68-1). These definitions are based on 6 age-specific vital signs and laboratory criteria (Table 68-2). The definition of sepsis requires an abnormal temperature or abnormal white blood cell count.

Table 68-1. International Consensus Definitions for Pediatric Sepsis

Infection	Suspected or proven infection by any pathogen OR a clinical syndrome associated with a high probability of infection

SIRS	2 out of 4 criteria, one of which must be abnormality of temperature or leukocyte count
	• Core temperature >38.5°C (101.3°F) or <36°C (96.8°F)
	• Leukocyte count elevated or depressed for age (not secondary to chemotherapy)
	    OR >10% immature neutrophils
	• Tachycardia (heart rate >2 SD above reference range for age in the absence of external stimulus, chronic drugs, or painful stimuli)
	    OR otherwise unexplained persistent elevation over a 0.5- to 4-h time period
	    OR children <1 y: bradycardia (mean HR ,10th percentile for age in absence of external vagus stimulus, beta-adrenergic blocking agents, or congenital heart disease)
	• Tachypnea (respiratory rate >2 SD above reference range for age) or mechanical ventilation for an acute process not related to underlying neuromuscular disease or anesthesia

Sepsis	SIRS in the presence of suspected or proven infection

Severe sepsis	Sepsis plus 1 of the following conditions:
	1. Cardiovascular organ dysfunction, defined as the following (despite >40 mL/kg of isotonic intravenous fluid in 1 h):
	  • Hypotension <5th percentile for the patient's age or systolic BP <2 SD below reference range for age
	    OR
	  • Need for vasoactive drug to maintain BP in normal range
	    OR
	  • 2 of the following conditions:
	    – Unexplained metabolic acidosis: base deficit >5 mEq/L
	    – Increased arterial lactate >2 times of upper limit of normal range
	    – Urine output <0.5 mL/kg/h
	    – Prolonged capillary refill >5 s
	    – Core-to-peripheral-temperature gap >3°C (5.4°F)
	2. ARDS as defined by the presence of a Pao_2/Fio_2 ratio ≤300 mm Hg, bilateral infiltrates on chest radiograph, and no evidence of left ventricular failure
	3. 2 or more other organ dysfunctions
	  Neurologic: acute change in mental status with GCS ≤11 or change of ≥3 from baseline
	  Hematologic: INR >2 OR platelet count <80,000 or decline by 50% from past 3 days
	  Renal: serum creatinine level ≥2 times upper limit for the patient's age or 2-fold increase from baseline
	  Hepatic: total bilirubin ≥4 mg/dL (not applicable for newborn)

Septic shock	Sepsis and cardiovascular organ dysfunction as defined previously

Abbreviations: ARDS, acute respiratory distress syndrome; BP, blood pressure; GCS, Glasgow Coma Scale; INR, international normalized ratio; SD, standard deviation; SIRS, systemic inflammatory response syndrome.

Adapted from Turner, DA, Cheifetz IM. Shock. In: Kliegman R, Nelson WE. *Nelson Textbook of Pediatrics.* 19th ed. Philadelphia, PA: Elsevier/Saunders; 2011:305–314, with permission.

Table 68-2. Age-Specific Vital Signs and Laboratory Variables for Pediatric Sepsis

Age Group	HR[a,b] (beats/min)	Respiratory Rate[b] (beats/min)	Leukocyte Count[a,b] (x 10^3/mm)	SBP[a] (mm Hg)
0 d–1 wk	>180 or <100	>50	>34	<65
1 wk–1 mo	>180 or <100	>40	>19.5 or <5	<75
1 mo–1 y	>180 or <90	>34	>17.5 or <5	<100
2–5 y	>140	>22	>15.5 or <6	<94
6–12 y	>130	>18	>13.5 or <4.5	<105
13–<18 y	>110	>14	>11 or <4.5	<117

Abbreviations: HR, heart rate; SBP, systolic blood pressure.
[a] Lower values are for the 5th percentile.
[b] Upper values are for the 95th percentile.
Modified from Goldstein B, Giroir B, Randolph A; International Consensus Conference on Pediatric Sepsis. International pediatric sepsis consensus conference: definitions for sepsis and organ dysfunction in pediatrics. *Pediatr Crit Care Med.* 2005;6(1):2–8, with permission.

Children with young age, other comorbidities, or both are at highest risk for sepsis. Some risk factors for sepsis include hospitalization, presence of indwelling devices, immunocompromised states (eg, immunodeficiency, malignancies, solid-organ transplantation), Hemoglobin SS disease, splenic dysfunction or asplenia, congenital heart disease, and burns. Neonates in general are at increased risk for infection because of their immature immune systems and require specialized evaluation and management, the details of which lie outside the scope of this chapter.

Causes

Infectious and noninfectious causes of SIRS must be considered when evaluating a child for possible sepsis. The differential diagnosis for sepsis and SIRS is extensive (Table 68-3).

The most frequently identified organisms causing severe sepsis in children in the United States are *Staphylococcus* species followed by *Streptococcus* species. Fungal infections are more common among children with other comorbidities. Primary bacteremia and respiratory causes comprise most severe sepsis in children.

Clinical Features

The earliest signs of sepsis are characterized by the triad of fever (or hypothermia), tachypnea, and tachycardia. Sepsis is a dynamic process due to the inflammatory response of the host. Sepsis begins as an infection and may lead to additional organ dysfunction and septic shock. As the severity of sepsis

Table 68-3. Differential Diagnosis of Systemic Inflammatory Response Syndrome

Infection	Metabolic-Endocrine
Bacteremia or meningitis (*Staphylococcus aureus, Streptococcus pneumoniae*, group A streptococci, *Haemophilus influenzae* type b, *Neisseria meningitidis*) Viral Illness (influenza, enteroviruses, herpes simplex virus, respiratory syncytial virus, cytomegalovirus, Epstein-Barr virus) Encephalitis (arboviruses, enteroviruses, herpes simplex virus) Rickettsiae (Rocky Mountain spotted fever, *Ehrlichia* species, Q fever) Syphilis Vaccine reaction (pertussis, influenza, measles) Toxin-mediated reaction (toxic shock, staphylococcal-scalded skin syndrome) Fungal infection Urinary tract infection Endocarditis	Adrenal Insufficiency (adrenogenital syndrome, corticosteroid withdrawal) Electrolyte disturbances (hyponatremia or hypernatremia; hypocalcemia or hypercalcemia) Diabetes insipidus Diabetes mellitus Inborn errors of metabolism (organic acidosis, urea cycle, carnitine deficiency, mitochondrial disorders) Hypoglycemia Reye syndrome
	Hematologic
	Anemia (sickle cell disease, blood loss, nutritional) Methemoglobinemia Splenic sequestration crisis Leukemia or lymphoma Hemophagocytic syndromes
Cardiopulmonary	**Neurologic**
Pneumonia Pulmonary emboli Heart failure arrhythmia Pericarditis Myocarditis	Intoxications (drugs, carbon monoxide, intentional or unintentional overdose) Intracranial hemorrhage Infant botulism Trauma (child abuse, accidental) Guillain-Barré syndrome Myasthenia gravis
Gastrointestinal	**Other**
Gastroenteritis with dehydration Volvulus Intussusception Appendicitis Peritonitis Necrotizing enterocolitis Hepatitis Hemorrhage Pancreatitis	Anaphylaxis (food, drug, insect sting) Hemolytic-uremic syndrome Kawasaki disease Erythema multiforme Hemorrhagic shock–encephalopathy syndrome Poisoning Toxic envenomation Macrophage activation syndrome

Modified from Turner DA, Cheifetz IM. Shock. In: Kliegman R, Nelson WE, eds. *Nelson Textbook of Pediatrics*. 19th ed. Philadelphia, PA: Elsevier/Saunders; 2011:305–314, with permission.

worsens in this dynamic process, it is common to see changes in mental status and signs of decreased perfusion. Low urine output is also a common sign of hypovolemia and decreased perfusion.

Mental status abnormalities vary on the basis of the developmental age of the patient and on the basis of the severity of illness. Signs of decreased or altered mental status may include irritability, inappropriate crying, drowsiness, confusion, and lethargy.

Changes in respiratory status are common and can vary depending on the severity of sepsis and the inciting cause. Primary respiratory sources of infection are a common cause of sepsis in children and therefore may present with more severe alterations in respiratory status in comparison to other causes. Signs and symptoms range from mild tachypnea to hypoxemia and grunting with impending respiratory failure.

Septic shock is typically categorized on the basis of warm shock and cold shock. Warm shock is defined by a high cardiac output and low systemic vascular resistance state; whereas cold shock is defined by a low cardiac output and high systemic vascular resistance state. The signs and symptoms of these two states vary greatly on the basis of the contrasting physiologic states. Warm shock is characterized by bounding peripheral pulses, vasodilation with flash capillary refill, and widened pulse pressure. In contrast, cold shock is characterized by diminished pulses, prolonged capillary refill greater than 3 seconds, and mottled cool extremities. Hypotension is often a late sign that may soon be followed by cardiovascular collapse and is not necessary for the diagnosis for septic shock. However, the presence of hypotension is confirmatory for the diagnosis of septic shock.

Evaluation and Management

Prompt recognition of sepsis is essential to early goal-directed therapy that has been shown to improve outcomes and reduce mortality. Well established, evidenced-based international guidelines are available for the evaluation and management of sepsis in infants and children. Septic shock is a dynamic process that requires ongoing reassessment of clinical status and appropriate titration or change in therapies.

The algorithm developed in 2002 and updated in the 2007 American College of Critical Care Medicine (ACCM) "Clinical Guidelines for Hemodynamic Support of Neonates and Children With Septic Shock" has been incorporated into the American Heart Association *Pediatric Advanced Life Support (PALS) Provider Manual* (Evidence Level I and Evidence Level III) (Figure 68-1). These guidelines call for the rapid, time-sensitive, stepwise execution of therapeutic interventions within 1 hour. In addition, the Surviving Sepsis Campaign "International Guidelines for the Management of Severe Sepsis and Septic Shock" has been instrumental in the review and grading of best practices for care of both adults and children with severe sepsis and septic shock. These guidelines were last updated in 2008 (Evidence Level I and Evidence Level III).

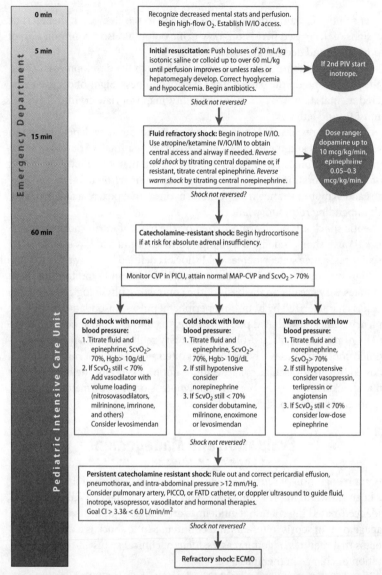

Figure 68-1. Algorithm for time-sensitive, goal-directed, stepwise management of hemodynamic support in infants and children (Evidence Level I and Evidence Level III).
Proceed to next step if shock persists. (1) First-hour goals: Restore and maintain heart rate thresholds, capillary refill ≤2 seconds, and normal blood pressure in the first hour/emergency department. Support oxygenation and ventilation as appropriate. (2) Subsequent intensive care unit goals: If shock is not reversed, intervene to restore and maintain normal perfusion saturation >70%, and CI > 3.3, < 6.0 L/min/m^2 in pediatric intensive care unit (PICU).

Abbreviations: CI, cardiac index; CRRT, continuous renal replacement therapy; CVP, central venous pressure; ECMO, extracorporeal membrane oxygenation; FATD, femoral arterial thermodilution; Hgb, hemoglobin; IM, intramuscular; IO, intraosseous; IV, intravenous; MAP, mean arterial pressure; PICCO, pulse contour cardiac output.

From Brierly J, Carcillo JA, Choong K, et al. Clinical practice parameters for hemodynamic support of pediatric and neonatal septic shock: 2007 update from the American College of Critical Care Medicine. *Crit Care Med.* 2009;37(2):666–688, with permission.

As with the initial evaluation of any patient, it is necessary to quickly perform a focused evaluation of the patient's airway, breathing, circulation, and neurologic status and to determine if the patient meets criteria for severe sepsis or septic shock. In the first 5 minutes, patients should be placed on 100% supplemental oxygen, vascular access must be obatined either via peripheral intravenous (PIV) or intraosseous (IO) access to begin fluid resuscitation, blood culture and serum glucose level must be obtained, and antibiotics must be started. Hypoglycemia should be promptly treated.

Supplemental oxygen typically via nasal cannula or face mask should be given to all patients with sepsis regardless of pulse oximetry saturation to maximize oxygen delivery. Intubation may be necessary for impending respiratory failure, for refractory shock not rapidly stabilized with fluids and peripherally administered inotropes, or for placement of central venous access and arterial monitoring. Intubation with ketamine is preferred over etomidate for sedation in children given that it has been shown to cause transient adrenal insufficiency. One dose of hydrocortisone should be given to patients that receive etomidate. Many drugs commonly given for intubation may cause hypotension and should be used with caution.

It is recommended that vascular access be obtained within the first 5 minutes of patient presentation. It may be difficult to obtain sufficient PIV access on an infant or child with severe sepsis or septic shock. The American Heart Association PALS guidelines support the early use of IO access if PIV access is not possible in the first 5 minutes or if additional access is necessary to rapidly administer the goal-directed therapies outlined in Figure 55-1. Sufficient vascular access must be quickly obtained to administer up to 60 mL/kg of fluids, empiric antibiotcs, and dopamine if indicated within the first hour of patient presentation. Inotropes may be given through PIV or IO access with careful monitoring for infiltration while central venous access is being obtained.

Hypovolemia is common in children with sepsis and often requires proportionately larger volumes of fluid relative to adults. Fluid boluses of isotonic crystalloid (normal saline or lactated Ringer's solution) should be given in rapid 20 mL/kg increments over 5 to 10 minutes to restore tissue perfusion (Table 68-4). The targeted goals of fluid resuscitation listed in Table 55-4 are varied and reflect improved perfusion and organ system function. These are appropriate for nearly all patients; central venous pressure measurements are not required but if available can further guide therapy. Infants and children with severe sepsis and septic shock may require ongoing total fluid resuscitation volumes as high as 100 to 200 mL/kg through repeated 20 mL/kg bolus infusions. Fluid boluses may be given via rapid infuser system or using a manual syringe-delivery system to increase speed of delivery.

Dopamine should be started either in addition to ongoing fluid resuscitation in children who have not improved following 60 mL/kg fluid or immediately with hypotension (Evidence Level II-2). Norepinephrine should be added to those with fluid and dopamine refractory warm shock, and epinephrine should be added to those with fluid and dopamine refractory cold shock.

Table 68-4. Fluid Therapy: Methods and Goals of Therapy (Level of Evidence II-2)

Fluids	Normal Saline; Lactated Ringer Solution
Methods	Rapid 20 mL/kg (IV, rapid infuser, manual syringe system)
Goals of therapy	1. Improvement in tachycardia 2. Urine output within reference range (>1 mL/kg/h) 3. Capillary refill <2 s 4. Mental status within reference range 5. CVP of 8–12 mm Hg

Abbreviations: CVP, central venous pressure; IV, intraveous.

Critical illness adrenal insufficiency is common among children with shock that is refractory to fluids and inotropic support.

The use of hydrocortisone in septic shock in children is controversial. The ACCM-PALS guidelines recommend empiric hydrocortisone (100 mg/m^2) be given to those with catecholamine resistant shock, purpura fulminans, or other risk factors for adrenal insufficiency, including those with prior steroid exposure or hypothalamic/pituitary abnormality (Evidence Level II-2). It is also recommended to give 1 dose of hydrocortisone to children that receive etomidate for intubation. Adrenocorticotopic hormone–stimulation testing should not be performed. Steroid therapy may be weaned when inotropic support is no longer needed. Hydrocortisone provides both glucocorticoid and mineralcorticoid effect.

Blood cultures should be obtained prior to starting antibiotics provided that they do not siginificantly delay antibiotic administration (Evidence Level I). Two or more blood cultures should be obatined, and at least 1 culture should be peripheral. Cultures from existing vascular access that has been in place for more than 48 hours should be obtained from each lumen and will help determine if the infection is a catheter-associated blood stream infection (Evidence Level I). Cultures from other sources including urine and cerebrospinal fluid should be obatined if clinically indicated. It is essential to try to identify the source of sepsis and to intervene accordingly. For example, sepsis secondary to septic arthritis or soft-tissue abscess requires drainage and debridement, whereas sepsis secondary to catheter-related bacteremia may require removal of vascular catheter depending on severity of illness and the inciting organsim (Evidence Level I).

Empiric intravous broad-spectrum antibiotics should be started immediately upon obtaining blood cultures and should be given within the first hour of patient presentation (Evidence Level I). Antibiotics should not be delayed in patients that cannot tolerate lumbar puncture. The selection of intial appropriate antibiotic therapy must take into consideration possible infection sources on the basis of history and physical examination, high risk conditions, history of prior infections, local resistance patterns, and speed of administration.

In a quality improvement process project for the implementation of these evidence-based guidelines for children with suspected sepsis, Cruz and Perry developed a shock protocol for the "Implementation of Goal-Directed Therapy for Children With Suspected Sepsis in the Emergency Department," with standardization of intial empiric antibiotic therapy for 2 groups of patients. High risk patients (with the exception of patients with asplenia) received piperacillin-tazobactam and gentamicin given at the same time via the same vascular access point, followed by vancomycin. All other patients, including those with asplenia, first received ceftriaxone over 3 minutes, then vancomycin and naficillin. Preprinted order sets improved efficiency and delivery of appropriate antibiotics.

This quality improvement process project helped to address some of the logistic barriers of implementation of the evidence-based guidelines for severe sepsis and septic shock. The main barriers that were identified were delay in recognition of patients with compensated septic shock and delays in implementation of resuscitative measures. Creation and utilization of a computerized triage tool that corrected heart rate for pyrexia and electronically alerted nursing staff if a patient fell outside of the age-appropriate reference range to consider activating the shock protocol. The protocol was also activated for the following reasons: fever (>38°C [100.4°F]) or hypothermia (<35.5°C [95.9°F]); ill appearance with: altered mental status or delay in capillary refill greater than 3 seconds; shock; or criteria met for being at high risk of sepsis. High risk patients were defined as having a history of malignancy, bone marrow transplantation, asplenia, solid-organ trasnplant, immunodeficiency, or central venous catheterization.

Protocol activation resulted in patients being taken to designated resuscitation rooms and notification of the attending to see the patient, of the transport team to assist emergency department staff with resuscitation, and of the pediatric intensive care unit of potential admission. In addition, a standardized graphic flow sheet was utilized to document progress of resuscitation alongside preprinted order sets (Table 68-5). The preprinted order sets included a bundled laboratory evaluation, chest radiograph, and empiric antibiotic regimen depeding on risk category. Fluids were administered via rapid infuser or manually via syringe to increase speed of delivery. Protocol implementation reduced triage time to first fluid administration from 56 to 22 minutes (P <.001) and triage time to first antibiotics from 130 to 38 minutes. (P <.001) (Evidence Level II-3).

Other recommendations from the Surviving Sepsis Campaign guidelines include blood transusion to achieve hemoglobin of 7 g/dL (Evidence Level I). It is recommended to trasnfuse red blood cells to a higher hemoglobin of 10 g/dL in refractory septic shock to obtain mixed venous oxygen saturation greater than or equal to 70% (Evidence Level III).

Infants, in particular, are at high risk for developing hypoglycemia, which requires prompt treatment. Hyperglycemia is also common in infants and children with severe sepsis and septic shock. In adults, it is recommended to aim to keep glucose near 150 mg/dL with validated insulin protocol. Improved glycemic control has been associated with improved outcomes in adults

Table 68-5. Preprinted Order Set for Shock Protocol

Category	Intervention	Expected Time Frame From Protocol Initiation	Notes
Nursing			
Vital-sign measurement	Supplemental oxygen; pulse oximetry; cardiopulmonary monitoring	5 min	Measure vital signs every 15 min
Vascular access	No anesthetic creams used; freezing sprays can be used	5–10 min	Physician notified if no access after 5 min
Strict monitoring of UOP, fluids administered	Foley catheter if not neutropenic	From onset	Vital-sign flow sheet
Blood pressure support			
Fluid resuscitation	20 mL/kg (maximum 1 L) IV up to 3 boluses; all boluses were given push-pull or via rapid infuser	15 min (to start of first bolus)	10 mL/kg boluses with cardiac conditions, BMT patients, and patients immediately after lung transplant
Vasoactive agents	Warm: norepinephrine; cold shock: dopamine ± epinephrine	Order with completion of third bolus	Order with completion of third bolus
Antibiotic therapy			
High risk (except asplenia)	Piperacillin-tazobactam, gentamicin, Vancomycin	30 min	Piperacillin-tazobactam and gentamicin given first, at same time via same line
Asplenia & immunologically normal hosts	Ceftriaxone, vancomycin, nafcillin	30 min	Ceftriaxone given first over 3 min, then vancomycin
Other medications			
Stress-dose steroids	Hydrocortisone 100 mg/m^2	30 min	No ACTH-stimulation testing performed

Laboratory, radiographic evaluation		
Screening laboratory tests	CBC; chemistries; liver panel; DIC panel; CRP; VBG with lactate; consider type and screen	10 min after received by laboratory	Sent via life-threatening laboratory system
Microbiology	Blood culture: peripheral and central (if applicable); urine culture, rapid RSV and influenza assays	...	All lumens of central lines cultured
Radiology	Portable chest radiograph	...	Able to be viewed in resuscitation room
Other			
Page primary services; page ICU	...	At time of protocol initiation; with completion of third bolus	ICU charge nurse receives page with each shock-protocol initiation

Abbreviations: ACTH, adrenocorticotopic hormone; BMT, bone marrow transplant; CBC, complete blood count; CRP, C-reactive protein; DIC, disseminated intravascular coagulation; ICU, intensive care unit; IV, intravenous; RSV, respiratory syncytial virus; UOP, urine output; VBG, venous blood gas.

From Cruz AT, Perry AM, Williams EA, Graf JM, Wuestner ER, Patel B. Implementation of goal-directed therapy for children with suspected sepsis in the emergency department. *Pediatrics*. 2011;127(3):e758–e766.

(Evidence Level I); there is currently no such data in children. There is concern over the development of hypoglycemia among children receiving insulin therapy for hyperglycemia. Frequent glucose monitoring should be performed if insulin is administered in infants and children with sepsis.

Deep venous thrombosis prophylaxis is recommended in post-pubertal children with severe sepsis. Low-dose unfractionated heparin or low-molecular weighted heparin may be used unless there is a contraindication, at which time compression stockings or intermittent compression devices should be used (Evidence Level II-2).

Outcomes for infants and children with severe sepsis and septic shock continue to improve with the implementation of the guidelines developed by the ACCM and Surviving Sepsis Campaign and adopted by PALS. Despite significant improvements in morbidity and morality, the most recent guidelines documented an increase in probability that children with septic shock relative to adults require larger volumes of fluid resuscitation, inotropic and vasoactive agent support, hydrocortisone for relative adrenal insufficiency, and extracorporeal membrane oxygenation for refractory shock (Evidence Level III). Early recognition and identification of infants and children in compensated and uncompensated septic shock is crucial in ensuring that they be given adequate treatment and fluid resuscitation to reverse volume depletion before hypotension.

Long-term Monitoring

Infants and children with pediatric sepsis should be seen by the primary care physician within 1 week of discharge following hospitalization for sepsis. It is important to evaluate the child's nutritional status, growth, and activity level while screening for superinfection and bacterial colonization associated with antibiotic therapy.

Hearing screening is recommended for infants or children that are at risk for hearing loss, including those that were treated with such ototoxic medications as aminoglycosides. Both hearing screening and neurodevelopment assessment should be performed on infants and children that are at risk for long-term neurologic sequelae from sepsis (ie, meningitis, prolonged states of hypoxia or poor perfusion, and extracorporeal membrane oxygenation support).

Suggested Reading

Brierley J, Carcillo JA, Choong K, et al. Clinical practice parameters for hemodynamic support of pediatric and neonatal septic shock: 2007 update from the American College of Critical Care Medicine. *Crit Care Med*. 2009;37(2):666–688

Carcillo JA, Fields AI; American College of Critical Care Medicine Task Force Committee. Clinical practice parameters for hemodynamic support of pediatric and neonatal patients in septic shock. *Crit Care Med.* 2002;30(6):1365–1378

Cruz AT, Perry AM, Williams EA, Graf JM, Wuestner ER, Patel B. Implementation of goal-directed therapy for children with suspected sepsis in the emergency department. *Pediatrics.* 2011;127(3):e758–e766

Dellinger RP, Levy MM, Carlet JM, et al. Surviving Sepsis Campaign: international guidelines for management of severe sepsis and septic shock: 2008. *Intensive Care Med.* 2008;34(1):17–60

European Society of Intensive Care Medicine, International Sepsis Foundation, Society of Critical Care Medicine. Surviving Sepsis Campaign Web site. http://www.survivingsepsis.org. Accessed January 13, 2015

Goldstein B, Giroir B, Randolph A; International Consensus Conference on Pediatric Sepsis. International pediatric sepsis consensus conference: definitions for sepsis and organ dysfunction in pediatrics. *Pediatr Crit Care Med.* 2005;6(1):2–8

Rivers E, Nguyen B, Havstad S, et al. Early goal-directed therapy in the treatment of severe sepsis and septic shock. *N Engl J Med.* 2001;345(19):1368–1377

Turner, DA, Cheifetz IM. Shock. In: Kliegman R, Nelson WE. *Nelson Textbook of Pediatrics.* 19th ed. Philadelphia, PA: Elsevier/Saunders; 2011:305–314

Watson RS, Carcillo JA, Linde-Zwirble WT, Clermont G, Lidicker J, Angus DC. The epidemiology of severe sepsis in children in the United States. *Am J Respir Crit Care Med.* 2003;167(5):695–701

CHAPTER 69

Shock

Nathan E. Thompson, MD, PharmD; Martin Wakeham, MD;
and Timothy E. Corden, MD

Key Points

- Shock is a result of organ dysfunction at the cellular level due to a lack of oxygen delivery, oxygen utilization, or both.

- Symptoms of shock are a result of organs "not getting what they need" to function (as in poor mentation or decreasing urine output) or compensatory mechanisms intended to increase oxygen delivery to "core" vital organs (as in increased heart rate and conservation of core perfusion evidenced by reduced peripheral pulses, prolonged capillary refill, or cool extremities).

- For all types of shock, initial therapy is directed at restoring oxygen delivery to tissues.

- Early goal-directed therapy in septic shock includes immediate fluid resuscitation, vasoactive agent use within the first hour for fluid refractory cases, and prompt use of antibiotics.

- Frequent reassessment of the patient undergoing treatment for shock is essential to appropriately guide ongoing therapy.

Overview

Shock is one of the most common critical conditions encountered in pediatrics and frequently presents for medical care in a community setting. Given the severe consequences of untreated shock, it is imperative that pediatricians, regardless of practice setting, be able to recognize the early signs of shock, initiate therapy, and arrange for decision-making support or transfer to an appropriate care center as needed. Rapid initiation of care can save lives.

Shock is the acute development of a dysfunctional metabolic imbalance at the cellular/tissue level due to an inability to deliver or utilize adequate biochemical substrates to meet metabolic demand resulting in organ dysfunction. Shock can be defined by the simple equation:

Metabolic Demand > Metabolic Substrate Delivery or Utilization

Failure to provide adequate tissue oxygenation is the primary biochemical determinant in the development of a shock state. Figure 69-1 depicts an idealized relationship of oxygen delivery (DO_2) versus tissue utilization or consumption of oxygen ($\dot{V}O_2$). The inflection point on the graph is referred to as the critical delivery point; keeping delivery of oxygen beyond this critical point keeps tissues well supplied and using efficient aerobic metabolism to produce 36 adenosine triphosphate units of energy for each molecule of glucose, with water and CO_2 as amenable by-products. When delivery is compromised, falling below the critical delivery point, tissue metabolism becomes hampered and forced into an anaerobic state, now only producing 2 adenosine triphosphate units for each glucose molecule, with lactic acid as a prominent by-product. As metabolic efficiency is reduced, so is organ function. The symptoms associated with shock are a direct result of organs not getting what is necessary to function properly and the body's attempt to compensate and preserve delivery to vital "core" structures. Mentation is altered (brain), gut motility is compromised (bowel), urine output is decreased (kidneys), extremities become cool, and peripheral pulses become weak as the body tries to shift perfusion to core vital organs. The above simple concept is valuable, as it helps explain where symptoms of shock derive from and forms the basis for treatment aimed at improving tissue DO_2.

The amount of oxygen delivered to tissue is directly related to cardiac output and oxygen content of arterial blood (Cao_2).

$$DO_2 = cardiac\ output \times Cao_2$$

$$Cardiac\ output = Heart\ rate \times Stroke\ volume$$
$$(which\ depends\ on\ preload,\ contractility,\ and\ afterload)$$

$$Cao_2 = (1.34 \times Hemoglobin \times Arterial\ oxygen\ saturation) + (0.003 \times Pao_2)$$

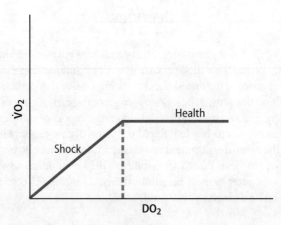

Figure 69-1. Oxygen consumption dependence on oxygen delivery—*idealized*.
Beyond critical delivery point (red line) tissues are content (ie, in a state of health); below inflection, cell metabolic demand is not being met; cells are in state of shock.

Although graphs and formulas can appear complicated, it is helpful to think about these integral concepts in terms of our attempts to help a patient who already manifests compensatory mechanisms. There are two methods to increase or improve DO_2: increase cardiac output or increase Cao_2 (Figure 69-2). We often affect cardiac output by addressing stroke volume via administering fluid to augment preload, increasing contractility by giving patients inotropes, and effectively manipulating afterload. Infants and young children are very efficient at increasing heart rate to augment cardiac output, which is the reason tachycardia is a hallmark symptom of shock in young children. Cao_2 can be increased by assuring adequate oxygenation with supplemental oxygen by mask or, if needed, mechanical ventilator assistance. Transfusion of additional red blood cells also increases Cao_2 via increased hemoglobin. These therapeutic manipulations of cardiac output or Cao_2 are directed at increasing DO_2 to critical tissues in an effort to return a patient to a point beyond the critical delivery inflection (see Figure 56-1) and to restore efficient tissue metabolism and organ function. Understanding these basic concepts is useful as a foundation to focus the appropriate evaluation and management of shock in pediatric patients.

Shock can result from a variety of conditions, but in general the cause can be classified into 1 of 4 categories: hypovolemic, distributive, cardiogenic, and obstructive. Any condition that increases the metabolic demand of tissues, such as fever, pain, or tachypnea, will contribute to the development and severity of the shock state. Regardless of the initial cause, prolonged untreated shock will progress to organ injury and death.

Unlike adults, children are frequently able to maintain an adequate systolic blood pressure (SBP) in the early stages of shock by increasing their heart rate and by increasing systemic vascular resistance (SVR), as demonstrated by delayed capillary refill and cool extremities. However, despite the child's ability

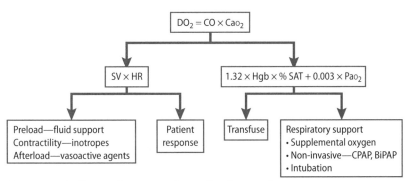

Figure 69-2. Delivery of oxygen: why we do what we do.
How clinical bedside care (red) relates to physiology of increasing oxygen delivery.
Abbreviations: BiPAP, bilevel positive airway pressure; CO, cardiac output; CPAP, continuous positive airway pressure; DO_2, delivery of oxygen; Hgb, hemoglobin; HR, heart rate; SV, stroke volume.

to maintain SBP during these early stages of "compensated" shock, organ perfusion is still impaired with inadequate DO_2 and other biochemical substrates (thus, blood pressure is not incorporated as part of the early diagnostic criteria). Normotensive or compensated shock will ultimately progress to hypotensive/uncompensated shock if left untreated. Hypotension is usually a late finding, typically occurring after other signs of end-organ injury, such as alterations in mental status and oliguria. Often no decrease in SBP will be noted until just prior to circulatory collapse. In summary, untreated shock will progress in the following predictable pattern:

Compensated Shock ⇨ *Organ Injury* ⇨ *Hypotensive Shock*
⇨ *Circulatory Collapse*

Given that blood pressure (BP) values within reference range are age dependent, the following general rule is useful to diagnose hypotension in children (aged 1–10 years):

Hypotension in SBP <70 mm Hg + (age × 2) mm Hg

Shock Phenotypes and Etiologies

The 4 types of shock phenotype and the most common underlying pathophysiology are depicted in Table 69-1. For assessment of severity of dehydration see Table 69-2.

The different types of shock have several overlapping features. Table 69-3 summarizes the potential etiologies of the 4 different categories. A stepwise approach to defining the form of shock is presented in Figure 69-3.

Evaluation

Early recognition of the signs and symptoms of shock allows for rapid, appropriate interventions and the prevention of progressive end-organ injuries. Tachycardia is uniformly an early, but nonspecific, clinical feature regardless of etiology of the shock. Children will augment their heart rate in an effort to increase cardiac output to compensate for diminished perfusion and inadequate metabolic substrate delivery. Other clinical features associated with shock including alterations in SVR, peripheral pulse intensity, and respiratory effort will vary based on underlying cause of the shock state. It is these variations in clinical findings that allow for timely determination of the category of shock and rapid implementation of appropriate medical interventions.

Table 69-1. The 4 Types of Shock Phenotype

Phenotype	Pathophysiology
Hypovolemic shock	• Most common cause of pediatric shock • Any condition that reduces intravascular blood volume to extent that cardiac output and tissue perfusion are impaired (decrease in preload and stroke volume) • Diarrhea/dehydration most common cause of hypovolemic shock worldwide (See Table 69-2 for assessment of severity of dehydration.)
Distributive shock	• Any alteration in the distribution of metabolic substrates to the tissue, usually from abnormalities in vascular tone • Sepsis: altered vascular tone with inappropriate reduction in SVR, causing increased pooling within vascular system (Cytokines cause increased capillary permeability; septic mediators reduce use of oxygen at cell level.) • Anaphylaxis: immunologic mediators (primarily histamine) from basophils and mast cells in response to allergen alter vascular tone • Neurogenic shock due to head or high cervical spinal injury—autonomic impairment and loss of vascular tone
Cardiogenic shock	• Myocardial dysfunction that impairs cardiac output to extent that metabolic demands of tissues cannot be met (primary pump failure) • Decrease in cardiac output most often related to a reduction in cardiac contractility and thus impaired stroke volume
Obstructive shock	• Mechanical obstruction that impairs blood flow to or from the heart • Tension pneumothorax: collapsed lung that increases intrathoracic pressure to impair venous return to the heart • Cardiac tamponade: increases external mechanical pressure on the heart and great vessels, impairing return to the heart • Pulmonary embolism: impairs blood flow leaving the right ventricle and reduces left ventricular stroke volume

Abbreviation: SVR, system vascular resistance.

The ongoing evaluation of shock is largely based on serial physical examination findings and vital sign assessments. Heart rate, BP, intensity and regional differentiation of pulses, capillary refill time, graded temperature of extremities, mental status, and urine output are all indices of cardiac output and compensatory adjustments that can be trended over time, both to determine progression of disease as well as effectiveness of interventions. Laboratory studies can help elucidate the etiology of shock, evaluate end-organ dysfunction, and aid in estimating Cao_2, delivery, and utilization to monitor metabolic biochemical markers, such as lactate acid levels, and to inform on the effect of therapy over

Table 69-2. Clinical Features of Dehydration in Pediatrics

Clinical Feature	Mild (4%–5% Impairment)	Moderate (6%–9% Impairment)	Severe (≥10% Impairment)
General condition	Alert, restless, thirsty	Drowsy, thirsty	Lethargic, limp, cold, mottled
Peripheral pulses	Normal	Rapid, weak	Rapid, weak, or absent
Respirations	Normal	Deep	Deep, rapid
Anterior fontanelle	Normal	Sunken	Very sunken
Eyes	Normal, tearing	Sunken, dry	Very sunken, dry
Mucous membranes	Moist	Dry	Very dry
Skin turgor	Pinch that retracts quickly	Pinch that retracts slowly	Tenting
Capillary refill	<2 s	3–4 s	>4 s
Urine output	Normal	Reduced	Absent

Table 69-3. Shock Phenotypes in Children and Most Common Etiologies Children

Category	Potential Etiologies
Hypovolemia	• Fluid/electrolyte loss: diarrhea, vomiting, diabetic ketoacidosis • Hemorrhage • Burns • Capillary leak syndromes • Sepsis
Distributive	• Sepsis • Anaphylaxis • Neurologic injury: head trauma, cervical spine trauma
Cardiogenic	• Congenital heart disease • Cardiomyopathy • Myocarditis • Arrhythmia • Toxins • Cardiac trauma • Sepsis

Obstructive	• Tension pneumothorax
	• Cardiac tamponade
	• Pulmonary embolism
	• Neonatal ductal-dependent malformations
	   – Critical aortic coarctation
	   – Critical aortic valve stenosis
	   – Hypoplastic left heart syndrome

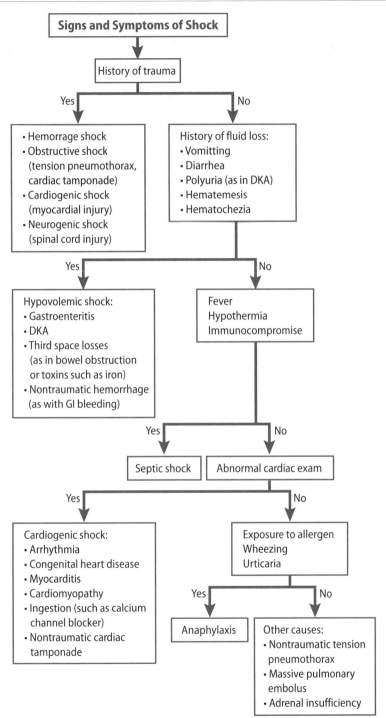

Figure 69-3. Approach to the classification of undifferentiated shock in children.

Abbreviations: DKA, diabetic ketoacidosis; GI, gastrointestinal.

Reproduced with permission from: Waltzman M. Initial evaluation of shock in children. In: UpToDate, Post TW (Ed), UpToDate, Waltham, MA. (Accessed on February 24, 2015.) Copyright © 2015 UpToDate, Inc. For more information visit www.uptodate.com.

time. Laboratory studies ideally obtained for the evaluation of the pediatric patient with shock are summarized in Table 69-4. When cardiogenic shock is suspected, brain natriuretic peptide, a marker for ventricular dilation, and cardiac troponin levels, a marker for ischemic injury, are also recommended as initial aids in diagnosis and for trending treatment response. The frequency of laboratory monitoring should correlate with the severity of illness, with the most critically ill children having studies obtained at shorter intervals.

Table 69-4. Laboratory Studies for Evaluation and Monitoring of Shock

Study	Use To
Arterial blood gas	• Evaluate acidosis. • Evaluate oxygenation. • Evaluate ventilation.
Complete blood count	• Evaluate for anemia. • Assess hydration. • Find evidence of infection. • Evaluate for DIC.
Coagulation studies: prothrombin time, partial thromboplastin time, fibrinogen, and D-dimers	• Evaluate for DIC.
Electrolyte, glucose, BUN, creatinine, liver enzymes, ionized calcium	• Evaluate acidosis. • Calculate anion gap. • Correct electrolyte derangements. • Correct hypoglycemia. • Evaluate liver perfusion. • Evaluate renal function and hydration status.
Lactate	• Evaluate acidosis.
Venous oxygen saturation[a]	• Assess tissue DO_2 and utilization.

Abbreviation: BUN, blood urea nitrogen; DIC, disseminated intravascular coagulation; DO_2, oxygen delivery.
[a] Available if central venous line in place; ideal sample, $Scvo_2$, SVC right atrial junction.

Septic Shock

Septic shock, or shock present in the setting of infection, typically can have features of distributive, hypovolemic, or cardiogenic dysfunction. Although the origin of a septic shock state begins with infection, it is the over-activation of a host's defense system in response to infection that leads to many of the clinical findings. This systemic response is referred to as *systemic inflammatory response syndrome*, or SIRS, a state that can be triggered by multiple conditions such as trauma and burns, as well as infection. Septic shock is also defined as SIRS plus shock in the presence of a clinical setting of proven or suspected infection. A diagnosis of SIRS requires 2 of the following 4 criteria:

- Temperature greater than 38.5°C (101.3°F) or less than 36 °C (96.8°F)
- Leukocytosis or leukopenia for the patient's age or greater than 10% immature neutrophils

- Tachycardia as defined by heart rate greater than 2 standard deviations above the normal range for the patient's age; for children younger than 1 year of age, bradycardia as defined by mean heart rate less than 10th percentile for age
- Tachypnea as defined by respiratory rate greater than 2 standard deviations above the normal range for the patient's age or acute respiratory failure requiring mechanical ventilatory support

The suspicion of infection with the concurrent absence of another potential etiology of SIRS is adequate to meet the diagnostic criteria for sepsis in children.

Management

When rendering assistance to critically ill or injured children, immediate attention to the ABCs is essential and necessary and helps achieve the primary goals of shock management—optimization of DO_2 to the tissue, reduction of overall metabolic demand when possible, and return of end-organ function. Many interventions should be provided as generalized management of shock regardless of underlying etiology. These interventions should be initiated promptly as soon as the shock state is identified. Early, aggressive interventions in children with shock are associated with improved outcomes. Ongoing resuscitation efforts should always be guided by reassessment of patient response to a given therapy.

Supplemental oxygen should be administered to all patients in shock to optimize the Cao_2 of the blood (a potential neonatal exception to the use of supplemental oxygen is the treatment of neonates with presumed ductal dependent conditions; goal arterial saturations of 75%–85% are acceptable, as increasing oxygen levels can promote ductal closure). In children found to be anemic, blood transfusion is important to increase Cao_2 and subsequent delivery. Interventions aimed at reducing metabolic demand, such as antipyretic therapy for the treatment of fever, should be considered. Respiratory support by bilevel positive airway pressure or invasive mechanical ventilation should be provided early in children exhibiting respiratory compromise (Evidence Level II-2). The pharmacologic agents typically used to improve tissue perfusion in the management of shock are summarized in Table 69-5.

Fluid resuscitation is often indicated to augment preload, subsequent stroke volume, and cardiac output, thereby leading to improved tissue perfusion in many forms of shock. Early fluid resuscitation should be performed with crystalloid solutions because of their wide availability and safety (Evidence Level I). Fluid should be administered by the fastest means available to reverse the shock state. Although intravenous fluid pumps or gravity are convenient methods for delivering fluid, these approaches may delay delivery of therapy in an emergent situation. A manual push-pull method with an in-line 3-way

Table 69-5. Pharmacologic Agents Used in the Management of Shock

Medication	Class	Effect	Dosing
Dobutamine	Inotrope	Increases heart rate Increases cardiac contractility	2–20 mcg/kg/min
Dopamine	Inotrope/ vasoconstrictor	Increases heart rate Increases cardiac contractility Increases SVR	5–15 mcg/kg/min (beta-adrenergic effects) ≥15 mcg/kg/min (alpha-adrenergic effects)
Epinephrine	Inotrope/ vasoconstrictor	Increases heart rate Increases cardiac contractility Increases SVR	0.1–1 mcg/kg/min
Norepinephrine	Vasoconstrictor/ inotrope	Primarily increases SVR Minor effect on heart rate and contractility	
Milrinone	Inotrope and vasodilator	Reduces afterload Improves cardiac contractility	0.5–0.75 mcg/kg/min
Vasopressin	Vasoconstrictor- cofactor	Endothelial cofactor to augment catecholamine effects	0.2–2 mU/kg/min

Abbreviation: SVR, systemic vascular resistance.

stopcock allows for rapid controlled fluid administration and will usually permit a 20 mL/kg fluid bolus to be delivered in less than 5 minutes regardless of patient size. Use of pressure bags may also expedite fluid delivery (Evidence Level I). Central vascular access may be needed for monitoring and ongoing resuscitation, but initial resuscitation efforts should not be postponed by waiting for central access to be obtained. If initial attempts at venous access are unsuccessful, intraosseous access should be promptly obtained to begin resuscitation efforts. Reassessment of condition is particularly important during and after fluid administration. Improvement in status is a good indicator for additional volume support, but further deterioration of condition may indicate shock due to cardiac failure in which additional fluid can contribute to worsening myocardial function. Additional defined interventions aimed at specific categories of shock are outlined in the following sections.

Hypovolemic Shock

Hypovolemic shock is potentially the most straightforward type of shock to treat. Therapy is directed at "filling up the tank," increasing preload, stroke volume, and ultimately cardiac output and DO_2 to tissues. Initially managed with the administration of 20 mL/kg of crystalloid fluid boluses (Evidence Level II-2), fluid boluses should be repeated as needed based on clinical response. Boluses should be administered rapidly over 5 to 10 minutes. The etiology of hypovolemia, hemorrhagic versus non-hemorrhagic, should be identified early on to aid in the determination of fluid type used for ongoing resuscitation. When hemorrhage is suspected, such as with trauma cases, it is recommended to use packed red blood cells as the fluid of choice if reassessment indicates continued need for fluid support beyond 40 mL/kg of crystalloid (O negative blood, universal donor as emergent source). In this circumstance, bleeding into potential hidden spaces (ie, pleural space, pelvis, abdomen, and bone) should be considered; surgery may be required to address ongoing hemorrhage. Inotropes are not commonly required for the management of hypovolemic shock except in cases of severe shock. In this case, vasoconstrictor therapy may be required until adequate fluid resuscitation is accomplished and control of ongoing fluid losses is achieved.

Distributive Shock

Septic Shock

The management of septic shock should follow an organized, goal-directed pathway (Figure 69-4). Once evidence of altered perfusion and end-organ dysfunction is recognized, supplemental oxygen is provided; vascular access, obtained. Initially, peripheral access is adequate to begin the resuscitation process. Repeated fluid boluses of 20 mL/kg of isotonic crystalloid should be administered rapidly. It is not uncommon for septic pediatric patients to require large amounts of fluid during resuscitation, even exceeding 100 mL/kg. Fluid support should be guided by reassessment after each bolus is administered; volume support should be halted if the patient develops signs of becoming fluid overloaded: hepatomegaly, cardiac gallop, or evidence of pulmonary edema—rales and increased work of breathing. Positive response to fluid efforts is indicated by resolving shock symptoms and improvement in organ perfusion and function indicated by heart rate trending toward the reference range for the patient's age, improving peripheral pulses, capillary refill less than 2 seconds, increase in urine output, and improving mental status (Evidence Level III). If shock remains unresponsive to fluid therapy after 3 fluid boluses or 60 mL/kg, central venous access is indicated. Presence of a venous central line allows for ongoing fluid support aided by measurement of central venous pressure (CVP) (adult protocols for early goal-directed therapy set a CVP of 8–12 mm Hg as a marker for appropriate volume resuscitation), administration of vasoactive agents, and measurement of central venous oxygen saturation ($Scvo_2$) values. If the child remains ill perfused with ongoing fluid support at or beyond 60 mL/kg, a vasoactive agent should be started within the first hour of therapy; dopamine or epinephrine are reasonable initial choices. If a central line is not available, vasoactive agents can be administered via a peripheral intravenous line with a carrier solution to augment delivery until central access is obtained. The carrier solution, unfortunately, may not lessen the chance of tissue injury from vasoactive drug infiltration; close monitoring of peripheral intravenous line site is advised. Antibiotic therapy should also be initiated promptly, ideally within the first hour of presentation, and laboratory values should be obtained early on to guide the correction of metabolic derangements, especially hypoglycemia and hypocalcemia. Patients with an inadequate response to initial fluid resuscitation and noted anemia (ie, hemoglobin less than 10 g/dL) should be considered candidates to receive packed red blood cell transfusion to increase O_2-carrying capacity and DO_2 to tissues.

Patients with persistent shock state not responding to initial fluid and vasoactive agents (known as catecholamine resistant shock) should receive hydrocortisone if they have risk factors for absolute adrenal insufficiency (ie, purpura fulminans, recent steroid use, history of hypothalamic-pituitary, or adrenal abnormalities) (Evidence Level III). Hydrocortisone should be delivered intermittently every 6 hours or continuously; a dosage range of 1 to 2 mg/m^2/day can be used for stress coverage (please note, sepsis steroid dose, beyond adrenal replacement, remains open). If time permits, a baseline cortisol level and a repeat level following low-dose adrenocorticotropic hormone stimulation test should be obtained. The results of the adrenocorticotropic hormone challenge and baseline cortisol levels can help guide the ongoing need for cortisol support. Cortisol supplement can usually be stopped in patients who are found later to be adrenal competent.

Preferably in a pediatric intensive care unit setting, further therapy including vasoactive agent selection and modification should be guided by the assessment of BP and physical examination findings as a proxy for SVR and Scvo$_2$ values as illustrated in the American College of Critical Care Medicine guidelines adopted by the American Heart Association (see Figure 56-4). In settings where invasive monitoring is not possible, clinicians can continue resuscitation efforts based on physical findings and noninvasive monitoring. Assistance from a tertiary care center to arrange transport and consultation with a pediatric critical care physician should be sought for these cases.

Reasonable samples for Scvo$_2$ can be obtained from a venous central line in the superior vena cava near the right atrium. Scvo$_2$ is used as a measure of oxygen/metabolic delivery to tissues and ability for tissues to use oxygen as an energy substrate. When healthy, having an Scvo$_2$ value of 70% indicates that tissue extraction of oxygen is being satisfied by current delivery of oxygen. When in ill health, values less than 70% indicate DO_2 may be inadequate and in need of augmentation. Values greater than 70% with ongoing clinical and laboratory findings indicative of septic shock may represent an inability of cells to use oxygen, resulting in greater amounts of oxygen leftover after tissue extraction; oxygen now appears on the venous side, raising venous saturation.

In septic children with warm peripheral extremities, bounding pulses, wide pulse pressure, typically low blood pressure and Scvo$_2$ greater than or equal to

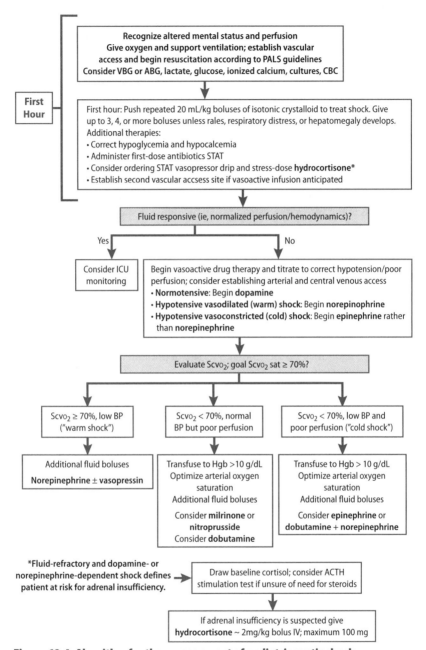

Figure 69-4. Algorithm for the management of pediatric septic shock.

Abbreviations: ABG, arterial blood gas; ACTH, adrenocorticotropic hormone; BP, blood pressure; CBC, complete blood count; Hgb, hemoglobin; ICU, intensive care unit; Scvo$_2$, central venous oxygen saturation; STAT, signal transducer and activator of transcription; VBG, venous blood gas.

From Kleinman ME, Chameides L, Schexnayder SM, et al. Part 14: pediatric advanced life support: 2010 American Heart Association Guidelines for Cardiopulmonary Resuscitation and Emergency Cardiovascular Care. *Circulation*. 2010;122(18 Suppl 3):S876–S908, with permission.

70% ("warm shock," low SVR) management should consist of additional fluid boluses and the initiation of a norepinephrine infusion in an effort to augment SVR and organ perfusion pressure (Evidence Level II-3). Children with poor perfusion, despite a normalized blood pressure and an Scvo$_2$ of less than 70%, may benefit from further titration of an inotropic agent such as dopamine or epinephrine and addition of a vasodilator/afterload-reducing agent such as milrinone or nitroprusside (Evidence Level II-3). Further fluid loading is typically required when starting an afterload-reducing agent. Children with an Scvo$_2$ of less than 70%, low blood pressure, and poor perfusion are considered to have "cold shock." These children can be managed with optimization of fluid support and with either further titration of an epinephrine infusion or the combination of norepinephrine and dobutamine (Evidence Level II-3). Regardless of the vasoactive agent chosen, the infusion should be titrated to achieve an adequate blood pressure and normalizing heart rate for the patient's age, physiologic Scvo$_2$, improved physical examination markers of perfusion such as improving distal pulses, capillary refill time, improved urine output, recovering mentation, and improvement in biochemical markers of perfusion (Evidence Level II-2). Early goal-directed therapy and adherence to guidelines has been shown to reduce the morbidity and mortality associated with pediatric sepsis (Evidence Level II-2). Although much of the above therapy ideally is optimized in a pediatric intensive care unit setting, the importance of early recognition and initial resuscitation at the site of presentation cannot be emphasized enough.

Some cases of pediatric shock are refractory to even meticulous goal-directed therapy. When confronted with refractory patients, clinicians must first review the cause and address all correctable circumstances that may have presented themselves: obstructive lesions (eg, pericardial tamponade, pneumothorax), adrenal insufficiency, untreated occult infection, and unaccounted for blood or fluid ongoing losses. After establishing a true refractory state, the use of mechanical circulatory support should be considered. Transfer to a tertiary pediatric center with extracorporeal membrane oxygenation (ECMO) capabilities for evaluation as an ECMO candidate should be considered (Evidence Level II-2).

Anaphylaxis

The management of anaphylaxis is aimed at inhibiting or counteracting the immunologic mediators causing the shock state. Epinephrine remains the primary pharmacologic agent in the management of anaphylaxis. Epinephrine (1:1000 concentration) is given by intramuscular injection into the anterolateral thigh region at 0.01 mg/kg (0.01 mL/kg) to a maximum dose of approximately 0.3 mg (0.3 mL) or by an auto-injector at the onset of severe allergic symptoms, such as hypotension or angioedema. Children weighing more than 30 kg may receive an adult auto-injector (at 0.3 mg). The pediatric auto-injector (at 0.15 mg) should be administered to children weighing 10 to 30 kg. Epinephrine may be repeated every 5 to 15 minutes if needed, regardless of what device is used for dose administration. Epinephrine should never be given subcutaneously for the management of anaphylaxis. The onset of action may not occur prior to the development of severe symptoms when delivered by the subcutaneous route.

A number of other interventions may be needed in the management of anaphylaxis following the administration of epinephrine. Upper airway edema can be a life-threatening symptom of anaphylaxis. Frequent and repeated airway and respiratory evaluations should be performed. An experienced provider skilled in airway management and endotracheal intubation should be available in case the patient's upper airway obstruction progresses. Crystalloid fluid boluses may be given repeatedly in anaphylactic shock to maintain blood pressure. As with the septic patient, fluid amounts in excess of 60 mL/kg may be required to address hypotension in the anaphylactic patient. Epinephrine (1:10,000 concentration), dopamine, or norepinephrine infusions are indicated for shock refractory to fluid resuscitation. The use of these vasoactive agents is directed at increasing the SVR back to a more physiologic appropriate level to allow for hemodynamic stability. Bronchospasm can be treated with albuterol aerosol therapy or a metered-dose inhaler. Some patients experience an episode of recurrence of anaphylaxis up to 72 hours after the initial event; this should be taken into consideration when making decisions for ongoing monitoring of patients even after apparent resolution of symptoms with therapy. The mediators of anaphylaxis can also be affected by the administration of corticosteroids and antihistamines, but these agents are in addition to and should not take the place of intramuscular epinephrine in acute management.

Neurogenic Shock

Neurogenic shock can be managed with the rapid administration of isotonic crystalloid fluid to fill the circulation void created by the loss of vascular tone. Vasopressors such as norepinephrine can be used in the management of fluid refractory hypotension. Norepinephrine will increase peripheral vascular tone, augmenting SVR, perfusion, and BP.

Cardiogenic Shock

The management of the child in cardiogenic shock is significantly different than managing children with other forms of shock in that aggressive fluid resuscitation may further exacerbate the child's condition. Children presenting with hypotension may require no or only modest fluid resuscitation. Frequently, children with cardiogenic shock have adequate or even excessive preload, and additional administration of fluid is not necessary. If cardiogenic shock is suspected and the clinician feels fluid administration is still indicated, the fluid should be given in a 5 to 10 mL/kg fluid bolus and given slowly along with reassessment of the patient's hemodynamics and respiratory findings for signs of worsening failure. Establishing central venous access early to determine the CVP can aid in fluid status determination. Children with hypotension and elevated filling pressures, detected by examination (eg, hepatomegaly, rales, gallop) or direct central line measurement, may benefit from inotropic support to augment cardiac contractility. Supplemental oxygen to support arterial saturation and DO_2 to the myocardium is an easily delivered first-line inotrope. Epinephrine, dobutamine, and dopamine are all acceptable infusion options for inotropic support in children with cardiogenic shock. Phosphodiesterase inhibitors, such as milrinone, are also useful agents for treating cardiac failure through directly increasing cardiac contractility and reducing afterload on the heart by reducing peripheral vascular resistance. The decision to use milrinone in the setting of cardiac failure and ill perfusion must be made with great care and appropriate monitoring (ie, respiratory and hemodynamic, preferably including an arterial line), as the vasodilator properties of the drug may exceed the inotropic effect on the heart, resulting in further hypotension. The loading dose of milrinone prior to starting an infusion is typically omitted in this setting. Early mechanical respiratory support with bilevel positive airway pressure or intubation may be employed to reduce energy expenditure, improve oxygenation, and reduce cardiac afterload. Close hemodynamic and respiratory monitoring is essential when initiating and optimizing cardiac supportive therapy.

Once the child with cardiogenic shock becomes normotensive, diuretics and vasodilators should be started. Diuretic therapy can unload the myocardium and improve contractility, ultimately helping to reduce pulmonary edema and hepatomegaly due to venous congestion. Afterload reduction with vasodilators can result in increased stroke volume. Phosphodiesterase inhibitors are a good option in this setting; nitroprusside is also an alternative.

Children with cardiogenic shock refractory to medical management may benefit from extracorporeal life support (ECLS) used as a bridge to recovery if the cause of shock is deemed to be reversible. This type of life support includes ECMO or a ventricular-assist device to maintain tissue homeostasis while the underlying etiology of cardiogenic shock is addressed. It is typically only available at a tertiary care center. Arrangements for patient transport should be made early in the disease course if ECLS is required for patient stabilization.

Obstructive Shock

In obstructive shock, early aggressive fluid resuscitation can be lifesaving. Multiple fluid boluses may be required to raise preload to a point that the mechanical pressure from the obstructive lesion can be overcome and cardiac output maintained. Rapid fluid administration can provide the time needed to arrange for more definitive therapies to correct the underlying cause of obstructive shock.

Obstructive shock caused by cardiac tamponade requires pericardiocentesis to relieve the excess fluid or air within the pericardial space. In an emergent situation, pericardiocentesis can be done with the use of anatomic landmarks. Ideally, the procedure is done under direct visualization with echocardiography. A catheter is often left in place to continue to drain the pericardial space following the initial evacuation of fluid.

If a tension pneumothorax is suspected as the etiology of shock, it should be initially managed with immediate needle decompression to the involved pleural space without waiting for a confirmatory chest radiograph if the child is decompensating. This lifesaving procedure can be performed quickly by inserting a 16- to 18-gauge catheter into the pleural space. The catheter should be inserted in the second intercostal space at the mid-clavicular line. If the pleural space is successfully decompressed, a gush of air should be heard or felt. The catheter (with needle removed) should be left in place until a chest tube can subsequently be placed for ongoing decompression.

Neonatal Obstructive Lesions

Neonates can present in shock secondary to left-sided congenital cardiac obstructive malformations after closure of a patent ductus arteriosus. Neonates presenting with findings that raise suspicion for ductal dependent lesions should be placed on a prostaglandin infusion as part of treatment for shock until echocardiography can clearly delineate the cardiac and vascular anatomy. Clinicians should also anticipate the potential need for mechanical ventilation to aid the distressed infant and address the possibility of prostaglandin induced apnea. Restoration of a ductal-flow murmur and increased lower body perfusion, including improved femoral pulses and increased urine output, are indicators of restored ductal flow. Fluid administration, correction of hypocalcemia, and inotropic support are also frequently necessary therapies in this setting.

Acknowledgement: The authors thank Ms Mary Cziner, Program Coordinator, Injury Research Center, Medical College of Wisconsin, for her thoughtful suggestions and editing of the chapter.

Suggested Reading

Brierley J, Carcillo JA, Choong K, et al. Clinical practice parameters for hemodynamic support of pediatric and neonatal septic shock: 2007 update form the American College of Critical Care Medicine. *Crit Care Med.* 2009;37(2):666–688

Carcillo JA, Davis AL, Zaritsky A. Role of early fluid resuscitation in pediatric septic shock. *JAMA.* 1991;266(9):1242–1245

Gorelick MH, Shaw KN, Murphy KO. Validity and reliability of clinical signs in the diagnosis of dehydration in children. *Pediatrics.* 1997;99(5):E6

Han YY, Carcillo JA, Dragotta MA, et al. Early reversal of pediatric-neonatal septic shock by community physicians is associated with improved outcome. *Pediatrics.* 2003;112(4):793–799

Kleinman ME, Chameides L, Schexnayder SM, et al. Part 14: pediatric advanced life support: 2010 American Heart Association Guidelines for Cardiopulmonary Resuscitation and Emergency Cardiovascular Care. *Circulation.* 2010;122(18 Suppl 3):S876–S908

Lane RD, Bolte RG. Pediatric anaphylaxis. *Pediatr Emerg Care*. 2007;23(1):49–56

Stoner MJ, Goodman DG, Cohen DM, Fernandez SA, Hall MW. Rapid fluid resuscitation in pediatrics: testing the American College of Critical Care Medicine guideline. *Ann Emerg Med*. 2007;50(5):601–607

Turner DA, Cheifetz IM. Shock. In: Kliegman RM, Stanton BF, Gemell JW, et al, eds. *Nelson Textbook of Pediatrics*. 19th ed. Philadelphia, PA: Saunders/Elsevier; 2011:305–314

CHAPTER 70

Snakebite

Marlie Dulaurier, MD, and Mary Jo Bowman, MD

Key Points

- Snake venom envenomation is a medical emergency. Envenomation is complex and not only affects the local bite site but can also involve multiple organ systems.

- Diagnosis and management are based on clinical signs and symptoms of envenomation, as well as identification of the snake.

- Good supportive care and initial management (with special attention to airway, breathing, and circulation) reduce subsequent morbidity and mortality.

- The efficacy of treatment is enhanced by prompt administration of sufficient quantities of the appropriate neutralizing antivenin in conjunction with aggressive supportive care in the intensive care unit.

Overview

Most snakebites are harmless and usually occur from nonpoisonous snakes. North America has 25 species of poisonous snakes, and most poisonous bites are delivered by pit vipers, which include rattlesnakes, moccasins, cotton mouths, and copperheads. Approximately 2,500 children each year experience a poisonous snakebite, and because of smaller limb size and less subcutaneous tissue, children usually receive a larger dose of venom per kilogram. As a result, the clinical course for children who receive poisonous snakebites is often more severe than the course of adults. Fortunately, death is rare.

Definitions

Classification of Poisonous Snakes

- In North America, the two families of venomous snakes are Elapidae and Viperidae (with subfamily Crotalidae).
- The subfamily Crotalidae (pit vipers) includes rattlesnakes (*Crotalus* and *Sistrurus* species), cottonmouths (*Agkistrodon* species), and copperheads (*Agkistrodon* species). The only native venomous snake in the family Elapidae is the coral snake.

- Coral snakes are relatively shy creatures, and bites are uncommon, accounting for less than 1% of venomous snakebites in the United States.

Identification of Poisonous Snakes

The characteristic features of the poisonous snakes include a triangular-shaped head, nostril heat-sensing pits, elliptical pupils, fangs, and subcaudal plates arranged in a single row (Figure 70-1).

The Crotalidae family (pit vipers) can be found in all regions of the country, with different species having varying habitats. Cottonmouths reside near swamps or rivers, copperheads are found in aquatic and dry environments, and rattlesnakes prefer dry grasslands and rocky hillsides.

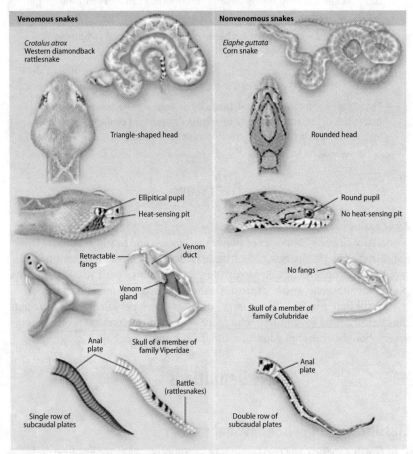

Figure 70-1. Comparison of venomous snakes (pit vipers) and nonvenomous snakes in the United States.

From Gold BS, Dart RC, Barish RA. Bites of venomous snakes. *N Engl J Med.* 2002;347(5):347–358, with permission.

All coral snakes belong to the family Elapidae, the Eastern coral snake (*Micrurus fulvius*) and the Texas coral snake (*Micrurus tener*) being the most common in the United States. The coral snake species in the United States are brightly colored with red, yellow, and black rings. The nonvenomous king snakes share the same colors but not in the same order. A common mnemonic to recall the order of bands is "red on yellow, kill a fellow; red on black, venom lack."

Cobras, mambas, and kraits are also members of the family Elapidae but are not indigenous to North America. However, private collectors and zoos are keeping these species, thus making bites by nonindigenous species more common.

Clinical Features

The most important factors needed in making a definitive diagnosis of snake venom poisoning are positive identification of the snake and clinical signs and symptoms of envenomation. It is critical to distinguish the bite from those caused by nonvenomous snakes, other animals, or objects.

The child or guardian may be able to identify the snake. If the child or guardian is unable to provide a positive identification of the offending snake, clinicians must rely solely on signs and symptoms of envenomation to make the diagnosis (Table 70-1). Approximately 25% of all pit viper bites and 50% of all coral snakebites in the United States do not result in envenomation and are considered "dry" bites.

Table 70-1. Characteristics of Elapidae and Crotalidae Bites

	Elapidae	Viperidae, Subfamily Crotalidae
Members	Coral snakes	Pit vipers (ie, rattlesnakes, cottonmouths, copperheads [moccasins])
Venom type	Neurotoxic	Cytotoxic
Signs	Bite is minimally painful.	Bite is painful immediately.
Time frame	Signs/symptoms of envenomation might be delayed up to 12 h.	Pain and swelling occur in minutes (usually within 30 to 60 min).
Symptoms	Mild drowsiness, cranial nerve palsies (manifested by conditions such as ptosis, diplopia, dysarthria, and dysphagia), weakness, paresthesia, dyspnea, seizures, or a combination thereof Can progress rapidly	At bite site: edema and ecchymosis; bullae development and tissue necrosis in severe cases Systemic: nausea, vomiting, diaphoresis, weakness, tingling around face, and muscle fasciculations
Causes of death	Respiratory failure (from diaphragmatic paralysis)	Hemorrhagic shock, coagulopathy, ARDS, and renal failure

Abbreviation: ARDS, acute respiratory distress syndrome.

Crotalidae Envenomation

Signs and symptoms of Crotalidae envenomation include the presence of fang marks, pain, edema, erythema, or ecchymosis of the bite site and adjacent tissues. Localized burning pain and early progressive edema around the bite site are common and are usually evident within 5 minutes following envenomation. Most pit viper envenomations are painful. Within 10 minutes, edema (proximal and distal to the bite site) develops. Edema is rarely delayed more than 30 minutes following envenomation, but in a few cases it may be delayed up to a few hours. Bullae may also be noted and can be serous or hemorrhagic in nature. Ecchymosis usually appears later in the course, approximately 3 to 6 hours after envenomation.

Systemic manifestations usually include nausea, vomiting, perioral paresthesia, tingling of the fingertips and toes, fasciculations, lethargy, and weakness. Patients may show concern over a rubbery, minty, or metallic taste. More severe systemic effects include altered mental status, severe tachycardia, tachypnea, respiratory distress, hypovolemic shock, metabolic acidosis, and hypotension. Coagulopathy is a frequent occurrence following bites by rattlesnakes.

Elapidae Envenomation

Snakes in the Elapidae family primarily produce a neurotoxic venom. This venom has a curare-like effect by blocking neurotransmission at the neuromuscular junction. Although the bite is minimally painful (the venom is not cytotoxic), lack of immediate symptoms does not mean that envenomation has not occurred. Clinicians must be perceptive in looking for signs of neurovascular dysfunction as well as impending respiratory failure from diaphragmatic dysfunction. Severe signs and symptoms can include hypersalivation, cyanosis, trismus, respiratory distress, pharyngeal spasm, tachycardia, and hypotension. These symptoms can progress rapidly leading to respiratory failure, cardiovascular collapse, and death.

Evaluation

It is important that clinicians evaluate the severity of envenomation. Multiple factors influence the severity of envenomation, including the species and size of the snake, the amount and toxicity of the venom injected, the location of the bite, first aid treatments performed, timing of definitive treatment, comorbid conditions, and the patient's unique susceptibility to the venom.

In recent years, first aid measures for snakebites have been radically revised to exclude methods that were found to worsen a patient's condition, such as tight (arterial) tourniquets, aggressive wound incisions, and ice (Evidence Level II-1).

The focus of first responders should be on ABCs. It is important to support airway and breathing, administer oxygen as needed, establish intravenous access, reduce and prevent excessive activity (ambulation should be refrained from as much as possible), and immobilize the bitten extremity.

Initial laboratory evaluation of the patient should include complete blood count with differential, coagulation studies (specifically, prothrombin time, activated partial thromboplastin time, and international normalized ratio), fibrinogen and split products, type and screen, serum chemistries, creatinine phosphokinase level, and urinalysis looking for myoglobinuria. Arterial blood gas or lactate level should be obtained in patients with systemic symptoms.

Management

The most important tenets of treatment of persons bitten by venomous snakes are aggressive supportive care and administration of antivenin (Figure 70-2). The onset of signs and symptoms can be delayed up to several hours; therefore, observation is vital to determine further care. First establish airway, breathing, and circulation; then obtain a quick history, which should include the time of the bite, events occurring around that, a description of the snake, first aid or home treatments used, past medical history, and allergies (specifically to horse or sheep products). The physical examination should be complete, with special attention paid to the cardiovascular, pulmonary, and neurologic systems. The bite site should be examined for bite marks or scratches. It is important to obtain circumferential measurements above and below the bite site, initially and then every 15 to 30 minutes thereafter. As swelling progresses, each new area should be time marked to aid in guiding the need for additional antivenin administration.

The need for antivenin in patients of pit viper bites is determined by envenomation severity (Table 70-2, Evidence Level II-1). Initially, mild presentations may progress to moderate or even severe presentations over the course of several hours. Determining envenomation severity is therefore a dynamic process.

Antivenin administration is given without regard to patient size and is based solely on degree of envenomation.

The current antivenin, approved by the US Food and Drug Administration in 2000 (CroFab, Savage), is a monovalent immunoglobulin fragment derived from sheep but purified to avoid other antigenic proteins. CroFab is made specifically from venom of Crotalidae family. No antivenin is currently available for Elapidae (coral snake) bites.

Even without antivenin available, most patients can be treated with sound supportive care. If airway management and respiratory support are adequate, excellent outcome is usually seen, although the course may be prolonged.

Snakes do not harbor *Clostridium tetani* in their mouths, but their bites may carry other bacteria, especially gram-negative species. Tetanus prophylaxis is recommended if the patient is not immunized (Evidence Level III).

Emergency Department and Hospital Management of Pit Viper Snakebite
Includes: Rattlesnakes, Copperheads, and Cottonmouths (Water Moccasins)

1   Assess Patient
- Mark leading edge of swelling and tenderness every 15–30 minutes
- Immobilize and elevate extremity
- Treat pain (IV opioids preferred)
- Obtain initial lab studies (protime, Hgb, platelets, fibrinogen)
- Update tetanus
- Contact poison control center (1-800-222-1222)

2   Check for Signs of Envenomation
- Swelling, tenderness, redness, ecchymosis, or blebs at the bite site, *or*
- Elevated protime; decreased fibrinogen or platelets, *or*
- Systemic signs, such as hypotension, bleeding beyond the puncture site, refractory vomiting, diarrhea, angioedema, neurotoxicity

None →

9   Apparent Dry Bite/No Bite
- Do not administer antivenom
- Observe patient ≥ 8 hours
- Repeat labs prior to discharge
- *If patient develops signs of envenomation, return to box 2*

↓ Present

3   Check for Indications for Antivenom
- Swelling that is more than minimal and that is progressing, *or*
- Elevated protime; decreased fibrinogen or platelets, *or*
- Any systemic signs

None →

10   Apparent Minor Envenomation
- Do not administer antivenom
- Observe patient 12–24 hours
- Repeat labs at 4–6 hours and prior to discharge
- *If patient develops progression of any signs of envenomation, return to box 3*

↓ Present

4   Administer Antivenom
- Establish IV access and give IV fluids
- Pediatric antivenom dose = adult dose
- Mix 4–6 vials of crotaine Fab antivenom (CroFab®) in 250 ml NS and infuse IV over 1 hour
  - For patients in shock or with serious active bleeding
    - Increase initial dose of antivenom to 8–12 vials
    - Call physician expert (see box 12)
- Initiate first dose of antivenom in ED or ICU
  - For suspected adverse reaction: hold infusion, treat accordingly, and call physician-expert
- Re-examine patient for treatment response within 1 hour of completion of antivenom infusion

5   Determine if Initial Control of Envenomation Has Been Achieved
- Swelling and tenderness not progressing
- Protime, fibrinogen, and platelets normal or clearly improving
- Clinically stable (not hypotensive, etc.)
- Neurotoxicity resolved or clearly improving

No →

11   Repeat Antivenom Until Inital Control is Achieved
- *If initial control is not achieved after 2 doses of antivenom, call physician expert (see box 12).*

↓ Yes

6   Monitor Patient
- Perform serial examinations
- Maintenance antivenom therapy may be indicated
  - **Read Box 13 (Maintenance antivenom therapy)**
- Observe patient 18–24 hours after initial control for progression of any venom effect
- Follow-up labs 6–12 hours after initial control and prior to discharge
- *If patient develops new or worsening signs of envenomation, administer additional antivenom per box 4*

7   Determine if Patient Meets Discharge Criteria
- No progression of any venom effect during the specified observation period
- No unfavorable laboratory trends in protime, fibrinogen, or platelets

↓ Yes

8   See Post-Discharge Planning (box 14)

Figure 70-2. Emergency department and hospital management of pit viper snakebite (includes rattlesnakes, copperheads, and cottonmouths [water moccasins]).

12 When to Call a Physician-Expert
Direct consultation with a physician-expert is recommended in certain high-risk clinical situations:
- **Life-threatening envenomation**
  Shock
  Serious active bleeding
  Facial or airway swelling
- **Hard to control envenomation**
  Envenomation that requires more than 2 doses of antivenom for initial control
- **Recurrence or delayed-onset of venom effects**
  Worsening swelling or abnormal labs (protime, fibrinogen, platelets, or hemoglobin) on follow-up visits
- **Allergic reactions to antivenom**
- **If transfusion is considered**
- **Uncommon clinical situations**
  Bites to the head and neck
  Rhabdomyolysis
  Suspected compartment syndrome
  Venom-induced hives and angioedema
- **Complicated wound issues**
If no local expert is available, a physician-expert can be reached through a certified poison center (1-800-222-1222) or the antivenom manufacturer's line (1-877-377-3784).

13 Maintenance Antivenom Therapy
- Maintenance therapy is additional antivenom given after initial control to prevent recurrence of limb swelling
  - Maintenance therapy is 2 vials of antivenom Q6H × 3 (given 6, 12, and 18 hours after initial control)
- Maintenance therapy may not be indicated in certain situations, such as
  - Minor envenomations
  - Facilities where close observation by a physician-expert is available.
- Follow local protocol or contact a poison center or physician-expert for advice.

14 Post-Discharge Planning
- Instruct patient to return for
  - Worsening swelling that is not relieved by elevation
  - Abnormal bleeding (gums, easy bruising, melena, etc.)
- Instruct patient where to seek care if symptoms of serum sickness (fever, rash, muscle/joint pains) develop
- Bleeding precautions (no contact sports, elective surgery or dental work, etc.) for 2 weeks in patients with
  - Rattlesnake envenomation
  - Abnormal protime, fibrinogen, or platelet count at any time
- Follow-up visits:
  - Antivenom not given:
    - PRN only
  - Antivenom given:
    - Copperhead victims: PRN only
    - Other snakes: follow up with labs (protime, fibrinogen, platelets, hemoglobin) twice (2–3 days and 5–7 days), then PRN

15 Treatments to Avoid in Pit Viper Snakebite
- Cutting and/or suctioning of the wound
- Ice
- NSAIDs
- Prophylactic antibiotics
- Prophylactic fasciotomy
- Routine use of blood products
- Shock therapy (electricity)
- Steroids (except for allergic phenomena)
- Tourniquets

16 Notes
- **All treatment recommendations in this algorithm refer to crotalidae polyvalent immune Fab (ovine) (CroFab®).**
- This worksheet represents general advice from a panel of US snakebite experts convened in May, 2010. No algorithm can anticipate all clinical situations. Other valid approaches exist, and deviations from this worksheet based on individual patient needs, local resources, local treatment guidelines, and patient preferences are expected. **This document is not intended to represent a standard of care.** For more information, please see the accompanying manuscript, available at www.biomedcentral.com.

Figure 70-2 *(cont)*

Abbreviations: ED, emergency department; Hgb, hemoglobin; ICU, intensive care unit; IV, intravenous; lab, laboratory; NS, normal saline; NSAID, nonsteroidal anti-inflammatory drug; PRN, as needed.

From Lavonas, Ruha AM, Banner W, et al. Unified treatment algorithm for the management of crotaline snakebite in the United States: results of an evidence-informed consensus workshop. *BMC Emerg Med.* 2011;11:2.

Table 70-2. Grading Scale for Severity of Snake Bites

Degree of Envenomation	Presentation	Treatment
0. None	Punctures or abrasions; some pain or tenderness at the bite	Local wound care, no antivenin
I. Mild	Pain, tenderness, edema at the bite; perioral paresthesia may be present	If antivenin is necessary, administer about 5 vials.[a]
II. Moderate	Pain, tenderness, erythema, edema beyond the area adjacent to the bite; often, systemic manifestations and mild coagulopathy	Administration of 5 to 15 vials of antivenin may be necessary.
III. Severe	Intense pain and swelling of entire extremity, often with severe systemic signs and symptoms; coagulopathy	Administer at least 15 to 20 vials of antivenin.
IV. Life-threatening	Marked abnormal signs and symptoms; severe coagulopathy	Administer at least 25 vials of antivenin.

[a] Because of their less potent venom, grade-I copperhead bites are usually not treated with antivenin.

From Juckett G, Hancox JG. Venomous snakebites in the United States: management review and update. *Am Fam Physician*. 2002;65(7):1367–1375, with permission.

Admission to the hospital is routine for most envenomation cases. For dry pit viper bites, observation in the emergency department for at least 8 to 10 hours is recommended. Coral snakebites should be observed for a minimum of 24 hours. Patients with severe envenomation will likely need care in the intensive care unit for invasive monitoring and airway protection.

Complications

Local wound complications may include infection. Severe rattlesnake envenomations can be associated with increased compartment pressures. Compartment syndrome is the most frequent complication of pit viper snakebite. The reaction to envenomation, such as extensive swelling, tense feeling, extreme tenderness or pain, and decreased sensation, might mimic true compartment syndrome. If there is concern for compartment syndrome, diagnosis requires objective evidence of compartment pressure elevations greater than 30 mm Hg measured with a Stryker handheld digital monitor (Stryker Corporation, Kalamazoo, Michigan).

If compartment pressures are found to be truly elevated, the first treatment should be administration of additional antivenin. This intervention should effectively reduce compartment pressures. After administration of antivenin, observation should occur for up to 4 hours with repeat of compartment pressures. If pressures are still elevated or the patient has vascular compromise, surgical intervention might be required. Surgical intervention primarily uses fasciotomy as a means of lowering elevated compartment pressure (Evidence Level III). Experts debate as to the efficacy of fasciotomy, as it does not prevent the progression of the envenomation, treat systemic symptoms, or prevent the need for additional antivenin. However, it is still considered to be routine practice in some parts of the United States. Evidence regarding the efficacy of surgical fasciotomy is sparse. Fasciotomy can make the course of treatment and recovery longer and is associated with multiple complications, including but not limited to nerve damage, disfiguring scars, contractures, and loss of limb function.

Antivenin can be lifesaving; however, it also may lead to immediate hypersensitivity (anaphylaxis, type I) and delayed hypersensitivity (serum sickness, type III) reactions and must be used with caution. Serum sickness usually occurs 7 to 21 days following treatment with antivenin. Signs and symptoms of serum sickness include fever, rash, arthralgias, urticaria, and lymphadenopathy. Treatment involves a tapering course of prednisone at 2 mg/kg/day (maximum dose of 60 mg/day) over a 7- to 10-day period (Evidence Level I).

Suggested Reading

Cheng AC, Seifert SA. Evaluation and management of coral snakebites. *UpToDate.* Waltham, MA: UpToDate; 2015

Cheng AC, Seifert SA. Management of Crotalinae (rattlesnake, water moccasin [cottonmouth], or copperhead) bites in the United States. *UpToDate.* Waltham, MA: UpToDate; 2014

Correa JA, Fallon SC, Cruz AT, et al. Management of pediatric snake bites: are we doing too much? *J Ped Surg.* 2014;49(6):1009–1015

Gold BS, Dart RC, Barish RA. Bites of venomous snakes. *N Engl J Med.* 2002;347(5): 347–356

Sasaki J, Khalil PA, Chegondi M. Coral snake bites and envenomation in children: a case series. *Pediatr Emerg Care.* 2014;30(4):262–265

Warrell DA. Venomous bites, stings, and poisoning. *Infect Dis Clin North Am.* 2012;26(2):207–223

CHAPTER 71

Trauma and Assessment of Injury

Laurie H. Johnson, MD

Key Points

- Trauma is a disease process with predictable patterns of injury; those injuries which are mild are easily treated in an outpatient setting.

- The initial assessment of the injured child includes a thorough and systematic examination to determine the location and extent of all possible injuries; the Advanced Trauma Life Support approach consists of a primary survey to identify any life-threatening injuries, stabilize the patient, and perform a complete examination called the secondary survey to identify all other injuries.

- Traumatic injuries are classified according to severity (ie, mild, moderate, or severe), type (ie, blunt or penetrating), and location.

- Many injuries require subspecialty consultation or follow-up. A thorough history and physical examination must be performed to identify and properly treat all injuries.

- Anticipatory guidance and injury prevention measures should be pursued whenever possible to most effectively decrease the burden of traumatic injuries in children.

Overview

Unintentional injuries result in a large percentage of pediatric morbidity and mortality. Injury mechanisms include but are not limited to falls, motor vehicle crashes, burns, pedestrians struck by motor vehicles, and recreational activities. The initial assessment of an injured child includes a thorough and systematic examination to determine the location and extent of all possible injuries. This allows the clinician to provide timely and appropriate treatment, as well as to accurately disposition the child for discharge to home, admission, or transfer to another facility for definitive care if necessary.

Injuries are classified according to severity, type, and location. Injuries are described as mild, moderate, or severe depending on the extent of the injury and can be either blunt or penetrating. The terms *multiple* or *local* refer to the number of body regions affected. For the purposes of evaluation of children by nonsurgically trained clinicians, multiple trauma can be defined as that which involves more than one area of the body (such as a facial laceration with an accompanying forearm fracture after a fall from a playground swing). Mild or minor injuries include local or multiple superficial lacerations, abrasions, contusions, sprains, and fractures from mechanisms that are sustained at low velocity with no or minimal force (such as a fall from standing height when walking). Minor injuries may also accompany more serious injuries, such as splenic laceration from a bicycle crash in which the patient sustains obvious abrasions and contusions to the face and extremities in addition to intra-abdominal injury from the handlebar striking the abdomen (Box 71-1).

Box 71-1. Classification/Characteristics of Trauma by Severity

Mild
History – Minimal force
Vital Signs – Normal
Local Findings – Superficial
Laboratory/Other Studies – Few to none

Moderate
History – Significant force
Vital Signs – Normal
Local Findings – Suspicious for internal injuries
Laboratory/Other Studies – Intermediate

Severe
History – Critical force
Vital Signs – Abnormal
Local Findings – Indicative of internal injuries
Laboratory/Other Studies – Many

Multiple challenges complicate the care of pediatric trauma patients. Young children have many unique characteristics which differentiate them from teenagers and adults, including differences in injury patterns as well as physiology. Because the developing pediatric skeleton is incompletely calcified and has multiple active growth centers, pediatric patients may sustain specific fractures that are initially occult or difficult to appreciate and may experience significant internal injuries without associated fractures. Children have a large surface-area-to-body-mass ratio, which can result in rapid heat loss even in ambient temperatures. The proportionally larger head and smaller body volume of the younger pediatric patient results in greater force from a traumatic mechanism being applied to underlying structures and organs than in the adult, often leading to multiple traumatic injuries in the child. Accordingly, younger pediatric patients who are not "adult-sized" have different patterns of injury than those seen in adults and "adult-sized" teens for a particular traumatic mechanism (Table 71-1).

Table 71-1. Injury Patterns Secondary to Common Mechanisms of Injury

Mechanism of Injury	Injury Pattern
Pedestrian struck	Low speed: lower extremity fractures
	High speed: multiple trauma, head/neck injuries, lower extremity fractures
Motor vehicle crash occupant	Restrained: chest/abdomen injuries, lower spine fractures
	Unrestrained: multiple trauma, head/neck/face injuries
Fall from a height	Low: upper extremity fractures
	Medium: head/neck injuries, upper/lower extremity fractures
	High: multiple trauma, head/neck injuries, upper/lower extremity fractures
Fall from a bicycle	Helmet worn: upper extremity fractures
	No helmet worn: head/neck/face injuries, upper extremity fractures
	Striking handlebar: intra-abdominal injuries

Modified from American College of Surgeons Committee on Trauma. *ATLS: Advanced Trauma Life Support for Doctors.* 8th ed. Chicago, IL: American College of Surgeons; 2008:227, with permission.

Also, young and nonverbal children may be difficult to accurately assess, as their communication skills are limited and they are often frightened by the traumatic event as well as efforts of the health care professionals who are trying to assist them. Optimization of parental presence, child life specialists, and distraction techniques can be of great value during the examination to facilitate determination of exact injuries in the young or anxious patient.

Initial Evaluation

A patient who has experienced a traumatic mechanism should be triaged according to the professional's initial impression of the type and extent of injury. Assessment of the pediatric trauma patient presenting to an emergency department follows the systematic approach of Advanced Trauma Life Support (ATLS) developed by the American College of Surgeons. Patients who seem to have only mild or minor local trauma may be triaged for further evaluation by a single clinician according to standard triage protocols. Those who have multiple trauma or have the possibility of moderate or severe trauma are best evaluated according to a tiered system of trauma activations. Activation criteria exist based on physiologic parameters, with the most critically injured patients receiving the highest level of activation, those with moderate injuries receiving mid-level activation, and those with milder injuries receiving lowest level activation. The size and exact composition of the team may differ among institutions. In hospitals designated as trauma centers, those in attendance at a trauma evaluation include one or more of the following: emergency medicine physician, surgeon, nurse, respiratory therapist, paramedic or patient care assistant, social services professional, pastoral care.

The goals of the ATLS systematic approach are to methodically complete a primary survey to identify any life-threatening injuries, stabilize the patient, reassess the components of the primary survey, and perform a more complete examination called the secondary survey to identify all other injuries (Table 71-2). The primary survey can be remembered by the first 5 letters of the alphabet (ABCDE) to assess the patient's airway (A), breathing (B), circulation (C), and disability (D) or level of consciousness and to expose (E) the patient. Once a deficiency has been identified, it should be addressed prior to advancing to the next letter of the mnemonic; for instance, if the patient does not have a secure airway, definitive steps must be made toward securing the airway prior to proceeding to the assessment of breathing.

Table 71-2. Advanced Trauma Life Support Systematic Approach

1.	• Primary survey ○ A—airway ○ B—breathing ○ C—circulation ○ D—disability or level of consciousness ○ E—expose patient for examination • Obtain concise history
2.	• Secondary survey ○ Thorough head-to-toe examination to identify all other injuries • Obtain more detailed history
3.	• Pertinent laboratory studies, radiographs, consultations

An initial, concise history should also be obtained, which can be remembered using the AMPLE mnemonic (Box 71-2). Historical details can be potentially obtained from the patient, the parent or family member, any bystanders or witnesses to the incident, and emergency medical services crew. A more thorough history can be obtained as the examination proceeds. The secondary survey begins once the primary survey has been successfully completed and is a thorough, head-to-toe physical examination in which the patient's entire body is examined for injury and pertinent laboratory studies, radiologic studies, and subspecialist consults are obtained as appropriate.

During the initial assessment of the injured patient, the ABCDE mnemonic can be quickly and easily applied in the mild or moderately injured patient. Observations of healthy respiratory effort and the ability of the patient to verbally respond (for a young patient to cry and the older patient to answer

Box 71-2. AMPLE Mnemonic (Emergency Scene)

A	Allergies
M	Medications
P	Past medical history
L	Last oral intake
E	Events leading up to the injury or illness

basic questions) are reassuring that the airway is intact and breathing is unlabored. This is confirmed by examination of a midline trachea with auscultation of breath sounds bilaterally, and maintenance of cervical spine immobilization is necessary until the neck can be more closely examined. To maintain proper neck immobilization in a patient with altered mental status while ensuring a patent airway, the airway should be opened using the chin-lift or jaw-thrust maneuvers. Circulation is then evaluated by palpating and noting the quality of the peripheral and central pulses.

The method of defining a trauma patient's disability or level of consciousness is by assessing and assigning a Glasgow Coma Scale (GCS) score (Table 71-3; a modified GCS for infants and young children can be found in Chapter 72, Table 72-3). This does not replace a complete neurologic exam that should be performed during the secondary survey but provides a rapid baseline in documenting normal mental status, which can be rapidly repeated and monitored for trends if the patient's status should change. Any patient who has respiratory symptoms/concerns or any alteration of mental status should have supplemental oxygen provided. A patient with bony complaints of the spine should remain lying supine with cervical spine immobilization until a complete evaluation can be performed. For this patient, evaluation of the patient's back or transfer of the patient from one location to another should occur via the "logroll" technique. In this technique, neutral anatomic spine alignment is maintained: one person maintains cervical spine immobilization while at least two other individuals control the body at the shoulders, hips, and extremities to roll the patient onto his side. Exposure of the patient occurs by removing garments as quickly as possible, being mindful of maintaining normothermia. Care should be taken to note in what environment the injury or injuries occurred to initiate appropriate treatment. For example, a motor vehicle crash into a water-filled ditch in winter might cause concern for hypothermia or aspiration, while the explosion of an aerosol can within a confined space would cause concern for possible inhalation injury in addition to any obvious cutaneous injuries.

Vital signs should be carefully monitored, and tachycardia (unrelated to age-appropriate crying), tachypnea, or hypotension should be addressed. If a patient does not have a reassuring primary survey, immediate actions should be taken for the patient to be transported by emergency medical services to the

Table 71-3. Glasgow Coma Scale[a]

	1	2	3	4	5	6
Eyes	Does not open eyes	Opens eyes in response to painful stimuli	Opens eyes in response to voice	Opens eyes spontane-ously	N/A	N/A
Verbal	Makes no sounds	Incompre-hensible sounds	Utters inappropri-ate words	Confused, disoriented	Oriented, converses normally	N/A
Motor	Makes no movements	Extension to painful (decer-ebrate response)	Abnormal flexion to painful stimuli (de-corticate response)	Flexion/withdrawal to painful stimuli	Local-izes painful stimuli	Obeys com-mands

[a] The lowest possible score (the sum) is 3 (deep coma or death), while the highest is 15 (fully awake and oriented). Derived from Teasdale G, Jennett B. Assessment of coma and impaired consciousness: a practical scale. *Lancet.* 1974;2:81–84.

nearest emergency department or trauma center. In an emergency department setting, life-threatening conditions are identified and treated in the primary survey. These include but are not limited to tension pneumothorax, penetrating chest wound, cardiac tamponade, flail chest with open pneumothorax, respiratory distress or difficulty, decreased or absent pulses, hemorrhage, a GCS of less than 8, or a rapidly deteriorating GCS. The details of these conditions and the appropriate treatments are beyond the scope of this chapter, but these represent important patient conditions that should be identified and treated as soon as possible.

Patients presenting to an outpatient setting should receive a similar evaluation on a smaller, less formal scale; the patient who is breathing spontaneously, has intact mental status that is appropriate for age, normal peripheral pulses, and no obvious moderate or severe injuries can then be carefully examined for all possible injuries. Treatments and any referrals to a subspecialist or emergency department are then based on the injuries identified. Patients with problems with airway/breathing/circulation, abnormal vital signs, or altered mental status or clinician concern for moderate or serious injuries due to mechanisms with a history of significant force should be transported by emergency medical services to an emergency department for prompt evaluation.

Detailed Evaluation and Basic Management

The secondary survey is the complete head-to-toe examination of the patient, the components of which can be utilized in any setting for a thorough examination of potential injuries. Several tenets of general management can be applied. Initial concern for intracranial or visceral injuries or any extensive, vigorously bleeding, or complicated wounds should initiate emergent transfer to an emergency department for further evaluation and definitive management. If a patient requires subspecialty consultation or transfer for further evaluation, the patient should remain *nil per os,* or "NPO," in the event of possible procedural sedation or pending operation. Obvious superficial wounds should be irrigated and dressed with clean bandages until definitive treatment occurs. Orthopedic injuries should be splinted in a position where pulses are intact and radiographs (multiple views) should be obtained. Details of wound and fracture management are discussed later in the chapter.

The entire head and neck should be visually examined for lacerations, abrasions, and puncture wounds. Puncture wounds of the skull should be carefully inspected, and any concern for violation of the skull should be pursued with a non-contrast computed tomography (CT) of the head. This modality is also necessary in assessing for skull fractures and moderate or severe traumatic brain injury, including epidural hematoma, subdural hematoma, subarachnoid hemorrhage, and diffuse axonal injury. Neck wounds should be meticulously examined for possible violation of the platysma, and the neck should be inspected for bruits, hematomas, and pulses. Suspicion for anything other than an obviously superficial wound of the dermis of the neck or for any other soft-tissue abnormalities warrants immediate surgical evaluation. While cervical spine injuries are rare in children, cervical spine immobilization should be maintained for any patient with altered mental status, significant facial injuries, sensory or motor subjective concerns, or objective neurologic deficits on examination, as well as in those patients with distracting injuries (such as long bone fractures, extensive wounds, suspected intra-abdominal or intrathoracic injuries). The cervical spine should be palpated for midline or paraspinal tenderness; midline tenderness calls for maintenance of cervical spine immobilization, while anterior-posterior, open mouth, and odontoid views are obtained to evaluate for bony injury. Abnormalities of cervical spine radiographs or abnormal neurologic examination findings call for immediate neurosurgical consultation, with strict maintenance of cervical spine immobilization.

According to the National Emergency X-Radiography Utilization Study (NEXUS) criteria, radiographs of the cervical spine may not be necessary in pediatric patients 8 years and older deemed to be at low risk for a cervical spine injury; there were too few patients younger than 2 years and too few cases of cervical spine injury in patients younger than 8 years to be able to extend these criteria to those populations with confidence. Low-risk patients are those who have the *absence* of the following: midline cervical tenderness to palpation, altered level of consciousness, evidence of intoxication, focal neurologic deficit, and distracting injury (Evidence Level II-2).

The skull and facial bones should be carefully palpated for tenderness, crepitus, and the possibility of underlying fractures (Figure 71-1). Motor and sensory deficits indicate nerve injury or entrapment and require referral for further evaluation. The temporomandibular joint and the mandible should be palpated for tenderness and assessed for malocclusion. Any examination findings suspicious for intracranial injury, skull fracture, or facial fracture other than a nasal fracture can be further evaluated by non-contrast CT. The nose should be examined for obvious deformity, presence of septal hematoma, and any bleeding or rhinorrhea (clear watery rhinorrhea may be suspicious for cerebrospinal fluid leak secondary to cribriform plate or temporal bone fracture). No imaging is indicated in suspected nasal fracture; patients should follow up within 4 to 5 days for reassessment of nasal deviation after the swelling has subsided. The tympanic membranes should be examined bilaterally to confirm they are intact with no hemotympanum present.

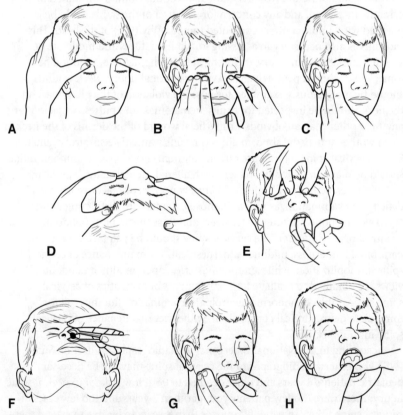

Figure 71-1. Examination for facial fractures.
A, Palpate supraorbital ridges, keeping patient's head steady. B, Palpate infraorbital ridges using index, middle, and ring fingers. C, Palpate the zygomatic arch. D, Palpate the infraorbital rims, zygomatic bodies, and maxilla. E, Examine nasal bone and maxilla for stability/displacement. F, Evaluate nasal septum and mucosa. G, Evaluate occlusion. H, Palpate mandible.

Pupil size, pupil reactivity, and extraocular movements should be assessed bilaterally. Pain with extraocular movements, periorbital tenderness to palpation, or a combination thereof can be further evaluated with orbital CT to evaluate for orbital fracture with entrapment; patients with orbital fractures should receive an evaluation by an ophthalmologist. With visual concerns or the possibility of eye injury, visual acuity should be elicited if the patient is verbal by assessing the patient's ability to count the number of the clinician's fingers held at varying distances. Near vision can be assessed using a standard vision chart or vision card; deviations of near vision unilaterally from the patient's baseline after injury warrant ophthalmologic consultation. With a history of eye trauma, the upper eyelid should be everted for the presence of a foreign body; fluorescein testing performed for corneal abrasion; and detailed inspection performed for hyphema. Suspicion of hyphema warrants an ophthalmology consultation, maintaining bed rest with the patient's head elevated at a 45-degree angle. Additional reasons to seek ophthalmology consultation include suspicion for ruptured globe, eye foreign bodies, and eyelid lacerations complicated by one of the following: accompanying full-thickness involvement of lid, ptosis, involvement of the tear drainage system, tissue avulsion, or eyeball injury.

The mouth and oral cavity should be inspected for injuries to the hard and soft palate. Lesions that have expanding hematomas, persistent bleeding, or associated neurologic deficits need immediate otolaryngological consultation. Dentition should be evaluated for absent or injured teeth; plain radiographs to evaluate for retained teeth fragments should be obtained if any teeth are chipped or avulsed or for any teeth or fragments that are not readily locatable. A diagram of tooth eruption schedules (Figure 71-2) can be consulted to determine if primary or permanent teeth are injured or affected. An avulsed permanent tooth should be rinsed with water or saline and gently re-implanted into the socket as soon as possible; if re-implantation is not immediately possible, the tooth should be placed in milk or one of the commercially available cell culture media to maintain the vitality of the tooth root.

The chest should be visually inspected for contusions or penetrating wounds, and the heart and lungs should be auscultated. Persistent tachypnea or tachycardia or abnormal oxygen saturation, even in the absence of obvious external injuries, should prompt immediate surgical evaluation.

The abdomen and pelvis should also be inspected visually as well as palpated; abdominal tenderness to palpation or contusions require transfer to an emergency department for further evaluation because of the possibility of solid-organ or hollow-viscous injury. Screening laboratory studies (of transaminases and amylase) for solid-organ injury should not be obtained in isolation, as they are not reliable for the detection of intra-abdominal injury, but should be combined with other diagnostic tests and physical examination findings (Evidence Level II-2). If there is any concern for pelvic stability (as assessed by gentle compression and distraction of the iliac wings), immediate surgical evaluation is required. The patient's back should be examined, including

Primary Teeth Eruption Chart

Primary Teeth

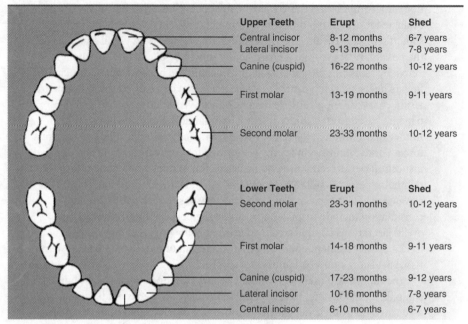

Upper Teeth	Erupt	Shed
Central incisor	8-12 months	6-7 years
Lateral incisor	9-13 months	7-8 years
Canine (cuspid)	16-22 months	10-12 years
First molar	13-19 months	9-11 years
Second molar	23-33 months	10-12 years

Lower Teeth	Erupt	Shed
Second molar	23-31 months	10-12 years
First molar	14-18 months	9-11 years
Canine (cuspid)	17-23 months	9-12 years
Lateral incisor	10-16 months	7-8 years
Central incisor	6-10 months	6-7 years

Figure 71-2. Primary and permanent tooth development.
From American Dental Association. Tooth eruption: the primary teeth. *J Am Dent Assoc.* 2005;136(11):1619.
Copyright © 2014 American Dental Association. All rights reserved. Reprinted with permission.

midline palpation of the thoracic, lumbar, and sacral spines. Midline tenderness to palpation of the spine in the post-trauma setting is investigated with anterior-posterior and lateral radiographs while maintaining spinal precautions. The perineum should be inspected for contusions, hematomas, lacerations, or urethral bleeding. Gross hematuria, or urinalysis with microscopic hematuria of 50 red blood cells per high power field, is indicative of genitourinary tract injury and should be further evaluated with a CT of the abdomen and pelvis. A rectal examination is necessary in patients with penetrating injuries or non-minor blunt torso injuries (such as a significant direct blow or deceleration) to evaluate sphincter tone, the presence of gross blood, and detection of possible pelvic fractures.

The extremities should be evaluated for integrity of pulses, motor function, and sensation. Peripheral pulses and detailed sensation testing should be documented in any injured extremity, and splinting of the injured extremity in a position with intact pulses should be performed prior to initiation of radiographs. Radiographs should be obtained from multiple angles, as a fracture may not be evident in a single view of the bone. Comparison radiographs of the unaffected side may be of benefit because of the variations in pediatric bone contour and configuration of the epiphyseal plate (Evidence Level III). Obvious deformities suspicious for fractures, dislocations, or both should be splinted and referred to an emergency department for further evaluation, as fractures with greater than 15 degrees of angulation and all dislocations require reduction and definitive immobilization. Open fractures are those with defects of the skin and soft tissue overlying the fracture site, and they require vigorous irrigation as well as skin flora antimicrobial prophylaxis and consultation with an orthopedist because of the risk of infection. Growth plate injuries are stratified according to the Salter-Harris classification, with increasing risk of growth disturbance as the classification number increases (Figure 71-3).

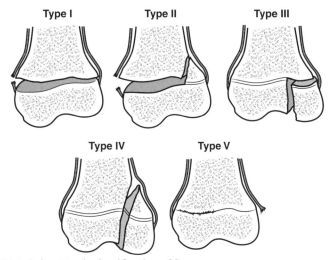

Figure 71-3. Salter Harris classification of fractures.

Any superficial wounds (eg, lacerations, abrasions, punctures) should be copiously irrigated with water or normal saline. All wounds should be locally explored for possible foreign bodies. Primary closure can be performed on facial lacerations for up to 24 hours post-injury and for up to 8 to 12 hours for other lacerations. Current methods for wound closure include tissue adhesive (ie, skin glue), adhesive tape, sutures, and staples. Puncture wounds, animal bites, and human bites should preferentially be left open because of the high risk for infection. Antimicrobial prophylaxis should be initiated for bites to aid in infection prevention. Penetrating foreign bodies should be left in place until complete evaluation of the wound can occur; those foreign bodies that are not obviously superficial and easily removable should be removed by a surgical subspecialist. Additional reasons for referral to a subspecialist include foreign bodies over fracture sites (considered open fractures, as mentioned above), wounds that are extensive or complicated (eg, devitalized tissue, tendon or nerve involvement), or those which present for treatment because of inability to perform primary closure due to the nature of the bite or a delay in seeking treatment. In addition to the historical factors surrounding the injury, the patient's tetanus status should be elicited and immunization provided as needed.

Suggested Reading

American College of Surgeons Committee on Trauma. *ATLS: Advanced Trauma Life Support for Doctors.* 8th ed. Chicago IL: American College of Surgeons; 2008

Chasm RM, Swencki SA. Pediatric orthopedic emergencies. *Emerg Med Clin North Am.* 2010;28(4):907–926

Fleisher GR, Ludwig S, eds. *Textbook of Pediatric Emergency Medicine.* 6th ed. Philadelphia, PA: Wolters Kluwer/Lippincott Williams & Wilkins; 2010

Mikrogianakis A, Valani R, Cheng A; Hospital for Sick Children. *The Hospital for Sick Children Manual of Pediatric Trauma.* Philadelphia, PA: Wolters Kluwer/Lippincott Williams & Wilkins; 2008

Schonfeld D, Lee LK. Blunt abdominal trauma in children. *Curr Opin Pediatr.* 2012;24(3):314–318

Shah BR, Lucchesi M, eds. *Atlas of Pediatric Emergency Medicine.* New York, NY: McGraw-Hill, Medical Publishing Division; 2006

Spiro DM, Zonfrillo MR, Meckler GD. Wounds. *Pediatr Rev.* 2010;31(8):326–334

Swischuk LE, Hernandez JA. Frequently missed fractures in children (value of comparative views). *Emerg Radiol.* 2004;11(1):22–28

Viccellio P, Simon H, Pressman BD, et al. A prospective multicenter study of cervical spine injury in children. *Pediatrics.* 2001;108(2):E20

CHAPTER 72

Traumatic Brain Injury

Elizabeth H. Mack, MD, MS

Key Points

- Traumatic brain injury is the most common cause of death and disability in children and adolescents, and in multisystem trauma the head is a commonly injured organ.

- Multiple mechanical forces (ie, acceleration and deceleration, rotational or torsional) at the moment of injury result in the primary injury; secondary injury leads to further morbidity and mortality.

- A variety of clinical scoring systems (Pediatric Trauma Score, Glasgow Coma Score, Pediatric Risk of Mortality III) are used to stratify risk and evaluate treatments in these children.

- Management priorities include
  - Hypertonic saline as first-line osmotherapy
  - Avoidance of hypoxia; providing normal ventilation
  - The risk/benefit of intracranial pressure monitoring and hypothermia are still under study in children with traumatic brain injury.
- Several past interventions (eg, corticosteroids) are no longer supported by research.

Overview

Traumatic brain injury (TBI) is the most common cause of death and disability in children and adolescents, and in multisystem trauma the head is commonly injured organ. The various mechanical forces (ie, acceleration and deceleration, rotational or torsional) at play at the moment of injury result in the primary injury. Secondary brain injury must be managed as well, though often it is more difficult to manage (Box 72-1).

The Monroe-Kellie doctrine states that when homeostasis of the skull contents (ie, venous and arterial volume, brain, and cerebrospinal fluid [CSF]) is disrupted, the brain is compliant until the intracranial pressure reaches a critical point. In addition, if the usual compensatory mechanisms are disturbed in the brain injury, the threshold for an increase in intracranial pressure will be lowered. Also, if drainage or reabsorption of the CSF is disrupted, further alteration in the threshold for an increase in intracranial pressure (ICP) occurs.

Box 72-1. Primary and Secondary Brain Injury

Primary Brain Injury
- Diffuse and focal axonal injury
- Diffuse and focal vascular compromise
- Brain contusion
- Brain laceration

Secondary Brain Injury
- Diffuse and focal hypoxic ischemia
- Diffuse and focal cerebral edema
- Intracranial hypertension
- Contra coup injury
- Hydrocephalus
- Seizures
- Coagulopathy, risk for further bleeding
- Hypo/hypernatremia

In general, the 3 major mechanisms of damage in TBI include focal hemorrhagic and non-hemorrhagic lesions affecting the cortical gray matter, diffuse axonal injury, and secondary injury including cerebral edema (see Table 72-2). Focal hemorrhages include epidural (typically due to arterial bleeding and presenting with short lucid interval then rapid decline), subdural (typically due to venous bleeding), subarachnoid, intraventricular, and intraparenchymal. Blunt trauma often results in associated skull fracture. Diffuse axonal injury results from shearing forces commonly acting on the gray-white interface and is thought to be the cause of many severe neurologic deficits. Inflicted TBI or abusive head trauma are other causes of TBI but are not within the scope of this chapter because of the differing mechanism of injury.

Several anatomic differences exist between adults and children that increase the risk and severity of injury in pediatric TBI. Primarily, the child's head is proportionally larger; the brain, less myelinated; and the cranial bones, thinner. Also, the child's body surface area is larger in comparison, leading to greater heat loss after injury, further complicating the course of TBI.

Evaluation

As with any trauma, the primary survey (known by its mnemonic ABCDE) must be conducted to assess airway, breathing, circulation, disability, and exposure. Resuscitation of the pediatric trauma patient is concurrent with the primary survey in a continuous cycle of assessment, intervention, and reassessment. Attention to the vital signs, primary survey, and aggressive resuscitation will ideally prevent further secondary brain injury. Suspicion and empiric management of cervical spine injury should accompany the primary survey.

The secondary survey involves the SAMPLE history (for symptoms, allergies, medications, past illnesses, last meal, and event/environment) as well as a complete head-to-toe physical examination. Physical examination findings suspicious for basilar skull fracture include mid-face instability, hemotympa-num, raccoon eyes, and Battle sign (ie, mastoid ecchymosis). If basilar skull fracture is suspected, care should be taken to avoid nasogastric tube placement.

Clinicians and researchers have debated over the proper trauma score to stratify risk and predict outcomes for the pediatric population. The Injury Severity Score and the Revised Trauma Score are in use but do not address children in particular. The Glasgow Coma Scale (GCS) is used to assess neurologic function following injury and has been modified for infants and young children (Table 72-1; for the unmodified GSC, see Chapter 71, Table 71-3). Patients with a GCS score of 13 to 15 are classified as having mild TBI; 9 to 12, moderate; and 3 to 8, severe. The Pediatric Risk of Mortality III and Pediatric Index of Mortality II focus on outcomes of all patients admitted to pediatric intensive care units. The Pediatric Trauma Score is acceptable for use in the field and for prediction of outcomes, as well as recognized by the American College of Surgeons Committee on Trauma and the American Pediatric Surgical Association Trauma Committee (Table 72-2).

Initial laboratory tests that should be considered are outlined in Box 72-2.

Management

Pediatric TBI consensus guidelines were published in 2003 and included a "critical pathway" to guide management. In 2012, the guidelines were updated and the critical pathway was removed. The 2012 guidelines adhered more strictly to evidence-based guidelines and, in fact, 25 articles considered in 2003 guidelines were removed in the most recent update because of weak design or unrelated patient populations.

Difficulties designing studies and summarizing the literature revolve around varying outcomes (in ICP, mortality, and Glasgow Outcome Scale Table 72-3), definitions (of fever, hypothermia, goal cerebral perfusion pressure, and goal ICP), ethical issues related to early intervention in such severe disease, the time-sensitive nature of the interventions necessary, selection criteria and bias for studies, and changing standard background therapy over time (in steroids, hyperventilation, ICP monitoring, hypothermia, and decompressive craniec-tomy), all of which confound results. The 2012 guidelines classify recommen-dations based mostly on randomized, controlled trials as Evidence Level I, prospective/retrospective data as Evidence Level II, and retrospective data as Evidence Level III (Table 72-4).

Table 72-1. Modified Glasgow Coma Scale for Infants and Children

Category	4 y–Adult	Child 1 y–4 y	Infant <1 y	Score
Motor	Follows commands	Normal spontaneous movement	Normal spontaneous movement	6
	Localizes pain	Localizes pain	Withdraws to touch	5
	Withdraws to pain	Withdraws to pain	Withdraws to pain	4
	Decorticate flexion	Decorticate flexion	Decorticate flexion	3
	Decerebrate extension	Decerebrate extension	Decerebrate extension	2
	None	None	None	1
Verbal	Oriented and alert	Oriented, speaks, interacts, social	Coos/babbles	5
	Disoriented	Confused speech, consolable, disoriented	Irritable cry, consolable	4
	Nonsensical speech	Inappropriate words, inconsolable	Cries persistently to pain	3
	Moans, incomprehensible	Incomprehensible, agitated	Moans to pain	2
	None	None	None	1
Eye opening	Spontaneous	Spontaneous	Spontaneous	4
	To voice	To voice	To voice	3
	To pain	To pain	To pain	2
	None	None	None	1

Derived from Teasdale G, Jennett B. Assessment of coma and impaired consciousness: a practical scale. *Lancet.* 1974;2:81–84.

Table 72-2. Pediatric Trauma Score

Points	+2	+1	−1
Size (kg)	>20	10–20	<10
Airway	Normal	Maintained	Unmaintained
SBP (mm Hg)	>90	50–90	<50
CNS	Awake	Obtunded	Coma
Open wound	None	Minor	Major
Skeletal trauma	None	Closed	Open/multiple

Abbreviations: CNS, central nervous system; SBP, systolic blood pressure.

Box 72-2. Initial Laboratory Tests Suggested in Severe Pediatric TBI

- Blood gas (CBG, VBG, or ABG)
- CBC
- BMP
- PT/INR, PTT
- CT head/neck and other imaging as indicated

Abbreviations: ABG, arterial blood gasses; BMP, basic metabolic panel; CBC, complete blood count; CBG, capillary blood gasses; CT, computed tomography scan; PT/INR, prothrombin time/international normalized ratio; PTT, partial thromboplastin time; TBI, traumatic brain injury; VBG, venous blood gasses.

Table 72-3. Glasgow Outcome Scale

Scale	Description
5 (good outcome)	Resumption of normal life; may be minor neurologic or psychological deficits (or both)
4 (moderately disabled)	Able to work in a sheltered environment and travel by public transportation
3 (severely disabled)	Dependent for daily support by reason of mental or physical disability (or both)
1 (persistent vegetative state)	Unresponsive and speechless for weeks or months until death
0 (death)	Not applicable

Derived from Jennet B, Bond M. Assessment of outcome after severe brain damage. *Lancet*. 1975;1(7905): 480–484.

Table 72-4. Guidelines for Management of Severe TBI

Aspect of Care	Evidence Level	Pediatric 2012 Guideline	Adult 2007 Guideline
Oxygenation and ventilation	I	None	None
	II	None	• Prophylactic hyperventilation (Pco_2 <25 mm Hg) is not recommended.
	III	• Consider avoiding prophylactic hyperventilation (Pco_2 <30 mm Hg) in first 48 h. • Consider advanced neuromonitoring for evaluation of cerebral ischemia if hyperventilation is used for refractory ICP.	• Hyperventilation is recommended as temporizing measure for reducing ICP. • Hyperventilation should be avoided in first 24 h when CBF is critically reduced. • If hyperventilation is used, jugular venous saturation or $Pbto_2$ is recommended to monitor oxygen delivery. • Oxygenation should be monitored and hypoxemia (Pao_2 <60 mm Hg, saturation <90 mm Hg) avoided.
Circulation	I	None	None
	II	None	• BP should be monitored and hypotension (SBP <90 mm Hg) avoided.
	III	None	None
CPP & ICP goals	I	None	None
	II	None	• Avoid attempts to get CPP >70 because of ARDS risk. • -ICP is <20–25.
	III	CPP 40–50 ICP <20	• Avoid CPP <50.
Osmotherapy	I	None	None
	II	• Consider HTS at 6.5–10 mL/kg for increased ICP.	• Use mannitol at 0.25–1 g/kg for increased ICP; maintain SBP >90 mm Hg.
	III	• Consider 3% NS at 0.1–1 mL/kg/h. Min dose needed to keep ICP <20; keep Osm <360.	• Restrict mannitol use prior to ICP monitoring for herniation or progressive deterioration not explained by extracranial cause.
Prevention of PTS	I	None	None
	II	• Prophylactic use of AED not recommended to prevent late PTS	• Prophylactic use of AED to prevent early PTS

Table 72-4 *(cont)*

Aspect of Care	Evidence Level	Pediatric 2012 Guideline	Adult 2007 Guideline
	III	• Consider prophylactic treatment with phenytoin to decrease early PTS.	None
Sedation, analgesia, neuromuscular blockade	I	None	None
	II	None	• Propofol infusion for ICP but not for mortality or outcome benefit • Prophylactic burst suppression with barbs not recommended • High dose barbs for refractory ICP (Watch hemodynamics.)
	III	• May consider etomidate but should consider adrenal suppression risk • May consider thiopental • Continuous propofol not recommended • Should consider high dose barbiturates with BP monitoring	None
Temperature control	I	None	None
	II	• Moderate hypothermia (32°C–33°C [89.6°F–91.4°F]) beginning early after severe TBI for 24 h only should be avoided. • Moderate hypothermia (32°C–33°C [89.6°F–91.4°F]) beginning within 8 h for up to 48 h should be considered to reduce ICP. • If hypothermia is induced, rewarm at rate 0.5 C/h.	None
	III	• Moderate hypothermia (32°C–33°C [89.6°F–91.4°F]) beginning early for 48 h may be considered.	• No mortality benefit • May be decreased mortality if hypothermia maintained >48 h • Prophylactic hypothermia associated with higher GOS

Table 72-4 *(cont)*

Aspect of Care	Evidence Level	Pediatric 2012 Guideline	Adult 2007 Guideline
Advanced monitoring and definitive therapy	I	None	None
	II	None	• ICP should be monitored in all patients with severe but salvageable TBI and abnormal CT.
	III	• Consider EVD to treat ICP +/- lumbar drain. • Perform decompressive craniectomy if early signs of neurologic deterioration or herniation or refractory ICP to medical management in early stages of elevated ICP. • ICP monitoring may be considered if severe TBI because successful ICP monitor-based management is associated with improved survival and neurologic outcome. • If brain oxygenation monitoring is used, consider maintaining P_{BTO_2} >10 mm Hg.	• ICP monitoring if severe TBI and normal CT if age >40 y, posturing, or SBP <90 mm Hg • Recommend use of jugular venous saturation >50%, P_{BTO_2} >15 mm Hg
Corticosteroids	I	None	• Steroids contraindicated because of increased mortality
	II	• Not recommended to decrease ICP or improve outcomes	None
	III	None	None
Nutrition	I	None	None
	II	• No evidence to support immunomodulatory diet to improve outcome	• Full nutrition replacement by day 7
	III	None	None

Abbreviations: AED, antiepileptic drug; ARDS, acute respiratory distress syndrome; BP, blood pressure; CBF, cerebral blood flow; CPP, cerebral perfusion pressure; CT, computed tomography scan; EVD, externalized ventricular drain; GOS, Glasgow Outcome Scale; HTS, hypertonic saline; ICP, intracranial pressure; NS, normal saline; Osm, osmolality; PTS, posttraumatic seizures; SBP, systolic blood pressure; TBI, traumatic brain injury.

Primary goals of management of severe TBI include (1) optimizing cerebral perfusion pressure; (2) optimizing oxygenation, ventilation, circulation; and (3) decreasing the cerebral metabolic rate of oxygen ($CMRO_2$). Though the 2012 guidelines no longer discuss the recommendation regarding specialized training and end-tidal carbon dioxide monitoring if pre-hospital intubation is to be performed, these concepts still seem reasonable. Cerebral blood flow is closely related to mean arterial pressure and $Paco_2$ and should be maintained within the optimal range. Intubation is generally recommended in the initial management of severe TBI. Clinicians should aim for normoventilation rather than hyperventilation (unless acutely herniating) and avoid hypoxia (Evidence Level III). It is recommended that cerebral perfusion pressure be maintained at 40 to 50 mm Hg and ICP less than 20 mm Hg (Evidence Level III), but it should be noted that the ICP monitor needs to be zeroed at the tragus and the arterial line zeroed at the right atrium with the head of the bed at 30 degrees. Hypertonic saline is now recommended as the first-line treatment in osmotherapy for intracranial hypertension, as it is correlated with better outcomes and is a safer choice than mannitol in hemodynamically unstable patients (Evidence Level II, III).

Reduction of $CMRO_2$ may involve seizure prevention and treatment, sedation, analgesia, neuromuscular blockade, and temperature control. Antiepileptic drugs are recommended for prevention of early but not late posttraumatic seizures (Evidence Level II, III). Sedation and analgesia are recommended, but the combination is not prescribed, though propofol is specifically not recommended (Evidence Level III). Early moderate (32°C–33°C [89.6°F–91.4°F]) hypothermia may be considered, and slow rewarming is recommended, though this guideline was published before the Cool Kids trial was stopped because of futility (Evidence Level II, III).

Techniques for advanced monitoring and definitive therapy have long been discussed as being useful for management, but little data support whether they have a positive effect on patient outcomes. Intracranial pressure monitoring can be useful in severe TBI if the patient is not coagulopathic and not brain dead (Evidence Level III). External ventricular drains can both monitor and treat elevated ICP by draining cerebral spinal fluid if ICP is elevated or drainage is blocked (Evidence Level III).

Other aspects of care in severe traumatic brain injury have been studied in children. Vasogenic edema is not seen in TBI and therefore corticosteroids are specifically not recommended for decreasing ICP or improving outcomes (Evidence Level II). No evidence supports an immunomodulatory formula to improve outcomes in pediatric TBI (Evidence Level II). In addition, the head of bed should be midline and elevated to allow maximal drainage through the jugular veins. Cervical spine injury should be assumed, even in the absence of supporting data on computed tomography, until the patient is awake enough to cooperate with the examination or magnetic resonance imaging is able to be obtained.

Long-term Monitoring

While intact neurologic outcome is certainly the goal of therapy, survivors of severe TBI often require close monitoring after discharge. Many need inpatient rehabilitation, aggressive outpatient rehabilitative services, or both. In addition to the primary and secondary brain injuries experienced early in the course, many patients develop cerebral atrophy in the year after injury. Comprehensive visual, auditory, speech/language, and neurocognitive evaluations should ideally be performed after the acute phase of injury. The medical home will need to coordinate with families, rehabilitative services, subspecialists, and school services to facilitate the reintegration of these childhood survivors with TBI back into their environment.

Suggested Reading

Avarello JT, Cantor RM. Pediatric major trauma: an approach to evaluation and management. *Emerg Med Clin N Am.* 2007;25(3):803–836

Brain Trauma Foundation, American Association of Neurological Surgeons, Congress of Neurological Surgeons. Guidelines for the management of severe traumatic brain injury. *J Neurotrauma.* 2007;24(Suppl 1):S1–S106

Cooper A. Early assessment and management of trauma. In: Ashcroft KW, Holcomb GW, Murphy JP, eds. *Pediatric Surgery.* Philadelphia, PA: Elsevier; 2005:168–184

Kochanek PM, Carney N, Adelson PD. Guidelines for the acute medical management of severe traumatic brain injury in infants, children, and adolescents. *Pediatr Crit Care Med.* 2012;13(1):S1–S82

Tasker R. Head and spinal cord injury. In: Nichols DG, ed. *Rogers' Textbook of Pediatric Intensive Care.* Philadelphia, PA: Lippincott Williams & Wilkins; 2008:887–911

Index

Page numbers in *italic* denote a figure, table, or box.